DIABETES AND CARDIOVASCULAR DISEASE

Etiology, Treatment, and Outcomes

ADVANCES IN EXPERIMENTAL MEDICINE AND BIOLOGY

DIABETES AND CARDIOVASCULAR DISEASE
Etiology, Treatment, and Outcomes

Edited by

Aubie Angel

Diabetes Research and Treatment Centre
Winnipeg, Canada

Naranjan Dhalla

St. Boniface Research Centre
Winnipeg, Canada

Grant Pierce

St. Boniface Research Centre
Winnipeg, Canada

Pawan Singal

St. Boniface Research Centre
Winnipeg, Canada

Kluwer Academic / Plenum Publishers
New York, Boston, Dordrecht, London, Moscow

Library of Congress Cataloging-in-Publication Data

Diabetes and cardiovascular disease: etiology, treatment, and outcomes/edited by Aubie Angel ... [et al.].
        p.   ; cm.
    Includes bibliographical references and index.
    ISBN 0-306-46637-6
      1. Diabetic angiopathies.   I. Angel, Aubie.
    [DNLM]:   1. Diabetes Mellitus—complications—Congresses.   2. Cardiovascular
Diseases—etiology—Congresses.   WK 835 D53347 2001]
    RC700.D5 D525 2001
    616.4′62—dc21

                                                                    2001041362

ISBN 0-306-46637-6

©2001 Kluwer Academic/Plenum Publishers, New York
233 Spring Street, New York, New York 10013

http://www.wkap.nl/

10   9   8   7   6   5   4   3   2   1

A C.I.P. record for this book is available from the Library of Congress

PREFACE

Diabetes and Cardiovascular Disease: from Molecular Processes to Health Policy

Diabetes and cardiovascular disease together account for the largest portion of health care spending compared to all other diseases in Western society, and the cost continues to increase because of parallel trends including an aging population and an increasing incidence of obesity. In North America, this is most relevant in our First Nations community and other ethnic groups, particularly recent immigrants from the Caribbean and the Indian Subcontinent. Despite expanding knowledge about the importance of insulin resistance in type 2 diabetes mellitus, and autoimmune factors that predispose to type 1 diabetes, etiologic risk factors for cardiovascular complications continue to increase. Much is known about the health risks of obesity, diabetes, hypertension and hyperlipidemia as causal factors in cardiovascular disease, and many of these risk factors can be addressed through a growing array of effective pharmacologic agents. It is also true that behavioral and nonpharmacological strategies are important for individuals and populations. These require behavioral interventions within the community and in individual households. However, our ability to transfer this knowledge and improve lifestyle appears to be rudimentary. It is possible to address this problem by identifying the myriad barriers to a better informed public. Overcoming these barriers will ensure more effective care in the community. In the first instance, an understanding of the causes of diabetes and its cardiovascular complications must be widely appreciated as this will serve as a foundation for evidence based care and wider acceptance of sound science. The International Conference on Diabetes and Cardiovascular Disease, held in Winnipeg in June, 1999, was organized to bring together a multi-disciplinary group of researchers dedicated to further understanding amongst researchers, care givers, and the managers of the health system. The invited speakers were asked to submit their work for publication which served as the basis of this book.

New drugs and nutritional strategies have been developed to improve glycemic control, body weight, and metabolic risk predictors of cardiovascular disease. New interventions, to be valid, require clinical trials in order to establish the effectiveness of specific treatments. These interventions must be tested within the community under ordinary living conditions to confirm their effectiveness. It is our hope that new knowledge reported here will shorten the interval between basic observation, hypothesis testing, clinical trials, and the introduction of new treatments in the community. This should help improve the general well being of society.

The importance of prevention of heart disease cannot be overstated. With heart-health promotion initiatives, communities can be helped by informed provincial and federal policy makers. The work reported here is a compilation of themes that span broad areas of research relevant to the care of individuals and communities burdened with the disease as well as the costs of health care. It should serve as a valuable reference text for decision makers.

The various chapters include subjects grouped according to major themes that include: 1) epidemiology of diabetes mellitus; 2) metabolic risk factors in diabetes and cardiovascular disease; 3) endothelial function in diabetes; 4) hypertension in diabetes mellitus; 5) cardiac lipid metabolism in diabetes; 6) cardiac function in diabetes; 7) glycemic control and improved cardiovascular function; 8) diabetes management; 9) health promotion in preventing diabetes and its complications; and 10) health policy and national strategies in diabetes. This information should be of interest to scientists studying the cause of diabetes, the clinician concerned with the care of patients with diabetes and cardiovascular disease, and policy makers who help decide priorities for government support.

Finally, we would like to take this opportunity to thank our sponsors and pharmaceutical partners for supporting the conference on which this book is based. We also thank the Institute of Cardiovascular Sciences, St. Boniface General Hospital, and the Diabetes Research and Treatment Centre of Winnipeg for assembling this body of knowledge for the benefit of the patients we serve.

Aubie Angel
Naranjan Dhalla
Grant Pierce
and
Pawan Singal

CONTENTS

EPIDEMIOLOGY AND GENETIC DETERMINANTS OF DIABETES MELLITUS

METABOLIC RISK FACTORS IN DIABETES AND CARDIOVASCULAR DISEASE

HYPERTENSION AND DIABETES MELLITUS

CARDIAC LIPID METABOLISM IN DIABETES

CARDIAC FUNCTION AND OXIDATIVE
STRESS IN DIABETES

GLYCEMIC CONTROL AND IMPROVED CARDIOVASCULAR FUNCTION

DIABETES MANAGEMENT— A MULTIDISCIPLINARY APPROACH

HEALTH PROMOTION IN PREVENTING
DIABETES AND ITS COMPLICATIONS

HEALTH POLICY AND NATIONAL
STRATEGIES IN DIABETES

TYPE 2 DIABETES IN YOUTH: A NEW EPIDEMIC

Heather Dean
University of Manitoba

INTRODUCTION

Youth with type 2 diabetes represent an increasing proportion of children referred to pediatric diabetes centers in North America (1-5). Since this is a disease recognized only in the past decade in this age group, there is urgency to understand the etiology of this age shift, develop gold standard diagnostic criteria, determine optimum treatment guidelines and understand the natural history of this disease in childhood and adolescence. Firstly, awareness of this disease is important because there are many physicians who still do not believe that type 2 diabetes can occur in children. Diagnosis is a problem because the diagnostic criteria for differentiating type 1 and type 2 diabetes in children are based on clinical findings which are hard to fit into epidemiological paradigms for "gold-standard" definitions. Treatment is a problem because lifestyle modification is difficult for adolescents who may not feel any symptoms and who do not understand the concepts of risk and prevention of long term complications. Treatment is also a problem because there are no long term studies of drug therapy in youth with type 2 diabetes and none of the oral hypoglycemic drugs are approved for use in youth under age 18 years. Finally the morbidity of classical microvascular complications of diabetes including end stage renal disease and blindness may be more significant in this group with early onset disease than the morbidity of stroke and heart disease in adult onset disease.

In the province of Manitoba and the region of northwestern Ontario, combined to form a geographical area of central Canada, type 2 diabetes occurs almost exclusively in aboriginal children. This report will focus on the experience with that population.
Epidemiology of this disease includes discussion of incidence, prevalence, diagnostic criteria, treatment and outcomes.

EPIDIMIOLOGY

The incidence of type 2 diabetes in youth in Manitoba is increasing. This is based on a referred population to the only tertiary care pediatric diabetes center in the province at Children's Hospital in Winnipeg. The number of cases has increased from 1-2 cases per year to 20 cases in 1998. The 20 new patients in 1998 represented 33% of all children with new onset diabetes referred to Children's Hospital that year.

The long term diabetes screening study of the Pima Indians living in the Gila River community in Arizona provided proof that this is a new disease and not simply better case

Diabetes and Cardiovascular Disease: Etiology, Treatment and Outcomes
Edited by Aubie Angel *et al.*, Kluwer Academic/Plenum Publishers, 2001

1

finding in youth(6). In the 3 decades between 1967 and 1996, the prevalence of diabetes in Pima Indian youth aged 10-14 years increased 4-fold from 0.5% to 2% and for youth aged 15-19 years, the prevalence doubled from 2% to 4%.

In Manitoba with a total population of 1.1 million people, the MINIMUM age specific point prevalence of type 2 diabetes in aboriginal youth aged 10-19 years increased from 0.1% (1/1000) to 0.22% (2.2/1000) from 1986 to 1998. Although the true prevalence of type 2 diabetes in youth in Manitoba is likely to be grossly underestimated by these figures because it is based on a referred population, the experience of increasing prevalence mirrors that of the Pima Indian youth. The reasons for this underestimation in prevalence are lack of population screening, lack of referral of the older affected asymptomatic teenagers and lack of standards for reporting this disease in children.

One of the challenges facing the epidimiologists in this field is standardization of the age groupings for describing the epidimiological trends. In type 1 diabetes the accepted age groupings are 5 year intervals starting at 0-4 years. Since most youth with type 1 diabetes are transferred to adult care at age 18 and gestational diabetes clouds the picture in late adolescence, most epidimiological data on type 1 diabetes refers to youth age 0-14 years. This cannot be used in type 2 diabetes since most of the affected youth are age 10-19 years. The problem of age referral bias exists also in the type 2 population so that a smaller proportion of the 16-19 year olds may be referred for pediatric care. In Manitoba in the 12 years 1986-1998 inclusive, there were 82 children referred to the diabetes clinic at Children's Hospital. The age-specific prevalence is 2.1/1000 and 2.3/1000 respectively for the 10-14 year olds and the 15-19 years olds. This likely represents the biases noted above and underestimates the prevalence especially in the older age group.

It is noteworthy that the affected female youths outnumber the affected males by at least 4:1 and 80% of the youth live in remote northern communities.

Another challenge for epidimiologists is the use of age of onset to determine type of diabetes. Most studies in adults that are based on administrative databases such as the Manitoba Burden of Illness study in 1993 (7) combined all cases of diabetes in adults regardless of the type and started counting cases at age 25 years and older. In studies using administrative databases, diabetes diagnosed under age 18 has been assumed to be type 1 diabetes. This is no longer accurate. In order for us to understand the natural history of type 2 diabetes in youth and to determine the effectiveness of interventions, it is imperative that epidimiologists and clinicians develop a standardized strategy to distinguish the type of diabetes in the hospital separation data and diagnosis coding.

There are 3 population studies of diabetes in Canada that are based on community screening and include children and adolescents. These studies provide the only evidence of prevalence of diabetes in this age group. The first study in 1993 in 2 communities in Quebec showed no cases of diabetes in the youth aged 15-19 years (8). The second population screening study was conducted in Sandy Lake, Ontario and included youth aged 10-19 years (9). The prevalence of diabetes was 4% in the females aged 10-19 years. The third population screening study was conducted in children aged 5-19 years in 1996-1997 in the remote northern Manitoba community of Ste Theresa Point (10). There were 2 youth in the community previously known to have diabetes. The screening study identified 6 more affected youth. All were obese females. The overall prevalence of diabetes in youth aged 5-19 years in this community was 1.1% (11/1000). This is approximately 5-fold higher than the estimated prevalence based on the referred population. The majority of the youth in the community were obese, males more than females (11). The female to male ratio of diabetes was 8:0 and the age-specific prevalence in adolescent females was 3.6% (10).

From an international perspective, type 2 diabetes is appearing as a new problem in Hispanic children in the southwestern United States (5) and African-American children in many states (3,4). Japanese children are also recently demonstrating this disease (12).

DIAGNOSIS

The clinical criteria used to diagnose type 2 diabetes in children include ethnic origin at high risk, body mass index greater than 85th %ile for age and gender, and a strong family history of type 2 diabetes (13). Most youth have relative lack of classical symptoms and few are less than 10 years of age at diagnosis. Many children have acanthosis nigricans of the neck and axilla (14).

TREATMENT

Intensive lifestyle modification is effective in lowering blood glucose levels in a few days. This has been shown in the summer camp setting (15,16). However there are huge barriers to maintaining these intensive healthy lifestyle patterns, especially in the remote northern communities in Canada. Other barriers include the high cost of food that must be transported to the communities by air cargo, the monopoly on food supply in the north, the short growing season for fresh garden vegetables, the reliance on local water transportation which means that groceries may not be available for several months of the year when the waterways are freezing or thawing, the frigid outside temperatures for 4-5 months of the year that making walking outside dangerous, the unpaved roads that make walking in good weather unbearable for the dust, the wildlife that affect personal safety, the lack of running water that causes reliance on commercial sugar containing liquids, the limited organized recreational opportunities especially for female teens, and the lack of adult role models that are committed to a healthy lifestyle of good nutrition and physical activity.

The drugs used in adults for type 2 diabetes have not been studied in children for efficacy or safety. The use of insulin in children with type 1 diabetes is well known; but the use of short term insulin treatment at diagnosis in youth with type 2 diabetes has not been systematically explored (17).

NATURAL HISTORY

The Pima Indians who develop diabetes in youth experience the complications of diabetes at an earlier age. The young adults aged 20-29 who developed type 2 diabetes during childhood, compared with young adults who developed type 2 diabetes during adulthood, have higher prevalence of hypertriglyceridemia, hypercholesterolemia, hypertension, and microalbuminuria (18). We assume that this natural history will apply to our aboriginal children with type 2 diabetes in Canada. In Manitoba, we have seen young adults with blindness, end-stage-renal disease, and infants with congenital anomalies in their 20s (16). The risk is further exaggerated by the higher rates of primary renal disease in this population. The risk of end stage renal disease in aboriginal children in Manitoba is 6x greater than children from other ethnic groups (19).

PRIMARY PREVENTION

There are many projects to prevent diabetes in aboriginal communities in Canada. Some involve the entire community and others are targeted to school aged children. Examples of large school based prevention projects are Kahnawake, Quebec (20), and Sandy Lake, Ontario (9). The strategies for primary prevention in the community will benefit and encourage those with diabetes to work on secondary prevention of complications. Early diagnosis of diabetes in asymptomatic individuals must be accomplished by community screening or case finding of persons at risk using fasting blood glucose levels according to clinical practice guidelines (21).

CONCLUSION

The prevalence of type 2 diabetes in aboriginal children is increasing and is 2-5 fold greater than type 1 diabetes in children in the general population. Based on experience in urban cities across North America, we expect that children from other high risk ethnic groups will also be diagnosed with type 2 diabetes in increasing numbers in the next decade. It is important to differentiate the types of diabetes in children as the 2 diseases have unique requirements for education, risk assessment in the family, treatment, family counselling, and long term outcome. Conventional education and management strategies used in children with type 1 diabetes have been unsuccessful in this population. The drugs used in adults for type 2 diabetes have not been studied in children for efficacy or safety. The use of insulin in children with type 1 diabetes is well known; the use of short term insulin treatment at diagnosis in youth with type 2 diabetes has not been systematically explored. Microvascular complications may represent the greatest morbidity of type 2 diabetes this disease in young adult life and the risk may be greater than in type 1 diabetes. This is a devastating disease and it's only just begun (22). Our society needs large scale, population-based diabetes primary prevention initiatives since diabetes is now a public health problem.

REFERENCES

1. H.J. Dean, R.L. Mundy, M.E. Moffatt, Non-insulin-dependent Diabetes Mellitus in Indian children in Manitoba, *Can Med Assoc J.* **147**, 52-57 (1992).
2. S.B. Harris, B.A. Perkins, E. Whalen-Brough, Non-Insulin Dependent Diabetes Melitus among First Nations' Children. New Entity among First Nations People of North Western Ontario, *Canadian Family Physician.* **42**, 869-876 (1996).
3. O. Pinhas-Hamiel, L.M. Dolan, S.R. Daniels, D. Standiford, P.R. Khoury, P. Zeitler, Increased incidence of non-insulin dependent diabetes mellitus among adolescents, *J Pediatrics.* **128**, 608-615 (1996).
4. C. Pihoker, S.Y. Scott, S.Y. Lensing, M.M. Cradock, J. Smith, Non-insulin-dependent diabetes mellitus in African-American youths of Arkansas, *Clinical Pediatrics.* **37**,   97-102 (1998).
5. N. Glaser, K.L. Jones. Non-insulin-dependent diabetes mellitus in children and Adolescents, *Advances in Pediatrics.* **43**, 359-381 (1996).
6. D. Dabelea, R.L. Hanson, P.H. Bennett, W.C. Knowler, D.J. Pettitt, Increasing Prevalence of type 2 diabetes in American Indian children, *Diabetologia.* **41**, 904- 910 (1998).
7. J. Blanchard, S. Ludwig, A. Wajda, H. Dean, K. Anderson, N. Depew, The Incidence and Prevalence of diabetes in Manitoba:1986-1991 Adults, *Diabetes Care.* **19**, 807-811 (1996).
8. H.F. Delisle, J.M. Ekoe, Prevalence of non-insulin-diabetes mellitus and impaired glucose tolerance in two Algonquian communities in Quebec, *Can Med Assoc J.* **148**, 41-47 (1993).
9. S.B. Harris, H.A. Gittelsohn, B.A. Gittelsohn, et al, The prevalence of NIDDM and associated risk factors in Native Canadian, *Diabetes Care.* **20**, 185-187 (1997).
10. H.J. Dean, T.K. Young, B. Flett, P. Wood-Steiman, Screening for type 2 diabetes in aboriginal children in northern Canada, *The Lancet.* **353**, 1523-1524 (1998).
11. K. Young, B. Flett, P. Wood-Steiman, H.J. Dean, Childhood Obesity in a population at high risk for type 2 diabetes, *J Pediatrics.* **136**, 365-369 (2000).
12. M. Owada, Y. Hanaoka, Y. Tanimoto, T. Kitagawa, Descriptive epidimiology of non-insulin-dependent diabetes mellitus detected by urine screening in school children in Japan, *Acta Pediatrica Jpn.* **32**, 716-724 (1990).
13. H.J. Dean, Diagnostic criteria for non-insulin-dependent diabetes mellitus in youth (NIDDM-Y), *Clinical Pediatrics.* **37**, 67-71 (1998).
14. C.A. Stuart, C.R. Gilkison, M.M. Smith, A.M. Bosma, B.S. Keenan, M. Nagamani, Acanthosis Nigricans as a risk factor for non-insulin-dependent diabetes mellitus, *Clinical Pediatrics.* **37**, 63-79 (1998).
15. K.A. Anderson, H.J. Dean, The effect of diet and exercise on a native youth with poorly controlled NIDDM, *Beta Release.* **14**, 105-106 (1990).

16. H.J. Dean, NIDDM-Y in First Nation children in Canada, *Clinical Pediatrics.* **37**, 89-96 (1998).
17. K.L. Jones, Non-insulin-dependent diabetes mellitus in children and adolescents:The therapeutic challenge, *Clinical Pediatrics.* **37**, 103-110 (1998).
18. A. Fagot-Campagna, W.C. Knowler, D.J. Pettitt, Type 2 diabetes in Indian Children: Cardiovascular Risk Factors at diagnosis and 10 years later, *Diabetes 47* (suppl 1):A605 (1998).
19. B. Bullock, B.D. Postl, M.R. Ogborn, Excess prevalence of nondiabetic renal disease in native American children in Manitoba, *Pediatr Nephrol.* **10**, 702-704 (1996).
20. A.C. Macaulay, G. Paradis, L. Potvin, E.J. Cross, C. Saad-Haddad, A. McComber, S. Desrosiers, R. Kirby, L.T. Montour, D.L. Lamping, N. Leduc, M. Rivard, The Kahnawake Schools Diabetes Prevention Project: Intervention, Evaluation, and Baseline results of a Diabetes Primary Prevention Program with a Native Community in Canada, *Preventive Medicine.* **26**, 779-790 (1997).
21. S. Meltzer, L. Leiter, D. Daneman, H.C. Gerstein, D. Lau, S. Ludwig, J.F. Yale, B. Zinman, D. Lillie, Clinical Practice Guidelines for the management of diabetes in Canada, *Can Med Assoc J.* **159**, S1-S29 (1998).
22. A.L. Rosenbloom, J. Joe, R.S. Young, W.E. Winter, Emerging epidemic of type 2 diabetes in youth, *Diabetes Care.* **22**, 345-354 (1999).

UNDIAGNOSED DIABETES
BURDEN AND SIGNIFICANCE IN THE CANADIAN POPULATION

T. Kue Young
Professor and Head
Department of Community Health Sciences
University of Manitoba
Winnipeg, Manitoba, Canada

INTRODUCTION

An individual is said to have undiagnosed diabetes if he/she has not been previously diagnosed as having diabetes, but whose plasma glucose levels satisfy established criteria for diabetes. The corollaries of this definition is that:
1. Individuals with undiagnosed diabetes can only be detected in a survey or screening setting where they are tested for plasma glucose levels and inquired about a past history of diabetes.
2. Once detected, such individuals are no longer undiagnosed.

In 1979 the National Diabetes Data Group created order out of the chaos of multiple definitions and criteria for diabetes. The NDDG criteria were later superseded by the World Health Organization criteria (1985). In 1997 the American Diabetes Association (ADA) proposed new criteria which differ from the WHO ones in requiring only the fasting plasma glucose (FPG) for diagnosis, instead of both the FPG and the 2-hour post-challenge level. Diabetes (DM) is defined as FPG ^{3} 7.0 mmol/L; impaired fasting glucose (IFG) as FPG ^{3} 6.1 and <7.0 mmol/L; and normoglycemia as FPG <6.1 mmol/L.

The change in criteria offers an unique opportunity to study the outcome of undiagnosed diabetes, if a cohort of people who would now be labeled as DM (under the 1997 ADA criteria) but would not be considered DM some years ago could be found. These people would not have been subjected to special clinical or lifestyle interventions. Such a cohort exists in Manitoba, and this paper describes a method to study the clinical outcomes of undiagnosed diabetes among members of the cohort.

METHODS

This study involves linkage of two datasets: the Manitoba Heart Health Survey (MHHS) and the Manitoba Health Services Insurance Plan (MHSIP). The MHHS was conducted on a representative sample of the Manitoba adult population (aged 18-74) during October 1989-February 1990. It involved interviews, clinical examinations, and laboratory tests, including FPG. The overall response rate was 77% resulting in a sample of 2,792 individuals. Details of the MHHS has previously been published (Gelskey et al 1994; Young

Diabetes and Cardiovascular Disease: Etiology, Treatment and Outcomes
Edited by Aubie Angel *et al.*, Kluwer Academic/Plenum Publishers, 2001

7

et al 1995). At the time of the survey, individuals with FPG ≥7.8 mmol (based on the 1985 WHO criteria) were notified of the results and suggested to seek medical attention. Individuals with FPG ≥ 7.0 but <7.8 were left alone – at that time they were not considered to have DM, but now they would be under the 1997 ADA criteria.

The MHSIP covers the total population of Manitoba and captures all claims submitted by physicians for reimbursements and all hospital discharges. A substantial body of epidemiological and health services research has resulted from the MHSIP database (Roos and Shapiro 1995), including studies on the burden of diabetes in the province (Young et al 1991, Blanchard et al 1996). The accuracy and quality of the database is well established (Roos and Nicol 1999).

MHHS and MHSIP were linked electronically using a scrambled personal health insurance number. The details of the linkage has been previously published (Robinson et al 1998; Muhajarine et al 1997).

The MHHS dataset was first analysed as a cross-sectional study investigating the prevalence and the metabolic correlates of the various categories of diabetes status. The linked dataset was then analysed as a cohort study to examine the health care utilization pattern of the various diabetes status categories between 1990 and 1998.

RESULTS

The prevalence of diagnosed DM, undiagnosed DM, IFG, and normoglycemia in Manitoba is shown in Fig.1.

Overall the prevalence of undiagnosed DM is 2.2%, compared to 4.5% for previously diagnosed DM and 9.0% for IFG. Undiagnosed DM thus accounts for 33% of all diabetes cases.

Undiagnosed DM cases can be compared to the other categories of diabetes status in terms of plasma lipids (HDL, LDL, triglycerides, total/ HDL ratio), obesity (body mass index and waist/hip ratio), and blood pressure (Table 1).

Undiagnosed DM cases tend to have a more unfavourable lipid profile, more obese and higher mean blood pressure than normo- glycemic individuals. There is no significant difference between undiagnosed and diagnosed DM, or between undiagnosed DM and IFG cases.

Health care utilization is analysed by multiple linear regression with mean physician-visits per person-year as the dependent variable, and age group, sex, and diabetes status as independent variables. For this analysis there are 5 groups:

Figure 1. Prevalence of diabetes and impaired fasting glucose in the Manitoba population.

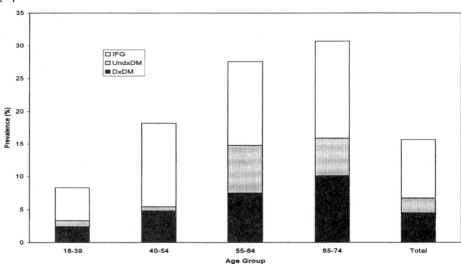

Table 1. Pairwise comparison of sex-specific, age-adjusted mean metabolic indicators

	Undx-DM vs Dx-DM		Undx-DM vs IFG		Undx-DM vs Normo	
	Male	Female	Male	Female	Male	Female
Total cholesterol	P>0.10	P>0.10	P>0.10	P>0.10	P>0.10	P>0.10
HDL-cholesterol	P>0.10	P>0.10	P>0.10	P>0.10	**P=0.038**	**P=0.037**
LDL-cholesterol	P>0.10	P>0.10	P>0.10	P>0.10	P>0.10	P>0.10
Triglycerides	P>0.10	P>0.10	P>0.10	P>0.10	**P=0.001**	**P<0.001**
Total/HDL ratio	P>0.10	P>0.10	P>0.10	P>0.10	**P=0.045**	**P=0.029**
Body mass index	P>0.10	P>0.10	P>0.10	P>0.10	**P=0.011**	**P=0.002**
Waist-hip ratio	P>0.10	P>0.10	P>0.10	P>0.10	**P=0.009**	**P=0.003**
Systolic blood pressure	P>0.10	P>0.10	P>0.10	P>0.10	**P=0.002**	**P<0.001**
Diastolic blood pressure	P>0.10	P>0.10	P>0.10	P>0.10	**P=0.009**	**P=0.001**

G-0 – normoglycemia [FPG<6.0 mmol/L]

G-1 – IFG [$6.0 \leq FPG < 7.0$]

G-2 – undiagnosed DM [$7.0 \leq FPG < 7.8$]

G-3 – undiagnosed DM [$FPG \geq 7.8$]

G-4 – diagnosed DM [self-report of past DM]

Note that both G-2 and G-3 are cases of undiagnosed DM at the time of the survey. G-3 cases, however, were notified of their "high" glucose values as an FPG of 7.8 was the cut-off point for DM at the time; they were likely to have been subjected to clinical/lifestyle interventions subsequent to the survey. G-2, on the other hand, remain unaware of their glucose values and not subject to any special interventions. Neither G-0 nor G-1 was notified of their glucose results.

G-2 have higher mean-MD-visits than G-0 [p=0.112] after controlling for age group and sex; similarly G-3 also have higher values than G-0 [p=0.086].

For hospitalization, multiple logistic regression was performed, with being hospitalized at least once during the study period as the outcome variable. Controlling for age group and sex, undiagnosed diabetes cases have an elevated risk of being hospitalized compared to normoglycemic individuals [G-2 compared to G-0, odds ratio = 1.23, 95% confidence interval 3.79, 0.40; G-3 compared to G-0, OR=2.07, 95%CI 6.87, 0.62; all DM vs non-DM, OR=1.88, 95% CI 3.17, 1.12]

DISCUSSION

This study demonstrates that undiagnosed diabetes represents a significant burden in the population and that it does carry important health risks as measured by metabolic indicators such as lipid profile, obesity indices, and blood pressure levels, as well as in long-term hospitalization and physician care.

The prevalence of diabetes and the distribution between diagnosed and undiagnosed cases are similar to data from the all-race population of the United States based on the NHANES-III survey (Harris et al 1998). The association of undiagnosed diabetes with various metabolic indicators on cross-sectional analysis is consistent with other reports in the literature (Harris 1993). The ability to follow a cohort of undiagnosed diabetes cases without clinical or lifestyle interventions represents a methodo-logic advance.

For the future, with a longer period of follow-up and the accumulation of more person-years of observation, the linked dataset is capable of more refined analyses using more specific clinical outcome indicators such as diagnoses of ischemic heart disease, stroke, chronic renal failure, etc, as well as medical procedures such as amputations and kidney dialysis. It will also allow an estimate of the time interval for progression to diagnosed diabetes.

REFERENCES

American Diabetes Association. Expert Committee on the Diagnosis and Classification of Diabetes Mellitus. Report. Diabetes Care 1997;20:1183-97.

Blanchard JF, Ludwig S, Wajda A, Dean H, Anderson K, Kendall O, Depew N. Incidence and prevalence of diabetes in Manitoba, 1986-1991. Diabetes Care 1996;19:807-811.

Gelskey DE, Young TK, Mandonald SM. Screening with total cholesterol: determining sensitivity and specificity of the National Cholesterol Education Program's guidelines from a population survey. J Clin Epidemiol 1994;47:547-53.

Harris MI, Goldstein DE, Flegal KM, Little RR, Cowie CC, Wiedmeyer HM, Eberhardt MS, Byrd-Holt DD. Prevalence of diabetes, impaired fasting glucose, and impaired glucose tolerance in U.S. adults. Diabetes Care 1998; 21:518-24.

Harris MI. Undiagnosed NIDDM: clinical and public health issues. Diabetes Care 1993; 16: 642-52.

Muhajarine N, Mustard C, Roos LL, Young TK, Gelskey DE. Comparison of survey and physician claims data for detecting hypertension. J Clin Epidemiol 1997;50:711-718.

Robinson JR, Young TK, Roos LL, Gelskey DE. Estimating the burden of disease: comparing administrative data and self reports. Med Care 1998;35:932-947.

Roos LL, Nicol JP. A research registry: Uses, development, and accuracy. J Clin Epidemiol 1999;52:39-47.

Roos NP, Shapiro E, eds. Health and Health Care: Experience with a Population-Based Health Information System. Med Care 1995;33 (Suppl):DS1-DS146.

World Health Organization. Expert Committee on Diabetes Mellitus. Second report. Geneva: WHO, 1985 [Tech Rep Ser No 727]

Young TK, Gelskey DE. Is non-central obesity metabolically benign? Implications for prevention from a population survey of Canadians. JAMA 1995;274:1939-1941.

Young TK, Roos NP, Hammerstrand KM. Esimated burden of diabetes mellitus in Manitoba according to health insurance claims: a pilot study. Can Med Assoc J 1991;144:318-324.

GENES, ENVIRONMENT AND DIABETES IN CANADIAN ABORIGINAL COMMUNITIES

Robert A. Hegele

Blackburn Cardiovascular Genetics Laboratory
John P. Robarts Research Institute
London, ON. Canada

INTRODUCTION

Mortality rates among aboriginal Canadians are higher than those in the general Canadian population[1-3]. This excess mortality is related to the increased risk of death from alcoholism, homicide, suicide and pneumonia in many native groups[1-3]. In contrast, some native groups have a markedly lower incidence of heart disease and certain types of cancer compared with the general Canadian population[4,5]. However, it has been suggested that the rapid cultural changes currently faced by many Canadian native groups may accelerate the development of "diseases of westernization", such as atherosclerosis and related conditions [5-8]. One factor that is inextricably linked to the anticipated rise of atherosclerosis in native Canadians is the emergence of diabetes mellitus as a health problem in certain native subgroups[9].

Recent estimates indicate that diabetes may be up to three times more prevalent in native than in non-native Canadian adults[3]. However, there is a wide range in the prevalence of diabetes amongst various aboriginal groups[9]. In a study of several aboriginal communities in Canada, it was found that the parallel of latitude and the language phylum were independent determinants of the wide variation in diabetes prevalence between groups[9]. Given that both geographical location and language are associated with other shared factors, such as genetic background[10], it is possible that genetic differences between aboriginal groups could contribute to the differences in the prevalence of diabetes between them.

My laboratory has been evaluating the genetic determinants of complex diseases and their intermediate phenotypes in Canadian aboriginal communities. These studies have provided an opportunity to compare and contrast the genetic and environmental attributes of two distinct aboriginal communities, which differ greatly in their prevalence of cardiovascular disease and diabetes. In particular, we have studied the genetics of the Oji-Cree of northwestern Ontario and the Inuit of Nunavut. The Oji-Cree have a frequency of non-insulin-dependent (type 2) diabetes of ~ 40%, which is among the world's highest[11], whereas the Inuit have a frequency of type 2 diabetes of <1% [9]. Other attributes of these groups are shown in Table1.

Diabetes and Cardiovascular Disease: Etiology, Treatment and Outcomes
Edited by Aubie Angel et al., Kluwer Academic/Plenum Publishers, 2001

Table 1. Some demographic attributes of the Oji-Cree and the Inuit

	Oji-Cree	Inuit
number of subjects	728	516
locale	Ontario, Sioux Lookout Zone	Keewatin, Northwest Territories
study name	Sandy Lake Health and Diabetes Project (SLHDP)	Keewatin Health Assessment Study (KHAS)
unit of study	Single reserve (Sandy Lake)	Eight communities
parallel of latitude	55th	60th to 70th
CHD prevalence *vs* the rest of Canada	3:1	1:2
diabetes prevalence *vs* the rest of Canada	5:1	1:3
absolute prevalence of diabetes or impaired glucose tolerance	40%	1%
average BMI	29.2 kg/m^2	25.8 kg/m^2
prevalence of smoking	27%	82%
current diet	Westernized processed food, high saturated fat, low fiber	traditional foods, with high n-3 fatty acids (marine animals)
activity level	relatively sedentary	relatively active

THE SANDY LAKE OJI-CREE

728 members (or 72% of eligible subjects) from the Sandy Lake reserve in northwestern Ontario were enrolled in a survey of diabetes and cardiovascular risk factors, called the Sandy Lake Health and Diabetes Project[11]. Sandy Lake is located at about the 55th parallel of latitude,

within the subarctic boreal forest. The community is isolated and is accessible only by air during most of the year. Historically, the ancestors of the contemporary residents of this region lived a nomadic, hunting-gathering subsistence typical of other Algonkian-speaking peoples of the northeastern subarctic. Since the development of the reservation and residential school systems, the lifestyle has changed from physically active to sedentary. Most members of the reserve now live in winterized cottages. Many community members have snowmobiles and automobiles. The primary food source has changed from wildlife with roots and berries to processed foods high in animal fats. The full details of the clinical, biochemical and genetic attributes of these subjects are described elsewhere [11-21].

THE KEEWATIN INUIT

516 randomly selected individuals from the Keewatin region, aged 18 to 80 years participated in a comprehensive health interview and examination survey, called the Keewatin Health Assessment Study[22,23]. The subjects came from eight communities situated on the western shore of Hudson Bay, between the 60th and 70th parallels of latitude. At the time of the survey, these communities still adhered to a relatively traditional lifestyle, including the consumption of arctic fish at least three times per week. Of great interest was the very high prevalence of cigarette smoking, approaching 80% of adult subjects[22,23]. Of the study participants, 92 reported themselves as being of European background. These 92 subjects were included as a contrast sample, in order to estimate allele frequencies from a reference, regional sample of subjects of European descent. The full details of the clinical, biochemical and genetic attributes of these subjects are presented elsewhere[24,25].

GENETIC "BURDEN" OF COMMON ALLELES FOR CARDIOVASCULAR DISEASE AND DIABETES

We wanted to estimate the genetic "burden of risk" for cardiovascular disease and diabetes in the Oji-Cree and the Inuit. Since there was no established method to evaluate the contributions from multiple "deleterious" alleles on these phenotypes, we devised a preliminary strategy to estimate such a burden. This involved comparing the frequencies of the "deleterious" allele from each marker system. Specifically, these were the *F5* Q506 allele (also called factor V Leiden)[25], *AGT* M174 and T235 alleles[18], *APOE* E4 allele (R112, R158)[16,17], *APOC3* -455C[16,17], *HL*-480C allele[27], *MTHFR* 677T allele[21], *PON1* R192 allele[16,17], *PON2* G148 allele[13,14], *PPPIR3* D allele[27], *FABP2* T54 allele[12], *HFE* Y282 allele[26] and *ADRB3* R64 allele[20]. The frequencies of the "deleterious" alleles in the control sample of white subjects from the Keewatin region, shown in Table 2, were each within the ranges of frequencies reported for other Caucasian populations[11-21,24-29]. All genotype frequencies in each population sample were found to not deviate significantly from the frequencies predicted by the Hardy-Weinberg equation.

There were many significant differences in allele frequencies between the aboriginal samples and between the aboriginal and regional white control samples (Table 2). First, compared to subjects of European origin, Oji-Cree had significantly different frequencies in

9 of the 13 alleles studied. In particular, compared to subjects of European origin, Oji-Cree had a higher frequency of *AGT* M174 and T235, *PON1* R192, and *ADRB3* R64 and a lower frequency of *F5* Q506, *HL* -480C, *MTHFR* 677T, *FABP2* T54 and *HFE* Y282.

Second, compared to subjects of European origin, the Inuit had significantly different frequency in 8 of the 13 alleles studied. In particular, compared to subjects of European origin, Inuit had a higher frequency of *AGT* T235, *APOE* E4, *PON1* R192, *FABP2* T54 and *ADRB3* R64, and a lower frequency of *F5* Q506, *MTHFR* 677T and *HFE* Y282.

Third, compared to the Inuit, the Oji-Cree had significantly different frequency in 5 of the 13 alleles studied. In particular, compared to the Inuit, the Oji-Cree had a higher frequency of *AGT* M174 and *MTHFR* 677T, and a lower frequency of *HL* -480C, *APOE* E4 and *FABP2* T54.

Thus, there were differences between Oji-Cree and Inuit, and between each aboriginal sample and subjects of European origin, in the frequencies of "deleterious" alleles of several

Table 2. Frequencies of "deleterious" alleles of candidate genes for diabetes and atherosclerosis in Oji-Cree, Inuit and subjects of European origin

		Oji-Cree	Inuit	Europeans
numbers of subjects:		724	175	92
gene	allele			
F5	Q506	0.003^*	0^*	0.024
AGT	T235	0.89^*	0.82^*	0.45
	M174	$0.38^{*,\#}$	0.08	0.11
APOE	E4	$0.11^{\#}$	0.23^*	0.13
HL	-480C	$0.45^{*,\#}$	0.60	0.68
APOC3	-455C	0.45	0.47	0.44
MTHFR	677T	$0.12^{*,\#}$	0.06^*	0.24
PON1	R192	0.77^*	0.70^*	0.35
PON2	G148	0.28	0.29	0.25
PPP1R3	deletion	0.28	0.33	0.29
FABP2	T54	$0.15^{*,\#}$	0.35^*	0.25
HFE	Y282	0.01^*	0^*	0.092
ADRB3	R64	0.40^*	0.30^*	0.080

legend: * allele frequency in the aboriginal group is significantly different from that in subjects of European origin ($P<0.05$); $^{\#}$ allele frequency in Oji-Cree is significantly different from that in Inuit ($P<0.05$); **abbreviations:** *F5*, gene encoding clotting factor V; *AGT*, gene encoding angiotensinogen; *APOE*, gene encoding apolipoprotein E; *HL*, gene encoding hepatic lipase; *APOC3*, gene encoding apolipoprotein CIII; *MTHFR*, gene encoding methylenetetrahydrofolate reductase; *PON1*, gene encoding serum paraoxonase; *PON2*, gene encoding paraoxonase-2; *PPP1R3*, gene encoding skeletal muscle regulatory G subunit of the glycogen-associated form of protein phosphatase 1; *FABP2* gene encoding intestinal fatty acid binding protein; *HFE*, hemochromatosis gene; *ADRB3*, gene encoding the beta-3-adrenergic receptor.

candidate genes for atherosclerosis and diabetes. It is possible that these inter-population differences in genetic architecture explain the differences in the prevalence of atherosclerosis and diabetes. This hypothesis can be tested more directly with different types of studies. However, the results are not fully consistent with the different prevalence of atherosclerosis and diabetes in Oji-Cree compared to Inuit and in Inuit compared to Canadians of European descent (Table 1).

For example, a simple tally of the alleles in Table 2 revealed an excess of "deleterious" alleles, compared to subjects of European origin, of 45% in Oji-Cree and 25% in Inuit. The higher frequency in both the Oji-Cree and Inuit of the "deleterious" alleles would suggest that both of these groups are genetically predisposed to atherosclerosis and/or diabetes and related phenotypes, compared to subjects of European origin. However, the present incidence of atherosclerosis and diabetes in the Inuit is low, whereas it is high in the Oji-Cree[5]. Several aspects of these disparities deserve comment at present.

First, the low prevalence of cardiovascular disease and diabetes in the Inuit compared to the rest of Canada was striking. This disparity is even more pronounced considering the high prevalence of cigarette smoking among the Inuit (Table 1). One explanation for this apparent paradox is that a potentially detrimental influence of the alleles has been overridden by a positive influence of the traditional Inuit lifestyle and diet[5]. If this were the true explanation, then westernization of the Inuit lifestyle could be expected to produce an increased expression of these diseases. The future prevalence of these diseases might even exceed the prevalence in the rest of Canada, given the excess of "deleterious" alleles in the Inuit. Alternatively, the genetic variants in Table 2 may have had little association with disease in the Inuit and other unmeasured genomic variants may have actually determined resistance to disease. Finally, it is possible that certain genetic variants, in particular *F5* Q506 and *MTHFR* 677T, were relatively more important determinants of the susceptibility to cardiovascular disease, and it was their lower prevalence that was the predominant factor underlying genetic resistance to disease compared with European subjects.

Second, the high prevalence of both diabetes and cardiovascular disease in the Oji-Cree compared the rest of Canada is notable (Table 1)[5]. One explanation for this observation is that it accurately reflects a detrimental influence of the alleles that were examined. In other words, the higher expression of these diseases resulted from a higher background of genetic susceptibility, in combination with recent deviation from the traditional Oji-Cree lifestyle and diet[11-21]. Indeed, the higher consumption of processed foods and "fast foods", bread and butter, and the lower consumption of vegetables, breakfast foods and hot meals were associated with an increased risk of diabetes in the Sandy Lake Oji-Cree[33,34]. Assuming this was a critical mechanism for disease initiation and progression, then it is possible that a simple reversion to a more traditional diet and lifestyle might have an impact upon the obesity and diabetes in these people. Alternatively, the studied variants may have had no association with disease, which was more related to other unmeasured variants.

Finally, the high prevalence of both diabetes and cardiovascular disease in the Oji-Cree compared to the Inuit deserves some reflection (Table 1)[5]. One explanation for the disparity in disease prevalence is that it accurately reflects significant differences in the genetic architecture between these two groups. Despite the fact that these are both aboriginal communities, there are several significant differences in the allele frequencies (Table 2). The explanation for the increased prevalence of these diseases among the Oji-Cree may simply be that there is a higher background of susceptibility in these people. There are also population-specific factors that could explain the difference. However, both groups had an excess of "deleterious" alleles compared to subjects of European origin (Table 2), and there were more differences in allele frequencies when each aboriginal group was compared to subjects of European origin than when they were compared to one another. This suggests that factors other than the alleles studied were the primary determinants of disease susceptibility.

Some of the differences between the Oji-Cree and the Inuit that could explain the differences in disease susceptibility are seen in Table 1. First, the Inuit live much further north than the Oji-Cree. This might serve to limit their exposure to the northward creep of noxious aspects of the North American lifestyle. This might also produce a greater adherence to a traditional diet and, along with greater physical activity, might result in lower body weight and less central obesity. Furthermore, there are some data to suggest that the impact of central obesity in the Inuit differs from non-Inuit. For example, in the Inuit, blood pressure and plasma lipoproteins are largely determined by the presence of central obesity, but carbohydrate tolerance and insulin sensitivity may not be. Thus, endogenous, perhaps genetic, differences could modulate the impact of obesity on health in the Inuit. The type of fat consumed might also be a key determinant in the expression of a particular metabolic phenotype. Whatever the mechanism, it will be important to monitor the impact of changing diet and physical activity on the prevalence of obesity and its sequelae in the Inuit.

A POPULATION-SPECIFIC GENETIC MARKER FOR TYPE 2 DIABETES IN OJI-CREE

The incidence of cardiovascular disease in the aboriginal population in Northern Ontario has tripled over the last 25 years[32]. A factor that is inextricably linked to this epidemic is the remarkably high prevalence of diabetes in these communities, which is a very recent phenomenon[9]. The Oji-Cree of Northern Ontario have a prevalence of non-insulin-dependent (type 2) diabetes of ~ 40%, which is among the world's highest[11], and is about 5 times higher than the prevalence of type 2 diabetes in the general Canadian population. It is somewhat remarkable that diabetes was virtually unknown as a medical diagnosis in these people as little as 60 years ago[11]. The rapid change in lifestyle is seen to be of primary importance in the recent diabetes epidemic[11]. However, the high population prevalence of diabetes suggests that there is some susceptibility among the aboriginals of northern Ontario.

For the last three years, we have searched for genetic determinants of type 2 diabetes among members of the Sandy Lake reserve. In the course of sequencing a variety of candidate genes, we identified a new variant in the *HNF1A* gene, namely G319S, in Ontario Oji-Cree with type 2 diabetes. The *HNF1A* gene product, HNF-1a, normally acts as a transcriptional activator of several hepatic genes[33,34]. S319 was absent from 1000 alleles taken from subjects representing six other ethnic groups, including the Inuit, suggesting that it is private for Oji-Cree. We observed a significantly increased relative risk of type 2 diabetes for both S319/S319 homozygotes and S319/G319 heterozygotes, who, respectively, had odds ratios of 18 (95% CI 2.1 to 150) and 2.0 (95% CI 1.4 to 2.7) compared with G319/G319 homozygotes. We also found a significant difference for the mean age-of-onset of type 2 diabetes, with G319/G319, S319/G319 and S319/S319 subjects affected in the fifth, fourth and third decades of life, respectively.

It is possible that *HNF1A* S319 is an allele of the "thrifty genotype"[35]. According to the "thrifty genotype" hypothesis, aboriginal people evolved a complement of genetic variants that provided for survival in a harsh environment, which was characterized by marked excursions in their energy intake, a pattern sometimes described as "feast or famine". The hypothesis proposed that such a complement of genetic variants encoded products that both efficiently utilized caloric energy for cellular metabolism and enabled the easy storage of excess energy for future use.

While such a metabolic framework might have been advantageous to natives in the context of a "feast or famine" pattern of subsistence, recent cultural changes have created a context of "feast and more feast" for some native groups. The propensity to more efficiently utilize caloric energy and to store the excess, which were advantageous in the context of "feast or famine", would be detrimental in the context of "feast and more feast". It is not yet clear whether the *HNF1A* S319 allele contributes to the "thrifty genotype" as the appropriate cellular biology and molecular experiments have not yet been done. However, given the complexity of factors such as the tissue distribution and large number of target genes for the *HNF1A* gene product, it will not be easy to derive the mechanism for developing diabetes from the results of reductionist *in vitro* experiments. It seems clear that *HNF1A* S319 was probably neutral at worst in the past, but is now strikingly associated with a detrimental phenotype in the context of obesity, inactivity and a high saturated fat diet in the Sandy Lake natives.

Assuming that the allele and genotype frequencies in Sandy Lake are representative of the ~16,000 aboriginal residents of northwestern Ontario, there may be as many as 200 and 3000 S319/S319 homozygotes and S319/G319 heterozygotes, respectively. Therefore, the *HNF1A* S319 allele may contribute considerably to diabetes morbidity amongst the native people in Northern Canada[33,34].

Even without fully understanding the cellular and molecular biology of *HNF1A* S319, the clinical collaborators for the Sandy Lake studies, Drs. Stewart Harris and Bernie Zinman, have begun an intervention strategy to delay the onset of diabetes in young Sandy Lake Oji-Cree. Such a strategy includes: 1) educating the community about diet and activity using anthropologically appropriate concepts, language and symbols; 2) identifying non-traditional foods that are associated with a lower risk of diabetes and providing education about finding, purchasing, preparing and consuming such products[30]; 3) encouraging prudent food choices from the traditional diet; 4) focussing these efforts towards younger adults and school-aged children[30,31]. It is also essential to plan that the community will eventually take control of administering such a prevention program. From the experience to date, such an effort will not succeed without community-wide understanding, acceptance and cooperation.

CONCLUSIONS: GENES, LIFESTYLE AND INTERVENTION

There are two main findings from the genetic studies outlined above. First, there is a high prevalence of "deleterious" alleles in samples taken from Canadian Oji-Cree and Inuit communities, compared with subjects of European origin. Second, there is a population-specific genetic marker, namely *HNF1A*, that is associated with type 2 diabetes in the Oji-Cree. The association of this genetic variant with diabetes in the Oji-Cree was very strong, but was specific only to those people.

The differences in disease prevalence between the Oji-Cree and Inuit could have been related to differences in the genetic backgrounds of these two groups, both with respect to the common variants in candidate genes and to the specific *HNF1A* G319S variant in the Oji-Cree. However, the findings also emphasize the pre-eminence of environmental factors, particularly the diet and level of activity, in determining disease susceptibility. The rapid change in the lifestyle of the Oji-Cree appears to have been a key factor that has unmasked their genetic susceptibility to diabetes. Furthermore, the differences in lifestyle between the Oji-Cree and Inuit probably contributed to the large differences in disease prevalence between these groups. This would suggest that it would be valuable to recommend, and also to assess the impact of, a return to a more traditional diet and lifestyle until the issue is clarified by future investigations.

Acknowledgments

The scientific collaborators for these studies included Drs. Kue Young, Bernard Zinman, Stewart Harris, Philip Connelly and Tony Hanley. The expert assistance of Henian Cao, Jian Wang, Carol Anderson, Matthew Ban and Doreen Jones are greatly appreciated. This work was supported by grants from the Medical Research Council of Canada (MA13430), the Canadian Diabetes Association, the Heart and Stroke Foundation of Ontario (#NA3628), and the Blackburn Group. Dr. Hegele is a Career Investigator of the Heart and Stroke Foundation of Ontario.

REFERENCES

1. F. Trovato. Mortality differentials in Canada 1951-1971: French, British and Indians. *Cult Med Psychiatry* 1988; 12: 459-477.
2. Y. Mao, B.W. Moloughney, R.M. Semenciw, H.I. Morrison. Indian reserve and Indian mortality in Canada. *Can J Pub Health* 1992; 83: 350-353.
3. H.L. MacMillan, A.B. MacMillan, D.R. Offord, J.L. Dingle. Aboriginal health. *CMAJ* 1996; 155:1569-1578.
4. T.K. Young. Mortality pattern of isolated Indians in northwestern Ontario. A 10 year review. *Public Health Rep* 1983; 98:467-475.
5. T.K. Young, M.E. Moffatt, J.D. O'Neil. Cardiovascular diseases in a Canadian Arctic population. *Am J Public Health* 1993; 83:881-887.
6. T.K. Young. Chronic diseases among Canadian Indians: towards an epidemiology of culture change. *Arctic Med Res* 1988; 47(I): 434-441.
7. T.K. Young. The Canadian north and the third world: is the analogy appropriate? *Can J Pub Health* 1983; 74: 239-241.
8. D. Steib, K. Davies. Health and development in the Hudson Bay/James Bay region. *Arctic Med Res* 1995; 54: 170-183.
9. T.K. Young, J. Reading, B. Elias, J.D. O'Neil. Type 2 diabetes mellitus in Canada's first nations: status of an epidemic in progress. *CMAJ* 2000; 163: 561-566.
10. T.K. Young, E.J. Szathmary, S. Evers B. Wheatley. Geographical distribution of diabetes among the native population of Canada: a national survey. *Soc Sci Med* 1990; 129-139.

11. S.B. Harris, J. Gittelsohn, A.J.G Hanley, A. Barnie, T.M.S. Wolever, J. Gao, A.Logan, B. Zinman B. The prevalence of NIDDM and associated risk factors in native Canadians. *Diabetes Care* 1997; 20:185-197

12. R.A. Hegele, S.B. Harris, A.J. Hanley, S. Sadikian, P.W. Connelly, B. Zinman. Genetic variation of intestinal fatty acid-binding protein associated with variation in body mass in aboriginal Canadians. *J Clin Endocrinol Metab* 1996; 81:4334-4337.

13. R.A. Hegele, P.W. Connelly, S.W. Scherer, A.J. Hanley, S.B. Harris, L.C. Tsui, B. Zinman. Paraoxonase-2 gene (PON2) G148 variant associated with elevated fasting plasma glucose in noninsulin-dependent diabetes mellitus. *J Clin Endocrinol Metab* 1997; 82:3373-3377.

14. R.A. Hegele, P.W. Connelly, S.W. Scherer, A.J. Hanley, S.B. Harris, L.C. Tsui, B. Zinman. Paraoxonase-2 G148 variant in an aboriginal Canadian girl with non-insulin-dependent diabetes. *Lancet* 1997; 350:785.

15. R.A. Hegele, B. Zinman, A.J. Hanley, S. Harris, P.W. Connelly. A common mtDNA polymorphism associated with variation in plasma triglyceride concentration. *Am J Hum Genet* 1997; 60:1552-1555.

16. R.A. Hegele, P.W. Connelly, A.J. Hanley, F. Sun, S.B. Harris, B. Zinman. Common genomic variants associated with variation in plasma lipoproteins in young aboriginal Canadians. *Arterioscler Thromb Vasc Biol* 1997; 17:1060-1066.

17. R.A. Hegele, P.W. Connelly, A.J. Hanley, F. Sun, S.B. Harris, B. Zinman. Common genomic variation in the APOC3 promoter associated with variation in plasma lipoproteins. *Arterioscler Thromb Vasc Biol* 1997; 17: 2753-2758.

18. R.A. Hegele, S.B. Harris, A.J. Hanley, F. Sun, P.W. Connelly, B. Zinman. Angiotensinogen gene variation associated with variation in blood pressure in aboriginal Canadians. *Hypertension* 1997; 29:1073-1077.

19. R.A. Hegele, S.B. Harris, A.J. Hanley, F. Sun, P.W. Connelly, B. Zinman. -6A promoter variant of angiotensinogen and blood pressure variation in Canadian Oji-Cree. *J Hum Genet* 1998;43:37-41.

20. R.A. Hegele RA, Harris SB, Hanley AJ, Azouz H, Connelly PW, Zinman B. Absence of association between genetic variation of the beta 3-adrenergic receptor and metabolic phenotypes in Oji-Cree. *Diabetes Care* 1998; 21:851-854.

21. R.A. Hegele, T.M. Wolever, A.J.Hanley, S.B. Harris, B. Zinman B. Methylenetetrahydrofolate reductase gene, dietary folate, NIDDM, and atherosclerosis in Canadian Oji-Cree. *Diabetes Care* 1998;21:322-323.

22. M.E.K. Moffatt, T.K Young, J.D. O'Neil JD. The Keewatin Health Assessment Study. *Arctic Med Res* 1993; 52: 18-21.

23. T.K. Young, Y.P. Nikitin, E.V. Shubinov, T.I. Astakhova, M.E.K. Moffatt, J.D. O'Neil. Plasma lipids in two indigenous arctic populations with low risk for cardiovascular diseases. *Am J Hum Biol* 1995; 7:223-236.

24. R.A. Hegele, T.K. Young, P.W. Connelly. Are Canadian Inuit at increased genetic risk for coronary heart disease? *J Mol Med* 1997; 75:364-370.

25. R.A. Hegele, C. Tully, T.K. Young, P.W. Connelly. V677 mutation of methylenetetra- hydrofolate reductase and cardiovascular disease in Canadian Inuit. *Lancet* 1997; 349:1221-1222.

26. D.R. Price, P.M. Ridker. Factor V Leiden mutation and the risks for thromboembolic disease: a clinical perspective. *Ann Int Med* 1997; 127:895-903.

27. R. Guerra, J. Wang, S.M. Grundy, J.C. Cohen. A hepatic lipase (LIPC) allele associated with high plasma concentrations of high density lipoprotein cholesterol. *Proc Natl Acad Sci USA* 1997; 94:4532-4537.

28. J. Xia, S.W. Scherer, P.T.W. Cohen, M. Majer, R.A. Norman, W.C. Knowler, C. Bogardus, M. Prochazka A common variant in PPPIR3 contributes to insulin resistance and type-2 diabetes. *Diabetes* 1998; 47:1519-1524.

29. A.T. Merryweather-Clarke, J.J. Pointon, J.D. Shearman, K.J.H. Robson. Global prevalence of putative haemochromatosis mutations. *J Med Genet* 1997; 34:275-278.

30. T.M. Wolever, S. Hamad, J. Gittelsohn, J. Gao, A.J. Hanley, S.B. Harris, B. Zinman. Low dietary fiber and high protein intakes associated with newly diagnosed diabetes in a remote aboriginal community. *Am J Clin Nutr* 1997; 66: 1470-1477.

31. J. Gittelsohn, T.M. Wolever, S.B. Harris, R. Harris-Giraldo, A.J.G. Hanley, B. Zinman. Specific patterns of food consumption and preparation are associated with diabetes and obesity in a native Canadian community. *J Nutr* 1998; 128: 541-547.

32. B. Shah, J.B. Hux. B. Zinman. Increasing rates of ischemic heart disease in the native population of Ontario, Canada. *Diabetes* 1999; A169.

33. R.A. Hegele, H. Cao, S.B. Harris, A.J. Hanley, B. Zinman. The hepatic nuclear factor-1alpha G319S variant is associated with early-onset type 2 diabetes in Canadian Oji-Cree. *J Clin Endocrinol Metab* 1999; 84:1077-82.

34. R.A. Hegele, H. Cao, A.J. Hanley, B. Zinman, S.B. Harris, C.M. Anderson. Clinical utility of HNF1A genotyping for diabetes in aboriginal Canadians. *Diabetes Care* 2000; 23:775-778.

35. J.V. Neel. The genetics of diabetes mellitus. *In* Early Diabetes. R. Camerini-Davalos, H.S. Cole (eds) 1970. Academic Press, Inc., Orlando, FLA, pp 3-10.

DIABETES IN SUB-SAHARAN AFRICA

Terry J. Aspray and Nigel Unwin

Department of Medicine, The Medical School
University of Newcastle upon Tyne, NE2 4HH,UK
and Department for International Development, British Government

THE BURDEN OF DIABETES IN AFRICA

Introduction

Diabetes mellitus represents a world-wide epidemic. The prevalence of diabetes mellitus is projected to increase between the years 1995 to 2010, by 87%, which represents 103 million new cases. In Africa as a whole, a doubling in the number of cases is expected, while in sub-Saharan Africa, a 2-3 fold increase in prevalence is projected for this period.[1]

Mechanisms Behind the Global Epidemic

Models of epidemiological and health transition predict that falling death rates from communicable diseases, particularly in childhood, contribute to demographic changes. An increase in numbers of survivors of childhood leads to a progressive "ageing" of the community, which is exaggerated by the control of fertility and smaller family size. There is an increase in health burden from chronic, non-communicable diseases (NCDs). This is already the case in established market economies.[2] The picture in middle-income countries is mixed, although NCDs are now recognised in some, such as Mauritius and the Caribbean as major health problems.[3][4] In low income countries, Murray and his team [5] report that chronic disease burden is projected to rise although infectious diseases will remain important for decades to come. However, the paucity of available data make such estimates difficult, especially in sub-Saharan Africa.[6] Recent research suggests that in urban and rural areas of sub-Saharan Africa, NCDs are important and in Tanzania, 15-34% of all deaths in adults, aged 15-59 years, are due to NCDs.[7] In sub-Saharan African countries, just as much as in established market economies, we need to estimate the future burden of chronic disease such as diabetes. The key elements for such estimates comprise:

Diabetes and Cardiovascular Disease: Etiology, Treatment and Outcomes
Edited by Aubie Angel et al., Kluwer Academic/Plenum Publishers, 2001

21

- Baseline disease rates
- Projected population growth
- Changes in population age structure
- Rates of urbanisation and likely lifestyle changes

Thus, our starting point is the use of published survey data, including age and sex specific prevalence and incidence figures for diabetes in representative countries. Figure 1 shows estimates available for over 35,000 subjects in eight different study populations between 1961 and 1989. However, the use of non-standard methodologies and differences between the study populations mean that these estimates of diabetes prevalence range from 0.2-5.7%.

Population growth and changes in age structure also influence future projections of disease prevalence. Estimates of these effects are difficult and in sub-Saharan Africa over recent years, a particular problem has been the estimation of the effect of deaths from HIV infection on chronic disease prevalence. However, AIDS mortality in young adults is likely to decrease the absolute numbers surviving into middle age, when diabetes and cardiovascular disease incidence increases.

The aetiololgy of type 2 diabetes is strongly influenced by aspects of "lifestyle". Overweight and obesity are important predictors of diabetes are with physical inactivity found to be a consistent risk factor in population studies. These lifestyle changes are associated with urban living and in Africa, a move from traditional to a modern "Western" lifestyle may be the most important factor with expansion of urban populations. Current projections are that the global population increase will be predominantly in cities at the expense of rural areas and this needs to be factored into any burden of disease model.

Figure 1. [Diabetes prevalence studies in sub-Saharan Africa: 1963-'89]

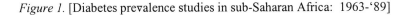

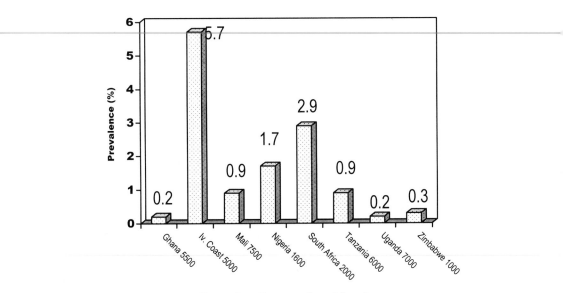

Country & no. of subjects

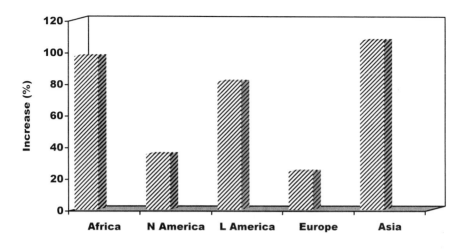

Figure 2. [Proportional increase in the number of people with diabetes 1995 to 2010]

Current Estimates of the Burden

Figure 2 shows world projections for diabetes prevalence in Africa, North and South America, Europe and Asia. These are relatively conservative estimates, particularly in low income countries, where they were based on baseline prevalence and demographic change alone. However, with an estimated world increase of 87%, the range is evident from 24% in Europe to 97% in Africa and 107% in Asia.

WORK FROM TANZANIA AND CAMEROON

Urban and Rural Differences in Diabetes Prevalence

Surveys performed in Tanzania over the past two decades have contributed greatly to our knowledge of diabetes and cardiovascular disease prevalence in urban and rural communities. Data from 1987 and 1989, confirm the low prevalence of diabetes in adults in rural areas at around 1%. The crude prevalence of hypertension in adults varies between 2.3% and 9.5% in rural areas but much of this difference can be attributed to differences in age structure between urban and rural communities. However, in our recently studies in urban (Dar es Salaam) and rural (Shari, Kilimanjaro) areas of Tanzania, a total of 1698 adults aged 15 years and over were recruited. Diabetes, overweight, obesity, and physical inactivity were significantly more prevalent in the urban area for both men and women. Diabetes prevalence in men from the city was 5.3%, which was 3.8% higher than in the rural area; similarly the urban female prevalence was 4.0%, which was 2.9% higher than the rural area. Using a definition of overweight as body mass index (BMI) greater than 25 kg/m^2, the difference in prevalence between urban and rural areas was 21.5% for men and 17.4% for women. Urban residents were also less physically active.

From these studies it has been possible to estimate the importance of likely determinants of diabetes risk. The population attributable fraction (PAF) is the proportion by which the disease in the entire population (for example, prevalence of diabetes) would be reduced in the absence of the "exposure"(for example overweight). Thus PAF is an estimate of the maximum benefit to be gained if it were possible to remove the exposure and we found that 64% of diabetes in men and 69% in women might be prevented if overweight were avoidable. The picture is thus of an more sedentary and overweight urban population with an increasing prevalence of diabetes and hypertension. Indeed 15% of urban me aged over 55 years were diabetic.

The Role of Urbanization

The adverse health effects of living in the city can be very rapid: with rural-to-urban Kenyan migrants showing a rise in blood pressure within 6 weeks of moving to the city.[8] The role of urbanisation in the aetiology of diabetes is an important component of the research agenda. We are currently studying adult migrants from rural areas who are followed up as they move to the city. Using a combined biomedical, genetic and socio-anthropological approach, we are attempting to "tease out" potential components of urbanisation with diet, exercise, biochemical risk factors, including lipid profiles, glucose tolerance and underlying genetic factors.

Improving the Treatment of NCDs in Africa

We are also concerned with developing appropriate and effective healthcare for adults with diabetes and other chronic diseases. The background to this work is important. A 5-year follow-up survey of 1250 newly-diagnosed cases of diabetes in Dar es Salaam, revealed a 29% mortality for those treated with insulin and a 16% mortality for those not requiring insulin. Moreover, of 124 deaths, which occurred in hospital, 54 were from potentially avoidable causes (e.g. keto-acidosis or infection).

Routine care available to Tanzanians with diabetes does not include glucose monitoring, other than urinalysis (when urine sticks are available). Equipment and drugs are often not available in the government health centres and screening eye and renal services are not developed.

In adult health service planning at district level, we are currently working to develop methods of rapidly evaluating services as well as developing evidence based guidelines for the treatment of chronic conditions in primary care. The work is underway in Tanzania, East Africa and Cameroon, Central West Africa. In 8 pilot clinics, guidelines for staff are being developed with training materials and structured patient records. The treatment protocols are simple and as inexpensive as possible: Drugs used for blood pressure control comprise thiazide diuretics and beta-blockers with glibenclamide, chlorpropamide and metformin used as first line hypoglycaemic agents. Simple screening for foot problems and impaired visual acuity, to identify cataract is included but not retinal screening, since retinal surgery is not available in the government service. Similar protocols have been developed for other chronic diseases: hypertension, asthma and epilepsy. New tools are also being developed for the evaluation of current services for adults with NCDs at district, region and national level. These includes methods to evaluate interventions, which are also being developed.

Causes of Adult Morbidity and Mortality in Africa

It is surprising how little is currently known about the causes of death of adults in sub-Saharan Africa. However, in Tanzania, for the past seven years, a demographic surveillance project has monitored all causes of adult death in a total study population of 300,000 people from two rural and one urban area. This study population is being expanded. All deaths are notified and the cause of death for each adult is assessed using a "verbal autopsy", developed and validated locally together with medical record tracing, where available. Some of the important findings of the adult morbidity and mortality project (AMMP) so far include the confirmation that, in adults aged 15-59 years, HIV/AIDS is the leading cause of death but that 15-30% of deaths are due to non-infectious disease. Mortality from stroke is seven times that in young adults in Europe. Male death rates are higher than female in most age groups and 90% of female deaths at reproductive age are **not** related to childbirth. There is a wealth of information in this surveillance study, which will help to develop strategies for the promotion of adult health in Tanzania. It is hoped that other African countries can use this research for information and methodological development.

SUMMARY

NCDs including diabetes, heart disease and stroke are global epidemics of the 21st century. The greatest burden on health will be in developing countries and sub-Saharan Africa is an area of major challenge: We are concerned with planning for the adult victims of the new epidemic and this includes the development of appropriate treatment. Therapy should be cost effective and evidence on the economics of treating chronic conditions in Africa is urgently required. Finally, health promotion, primary prevention and health screening strategies for chronic diseases such as diabetes, stroke and coronary heart disease are required.

ACKNOWLEDGEMENTS

Much of the material presented was inspired by the late Prof. Donald McLarty. Drs Ferdinand Mugusi, Henry Kitange, Prof. Jean-Claude Mbanya and their teams in Tanzania and Cameroon continue to combine clinical service development with research, in very difficult circumstances. Prof. George Alberti and Dr Nigel Unwin co-ordinate the NCD research programme at Newcastle University, UK.

The Department for International Development of the British Government funds the Essential NCD Health Intervention Project, **ENHIP** and Adult Morbidity and Mortality Project, **AMMP**; The Wellcome Trust funds the Rural to Urban Migration study in Tanzania and The European Union funds Action on NCDs in sub-Saharan Africa, **ANSA**).

REFERENCES

1. Amos AF, McCarty DJ, Zimmet P. The rising global burden of diabetes and its complications: estimates and projections to the year 2010. Diabetic Medicine 1997;14(5):S1-85.
2. Unwin N, Mugusi F, Aspray T, Whiting D, Edwards R, Mbanya JC, et al. Tackling the emerging pandemic of non-communicable diseases in sub-Saharan Africa: the essential NCD health intervention project. Public Health 1999;113:141-146.
3. Tuomilheto J, Li N, Dowse G, Gareeboo H, Chitson P, Fareed D, et al. The prevalence of coronary heart disease in the multi-ethnic and high diabetes prevalence population of Mauritius. Journal of Internal Medicine 1993;233:187-194.
4. PAHO. Health conditions in the Caribbean. Washington, D.C.: Pan American Health Organisation, 1997.
5. Murray CJL, Lopez AD. Mortality by cause for eight regions of the world: global burden of disease study. Lancet 1997;349:1269-1276.
6. Aspray TJ, Kitange, H., Setel, P., Unwin, N.C., Whiting, D. Disease burden in sub-Saharan Africa. Lancet 1998;351:1208-1209.

7. Adult Morbidity and Mortality Project (AMMP). Policy implications of adult morbidity and mortality. End of phase 1 report. Dar es Salaam: DfID(UK)/United Republic of Tanzania, 1997.
8. Poulter NR, Khaw KT, Hopwood BEC, Mugambi M, Peart WS, Rose G, et al. The Kenyan Luo migration study: observation on the initiation of a rise in blood pressure. British Medical Journal 1990;300:967-972.

CORONARY HEART DISEASE AND RISK FACTORS IN ASIAN INDIANS

Manisha Chandalia[1] and Prakash C. Deedwania[2]

[1]Department of Internal Medicine, University of Texas Southwestern Medical Center, and Department of Veterans Affairs Medical Center, Dallas, TX

[2]Cardiology Division, Department of Medicine, UCSF School of Medicine, Fresno, CA

INTRODUCTION

Traditionally individuals living in the Indian subcontinent (India, Pakistan, and Bangladesh) were considered to have a low prevalence of coronary heart disease (CHD). However, recent epidemiological studies have shown that Asian Indians who have migrated to western countries as well as those living in urban areas of the Indian subcontinent have a higher prevalence of CHD than do Caucasians of European ancestry[1-7]. This apparent excess of CHD could relate to environmental or genetic factors. Since lifestyle, including different levels of exercise, is shown to affect risk factors for CHD in Caucasians, it is likely that the adoption of the western lifestyle by Indians living in the urban areas of the Indian subcontinent or migrants to western countries could increase their risk for CHD. Asia is undergoing unprecedented economic growth, technological advances, and urbanization resulting in westernization of diet and reduction in physical activity. With these changes, it is likely that the prevalence of traditional risk factors for heart disease like hypercholesterolemia, hypertension and diabetes will increase. As a consequence, it is expected that CHD and morbidity and mortality associated with it will increase exponentially in the near future. A two-fold increase in the number of deaths related to CHD has been projected from year 1985 to year 2015. In men, the projected death rates per 100,000 population are 145 in 1985 and 253 in 2000 and 295 in 2015, while in women, the projected rates are 126, 204 and 239, respectively[8,9]. CHD is likely to account for at least 33.5% of total deaths by the year 2015 and would replace infectious disease as a number one killer in Indians.

Similarly alarming figures for CHD are reported for Asian Indians who have migrated to western countries[1]. During 1979-83, age-standardized CHD mortality was 40% higher in men and women of Indian subcontinent extraction compared to the general population of England and Wales, irrespective of social class or religious group[7]. The decrease in CHD mortality rates experienced by most of the western world over the past two decades contrasts sharply with the increase in CHD mortality in westernized Asian Indians[1,10]. Among UK-based Asian Indians, CHD mortality increased by 6% in men and 13% in women in the decade from 1970 to 1980. Excess mortality from CHD in Asian Indians is especially striking

Diabetes and Cardiovascular Disease: Etiology, Treatment and Outcomes
Edited by Aubie Angel et al., Kluwer Academic/Plenum Publishers, 2001

27

in young men[11]. This excess mortality could be explained by a higher prevalence of traditional risk factors for CHD in Asian Indians, compared to Caucasians. Alternatively, other risk factors may have a major role in Asian Indian CHD morbidity and mortality.

ROLE OF TRADITIONAL RISK FACTORS FOR CHD IN ASIAN INDIANS

The epidemiological studies comparing the rural and urban population of western India (Rajasthan and Haryana) showed that CHD was more prevalent in urban areas compared to rural areas in both men and women (men 6.0% vs 3.4%; women 10.5% vs 3.7%, respectively)[12-15]. The prevalence of hypertension, diabetes mellitus, obesity, truncal obesity, physical inactivity and increased levels of total cholesterol and LDL cholesterol were higher in the urban population compared to the rural population. However, smoking was more prevalent in rural men[16]. Thus it appears that an increase in the traditional risk factors of CHD in urban population compared to rural population is responsible for the increased prevalence of CHD in India. The increase in the risk factors can be attributed to adaptation of western lifestyle. However, when comparison is made between migrant Asian Indians and Caucasians of European ancestry in the country of migration, the picture is not clear any more.

The measurements of CHD risk factors, i.e., smoking, elevated serum cholesterol, hypertension and obesity, are no more common in Asian Indians than in Caucasians[17-19]. National household survey data in Britain show lower smoking rates in South Asian men than in the general population[20]. Similarly, two studies in which blood pressure in South Asians and Europeans in England was compared directly did not find blood pressure to be higher in South Asians[21,22]. In northwest London mean blood pressure was similar in Indians and Europeans[21]. Thus, levels of smoking and hypertension do not account for the high CHD rates in South Asians migrants. Similarly, in North-West London and in East London, plasma cholesterol was 0.7 mmol/l lower in South Asian men and women than in Europeans, in contrast to local mortality data which showed higher rates in South Asians[6,21,22]. Neither the levels of serum cholesterol prevailing in the home countries nor the levels in migrants to Britain appear to explain the high CHD mortality of South Asians in England and Wales. Low plasma levels of high-density lipoprotein (HDL) cholesterol and high levels of triglyceride are predictors of CHD risk in prospective studies. South Asian migrants have been found to have fairly consistently low HDL-cholesterol in studies from Britain, the USA and other countries[1]. However, low HDL-C alone can not explain the high prevalence of CHD in this group. The dietary fat intake among South Asian migrants to Britain has also been studied. In two studies, one using household food inventories[6] and the other weighed intakes[21] Gujaratis on North-West London were found to have low dietary saturated fat intakes and high polyunsaturated fat intakes compared with the British average. Total fat intake was similar to the levels in the British Population. Ghee, prepared by heating butter to drive off the water, is traditionally used in North Indian cooking. One analysis has shown that 12% of the sterol in ghee obtained from commercial and home-prepared sources was in the form of cholesterol oxides, which are not found in ordinary butter[23]. Since there is evidence from animal studies that cholesterol oxides are more atherogenic than pure cholesterol[24], the presence of these compounds in ghee was suggested as a possible cause of high CHD rates in South Asians in Britain and Trinidad. However, ghee is not widely used by Indians in Trinidad or London.

ROLE OF EMERGING RISK FACTORS FOR CHD IN ASIAN INDIANS :

Lp(a) concentrations are determined by genetic polymorphism rather than environmental influences, and high Lp(a) levels are thought to be important risk factors for CHD, especially when accompanied by increased levels of LDL cholesterol.

In one study, raised levels of Lp(a) were noted in both migrant Punjabis to UK and their siblings in India compared to native UK population[25]. Similarly, impaired endothelial function in healthy Asian Indians compared to Caucasians of European ancestry has been implicated in one study, implicating genetic or other novel risk factors, not accounted for by the major CHD risk factors, modulating endothelial function in Asian Indians with increased susceptibility to CHD[26]. Several other emerging risk factors for CHD, such as homocysteine, fibrinolytic parameters, neurohormones, markers of infections etc are being studied and compared in various ethnic populations and may shed some light on probable causes for difference in incidence and prevalence of CHD in these ethnic groups[27].

ROLE OF DIABETES AND INSULIN RESISTANCE IN CHD IN ASIAN INDIANS

One of the factors leading to premature CHD in this population may be a concomitant propensity to type 2 diabetes[22,28-31]. The prevalence of type 2 diabetes among Asian Indians is much higher than would be anticipated from their degree of obesity as opposed to marked obesity and type 2 diabetes in the Native American population in Arizona[6,30]. However, most cases of premature CHD occur in the absence of diabetes in Asian Indian population living in urban settings or having migrated to western countries. Therefore, other factors may play an important role in the high prevalence of CHD in Asian Indians.

One hypothesis has been proposed that could account for the high frequency of type 2 diabetes, low HDL cholesterol, high triglyceride and premature CHD in Asian Indians. This hypothesis observes that Asian Indians are susceptible to a generalized metabolic condition commonly referred to as insulin resistance syndrome[1]. Prolonged insulin resistance confers an increased risk for the development of type 2 diabetes, which is an independent risk factor for CHD. In addition, insulin resistance is often accompanied by other risk factors, e.g., dyslipidemia and hypertension (Fig. 1). Finally, it is possible that insulin resistance affects CHD risk status through other mechanisms that are independent of the established risk factors.

Recent reports indicate that Asian Indians in urban settings are more insulin

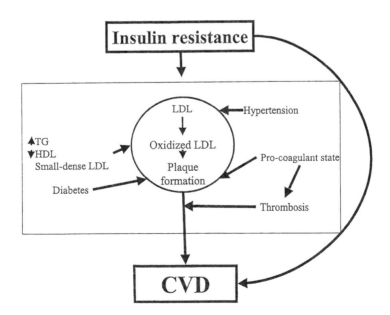

Figure 1. Schematic representation of the possible role of insulin resistance on development of cardiovascular disease (CVD).

resistant than matched Caucasian controls, with increased frequency of fasting hyperinsulinemia, hyperinsulinemic response to an oral glucose challenge, abnormal steady state concentration of glucose during an insulin suppression test with somatostatin and euglycemic-hyperinsulinemic clamp technique[22,30-34].

One factor contributing to insulin resistance is obesity. Very obese persons are almost uniformly insulin resistant[35-37]. Asian Indians they have been reported to have insulin resistance in the urban setting with only mild obesity[19,22,28-30]. Urban lifestyle with accompanying mild obesity and limited physical activity may be enough to induce insulin resistance in this population. Furthermore, studies in Caucasians have revealed that a moderate degree of obesity can lead to insulin resistance when fat is accumulated predominantly in the truncal region[38-42]. Truncal obesity can be identified clinically as an increase in waist circumference or an increase in truncal skinfold thickness. Individuals with abnormal fat distribution, characterized by a high waist-to-hip circumference ratio or a high truncal-to-peripheral-skinfolds-thickness ratio appear to be predisposed to developing insulin resistance[43]. The mechanistic basis of the association between truncal obesity and insulin resistance is unknown. Some investigators maintain that visceral fat is the compartment of adipose tissue most tightly linked with insulin resistance[40-42]. However, recent studies indicate that subcutaneous fat in the trunk is even better correlated with insulin sensitivity than is visceral or intraperitoneal fat[44-46]. The mechanism underlying this association is not know, although Jensen et al.[47] have shown that patients with upper body obesity (truncal obesity) have higher levels of nonesterified fatty acids (NEFA) than do those with lower body obesity. These high NEFA could lead to an increased fatty acid content of muscle and to inhibition of glucose oxidation[48].

Several reports have indicated that Asian Indians are susceptible to developing truncal obesity. The increased upper body obesity is reflected in reports of increased waist to hip

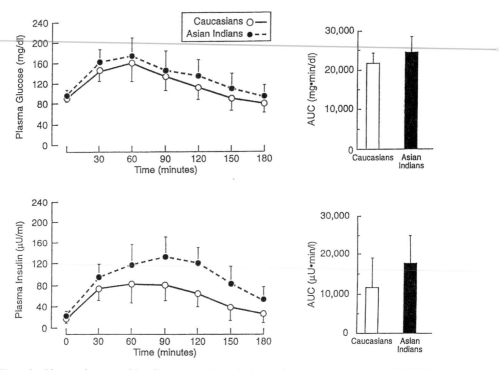

Figure 2. Plasma glucose and insulin concentrations during oral glucose tolerance test (OGTT) in Asian Indian and Caucasian men. The area under the curve for glucose and insulin during OGTT is represented with dark bars for Asian Indians and with open bars for Caucasians. The error bars represent standard deviation. (Reproduced with permission of ref. 32.)

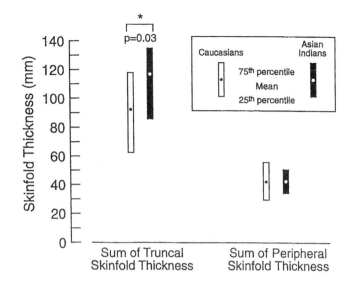

Figure 3. Sum of truncal (chest, mid-axillary, subscapular, abdominal and suprailiac) and peripheral (biceps, triceps, thigh and calf) skinfolds thickness in Asian Indians (dark bars) and Caucasian men (open bars). The bars indicate 25th and 75th percentile values and the circles represent the group mean. (Reproduced with permission of ref. 32.)

ratios and increased Truncal skinfold thickness in Asian Indians compared to other populations[19,34,49].

Chandalia et al.[32] compared 23 Caucasians of European ancestry with 21 Asian Indian healthy volunteers living in United states. General characteristics including age, BMI, fasting plasma glucose and LDL-Cholesterol were matched in both the groups. Only HDL-cholesterol was lower in Asian Indians compared to Caucasians (32+7 Vs 37+10; p=0.02, respectively). Anthropometric measurements including skinfolds thickness at truncal and peripheral sites, body composition, oral glucose tolerance test and euglycemic hyperinsulinemic clamp study were performed on all of the volunteers. The mean plasma glucose and insulin concentrations were higher in the Asian Indian group at all time points during OGTT (Fig. 2). The area under the curve for both plasma glucose and insulin were significantly higher in the Asian group. There were no differences in the percentage of total body fat mass between the two groups. However, the sums of truncal skinfolds were significantly higher in Asian Indians compared to Caucasians, and truncal-to-peripheral-skinfolds-thickness ratio were higher in Asian Indians (Fig. 3). During euglycemic hyperinsulinemic clamp study, the rate of glucose disposal was significantly lower in Asian Indians than in Caucasians. Furthermore, the insulin sensitivity index in the Asian Indians remained significantly lower than that in the Caucasians after adjustment for both total body fat and truncal skinfold thickness (p=0.04) (Fig. 4).

One of the most interesting observations of the study by Chandalia et al.[32] was a strong tendency for insulin resistance in lean Asian Indians. The study findings strongly suggest that Asian Indian men living in United States have relatively low insulin sensitivity even when their body fat content is in normal range compared to age- and body-fat-matched Caucasians. Whether the mechanism responsible for the low insulin sensitivity in Asian Indians is hereditary remains to be determined. However, it appears that the predisposition to insulin resistance and its metabolic abnormalities is genetically determined with environmental factors with westernization leading to further deleterious effects. No genetic marker for this condition in Asian Indians has been identified yet.

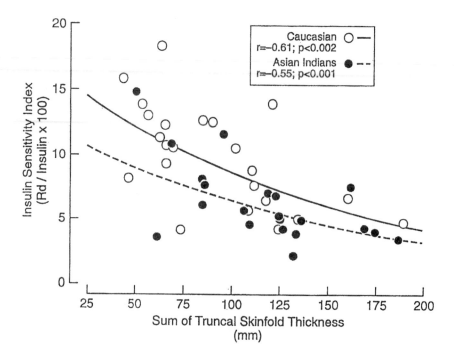

Figure 4. The relationship of insulin sensitivity index (Rd value divided by plasma insulin concentrations, during euglycemic-hyperinsulinemic clamp study at 20 mU/m2 min insulin infusion rate) and total body fat mass in Asian Indians and Caucasian men. Pearson product-moment analysis was used for computing the correlation coefficient (r) using insulin sensitivity index as dependent variable. The best-fit regression curves for Asian Indians and Caucasians are represented by interrupted and solid lines, respectively. (Reproduced with permission of ref. 32.)

THERAPEUTIC ASPECTS AND PUBLIC HEALTH IMPLICATIONS

From the foregoing, it is clear that whatever the mechanism underlying the excessive insulin resistance in Asian Indians, it may have a major impact in morbidity and mortality secondary to CHD in this population in the next century. The projected figures of increasing prevalence of CVD in the Asian Indian population call for the need of immediate intervention. Public and health care professional education to increase awareness and aggressive treatment of known CVD risk factors seems mandatory. One approach to decrease the risk for CHD in Asian Indians will be to manage traditional risk factors more aggressively for both primary and secondary prevention and to begin screening and treatment at an earlier age in Asian Indians. Besides LDL-C, particular attention must be directed to HDL-C and triglyceride since these are more often abnormal in Asian Indians. Other traditional risk factors should be also modified with aggressive management of blood pressure, lifestyle modification and smoking cessation. As moderate weight gain can lead to more significant increase in insulin resistance and overt diabetes in Asian Indians, awareness and education to prevent a sedentary lifestyle and weight gain may play an important role in prevention. Further research on the role of emerging risk factors on CVD in Asian Indians should be promoted to better focus our target of therapy. With increasing insight into the mechanism of insulin resistance and its role in CHD, and the availability of drugs for modifying insulin sensitivity, an exciting possibility exists in future for intervention and treatment of insulin resistance and, thus, prevention of CHD and diabetes.

REFERENCES

1. P. M. McKeigue, G. J. Miller, M. G. Marmot, Coronary heart disease in south Asians overseas: a review, *J Clin Epidemiol* **42**, 597-609 (1989).
2. S. G. Sarvotham, J. N. Berry, Prevalence of coronary heart disease in an urban population in northern India, *Circulation* **37**, 939-953 (1968).
3. B. D. Dewan, K. C. Malhotra, S. P. Gupta, Epidemiological study of coronary heart disease in rural community in Haryana, *Indian Heart J* **26**, 68-78 (1974).
4. H. T. Pedoe, D. Clayton, J. N. Morris, W. Bridgen, L. McDonald, Coronary heart-attacks in East London, *Lancet*, **2**, 833-838 (1975).
5. S. L. Chadha, S. Radhakrishnan, K. Ramachandran, U. Kaul, N. Gopinath, Epidemiological study of coronary heart disease in urban population of Delhi, *Indian J Med Res* **92**, 424-430 (1990).
6. P. M. McKeigue, M. G. Marmot, A. M. Adelstein, S. P. Hunt, M. J. Shipley, S. M. Butler, R. A. Riemersma, P. R. Turner, Diet and risk factors for coronary heart disease in Asians in northwest London, *Lancet* **2**, 1086-1090 (1985).
7. R. Balarajan, Ethnic differences in mortality from ischaemic heart disease and cerebrovascular disease in England and Wales, *BMJ* **302**, 560-564 (1991).
8. K. S. Reddy, Cardiovascular diseases in India, *WHO Stat Q* **46**, 101-107 (1993).
9. R. Gupta, S. Singhal, Coronary heart disease in India (Letter), *Circulation* **96**, 3785 (1997).
10. M. G. Marmot, Coronary heart disease: rise and fall of a modern epidemic, in *Coronary heart disease epidemiology: from aetiology to public health*, M. G. Marmot, P. Elliot, eds., Oxford University Press, Oxford (1992).
11. B. Williams. Westernized Asians and cardiovascular disease: nature or nurture? *Lancet* **345**, 401-402 (1995).
12. R. Gupta, H. Prakash, S. Majumdar, S. C. Sharma, V. P. Gupta. Prevalence of coronary heart disease and coronary risk factors in an urban population of Rajasthan, *Indian Heart J* **47**, 331-338 (1995).
13. R. Gupta, H. Prakash, V. P. Gupta. Prevalence and determinants of coronary heart disease in a rural population of India, *J Clin Epidemiology* **50**, 203-209 (1997).
14. S. P. Gupta, K. C. Malhotra. Urban-rural trends in epidemiology of coronary heart disease. *J Assoc Physicians Ind* **23**, 885-892. (1975).
15. K. S. Reddy, P. Shah, U. Shrivastava, Coronary heart disease risk factor in an industrialized population of north India (Abstract), *Can J Cardiol* **13**(Suppl B), 26B (1997).
16. R. Gupta, V. P. Gupta. Urban rural differences in coronary risk factors do not fully explain greater urban coronary heart disease prevalence, *J Assoc Physicians Ind* **45**, 683-686 (1997).
17. G. L. Beckles, G. J. Miller, B. R. Kirkwood, S. D. Alexis, D. C. Carson, N. T. Byam, High total and cardiovascular disease mortality in adults of Indian descent in Trinidad, unexplained by major coronary risk factors, *Lancet* **1**, 1298-1301 (1986).
18. G. J. Miller, G. L. Beckles, G. H. Maude, D. C. Carson, S. D. Alexis, S. G. Price, N. T. Byam, Ethnicity and other characteristics predictive of coronary heart disease in a developing community: principal results of the St James Survey, Trinidad, *Int J Epidemiol* **18**, 808-817 (1989).
19. P. M. McKeigue, B. Shah, M. G. Marmot, Relation of central obesity and insulin resistance with high diabetes prevalence and cardiovascular risk in South Asians, *Lancet* **337**, 382-386 (1991).
20. R. Balarajan, P. Yuen, British smoking and drinking habits: variation by country of birth, *Commun Med* **8**, 237-239 (1986).
21. G. J. Miller, S. Kotecha, W. H. Wilkinson, H. Wilkes, Y. Stirling, t. A. Sanders, A. Broadhurst, J. Allison, T. W. Meade, Dietary and other characteristics relevant for coronary heart disease in men of Indian, West Indian and European descent in London, *Atherosclerosis* **70**, 63-72 (1988).
22. P. M. McKeigue, M. G. Marmot, Y. D. Syndercombe Court, D. E. Cottier, S. Rahman, R. A. Riemersma, Diabetes, hyperinsulinaemia, and coronary risk factors in Bangladeshis in east London, *Br Heart* **60**, 390-396 (1988).
23. M. S. Jacobson, Cholesterol oxides in Indian Ghee, Possible cause of unexplained high risk of atherosclerosis in Indian Immigrant populations, *Lancet* **2**, 656-658 (1987).
24. H. Imai, N. T. Werthenssen, C. B. Taylor, K. T. Lee, Angiotoxicity and arteriosclerosis due to contaminants of USP grade cholesterol, *Arch Pathol Lab Med* **100**, 565-572 (1976).
25. D. Bhatnager, I. S. Anand, P. N. Durrington, D. J. Patel, G. S. Wander, M. I. Mackness, F. Creed, B. Tomenson, Y. Chandrashekhar, M. Winterbotham, R. P. Britt, J. E. Keil, J. S. Sutton, Coronary risk factors in people from the Indian subcontinent living in West London and thrie siblings in India, *Lancet* **345**, 405-409 (1995).
26. J. C. Chambers, A. McGregor, J. Jean-Marie, J. S. Kooner, Abnormalities of vascular endothelial function may contribute to increased coronary heart disease risk in UK Indian Asians. *Heart* **81**, 501-504 (1999).
27. S. S. Anand, S. Yusuf, V. Vuksan, S. Devanesen, P. Montague, L. Kelemen, L. Bosch, C. Sigouin, K. K.

Teo, E. Lonn, H. C. Gerstein, R. A. Hegele, M. McQueen, The study of health assessment and risk in ethnic groups (SHARE): rationale and design. The SHARE investigators, *Can J Cardiol* **14**, 1349-1357 (1998).

28. A. Ramachandran, M. V. Jali, V. Mohan, C. Snehalatha, M. Viswanathan, High prevalence of diabetes in an urban population in south India, *BMJ* **297**, 587-590 (1988).

29. A. Ramachandran, C. Snehalatha, D. Dharmaraj, M. Viswanathan, Prevalence of glucose intolerance in Asian Indians. Urban-rural difference and significance of upper body adiposity, *Diabetes Care* **15**, 1348-1355 (1992).

30. P. M. McKeigue, T. Pierpoint, J. E. Ferrie, M. G. Marmot, Relationship of glucose intolerance and hyperinsulinaemia to body fat pattern in south Asians and Europeans, *Diabetologia* **35**, 785-791 (1992).

31. H. M. Mather, H. Keen, The Southall Diabetes Survey: prevalence of known diabetes in Asians and Europeans, *Br Med J* (Clin Res Ed) **291**, 1081-1084 (1985).

32. M. Chandalia, N. Abate, A. Garg, J. Stray-Gundersen, S. M. Grundy, Relationship between generalized and upper body obesity to insulin resistance in Asian Indian men, *J Clin Endocrinol Metab* **84**, 2329-2335 (1999).

33. T. M. Knight, Z. Smith, A. Whittles, P. Sahota, J. A. Lockton, G. Hogg, A. Bedford, M. Toop, E. E. Kernohan, M. R. Baker, Insulin resistance, diabetes, and risk markers for ischaemic heart disease in Asian men and non-Asian in Bradford, *Br Heart J* **67**, 343-350 (1992).

34. A. Laws, J. L. Jeppesen, P. C. Maheux, P. Schaaf, Y. D. Chen, G. M. Reaven, Resistance to insulin-stimulated glucose uptake and dyslipidemia in Asian Indians, *Arteriosclerosis and Thrombosis* **14**, 917-922 (1994).

35. C. Bogardus S. Lillijoia, D. M. Mott, C. Hollenbeck, G. M. Reaven GM, Relationship between degree of obesity and in vivo insulin action in man, *Am J Physiol* **248**, E286-291 (1985).

36. H. Yki-Jarvinen, V. A. Koivisto, Effects of body composition on insulin sensitivity, *Diabetes* **32**, 965-969 (1983).

37. R. A. DeFronzo RA, Insulin secretion, insulin resistance, and obesity, *International Journal of Obesity* **6**, 73-82 (1982).

38. A. H. Kissebah, N. Vydelingum, R. Murray, D. J. Evans, A. J. Hartz, R. K. Kalkhoff, P. W. Adams, Relation of body fat distribution to metabolic complications of obesity, *J Clin Endocrinol Metab* **54**, 254-260 (1982).

39. S. B. Pedersen, J. D. Borglum, O. Schmitz, J. F. Bak, N. S. Sorensen, B. Richelsen, Abdominal obesity is associated with insulin resistance and reduced glycogen synthetase activity in skeletal muscle, *Metabolism* **42**, 998-1005 (1993).

40. D. Sparrow, G. A. Borkan, S. G. Gerzof, C. Wisniewski, C. K. Silbert, Relationship of fat distribution to glucose tolerance. Results of computed tomography in male participants of the Normative Aging Study. *Diabetes* **35**, 411-415 (1986).

41. M. Krotkiewski, P. Bjorntorp, L. Sjostrom, U. Smith, Impact of obesity on metabolism in men and women. Importance of regional adipose tissue distribution, *J Clin Invest* **72**, 1150-1162 (1983).

42. J. P. Despres, S. Moorjani, M. Ferland, A. Tremblay, P. J. Lupien, A. Nadeau, S. Pinaul, G. Theriault, C. Bouchard, Adipose tissue distribution and plasma lipoprotein levels in obese women. Importance of intra-abdominal fat, *Arteriosclerosis* **9**, 203-210 (1989).

43. H. Lundgren, C. Bengtsson, G. Blohme, L. S. Lapidus, L. Jostrom, Adiposity and adipose tissue distribution in relation to incidence of diabetes in women: results from a prospective population study in Gothenburg, Sweden, *Int J Obesity* **13**, 413-423 (1989).

44. N. Abate, A. Garg, R. M. Peshock, J. Stray-Gundersen, S. M. Grundy, Relationships of generalized and regional adiposity to insulin sensitivity in men, *J Clin Invest* **96**, 88-98 (1995).

45. N. Abate, A. Garg, R. M. Peshock, J. Stray-Gundersen, B. Adams-Huet, S. M. Grundy, Relationship of generalized and regional adiposity to insulin sensitivity in men with NIDDM, *Diabetes* **45**, 1684-1693 (1996).

46. B. H. Goodpaster, F. L. Thaete, J. A. Simoneau, D. E. Kelley, Subcutaneous abdominal fat and thigh muscle composition predict insulin sensitivity independently of visceral fat, *Diabetes* **46**, 1579-1585 (1997).

47. M. D. Jensen, M. W. Haymond, R. A. Rizza, P. E. Cryer, J. M. Miles, Influence of body fat distribution on free fatty acid metabolism in obesity, *J Clin Invest* **83**, 1168-1173 (1989).

48. P. J. Randle, Garland PB, Hales CN, Newsholme EA. The glucose-fatty acid cycle. Its role in insulin sensitivity and the metabolic disturbances of diabetes mellitus, *Lancet* **1**, 785-789 (1963).

49. R. B. Singh, M. A. Niaz, P. Agarwal, R. Beegum, S. S. Rastogi, N. K. Singh, Epidemiologic study of central obesity, insulin resistance and associated disturbances in the urban population of North India, *Acta Cardiol* **50**, 215-225 (1995).

THE PLASMA GLUCOSE LEVEL - A CONTINUOUS RISK FACTOR FOR VASCULAR DISEASE IN BOTH DIABETIC AND NON-DIABETIC PEOPLE

Hertzel C. Gerstein

Division of Endocrinology and Metabolism
Department of Medicine, McMaster University and
The Preventive Cardiology and Therapeutics Research Program
Hamilton Civic Hospitals Research Center
Hamilton, Ontario Canada

INTRODUCTION AND DEFINITION OF A RISK FACTOR

In epidemiologic studies, a risk factor is a measured variable that is associated with a subsequent risk of an adverse clinical outcome. Examples or different types of risk factors include demographic measurements (e.g. age and gender), clinical measurements (e.g. waist circumference or blood pressure), biochemical measurements (e.g. plasma glucose or cholesterol), exposures to drugs or environmental factors (e.g. smoking or radiation), or exposure to diseases (e.g. diabetes or hypertension). Risk factors may be both discrete (either present or absent) or continuous. An example of a discrete risk factor is the presence or absence of diabetes and an example of a continuous risk factor is the plasma glucose level.

A modifiable risk factor is one which if decreased or eliminated leads to a decrease or delay in the development of the outcome of interest. For example, smoking is a modifiable discrete risk factor for lung cancer - individuals who stop smoking have a lower subsequent incidence. Similarly, albuminuria is a modifiable continuous risk factor for renal failure - decreasing the albumin excretion rate in people with nephropathy (with various interventions) reduces the incidence of renal failure.

Finally, despite the fact that all causal factors are also risk factors, the converse is clearly not true. The majority of risk factors identified in epidemiologic studies are not causal factors. For example, the waist circumference clearly does not cause cardiovascular disease. It is extremely difficult in epidemiologic research to separate causal factors from risk factors. This discussion will therefore focus on plasma glucose as a risk factor for cardiovascular disease (CVD), and does not discuss its role as a possible causal factor for CVD.

DIABETES AS A RISK FACTOR

It has been known for many years that the presence of diabetes is an important risk factor for the development of serious chronic illnesses. Indeed, the glucose thresholds that separate diabetic from non-diabetic individuals were chosen on the basis of epidemiologic

Diabetes and Cardiovascular Disease: Etiology, Treatment and Outcomes
Edited by Aubie Angel et al., Kluwer Academic/Plenum Publishers, 2001

studies in which individuals above the diabetic glucose threshold had a much higher risk of developing eye and kidney disease than individuals below the threshold [1]. These thresholds therefore identify glucose levels above which individuals are at risk for eye and kidney disease. Most precisely, diabetes mellitus is a metabolic disorder characterized by hyperglycemia, that is associated with a high subsequent risk of eye and kidney disease. Indeed, although it is also associated with a high subsequent risk of nerve, CV and other diseases, the glycemic thresholds and definition of diabetes are not based on risks for these other problems.

DIABETES AS A RISK FACTOR FOR CARDIOVASCULAR DISEASE

Several epidemiologic studies have shown repeatedly that individuals with diabetes have a higher risk of cardiovascular disease in individuals without diabetes. These suggest that men have a 2-3 fold higher risk of cardiovascular mortality and women have a 4-5 fold higher risk of cardiovascular mortality than their non-diabetic counterparts [2,3,4,5,6,7]. Therefore, diabetes is a discrete risk factor for cardiovascular disease.

Whether or not the plasma glucose level is a risk factor for cardiovascular disease in diabetic individuals has not been clear until recently. Several large epidemiologic studies have now consistently shown that in individuals with diabetes, the risk of CVD rises with the degree of glycemia. Therefore, not only is diabetes a discrete risk factor for CVD, but in patients with diabetes, the plasma glucose level is a continuous risk factor for CVD.

GLUCOSE LEVEL AND THE RISK FOR
CARDIOVASCULAR DISEASE IN NON-DIABETIC PEOPLE

As noted above, the glycemic thresholds for diabetes were based on the risk for eye and kidney disease and not for CV disease. There is therefore no *a priori* reason that these thresholds should have any particular significance with regard to CV outcomes. That is, if hyperglycemia is a risk factor for CV disease, the risk may start to become apparent at either higher or lower levels. In fact, accumulating evidence suggests that lower levels are clearly an unrecognized CV risk factor.

The possibility that plasma glucose levels well below the diabetic cut-offs are a risk factor for CVD was first suggested by the Whitehall study in which a 2 hour capillary glucose after a 50 gram glucose load that was greater than 95 mg/dl (5.3 mmol/l) was associated with a markedly increased 7 ½ year CHD mortality [8]. Since that time, some, but not all prospective epidemiologic studies have shown a similar relationship between the glucose level and cardiovascular disease in non-diabetic individuals.

To get a more balanced view of the relationship between non-diabetic glucose levels and CV risk, we performed a systematic overview and meta-regression analysis of all of the prospective cohort studies that recorded CV outcomes according to baseline glucose levels [9]. All of the relevant studies published between 1966 and 1996 that include non-diabetic participants who were not selected on the basis of pre-existing disease, and that reported data in 3 or more quantiles were retrieved. These studies were categorized into those dealing with fasting and postprandial glucose levels and abstracted. The data from each study was modeled using an exponential model and the beta coefficients of each model were meta-analyzed. A plasma glucose level of 4.2 mmol/l was arbitrarily set at a relative risk of 1 before starting the analysis.

Twenty studies including 95,783 people (94% male) and comprising 1,193,231 person years of follow-up were retrieved and analyzed. Taken together, these studies showed that there was a clear exponential relationship between the fasting and postprandial glucose and cardiovascular events. A postprandial glucose of 7.8 mmol/l was associated with a relative risk of 1.58 (1.19-2.10). A fasting glucose of 6.1 mmol/l was associated with a relative risk of 1.33 (1.06-1.67).

When subjects with glucose levels that indicated undiagnosed diabetes were removed (i.e. those in the top quantile) and the analysis was repeated, the data were still significant for the postprandial glucose levels. This synthesis of the literature strongly suggests that glucose is a continuous risk factor for cardiovascular disease and that the postprandial glucose may be a more important determinant than the fasting glucose. Although these data were unadjusted, several of the abstracted studies did adjust the relationship between glucose and cardiovascular disease for other risk factors including age, blood pressure, weight, lipids and smoking.

Subsequent to completion of this analysis, several other studies reported a relationship between baseline glucose and subsequent cardiovascular disease in non-diabetic individuals. For example, a combined analysis of 3 large epidemiologic studies [10] showed that for non-diabetic individuals, 2 hour postprandial glucose levels in the 80th to 90th percentile increased the risk of all cause mortality by 15% after age adjustment.

To confirm the importance of non-diabetic levels of glucose as a risk factor for cardiovascular disease, data from a case controlled study of 300 South Asians following their first MI and 300 match controls were subsequently analyzed. Cases had a glucose tolerance test 10 days after admission if they did not have a history of diabetes, and had lipids measured within 24 hours of admission. The odds of a myocardial infarction increased with glucose quartile even after subjects with diabetes, impaired glucose tolerance and impaired fasting glucose were excluded. After excluding participants with impaired fasting glucose, Individuals with a fasting glucose between 5.21 mmol/l and 6.3 were 2.7 times more likely to be cases than individuals with fasting glucose less than 4.7 mmol/l (95% confidence interval 1.5-4.8). Postprandial glucose was an independent determinant of status as a case even after controlling for waist to hip ratio, cholesterol to HDL ratio, triglyceride, hypertension and smoking [11].

Taken together, these data all strongly support the hypothesis that non-diabetic glucose levels are a continuous risk factor for CVD. They do not identify a threshold (if indeed there is one) above which the risk begins to increase, but suggest that it is clearly lower than the threshold currently used to identify individuals with impaired glucose tolerance. They also strongly support the hypothesis that the postprandial glucose may be a more sensitive indicator of CV risk than the fasting glucose [12].

IS GLUCOSE A MODIFIABLE RISK FACTOR FOR CARDIOVASCULAR DISEASE?

There is accumulating evidence that in patients with type 2 diabetes, glucose control is likely to prevent cardiovascular disease. The UKPDS demonstrated a significant 39% relative risk reduction (95%CI 11,59) for myocardial infarction when metformin was used for glucose lowering in obese patients [13]; the UKPDS also demonstrated a marginally significant 16% relative risk reduction for myocardial infarction (95% CI 0,29) when either sulfonylureas or insulin were used to lower glucose levels [14]. The Kumamoto study [15] also showed that glucose lowering with insulin led to a relative risk reduction of 46% (albeit statistically nonsignificant). The DIGAMI study [16,17] showed that insulin use after a myocardial infarction reduced mortality by 29% (95% CI 4,51). The only study with any results in the opposite direction is the feasibility arm of the VACS DM study, in which individuals given intensified therapy had a nonsignificant 40% relative risk increase in cardiovascular events [18]. Neither this study nor the Kumamoto study were powered to detect effects on CV outcomes. Nevertheless, the studies reviewed above support the hypothesis that glucose lowering does indeed lead to lower CV outcomes in patients with type 2 diabetes.

Similar conclusions may apply to patients with type 1 diabetes. This was demonstrated in a recent systematic overview of all of the randomized trials of intensified insulin therapy, in which cardiovascular outcomes were measured [19]. Intensified insulin therapy led to a 45% relative risk reduction in the number of CV events (95%CI 12,65), and to a nonsignificant decrease of 28% in the number of patients developing a first event.

Whether or not the glucose lowering can prevent cardiovascular disease in nondiabetic people with dysglycemia (i.e. elevated glucose levels) is unknown. However, interventions that have been clearly shown to reduce cardiovascular risk also all decrease glucose levels (diet, exercise, weight loss, smoking cessation and ACE inhibitors).

CONCLUSION AND IMPLICATIONS

Up to 50% of non-diabetic males in the United States have a 2 hour plasma glucose > 5.9 mmol/l [20] and up to 49% of middle-aged men will develop CV disease[21]. If glucose is a modifiable cardiovascular risk factor in these individuals, then strategies to lower glucose may have a profound impact on the rate of cardiovascular disease in the community.

The plasma glucose is therefore a continuous risk factor for CVD. Studies to date support the hypothesis that strategies to lower glucose will reduce cardiovascular risk. This hypothesis can be tested in clinical trials of individuals with dysglycemia [22,23].

REFERENCES

1. Expert Committee on the Diagnosis and Classification of Diabetes Mellitus. Report of the Expert Committee on the Diagnosis and Classification of Diabetes Mellitus. Diabetes Care 1997; 20:1183-1197.
2. Stamler J, Vaccaro O, Neaton JD, Wentworth D. Diabetes, other risk factors, and 12-yr cardiovascular mortality for men screened in the Multiple Risk Factor Intervention Trial. Diabetes Care 1993; 16:434-444.
3. Kannel WB, McGee DL. Diabetes and cardiovascular disease. The Framingham study. JAMA 1979; 241:2035-2038.
4. Fuller JH, Shipley MJ, Rose G, Jarrett RJ, Keen H. Mortality from coronary heart disease and stroke in relation to degree of glycemia: the Whitehall study. Br Med J Clin Research Ed 1983; 287:867-870.
5. Barrett-Connor E, Cohn BA, Wingard DL, Edelstein SL. Why is diabetes mellitus a stronger risk factor for fatal ischemic heart disease in women than in men? The Rancho Bernardo Study. JAMA 1991; 265:627-631.
6. Goldbourt U, Yaari S, Medalie JH. Factors predictive of long-term coronary heart disease mortality among 10059 male Israeli civil servants and municipal employees. A 23 year mortality follow-up in the Israeli Ischemic Heart Disease Study. Cardiology 1993; 82:100-121.
7. Manson JE, Coldlitz GA, Stampfer MJ, Willett WC, Krolewski AS, Rosner B, et al. A prospective study of maturity-onset diabetes mellitus and risk of coronary heart disease and stroke in women. Arch Int Med 1991; 151:1141-1147.
8. Fuller JH, Shipley MJ, Rose G, Jarrett RJ, Keen H. Coronary-heart-disease risk and impaired glucose tolerance. The Whitehall study. Lancet 1980; 8183:1373-1376.
9. Coutinho M, Gerstein HC, Wang Y, Yusuf S. The relationship between glucose and incident cardiovascular events. A metaregression analysis of published data from 20 studies of 95,783 individuals followed for 12.4 years. Diabetes Care 1999; 22:233-240.
10. Balkau B, Shipley M, Jarrett RJ, Pyorala K, Pyorala M, Forhan A, et al. High blood glucose concentration is a risk factor for mortality in middle-aged nondiabetic men. Diabetes Care 1998; 21:360-367.
11. Gerstein HC, Pais P, Pogue J, Yusuf S. Relationship of glucose and insulin levels to the risk of myocardial infarction: a case-control study. J Am Coll.Cardiol. 1999; 33:612-619.
12. Haffner SM. The importance of hyperglycemia in the nonfasting state to the development of cardiovascular disease. Endocrine Reviews 1998; 19:583-592.
13. UK Prospective Diabetes Study (UKPDS) Group. Effect of intensive blood glucose control with metformin on complications in overweight patients with type 2 diabetes (UKPDS 34). Lancet 1998; 352:854-865.
14. UK Prospective Diabetes Study (UKPDS) Group. Intensive blood-glucose control with sulphonylureas or insulin compared with conventional treatment and risk of complications in patients with type 2 diabetes (UKPDS 33). Lancet 1998; 352:837-853.
15. Ohkubo Y, Kishikawa H, Araki E, Miyata T, Isami S, Motoyoshi S, et al. Intensive insulin therapy prevents the progression of diabetic microvascular complications in Japanese patients with non-insulin-dependent diabetes mellitus: a randomized prospective 6-year study. Diab Res Clin Pract 1995; 28:103-117.

16. Malmberg K, Ryden L, Efendic S, Herlitz J, Nicol P, Waldenstrom A, et al. Randomized trial of insulin-glucose infusion followed by subcutaneous insulin treatment in diabetic patients with acute myocardial infarction (DIGAMI study): Effects on mortality at 1 year. J Am Coll Cardiol 1995; 26:57-65.

17. Malmberg K, DIGAMI Study Group. Prospective randomised study of intensive insulin treatment on long term survival after acute myocardial infarction in patients with diabetes mellitus. Br Med J 1997; 314:1512-1515.

18. Abraira C, Colwell JA, Nuttall F, Sawin CT, Henderson W, Comstock JP, et al. Cardiovascular events and correlates in the veterans affairs diabetes feasibility trial. Arch Intern Med 1997; 157:181-188.

19. Lawson M, Gerstein HC, Tsui E, Zinman B. Effect of intensive therapy on early macrovascular disease in young individuals with type 1 diabetes. A systematic review and meta-analysis. Diabetes Care 1999; 22:(Suppl.2)B35-B39

20. Cowie CC, Harris MI. Physical and metabolic characteristics of persons with diabetes. In: Harris MI, Cowie CC, Stern MS, Boyko EJ, Reiber GE, Bennett PH, editors. Diabetes in America. NIH Publication No. 95-1468. 2nd ed. National Institutes of Health, 1995:117-164.

21. Lloyd-Jones DM, Larson MG, Beiser A, Levy D. Lifetime risk of developing coronary heart disease. Lancet 1999; 353:89-92.

22. Gerstein HC, Yusuf S. Dysglycaemia and risk of cardiovascular disease. Lancet 1996; 347:949-950.

23. Gerstein HC. Dysglycaemia: a cardiovascular risk factor. Diabetes Res.Clin Pract. 1998; 40 Suppl:S9-14.

MODIFIED LIPOPROTEINS AND CARDIOVASCULAR RISK

Waleed Aldahi, Jiri Frohlich

Healthy Heart Program
St. Paul's Hospital
University of British Colombia
Vancouver, B.C.

BACKGROUND

It is generally accepted that LDL is the source of cholesterol accumulating in atherosclerotic lesions[1,2]. The precise mechanism of this accumulation remains to be It is generally accepted that LDL is the source of cholesterol accumulating in elucidated. Modified LDL, the subject of this article, is evolving as a significant link between lipoproteins and atherosclerosis[3].

In the early 1980's Brown and Goldstein[4] noted that monocytes incubated with native LDL do not take up excess cholesterol and do not form foam cells. On the other hand, when native LDL was modified either by pre-incubation with endothelial cells, acetylation or malondialdehyde conjugation[5], it was avidly taken into the cells resulting in the formation of foam cells, a substrate of fatty streaks (the first stage of atherosclerosis)[5,6] (Table 1). Subsequently various other modifications of LDL that result in its uptake by macrophages and formation of foam cells have been described (Table 2).

This uptake of modified LDL by macrophages is not mediated by the native LDL receptors. The existence of different types of receptors for LDL was predicted based on the fact that patients with familial hypercholesterolemia lack LDL receptors but accumulate LDL-cholesterol in macrophages that are the substrate of atherosclerotic lesions[5]. Subsequently, a new receptor that recognizes acetyled LDL, namely Scavenger receptor A (SRA) was identified[13]. Unlike the native LDL receptor, the SRA is not regulated by intracellular cholesterol content, the key factor in the formation of foam cells[13,14].

OXIDATIVE MODIFICATION HYPOTHESIS

The oxidative modification hypothesis of atherosclerosis has been formulated over the past 20 years[14,15]. Briefly, this hypothesis suggests that oxidation of the native LDL particles by either endothelial cells, monocytes, macrophages or smooth muscle cells first leads to the formation of minimally oxidized LDL (MM-LDL) molecules (not taken up by scavenger receptors of the macrophages) that induces production of monocyte colony stimulating factor (M-CSF) and monocyte chemoattracting protein one (MCP-1)[4,14,15]. Presence of these chemoattractants in subendothelial space results in recruitment of

Diabetes and Cardiovascular Disease: Etiology, Treatment and Outcomes
Edited by Aubie Angel *et al.*, Kluwer Academic/Plenum Publishers, 2001

41

Table 1. Stages of atherosclerosis

1. Itima media thickening
2. Migration of circulating monocytes into the sub-intimal space
3. Uptake of modified LDL by macrophages,
   formation of foam cells, and development of fatty streaks,
   the earliest stage of atherosclerosis.
4. Intermediate lesion with a fibrous cap formed by smooth muscle
   replication
5. Complicated plaque (fibrosis and necrosis)

Table 2. Types of LDL modifications

Type	Reference
1. Oxidative Modifications	
• Acetylation	(4)
• Malondialdehyde conjugation	(7)
• Metal ions and hydroxy radicals	(8)
• Incubation with endothilial cells, Smooth muscle cells, monocytes or macrophages	(9)
2. Alternative Modifications	
• Self aggregation (uptakeby native LDL receptor)	(10)
• Complex with macromolecules,	(11)
- protoglycans & matrix proteins	
- Immune complexes	(12)

monocytes, further increase in endothelial permeability and, inside the arterial wall, in differentiation of monocytes to macrophages[16-18].

The accumulated monocytes/macrophages may further increase oxidation of LDL by production of more negatively charged apo B on the surface of LDL and recognition of the oxidized LDL by scavenger receptors of macrophages resulting in further increase its uptake by macrophages and ultimately formation of foam cells[5,14-20] (Figure 1).
While the physiologically relevant mechanisms for LDL oxidation in-vivo are not yet identified, several possible pathways have been proposed[21,22]. It is generally accepted that oxidation of LDL involves 3 phases[5,14,19]. The Lag phase where the polyunsaturated fatty acids (PUFAs) of the surface phospholipids of LDL undergo free radical-mediated peroxidative modification (abstraction of hydrogen atom)[18-20] in which lipooxygenases and myeloperoxidases play a major role[5,14,19,23-25], while the endogenous antioxidants suppress this process. The second phase, Propagation phase, involves the formation of lipid peroxides by the abstraction of a second hydrogen atom from a different PUFA and formation of double bonds. During this phase there is extensive conversion of lecithin to lysolecithin catalyzed by phospholipase A2 , an enzyme present in LDL[5,19]. Finally, decomposition phase results in the formation of aldehydes and ketones.[5,19,26] .

42

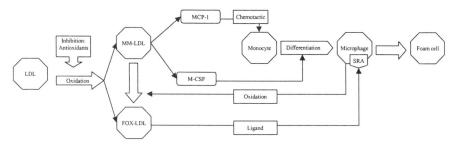

Figure 1. Mechanism of foam cell formation by cellular uptake of oxidized LDL

Table 3. Characteristics of oxidized LDL

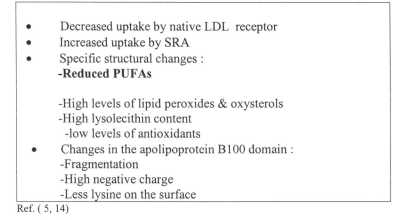

- Decreased uptake by native LDL receptor
- Increased uptake by SRA
- Specific structural changes :
  -Reduced PUFAs

  -High levels of lipid peroxides & oxysterols
  -High lysolecithin content
  -low levels of antioxidants
- Changes in the apolipoprotein B100 domain :
  -Fragmentation
  -High negative charge
  -Less lysine on the surface

Ref. (5, 14)

As the modified LDL loses its lysine residues, as a result of fatty acid fragmentation, it is less recognizable by the native LDL receptors. Subsequently, a modified fragment of apoprotein B forms the epitope that reacts with SRA[5,14,19]. The characteristics of oxidized LDL molecule are summarized in Table 3.

Small LDL particle sizes are more susceptible to oxidative stress compared to larger ones. Several other potential factors are under investigation[27].

Depending on the presence and concentration of metal ions in the incubation medium[8] monocytes *in vitro* can have either antioxidant or pro-oxidant activity. It is of interest to speculate that these findings may relate to the iron load hypothesis of atherosclerosis[28,29]. Several authors suggested a relation between the total body iron load and progression of atherosclerosis[30]. Also, an iron deficient diet significantly decreased the atherosclerotic lesions in apo E-KO mice[31] .

Roset et al[32] and Tuomainen et al[33] recently showed in a well designed studies an increased risk of myocardial infarction in carriers of the hemochromatosis gene HFE (Cys282Tyr mutation). This suggests that iron could have an important clinical role in ischeamic heart disease that needs to be investigated further . On the other hand, the findings of low levels of both Iron and Copper oxidative products in human fatty streaks and intermediate atherosclerotic lesions make their role in the initial stages of atherosclerosis less certain[24].

In summary, it is the oxidized, not the native LDL, that is atherogenic. The major reason for this distinction is the difference in the route of uptake of these molecules: while the native LDL is taken up by apo B-E LDL receptors that are subject to a feedback regulation, i.e. when the concentration of cholesterol inside the cell increases the

Table 4. Candidate oxLDL Receptors on the Macrophage (modified from reference 20)

• AcLDL-R (SRA-I and SRA-II)
• CD36
• Fc receptor
• Macrosialin
• Others?

Table 5. Effects of Oxidized LDL

1. Minimally Oxidized LDL
    • Recognized by native LDL recepors (36)
    • Stimulate release of M-CSF from endothelial cells which induces differentiation of monocytes into macrophages with increased SRA expression (16,18)
    • Induces leukocyte-endothelial cell adhesion (21)
    • Increases adherence & penetration of monocytes by **stimulating MCP-1 production by endothelial cells (15)**
 	
2. Fully Oxidized LDL
    • Major ligand for SRA leading to foam cell formation (13)
    • Chemotactic for monocytes & T-lymphocyts (37)
    • Inhibits the motility of tissue macrophages(21)
    • Cytotoxic to endothelial cells in vivo(21)
    • A mitogen for macrophages and smooth muscle cells (38)
    • Inhibits NO mediated vasodilatation (39)
    • Stimulates the expression of IL-1 gene in the arterial walls wich induce smoth muscle cell proliferation (21)
    • Stimulates PAI-1 production(5)
    • Inhibits lysosomal proteases (14,40,41)

production of these receptors is shut off, the scavenger receptors (Table 4) that take up oxidized LDL do not have this feedback regulation and continue to accept oxidized LDL despite an excess of cholesterol inside the cell[3].

INTERACTIONS OF OXIDIZED LDL (OXLDL)

In addition to its direct toxicity the oxLDL interacts with CD36 (expression of which is increased in macrophages)[34], cell surface differentiation markers such as HLA-DR[35] and the receptors outlined in Table 4.

The degree of oxidation of LDL results in its different biological activities. While the MM-LDL primarily stimulates production of the chemoattractants mentioned above, the accumulation of fully oxidized LDL (FOX-LDL) results in the production of foam cells. Table 5 summarizes the effects of minimally and fully oxidized LDL.

Recently, the effects of oxLDL on endothelial function response have been investigated [42-44]. Depending on the degree of LDL oxidation there is a decrease in vasodilatation secondary to increased blood flow to the forearm. Decreased production of nitric oxide is the likely mechanism of this deleterious action of oxidized LDL on endothelial function[45].

OXIDIZED LDL AND ATHEROSCLEROSIS

A number of studies relate plasma LDL susceptibility to oxidation (and also lower plasma antioxidant concentration) to atherosclerosis in both men and animals[46-49]. It has been shown that a significant drop in the antioxidant (vitamin E, beta-carotene, lycopene, etc) levels in LDL molecule is needed before it undergo oxidative modification[50]. Furthermore, a recent study demonstrated an increased concentration of 7 β-hydroxy cholesterol, a marker of LDL oxidation, in Lithuanian men (who are 2-3 times more likely to develop CAD than Swedish men) compared to Swedish men with similar other risk factors[51]. Interestingly, in these subjects there were no differences in α-tocopherol content of plasma lipids, or blood pressure. Some of these above observations led to trials of antioxidant in experimental animals and men. Several studies of supplementation with beta-carotene, a weak antioxidant, showed no significant effects on cardiovascular end points[52,53]. Furthermore, it has been shown that increased intake of beta-carotene may confer additional cardiovascular risk[54].

Several epidemiological studies with vitamin E provided a reasonable evidence to support the hypothesis that links vitamin E to coronary arteriosclerosis[55]. A prospective non-randomized trial by Hodis et al[56] showed (in the vitamin E arm of the study) that patients taking 100 IU/day or more of supplemental vitamin E had decreased coronary lesion progression compared to those with lower vitamin E intake (p=0.04). The subjects were men with previous coronary artery bypass graft surgery.

Table 6. Randomized controlled trials of vitamin E in coronary artery disease

Study	Subjects	n	Followup per year	Dose IU/day	Outcome	Limitations
ATBC (54)	Finish male smokers with no IHD	29133	6.1	50	No effect on coronary mortality	- Short follow up - Low dose - subjects are all Finish & smokers
CHAOS (57)	Men & women with CAD in UK	2002	1.4	800 and 400	- no difference in overall mortality -RR,0.53(95% CI,o.34-o.83) for combined non-fatal MI and cardiovascular death in vitamin E gruop. -Increased non-cardiac death in treatment goop??.	-lack of information about the severity of CAD - Gender, blood pressure and serum lipids are not equal between the groups at baseline - 2 different doses of vitamin E
GISSI prevention study (58,59)	Mediterranean men and women with recent MI (3 months)	1172	3.5	300	Preliminary results showed a statistically non significant reduction (4.7%) in mortality	

CI indicates confidence interval; CAD, coronary artery disease; MI, myocardial infarction; RR, relative risk.

However, two large prospective randomized double blind trials of vitamin E have been completed and showed no evidence of benefit from supplemental vitamin E. A summary of vitamin E randomized trials is shown in Table 6.

The alpha-tocopherol, beta carotene cancer prevention study (ATBC)[54] showed, by several analysis of the initial data[60,61], that vitamin E supplements (50 IU/day) have no effect on the occurrence of major coronary events. On the contrary, the combination of alpha-tocopherol and beta-carotene resulted in increased mortality.

On the other hand, The Cambridge heart antioxidant study (CHOAS)[57] showed that higher doses (400-800 IU/day) of vitamin E significantly decrease the risk of combined end points of cardiovascular death and non-fatal myocardial infarction (MI) by 47% (p= 0.005) compared to the placebo group. However, there is no difference in the overall mortality. Recently, preliminary results of the Heart Outcome Prevention Evaluation Study (HOPE)[62] and the Gruppo Italiano per lo Studio della Sopravvivenza nell`Infarto (GISSI- Prevention) study[59] showed no beneficial effects of vitamin E in prevention of CAD.

CONCLUSION

Oxidation of LDL results first in the formation of LDL species that induce migration of monocytes to subendothelial space and their differentiation into macrophages. At higher degrees of oxidation LDL interacts with specific scavenger receptors on the surface of macrophages, a process that results in the formation and accumulation of foam cells.

Despite many unanswered questions, the oxidative modification hypothesis remains a reasonable explanation of the initial stages of atherogenesis[20]. One of the big challenges for the next millennium is to standardize oxidized LDL measurement and correlate it quantitatively with the assessment of atherosclerosis.

While antioxidants appear to be a logical therapy for prevention of atherosclerosis, there is at present no convincing evidence of their effectiveness. Routine use of antioxidants is not advisable at this stage[63].

REFERENCES

1. Heinecke JW. Oxidants and antioxidants in the pathogenesis of atherosclerosis : Implications for oxidized low density lipoprotein hypothesis. Atherosclerosis, 1998. 141: 1-15.
2. Navab, M; Berliner, JA; Watson, AB. et al . The yin and yang of oxidation in the development of the fatty streaks. A review based on the 1994 George Lyman Duff Memorial lecture. Arteriosclerosis . Thromb. Vasc. Biol. July 1996. 16 (7): 831-842.
3. Steinberg,D. and Witzman, JL . Lipoproteins and atherogenesis: current concepts. JAMA. 1990, 264: 3047-3052.
4. Brown, M.S. and Goldstien J. A receptor mediated pathway for cholesterol homeostasis. L. Science. 1986, 232: 34-47.
5. Witzman JL and Steinberg D. Role of oxidized low-density lipoprotein in atherogenesis. J. Clin. Invest. December 1991. Volume 88, Pages : 1785-1792
6. Hegele, R.A. The pathogenesis of atherosclerosis. Clinica. Chimica. Acta. 1996. 246: 21-38.
7. Fogelman ,A.M.; Schechter,J.S.; Hokom, M.; et al . Malondialdehyde alteration of low density lipoprotein leads to cholesterol accumulation in human monocyte-macrophages. Proc. Natl. Acad. Sci. U.S.A. . 1980, 77: 2214-2218.
8. Heinecke ,J.W.; Rosen, H.; Chait,A. Iron and copper promote modification of low-density lipoprotein by human arterial smooth muscle cells in culture. J. Clin. Invest. . 1987, 74: 1890-1894.
9. Henriksen, T.; Mahoney, E.M.; Steinberg, D. Enhanced degradation of low-density lipoprotein previously incubated with cultured endothelial cells: recognition by receptors for acetylated low-density lipoproteins. Proc. Natl. Acad. Sci. U.S.A.. 1981. 78: 6499-6503.
10. Khoo, J.S.; Miller, E.; Mcloughlin, P.; Steinberg,D.. Enhanced macrophages uptake of low-density lipoprotein after self aggregation. Arteriosclerosis. 1988, 8: 348-58.
11. Hurt,E.; Camijo, G. . Effect of arterial protoglyns on the interaction of low-density lipoprotein with human monocyte-derived macrophages. Atherosclerosis. 1987, 67: 115-126.

12. Horkko, S.; Miller, E.; Dudl, E. et al . Antiphospholipid antibodies are directed against epitopes of oxidized phospholipids. Recognition of cardiolipin by monoclonal antibodies to epitopes of oxidized low-density lipoprotein. J. Clin. Invest. .Aug. 1986. 98 (3): 815-25.

13. Kodama, T; Freeman, M.; Rohrer, L. et al. Type 1 macrophage scavenger receptor contains alpha-helical and collagen like coiled coils. Nature. Feb. 8th 1990. 343 (6258): 513-5.

14. Steinberg, D. . Low-density lipoprotein oxidation and its pathobiological significance. The journal of biological chemistry. Aug. 22nd 1997. Vol. 272, No. 34 : 20963-20966.

15. Cushing, SD; Berliner, JA; Valente, AJ, etal. Minimally modified low-density lipoprotein induces monocyte chemotactic protein 1 in human endothelial cells and smooth muscle cells. Proc. Natl. Acad. Sci. U.S.A. July 1990. 87 (13): 5134-8.

16. Steinberg, D.; Parthasarathy, T.E.; Carew,J. D. et al. Beyond cholesterol: Modifications of low-density lipoprotein that increase its atherogenecity. N. E. J. Med. 1989. 320: 915-924.

17. Witztum, Joseph L. The oxidation hypothesis of atherosclerosis [Free radicals and antioxidants]. The Lancet. 17 sept. 1994. Vol. 344 (895): 793-795.

18. Lee, C.; Sigari, F.; Segrado, T. et al. All ApoB-containing lipoproteins induce monocyte chemotaxis and adhesion when minimally modified: Modulaton of lipoprotein bioactivity by platelet-activating factor acetylhydrolase [Atherosclerosis and Lipoproteins]. Arterioscler. Thromb. Vasc. Biol. June 1999, 19 (6):1437-1446.

19. Jialal, I. Evolving lipoprotein risk factors : lipoprotein (a) and oxidized low-density lipoprotein. Clinical Chemistry. 1998. 44: 8(B); 1827-1832.

20. Steinberg, D. Oxidative modification of low-density lipoprotein and atherosclerosis. Lewis A. Conner memorial lecture. Circulation. Feb. 18th 1997. Vol 95 (4) : 1062-1071.

21. Steinberg, D. Low-density lipoprotein oxidation and its pathological significance. J. Biol. Chem. Aug.22nd 1997. 272 (34): 20903-6.

22. Ross, R. The pathogenesis of atherosclerosis: A prospective for the 1990`s. Apr.29th 1993. 362 (6423): 801-9.

23. Esterbauer, H.; Wag, G.; Puhl, H. Lipid peroxidation and its role in atherosclerosis. Br. Med. Bull. July 1993. 49 (3): 566-76.

24. Heinecke, J. W. Mechanism of oxidative damage of low-density lipoprotein in human atherosclerosis. Current Opinion in Lipidology. 1997. 8: 268-274.

25. Esterbauer, H.; Gebicki, J.; Puhl, H.; Jurgens, G. The role of lipid peroxidation and oxidation in the oxidative modification of low-density lipoprotein. Free Radical Biol. Med. 1992; 13: 341-90.

26. Jurgens, G.;Hoff, H. F.; Chisolm III, G. M.; Esterbauer, H. Modification of human serum low-density lipoprotein by oxidation: Characterization and pathophysiological implications. Chem. Phys. Lipids. 1987; 45: 315-316.

27. Superko, H. R. Small dense low-density lipoprotein subclass pattern B: Issues for clinicians. Current atherosclerosis reports. July 1999, Vol.1, No.1: 50-57.

28. Sullivan, J. L. Iron versus cholesterol: prospectives on the iron and heart disease debate. J Clin. Epidemiol. 1996; 49: 1345-1352.

29. Lee, F.Y.; Lee, T. S.; Pan, C. C. et al. Colocalization of iron and ceroid in human atherosclerotic lesions. Atherosclerosis. 1998; 138:281-288.

30. Gillum, R. F. Body iron stores and atherosclerosis. Circulation 1997; 96: 3261-3263.

31. Lee, T. S.; Shiao, M. S.; Pan, C. C.; chau, L. Y. Iron deficient diet reduces atherosclerotic lesions in Apo E-deficient mice. Circulation. 1999; 99: 1222-1229.

32. Roset, M.; Van der Schouw, Y. T.; de Valk, B. et al. Heterozygosity for a hereditary hemochromatosis gene is associated with cardiovascular death in women. Circulation. 1999; 100:1268-1273.

33. Tuomainen, T.; Kontula, K.; Nyyssönen, K. et al . Increased risk of acute myocardial infarction in carriers of the hemochromatosis gene Cyst282Tyr mutation: a prospective cohort study in men in eastern Finland. Circulation. 1999; 100: 1274-1279.

34. Acton, S. L.; Scherer, P. E.; Lodish, H. F.; Krieger, M. Expression cloning of SR-BI, a CD36-related class B scavenger receptor. J. Biol. Chem. Aug. 19th 1994; 269 (33): 21003-21009.

35. Frostegard, J.; Nilsson, J.; Hargerstrand, A. et al. Oxidized low-density lipoprotein induces differentiation and adhesion of human monocytes and the monocytic cell line U937. Proc. Natl. Acad. Sci. U.S.A. Feb. 1990; 87 (3): 904-8.

36. Berliner, J. A.; Navab, M.; Fogelman, A. M. et al. Atherosclerosis: basic machanisms, oxidation, inflamation and genetics. Circulation 1995; 91: 2488-96.

37. Quinn, M. T.; Parthasarathy, S.; Fong, L. G.; Steinberg, D. Oxidatively modified low-density lipoprotein. A potential role in recruitment and retention of monocyte/macrophages during atherogenesis. Proc. Natl. Acad. Sci. U.S.A. May 1987; 84 (9): 2995-8.

38. Chatterjee, S. Ghosh, N. Oxidized low-density lipoprotein stimulates aortic smooth muscle proliferation. Glycobiology. Apr. 1996; 6 (3): 303-11.

39. Kugiyama, K.; Kerns, S. A.; Morrisett, J. D. et al. Impairment of endothilium-dependant arterial relaxation by lysolecithin in modified low-density lipoproteins. Nature. Mar. 8th 1990; 344(6262): 160-2.

40. Hoppe, G.; O`Neil, J.; Hoff, H. F. Inactivation of lysosomal proteases by oxidized low-density lipoprotein is partially responsible for its poor degradation by macrophages. J. Clin. Invest. 1994; 94: 1506-1512.

41. O`Neil, J.; Hoppe, G.; Sayre, L. M.; Hoff, H. F. Inactivation of cathepsin B by oxidized low-density lipoprotein involves complex formation induced by binding of putative reaction sites exposed at low PH to thiols on the enzyme. Free Radical. Biol. Med. 1997; 23: 215-225.

42. Harrison, D. G. Cellular and molecular mechanisms of endothelial cell dysfunction. J. of Clin. Invest. Nov.1st 1997; Vol. 100 (9): 2153-2157.

43. Posch, K.; Simecek, S.; Wascher, T. C. et al. Glycated low-density lipoprotein attenuates shear stress-induced nitric oxide synthesis by inhibition of shear stress-activated L-arginine uptake in endothelial cells. Diabetes. June 1999; 48 (6): 1331-7.

44. Ito, A.; Tsao, Ps.; Adimoolam, S.; Kimoto, M. et al. Novel mechanisms for endothelial dysfunction: dysregulation of dimethylarginine dimethyle aminohydrolase. Circulation. June 22nd 1999; 99 (24): 3092-5.

45. Stroes, E.; de Bruin, T.; de Valk, H. et al. NO activity in familial combined hyperlipidemia: potential role of cholesterol remnants. Cardiovascular Research. Dec. 1997; 36 (3): 445-52.

46. Salonen, J.; Nyyssönen, K. Salonen, R. et al. Lipoprotein oxidation and progression of carotid atherosclerosis. Circulation. 1997; 95: 840-845.

47. Yla-Herttuala, S.; Palinski, W. Rosenfeld, ME. Et al. Lipoproteins in normal and atherosclerotic aorta. Eur. Heart J. 1990; 11 (suppE): 88-99.

48. Yla-Herttuala, S.; Palinski, W. Rosenfeld, ME. Et al. Evidence for the presence of oxidatively modified low-density lipoprotein in atherosclerotic lesions of rabbit and man. J. Clin. Invest. 1989; 84: 1086-1095.

49. Palinski, W.; Rosenfeld, ME.; Yla-Herttuala, S. et al. Low-density lipoprotein undergoes oxidative modification in vivo. Proc. Natl. Acad. Sci. U.S.A. Feb. 1989; 86 (4): 1372-6.

50. Esterbauer, H.; Rothender, M.; Striegl, G. et al. Vitamin E and other lipophilic antioxidants protect low-density lipoprotein against oxidation. Fat. Sci. Technol. 1989: 9183-24.

51. Zieden, B; Kaminskas, A.; Kristenson, M. et al. Increased plasma 7 beta-hydroxycholesterol concentrations in a population with a high risk for cardiovascular disease. Arteriosclerosis, Thrombosis and Vascular Biology. Apr. 1999; 19 (4): 967-71.

52. Omenn, GS; Goodman, GE; Thornquist, MD, et al. Effects of a combination of beta-carotene and retinol on lung cancer and cardiovascular disease. N.E. J. Med. 1996; 334: 1150-55.

53. Hennekens, CH; Buring, JE; Manson, JE, et al. Lack of effect of long term supplementation with beta-carotene on the incidence of malignant neoplasmes and cardiovascular disease. N.E. J. Med. 1996;334: 1145-49.

54. Rapola, JM; Virtamo, J; Haukka, JK, et al. Effects of vitamin E and beta-carotene on the incidence of angina pectoris: a randomized double blind controlled trial. JAMA. 1996; 275: 693-8.

55. Spencer, AP; Carson, DS; Crouch, MA. Vitamin E and coronary artery disease. Archives of Internal Medicine. 1999; Vol. 159 (12): 1313-1320.

56. Hodis, HN; Mack, WJ; LaBree, L, et al .Serial coronary angiographic evidence that antioxidant vitamin intake reduces progression of coronary artery atherosclerosis. JAMA. 1995; 273: 1849-1854.

57. Stephens, N. G.; Parsons, A.; Schofeild, P. M.; et al. Randomized controlled trial of vitamin E in patients with coronary disease: Cambridge Heart Antioxidant Study (CHAOS). The Lancet. March 23rd 1996. Vol. 347: 781-786.

58. Marchioli, R.; Di Pasquale, A. I1 quadro di riferimento biochimico, farmacologico, epidemiologico del GISSI-prevenzione. G Ital Cardiol . 1993; 23: 933-64.

59. Ballantyne, C. M. Reducing atherothrombotic events in high-risk patients: recent data on therapy with statins and fatty acids. Current atherosclerosis reports. July 1999; Vol.1 No.1: 6-8.

60. Rapola, JM; Virtamo, J; Ripatti, S.; et al. Effects of alpha-tocopherol and beta-carotene supplementations on symptoms, progression and prognosis of angina pectoris. Heart. 1998; 79: 454-458.

61. Rapola, JM; Virtamo, J; Ripatti, S.; et al. Randomized trial of alpha-tocopherol and beta-carotene supplements on incidence of major coronary events in men with previous myocardial infarction. The Lancet. 1997; 349: 1715-1720.

62. The Hope study investigators. The HOPE (Heart Outcomes Prevention Evaluation) study. Can. J. Cardiol. Feb. 1996; 12 (2): 127-37.

63. Lonn, E. M.; Yusuf, S. Evidence based cardiology: Emerging approaches in preventing cardiovascular disease. BMJ. May 1st 1999. Vol. 318 (7194): 1337-1341.

ADVANCES IN LIPID-LOWERING THERAPY IN ATHEROSCLEROSIS

Jean Davignon

Hyperlipidemia and Atherosclerosis Research Group
Clinical Research Institute of Montreal
110 Pine Avenue West
Montreal, Quebec
H2W 1R7

EVOLVING CONTEXT FOR DRUG THERAPY OF DYSLIPIDEMIA

The treatment of atherosclerosis using lipid-lowering drugs has evolved markedly over the past decade. It has been driven by the results and implications of major clinical trials. There has been a paradigm shift in the last decade from stable coronary lesions of high-grade stenosis to unstable plaques of low-grade stenosis. These vulnerable culprit lesions are characterized by a large lipid core, rich in foam cells with a thin fibrous cap, rich in activated macrophages and inflammatory cells, and poor in smooth muscle cells[1,2]. The majority of myocardial infarctions arise from these plaques. Whereas stable, high-grade lesions allow for collateral circulation networks to form, culprit lesions are prone to rupture, hemorrhage and cause thrombus formation. There has also been renewed interest in the important contribution of endothelial dysfunction to impair myocardial perfusion in coronary artery disease (CAD)[3]. An acetylcholine infusion in normal arteries induces an endothelial-derived, nitric oxide-mediated vasodilation. In the presence of cardiovascular risk factors (i.e., hypercholesterolemia, smoking, hypertension, diabetes)[4] or CAD, intra-arterial acetylcholine induces a vasoconstriction which is inhibited by L-arginine analogues such as L-NMMA (N^ω-Nitroso-Mono-Methyl-Arginine). More attention is being given to the inflammatory component of atherosclerosis[5], which is assessed by plasma measurement of inflammatory markers such as C-reactive protein (CRP)[6], IL-6[7,8], or serum amyloid-A protein (SAA)[9]. Methods have been developed to measure local changes in heat produced by the inflammatory reaction over atherosclerotic plaques. Using a highly sensitive special thermography catheter, Stefanadis et al.[10] have shown a significant increase in thermal heterogeneity of human atherosclerotic plaques studied by intravascular ultrasound (IVUS) in arteries from patients with unstable angina or myocardial infarction, as compared to those of controls or of subjects with stable plaques. They observed a correlation between plasma levels of CRP and increase in heat differences between plaque areas and normal adjacent areas.

Without minimizing the importance of LDL-cholesterol (LDL-C) concentration and the need to reduce it, there has been renewed interest in the role of triglyceride-rich

Diabetes and Cardiovascular Disease: Etiology, Treatment and Outcomes
Edited by Aubie Angel *et al.*, Kluwer Academic/Plenum Publishers, 2001

49

lipoproteins in the etiology of CAD[11], which has been enhanced by the emergence of results from angiographic trials with fibrates, demonstrating reduced lesion progression and reduced incidence of CAD associated with a reduction in plasma triglyceride, an increase in HDL-cholesterol (HDL-C), and little effect on LDL-C[12]. Revision of previous dogmas[13] and new epidemiological evidence indicating an independent contribution of total plasma triglyceride concentration to CAD risk account in part for this resurgence of interest. These include the meta-analysis of Hokanson and Austin[14], the results of the Copenhagen Male Study[15] and those of the European Concerted Angina Trial (ECAT)[16]. One of the most compelling demonstrations of the relationship between plasma triglyceride levels and atherogenesis was made evident in the MARS trial, where small lesion progression correlated with markers of triglyceride-rich lipoproteins (TRL), especially apolipoprotein CIII in VLDL, even though there was a marked reduction of LDL-C by 80 mg per day of lovastatin[17]. It is fully recognized however that many other cardiovascular risk factors tend to cluster with hypertriglyceridemia, including high plasma levels of procoagulant factors (PAI-1, factor VIIa), remnant lipoproteins, small dense LDL, insulin resistance (especially in obese subjects), increased postprandial lipemia and low plasma HDL-C concentrations. It has also recently been recognized that TRL remnants in the circulation impair endothelial function[18] as it had been shown before for LDL-C[19]. Finally, interest has focused in recent years on the **pleiotropic effects** (i.e., multiple actions in different systems) of lipid-lowering drugs[20,21] and has brought a new dimension to the major therapeutic agents currently in use. This review will focus on the most widely prescribed lipid-lowering agents, fibrates and statins[22-25].

ADVANCES IN THE USE OF FIBRATES

Until recently there was a dearth of information regarding the performance of fibrates in CAD prevention and atherosclerosis progression in **clinical trials**. Several years ago, the Helsinki Heart Study **(HHS)** demonstrated that gemfibrozil administration was useful in the primary prevention of CAD. It showed, in particular, that a group of subjects at very high risk, those with a high LDL/HDL (≥5.0) ratio and a high plasma triglyceride concentration (≥2.3 mmol/L) benefited most (a 71% reduction in CAD composite endpoints)[26]. Since then, several clinical trials using fibrates have been completed. An angiographic trial using gemfibrozil, **LOCAT** (Lopid Coronary Angiography Trial), conducted in post-coronary artery bypass graft men (n = 395) with low HDL-C (≤1.01 mmol/L) and average LDL-C (≤4.5 mmol/L) showed significantly less narrowing in 32 months of average follow-up in minimum lumen diameter and average diameter of coronary segments as compared to placebo treated subjects. These results, achieved primarily with reductions in triglycerides (-36%) and increase in HDL-C (+21%) were comparable to those observed in trials conducted with statins[27]. **BECAIT** (Bezafibrate Infarction Prevention Study) conducted with bezafibrate (200 mg three times a day) in a selected group of men at high risk (n = 92) who had their first myocardial infarction before the age of 45 years, showed not only an improvement in coronary percentage stenosis and atherosclerosis progression, but also a 72% reduction in cumulative event rates over five years[12]. The treatment had no effect on LDL-C, lowered triglycerides 31%, VLDL-C 36%, fibrinogen 12% and raised HDL-C 9%. The **BIP** (Bezafibrate Infarction Prevention) study is a five-year, secondary prevention trial conducted in Israel, in 3090 CAD patients with low HDL-C, equally distributed between 400 mg bezafibrate-SR and placebo[28]. Preliminary data presented in Vienna in 1998, showed that a subset of subjects with hypertriglyceridemia treated with bezafibrate (n = 234) had a 40% reduction in combined primary endpoints (fatal and non-fatal myocardial infarction) as compared to subjects on placebo (n = 225). Overall in this study, LDL-C, triglycerides and fibrinogen were reduced respectively 6.2, 18.7 and 8.7%, and HDL-C was increased by 15.4%. The **VA-HIT**

(Veteran's Administration-HDL Intervention Trial) was another double-bind, randomized, placebo-controlled, secondary prevention trial in patients with low HDL-C (≤ 1.0 mmol/L), low LDL-C (≤ 3.6 mmol/L) and triglycerides ≤ 3.4 mmol/L[29]. Half of the 2531 men with CAD were randomized to gemfibrozil SR 1200 mg/day or placebo; preliminary results were presented at the 71st Scientific Sessions of the American Heart Association in November 1998. Total cholesterol and triglycerides were reduced by 2.8 and 24.5% respectively, and HDL-C was increased 7.5% after an average follow-up of 5.1 years. There was no significant effect on LDL-C. This resulted in a 22% reduction in combined fatal and non-fatal myocardial infarction (p = 0.006). In this trial, individuals both with triglycerides below or above 2.3 mmol/L benefited to the same extent. Finally, the three-year **SENDCAP** (St. Mary's, Ealing, Northwick Park Diabetes Cardiovascular Disease Prevention) study carried out in 164 subjects with type 2 diabetes showed that treatment of dyslipidemia with bezafibrate-SR 400 mg resulted in a significant reduction in cumulative CAD event rate[30]. The cumulative incidence was 23% in the placebo group compared to 7% in the treatment group (p<0.01). This study is the first of its kind in diabetes and an encouraging finding that awaits confirmation from ongoing larger clinical trials.

Major advances have been made in our understanding of the **mechanism of action of fibrates**. The discovery that many of the effects of fibrates are mediated by the peroxisome proliferator activated receptor alpha (PPARα) pathway constitutes a major breakthrough[31,32]. Fibrates after crossing the cell membrane bind in the cytoplasm to the PPARα which is a member of the nuclear receptor superfamily. The fibrate-PPARα complex enters the nucleus to interact with the 9-cis retinoic acid receptor (RXR) which binds in association with a nuclear factor (HNF4) to the peroxisome proliferator response element (PPRE) and alters the transcription of target genes, mainly involved in lipid and lipoprotein metabolism. Thus, the transcription of the apoAI[33-35], apoAII[36] and lipoprotein lipase genes[37] are enhanced, while that of apoCIII is repressed[38,39]. These effects account for the strong triglyceride-lowering and HDL-raising effects of fibrates. Thanks to further studies carried out at the Pasteur Institute in Lille, the marked difference between rats and humans with regards to the PPARα pathway and lipoprotein metabolism has been explained[40]. In humans, there is no induction of peroxisome proliferation via this pathway and apoAI transcription is enhanced by fibrates. In rats, peroxisome proliferation is enhanced and apoAI transcription is inhibited. The latter has been attributed to an inactive PPRE in the promoter of the apoAI gene in rats, in contrast to humans where this site is active. In rats, fibrates induce the transcription of transcription factor REV-erbα, which interacts with a REV-responsive element REV-RE to repress the transcription of apoAI. This REV-RE is inactive in man while the human PPRE is sensitive to the fibrate-induced effect of PPARα (the apoAI gene). Fatty acid β-oxidation is enhanced by fibrates through the PPARα pathway in both rats and humans thereby affecting triglyceride formation and VLDL secretion. A large variety of genes have PPREs, which involve many diverse biological functions including fatty acid binding and transport, acyl-CoA synthesis, ketogenesis, as well as gluconeogenesis and glyceroneogenesis. Drugs are being designed to improve the selectivity and the potency of the fibrates by interaction with the PPARα system. Staels et al.[7] have presented evidence that fibrates have potential anti-inflammatory effects. They have shown that the activation of human aortic smooth muscle cells is inhibited by fibrate-mediated PPARα activation. Specifically, they demonstrated that IL-1β-mediated IL-6 and 6-keto-PGF-1α induction is inhibited in a dose-dependent manner by Wy14643, another member of the fibrate class. They demonstrated also that fibrates inhibit in a dose-dependent manner the increased gene expression of cyclooxygenase-2 (COX-2) induced by IL-1β. COX-2 plays a role in inflammation as a key enzyme involved in the production of prostaglandins from arachidonic acids. In support of an effect of fibrates on inflammatory response, fenofibrate was found to reduce plasma C-reactive protein, fibrinogen and IL-6 in CAD patients[7]. These new findings illustrate the pleiotropic actions of fibrates some of which may also reduce plasminogen activator inhibitor-1 (PAI-1)[41,42], inhibit restenosis post-angioplasty[43] and improve exercise-induced vasomotion in normal and stenotic coronary arteries[44]. These add up to the wide range of lipoprotein effects of this class of drugs, which include lowering plasma triglycerides in both the fasting and the postprandial states, increasing HDL-C, shifting the atherogenic small dense LDL towards larger more buoyant particle sizes and modestly reducing plasma Lp(a) levels[25].

ADVANCES IN THE USE OF STATINS

Many of the advances in statin research have confirmed the notion that besides major class effects, there are also effects that are specific to individual members of the class. The **pharmacokinetic properties** in particular differ substantially from statin to statin, and differences in metabolism by the cytochrome P450 (CYP) enzyme system are particularly relevant to clinical practice. Most statins use the CYP3A4 enzyme system for detoxification. This is the case for lovastatin, simvastatin, atorvastatin and cerivastatin. Some of these have alternate mechanisms of detoxification such as 2D6 for simvastatin and 2C8 for cerivastatin. On the other hand, fluvastatin does not require metabolism by the CYP3A4 system and is detoxified mainly by CYP2C9 and CYP2D6. Pravastatin in contrast does not depend on P450 enzymes for catabolism as the molecule is already hydroxylated. These considerations are important to avoid drug interaction with the many agents detoxified by the CYP3A4 system (>50%). Many substances are substrates for, or inhibitors of the CYP3A4 system. These include for instance cyclosporin and itraconazole (both substrates and inhibitors), and substances as varied as erythromycin, azythromycin, astemizole, terfenadine, diltiazem, nifedipine, cisapride, triazolam, warfarin, nefazodone, triazolam, alprazolam, metformin, quinidine and grapefruit juice[45-47]. Lack of recognition of these potential interactions may lead to development of myopathy and occasionally rhabdomyolysis in cases of multiple drug combinations. Such a hazardous interaction was responsible for the early withdrawal of mibefradil, a promising calcium channel blocker due to reports of an increased frequency of *torsades de pointe*, rhabdomyolysis and death following combination therapy with simvastatin[48,49].

Many of the advances in our knowledge of the clinical utility of statins stem from the results of **five major clinical trials** which have involved 30817 subjects[50]. These include secondary prevention trials (4S, LIPID, CARE) and primary prevention trials (WOSCOPS, AFCAPS/TexCaps). Important lessons for the practice of medicine have been learned from the results of such studies. Some of these studies clearly indicated that patients with type 2 diabetes benefit from statin therapy with moderate[51] to large[52] reductions in CAD risk. The large **AFCAPS/TexCaps** (Air Force/Texas Coronary Atherosclerosis Prevention Study), one of the most recent outcome trials, emphasizes the importance of low HDL-C as a CAD risk factor in individuals at low risk[53]. It demonstrated that lovastatin therapy (40 mg/day) in subjects with low HDL-C concentrations (n = 3304) but otherwise at low CAD risk (only 17% had more than two risk factors) achieved a 37% reduction in major coronary events (fatal and non-fatal MI, sudden deaths or unstable angina), as compared to the placebo group (n = 3301) after 5.2 years of follow-up. This result was achieved with a reduction in total cholesterol, LDL-C and triglycerides of 18.4%, 25% and 15% respectively, associated with a 6% increase in HDL-C. There was also a 33% reduction in revascularization procedures and 35% reduction in fatal and non-fatal MI. According to the NCEP adult treatment panel guidelines, 83% of the patients included in the study would not have been considered eligible for drug treatment. These results stress the major benefit derived from statin therapy in low risk individuals in the prevention of CAD mortality and the importance of plasma HDL-C concentrations in the risk equation. In the angiographic **LCAS** (Lipoprotein and Coronary Atherosclerosis Study) trial the plasma HDL-C concentration was found to markedly influence the benefit of fluvastatin therapy (40 mg/day) on coronary lesion progression. Subjects in whom coronary atherosclerosis progressed more and who responded best to fluvastatin therapy had low HDL concentrations ($\leq$ 0.9mmol/L) at the outset compared to those who had levels $\geq$ 0.9 mmol/L. This was further reflected in a statistically significant improvement in the probability of event free survival (p = 0.002) in the subset of patients with low HDL over 2.5 years.

With the development of highly efficacious third generation molecules the **triglyceride-lowering property of statins** has become obvious and has emerged as a class effect[25,54]. Although not as strong as that exhibited by fibrates[55], it remains especially attractive because of its association with a strong LDL-C lowering effect and a large impact on the total cholesterol/HDL-C ratio[56]. The triglyceride lowering is a function of baseline triglycerides and appears to be commensurate with the potency of the statin to reduce LDL-C[54,57]. It has become evident as well that the cardiovascular benefits associated with statin therapy are in part due to **pleiotropic effects** affecting a wide range of different systems, and in many instances operating beyond the benefit derived from plasma lipid reduction[20,21]. Several arguments militate in favor of their existence including early separation in the survival curves between placebo and treatment groups in 4S, WOSCOPS and AFCAPS/TexCAPS, benefits beyond those predicted from the Framingham model in WOSCOPS[58], and the beneficial effect of LDL-C reduction by statins on stroke incidence even though LDL-C is not highly predictive of this condition[59]. One of the most significant advances in this area is the demonstration that myocardial perfusion can be rapidly improved in hypercholesterolemic patients following short-term aggressive lipid-lowering with a statin combined with cholestyramine and dietary management, as demonstrated by positron emission tomography scanning[60]. Such findings further support the numerous studies demonstrating the benefit of statin therapy on endothelial dysfunction[61-63]. This emergent class effect is now fully recognized. It is in part related to cholesterol reduction, but also ascribed to a direct effect on nitric oxide (NO) production demonstrated *in vitro*[64,65] and *in vivo*[19], to a reversal of the inhibitory effect of oxidized lipoproteins on endothelial constitutive NO synthase (ecNOS)[66], and can take place independently of LDL-C reduction *in vivo*[67]. Acute improvement in myocardial perfusion following treatment with statins could also be attributed in part to their inhibitory effect on endothelin production[68], ability to reduce plasma viscosity and improve erythrocyte deformability which is impaired in hypercholesterolemic subjects[69]. Among the other pleiotropic effects of statins that may have clinical relevance, one should mention their antioxidant properties[70-73], their ability to improve survival and reduce graft rejection after cardiac transplantation[74,75], and their inhibitory effect on platelet aggregation, PAI-1, and thromboxane production[76]. Some pleiotropic effects are specific to a statin type. For instance the inhibitory effect of statins on tissue factor transcription and production by macrophages[77] and on cell proliferation[78] are properties of lipophilic but not of hydrophilic statins. Their anti-carcinogenic properties related to their ability to induce apoptosis and inhibit cell proliferation have been confirmed in many cell culture experiments and animal models[20,79], including melanoma[80]. It is tempting to relate these findings to the significant reduction in melanoma frequency observed in the AFCAPS/TexCAPS trial (24/3301 in the placebo group versus 11/3304 in the treatment group, p=0.028)[53]. Conversely, the limited ability of a hydrophilic statin to penetrate muscle cells as compared to lipophilic statins is associated with a reduced likelihood of inducing muscle damage as shown in several animal experimental models[81-83].

Several **promising emergent properties** have been uncovered recently. One is the anti-inflammatory effects of statins postulated from the results of a nested case-control study in the CARE trial. Ridker and coworkers[9] observed that pravastatin was most effective at reducing the relative risk of recurrent events in subjects who manifested signs of inflammation with serum amyloid A protein and C-reactive protein above the 90th percentile. Compared to the placebo group, those with signs of inflammation had a higher risk but responded better to pravastatin in terms of risk reduction (-54% vs. -25%, p for trend <0.005). Interestingly, at baseline, these two subsets of patients matched for age and sex had similar levels of LDL-C, HDL-C and triglycerides. Another small study reported recently that circulating pro-inflammatory cytokines such as IL-6 and TNFα may be lowered by short-term statin therapy[8]. Another emerging property of major interest is a plaque stabilization effect. For instance it has been shown in the hypercholesterolemic WHHL rabbit that cerivastatin has the ability to reduce matrix metalloproteinase (MMP) 1, 3 and 9 in atherosclerotic lesions. These enzymes produced mainly by macrophages weaken the fibrous cap thereby enhancing the vulnerability of the plaque. Statin treatment is also accompanied by a reduced macrophage population, an increased collagen content and a reduction in tissue factor production. The first demonstration that statins might induce plaque stabilization in humans was shown recently by Crisby et al.[84]. In an open prospective study, patients scheduled for carotid endarterectomy with similar extent of carotid stenosis (>70% diameter reduction) were assigned to receive or not 40 mg of pravastatin for three months before surgery was performed. Using immunochemical and histochemical techniques, carotids from treated patients had significantly less lipids and oxidized LDL in their plaques than controls. Furthermore, there was a significant reduction in the number of macrophages and T-cells and less apoptosis, but as expected no change in smooth muscle cell number. The discovery of new statin pleiotropic effects has increased rapidly and steadily over the past few years. The clinical relevance of many of these has not been established, but some are opening new avenues of research and have far reaching potential and consequences. This is the case for the discovery that lovastatin improves renal blood flow, increases glomerular filtration rate and reduces proteinuria in the rat five-sixth nephrectomy model of renal insufficiency[85]. It is also the case for the observation that lovastatin and simvastatin are potent promoters of bone formation by stimulating osteoblast morphogenic protein-2 transcription[86]. These are exciting developments and one might see the day when statins will be prescribed for their non-lipid effects.

SUMMARY AND CONCLUSIONS

The accrued evidence that lipid-lowering therapy limits the progression of atherosclerosis and reduces CAD events is overwhelming. The focus has been on LDL-C reduction with statins, but recent evidence also stresses the importance of raising HDL-C and reducing triglyceride-rich lipoproteins (TRL). Treatment should take into account the type of dyslipidemia, combination therapy, drug interactions and pleiotropic effects of drugs (multiple effects in different systems). Statins and fibrates are the most widely prescribed. Fibrates have a major impact on plasma TRL and HDL-C levels. They enhance lipoprotein lipase, apoAI and apoAII transcription and reduce that of apoCIII. The discovery that their multiple actions are in large part mediated by the PPARα pathway is a breakthrough. Fibrates also lower plasma fibrinogen and plasma viscosity but their ability to inhibit smooth muscle cell activation is one of their most promising pleiotropic effects. Statins are safe and potent LDL-C-lowering agents but also lower TRL and raise HDL. Their pleiotropic effects are numerous, and include vasodilatory, anti-thrombotic, antioxidant, anti-proliferative, anti-inflammatory and plaque stabilizing properties. Many findings make a case for their early use in CAD to improve myocardial perfusion after a myocardial infarction, and they are indicated in heart transplant recipients to improve survival and reduce graft rejection. Fibrates and statins have complementary lipid modifying and pleiotropic effects so that their combination, carried out with caution to avoid potential untoward effects, should provide the highest cardiovascular benefit. This hypothesis is currently being tested in the Lipid in Diabetes Study (LDS), an outcome trial comparing monotherapy with fenofibrate and cerivastatin to combination therapy conducted in England.

REFERENCES

1. P. Libby, Molecular bases of the acute coronary syndromes. [Review] [49 refs], *Circulation*, 91:2844-2850 (1995).
2. R.T. Lee, P. Libby, The unstable atheroma, *Arterioscler. Thromb. Vasc. Biol.*, 17:1859-1867 (1997).
3. H. Drexler, B. Hornig, Endothelial dysfunction in human disease, *J. Mol. Cell. Cardiol.*, 31:51-60 (1999).
4. J.A. Vita, C.B. Treasure, E.G. Nabel, et al., Coronary vasomotor response to acetylcholine relates to risk factors for coronary artery disease [see comments], *Circulation*, 81:491-497 (1990).
5. R. Ross, Mechanisms of disease - Atherosclerosis - An inflammatory disease, *New Engl. J. Med.* 340:115-126 (1999).
6. P.M. Ridker, R.J. Glynn, C.H. Hennekens, C-Reactive protein adds to the predictive value of total and HDL cholesterol in determining risk of first myocardial infarction, *Circulation*, 97:2007-2011 (1998).
7. B. Staels, W. Koenig, A. Habib, et al., Activation of human aortic smooth-muscle cells is inhibited by PPARα but not by PPARgamma activators, *Nature*, 393:790-793 (1998).
8. R.S. Rosenson, C.C. Tangney, L.C. Casey, Inhibition of proinflammatory cytokine production by pravastatin, *Lancet*, 353:983-984 (1999).
9. P.M. Ridker, N. Rifai, M.A. Pfeffer, et al., Inflammation, pravastatin, and the risk of coronary events after myocardial infarction in patients with average cholesterol levels Inflammation, pravastatin, and the risk of coronary events after myocardial infarction in patients with average cholesterol levels, *Circulation*, 98:839-844 (1998).
10. C. Stefanadis, L. Diamantopoulos, C. Vlachopoulos, et al., Thermal heterogeneity within human atherosclerotic coronary arteries detected in vivo - A new method of detection by application of a special thermography catheter, *Circulation*, 99:1965-1971 (1999).
11. J. Davignon, J.S. Cohn. Triglycerides: A risk factor for coronary heart disease, *Atherosclerosis*, 124:S57-S64 (1996).
12. C.G. Ericsson, A. Hamsten, J. Nilsson, L. Grip, B. Svane, U. De Faire, Angiographic assessment of effects of bezafibrate on progression of coronary artery disease in young male postinfarction patients, *Lancet*, 347:849-853 (1996).
13. M.A. Austin, Plasma triglyceride as a risk factor for coronary heart disease - The epidemiologic evidence and beyond, *Am. J. Epidemiol.*, 129:249-259 (1989).
14. J.E. Hokanson, M.A. Austin, Plasma triglyceride level is a risk factor for cardiovascular disease independent of high-density lipoprotein cholesterol level: a meta-analysis of population based prospective studies, *J. Cardivasc. Risk*, 3:213-219 (1996).
15. J. Jeppesen, H.O. Hein, P. Suadicani, F. Gyntelberg, Triglyceride concentration and ischemic heart disease - An eight- year follow-up in the Copenhagen Male Study, *Circulation*, 97:1029-1036 (1998).
16. I. Bolibar, S.G. Thompson, A. Von Eckardstein, M. Sandkamp, G. Assmann, Dose-response relationships of serum lipid measurements with the extent of coronary stenosis: Strong, independent, and comprehensive, *Arterioscler. Thromb. Vasc. Biol.*, 15:1035-1042 (1995).
17. H.N. Hodis, W.J. Mack, S.P. Azen, et al., Triglyceride- and cholesterol-rich lipoproteins have a differential effect on mild/moderate and severe lesion progression as assessed by quantitative coronary angiography in a controlled trial of lovastatin, *Circulation*, 90:42-49 (1994).
18. K. Kugiyama, H. Doi, T. Motoyama, et al., Association of remnant lipoprotein levels with impairment of endothelium-dependent vasomotor function in human coronary arteries, *Circulation*, 97:2519-2526 (1998).
19. S. John, M. Schlaich, M. Langenfeld, et al., Increased bioavailability of nitric oxide after lipid-lowering therapy in hypercholesterolemic patients - A randomized, placebo- controlled, double-blind study, *Circulation*, 98:211-216 (1998).
20. J. Davignon, The pleiotropic effects of drugs affecting lipid metabolism. In: B. Jacotot, D. Mathé, J.C. Fruchart, eds. *Atherosclerosis XI. Proceedings of the IXth International Symposium on Atherosclerosis*, held in Paris, France on 5-9 October 1997, Elsevier Science Pte Ltd., Singapore (1998).
21. J. Davignon, Methods and endpoint issues in clinical development of lipid- acting agents with pleiotropic effects, *Am. J. Cardiol.*, 81:17F-23F (1998).
22. J. Davignon, Fibrates: A review of important issues and recent findings, *Can. J. Cardiol.*, 10:61B-71B (1994).
23. J. Davignon, M. Montigny, R. Dufour, HMG-CoA reductase inhibitors: a look back and a look ahead, *Can. J. Cardiol.*, 8:843-864 (1992).
24. M. Farnier, J. Davignon, Current and future treatment of hyperlipidemia: The role of statins, *Am. J. Cardiol.* 82:3J-10J (1998).
25. J. Davignon, Advances in drug treatment of dyslipidemia: Focus on atorvastatin, *Can. J. Cardiol.*, 14:28B-38B (1998).

26. V. Manninen, L. Tenkanen, P. Koskinen, et al., Joint effects of serum triglyceride and LDL cholesterol and HDL cholesterol concentrations on coronary heart disease risk in the Helsinki Heart Study: Implications for treatment, *Circulation*, 85:37-45 (1992).

27. M.H. Frick, M. Syvänne, M.S. Nieminen, et al., Prevention of the angiographic progression of coronary and vein- graft atherosclerosis by gemfibrozil after coronary bypass surgery in men with low levels of HDL cholesterol, *Circulation*, 96:2137-2143 (1997).

28. U. Goldbourt, S. Behar, H. Reicher-Reiss, et al., Rationale and design of a secondary prevention trial of increasing serum high-density lipoprotein cholesterol and reducing triglycerides in patients with clinically manifest atherosclerotic heart disease (the bezafibrate infarction prevention trial), *Am. J. Cardiol.*, 71:909-915 (1993).

29. V. Papademetriou, P. Narayan, H. Rubins, D. Collins, S. Robins, HIT Investigators. Influence of risk factors on peripheral and cerebrovascular disease in men with coronary artery disease, low high-density lipoprotein, cholesterol levels, and desirable low-density lipoprotein cholesterol levels, *Am. Heart J.*, 136:734-740 (1998).

30. R.S. Elkeles, J.R. Diamond, C. Poulter, et al., Cardiovascular outcomes in type 2 diabetes - A double-blind placebo-controlled study of bezafibrate: the St. Mary's, Ealing, Northwick Park Diabetes Cardiovascular Disease Prevention (SENDCAP) Study, *Diabetes Care*, 21:641-648 (1998).

31. K. Schoonjans, B. Staels, J. Auwerx, Role of the peroxisome proliferator-activated receptor (PPAR) in mediating the effects of fibrates and fatty acids on gene expression. [Review] [193 refs], *J Lipid Res*, 37:907-925 (1996).

32. B. Staels, J. Dallongeville, J. Auwerx, K. Schoonjans, E. Leitersdorf, J.G. Fruchart, Mechanism of action of fibrates on lipid and lipoprotein metabolism, *Circulation*, 98:2088-2093 (1998).

33. N. Vu-Dac, K. Schoonjans, B. Laine, J.-C. Fruchart, J. Auwerx, B. Staels, Negative regulation of the human apolipoprotein A-I promoter by fibrates can be attenuated by the interaction of the peroxisome proliferator-activated receptor with its response element, *J. Biol. Chem.* 269:31012-31018 (1994).

34. L. Berthou, N. Duverger, F. Emmanuel, et al. Opposite regulation of human versus mouse apolipoprotein A-I by fibrates in human apolipoprotein A-I transgenic mic, *J. Clin. Invest.*, 97:2408-2416 (1996).

35. M. Kockx, H.M.G. Princen, T. Kooistra, Studies on the role of PPAR in the fibrate-modulated gene expression of apolipoprotein A-I, plasminogen activator inhibitor 1, and fibrinogen in primary hepatocyte cultures from cynomolgus monkey, *Ann. NY Acad. Sci.*, 804:711-712 (1996).

36. L. Berthou, R. Saladin, P. Yaqoob, et al., Regulation of rat liver apolipoprotein A-I, apolipoprotein A-II and acyl-coenzyme A oxidase gene expression by fibrates and dietary fatty acids, *Eur. J. Biochem.*, 232:179-187 (1995).

37. B. Staels, K. Schoonjans, J.C. Fruchart, J. Auwerx, The effects of fibrates and thiazolidinediones on plasma triglyceride metabolism are mediated by distinct peroxisome proliferator activated receptors (PPARs), *Biochimie*, 79:95-99 (1997).

38. B. Staels, N. Vu-Dac, V.A. Kosykh, et al., Fibrates downregulate apolipoprotein C-III expression independent of induction of peroxisomal acyl coenzyme A oxidase. A potential mechanism for the hypolipidemic action of fibrates, *J. Clin. Invest.*, 95:705-712 (1995).

39. R. Hertz, J. Bishara-Shieban, J. Bar-Tana, Mode of action of peroxisome proliferators as hypolipidemic drugs. Suppression of apolipoprotein C-III, *J. Biol. Chem.* 270:13470-13475 (1995).

40. N. Vu-Dac, S. Chopin-Delannoy, P. Gervois, et al., The nuclear receptors peroxisome proliferator-activated receptor α and Rev-erbα mediate the species-specific regulation of apolipoprotein A-I expression by fibrates, *J. Biol. Chem.*, 273:25713-25720 (1998).

41. J. Arts, M. Kockx, H.M.G. Princen, T. Kooistra, Studies on the mechanism of fibrate-inhibited expression of plasminogen activator inhibitor-1 in cultured hepatocytes from cynomolgus monkey, *Arterioscler. Thromb. Vasc. Biol.,* 17:26-32 (1997).

42. J.I. Zambrana, F. Velasco, P. Castro, et al., Comparison of *bezafibrate* versus *lovastatin* for lowering plasma insulin, fibrinogen, and plasminogen activator inhibitor-1 concentrations in hyperlipemic heart transplant patients, *Am. J. Cardiol.*, 80:836-840 (1997).

43. S. Ishiwata, S. Nakanishi, S. Nishiyama, A. Seki, Prevention of restenosis by bezafibrate after successful coronary angioplasty, *Coronary Artery Dis.*, 6:883-889 (1995).

44. C. Seiler, T.M. Suter, O.M. Hess, Exercise-induced vasomotion of angiographically normal and stenotic coronary arteries improves after cholesterol-lowering drug therapy with bezafibrate, *J. Am. Coll. Cardiol.*, 26:1615-1622 (1995).

45. U. Christians, W. Jacobsen, L.C. Floren, Metabolism and drug interactions of 3-hydroxy-3-methylglutaryl coenzyme A reductase inhibitors in transplant patients: Are the statins mechanistically similar?, *Pharmacol. Ther.*, 80:1-34 (1998).

46. B.A. Hamelin, J. Turgeon, Hydrophilicity/lipophilicity: relevance for the pharmacology and clinical effects of HMG-CoA reductase inhibitors, *Trends Pharmacol. Sci.*, 19:26-37 (1998).

47. J.J. Lilja, K.T. Kivistö, P.J. Neuvonen. Grapefruit juice-simvastatin interaction: Effect on serum concentrations of simvastatin, simvastatin acid, and HMG-CoA reductase inhibitors, *Clin.Pharmacol.Ther.*, 64:477-483 (1998).

48. D. Schmassmann-Suhijar, R. Bullingham, R. Gasser, J. Schmutz, W.E. Haefeli, Rhabdomyolysis due to interaction of simvastatin with mibefradil, *Lancet*, 351:1929-1930 (1998).

49. T. Prueksaritanont, B. Ma, C. Y. Tang, et al., Metabolic interactions between mibefradil and HMG-CoA reductase inhibitors: an *in vitro* investigation with human liver preparations, *Br. J. Clin. Pharmacol.*, 47:291-298 (1999).

50. M. Kornitzer, Primary and secondary prevention of coronary artery disease: a follow-up on clinical controlled trials, *Curr. Opin. Lipidol.*, 9:557-564 (1998).

51. R.B. Goldberg, M.J. Mellies, F.M. Sacks, et al. Cardiovascular events and their reduction with pravastatin in diabetic and glucose-intolerant myocardial infarction survivors with average cholesterol levels - Subgroup analyses in the cholesterol and recurrent events (CARE) trial, *Circulation*, 98:2513-2519 (1998).

52. K. Pyörälä, T.R. Pedersen, J. Kjekshus, O. Faergeman, A.G. Olsson, G. Thorgeirsson, Cholesterol lowering with simvastatin improves prognosis of diabetic patients with coronary heart disease - A subgroup analysis of the Scandinavian Simvastatin Survival Study (4S), *Diabetes Care*, 20:614-620 (1997).

53. J.R. Downs, M. Clearfield, S. Weis, et al., Primary prevention of acute coronary events with lovastatin in men and women with average cholesterol levels - Results of AFCAPS/TexCAPS, *JAMA*, 279:1615-1622 (1998).

54. E.A. Stein, M. Lane, P. Laskarzewski, Comparison of statins in hypertriglyceridemia, *Am. J. Cardiol.*, 81:66B-69B (1998).

55. T.C. Ooi, T. Heinonen, P. Alaupovic, et al., Efficacy and safety of a new hydroxymethylglutaryl-coenzyme a reductase inhibitor, atorvastatin, in patients with combined hyperlipidemia: Comparison with fenofibrate, *Arterioscler. Thromb. Vasc. Biol.*, 17:1793-1799 (1997).

56. R.G. Bakker-Arkema, M.H. Davidson, R.J. Goldstein, et al., Efficacy and safety of a new HMG-CoA reductase inhibitor, atorvastatin, in patients with hypertriglyceridemia, *JAMA*, 275:128-133 (1996).

57. E. Stein, Cerivastatin in primary hyperlipidemia: A multicenter analysis of efficacy and safety, *Am. J. Cardiol.*, 82:40J-46J (1998).

58. C.J. Packard, J. Shepherd, S.M. Cobbe, et al., Influence of pravastatin and plasma lipids on clinical events in the West of Scotland Coronary Prevention Study (WOSCOPS), *Circulation*, 97:1440-1445 (1998).

59. H.C. Bucher, L.E. Griffith, G.H. Guyatt, Effect of HMGcoA reductase inhibitors on stroke - A meta-analysis of randomized, controlled trials, *Ann. Intern. Med.*, 128:89-95 (1998).

60. K.L. Gould, J.P. Martucci, D.I. Goldberg, et al., Short-term cholesterol lowering decreases size and severity of perfusion abnormalities by positron emission tomography after dipyridamole in patients with coronary artery disease: A potential noninvasive marker of healing coronary endothelium, *Circulation*, 89:1530-1538 (1994).

61. K. Egashira, Y. Hirooka, H. Kai, et al., Reduction in serum cholesterol with pravastatin improves endothelium-dependent coronary vasomotion in patients with hypercholesterolemia, *Circulation*, 89:2519-2524 (1994).

62. T.J. Anderson, I.T. Meredith, A.C. Yeung, B. Frei, A.P. Selwyn, P. Ganz, The effect of cholesterol-lowering and antioxidant therapy on endothelium-dependent coronary vasomotion, *New Engl. J. Med.*, 332:488-493 (1995).

63. G. O'Driscoll, D. Green, R.R. Taylor, Simvastatin, an HMG-coenzyme A reductase inhibitor, improves endothelial function within 1 month, *Circulation*, 95:1126-1131 (1997).

64. R.P. Brandes, A. Behra, C. Lebherz, R.H. Böger, S.M. Bode-Böger, A. Mügge, Lovastatin maintains nitric oxide - but not EDHF-mediated endothelium-dependent relaxation in the hypercholesterolemic rabbit carotid artery, *Atherosclerosis*, 142:97-104 (1999).

65. W.H. Kaesemeyer, R.B. Caldwell, J.Z. Huang, R.W. Caldwell. Pravastatin sodium activates endothelial nitric oxide synthase independent of its cholesterol-lowering actions, *J. Am. Coll. Cardiol.*, 33:234-241 (1999).

66. U. Laufs, V. La Fata, J. Plutzky, J.K. Liao, Upregulation of endothelial nitric oxide synthase by HMG CoA reductase inhibitors, *Circulation*, 97:1129-1135 (1998).

67. J.K. Williams, G.K. Sukhova, D.M. Herrington, P. Libby, Pravastatin has cholesterol-lowering independent effects on the artery wall of atherosclerotic monkeys, *J. Am. Coll. Cardiol.*, 31:684-691 (1998).

68. O. Hernández-Perera, D. Pérez-Sala, J. Navarro-Antolín, et al., Effects of the 3-hydroxy-3-methylglutaryl-CoA reductase inhibitors, atorvastatin and simvastatin, on the expression of endothelin-1 and endothelial nitric oxide synthase in vascular endothelial cells, *J. Clin. Invest.*, 101:2711-2719 (1998).

69. M. Kohno, K. Murakawa, K. Yasunari, et al., Improvement of erythrocyte deformability by cholesterol-lowering therapy with pravastatin in hypercholesterolemic patients, *Metabolism*, 46:287-291 (1997).

70. M. Aviram, G. Dankner, U. Cogan, E. Hochgraf, J.G. Brook, Lovastatin inhibits low-density lipoprotein oxidation and alters its fluidity and uptake by macrophages: In vitro and in vivo studies, *Metabolism*, 41:229-235 (1992).

71. H.A. Kleinveld, P.N. Demacker, A.F. De Haan, A.F. Stalenhoef. Decreased in vitro oxidizability of low-density lipoprotein in hypercholesterolaemic patients treated with 3-hydroxy-3- methylglutaryl-CoA reductase inhibitors, *Eur J Clin Invest*, 23:289-295 (1993).

72. R. Salonen, K. Nyyssönen, E. Porkkala-Sarataho, J.T. Salonen, The Kuopio Atherosclerosis Prevention Study (KAPS): Effect of pravastatin treatment on lipids, oxidation resistance of lipoproteins, and atherosclerotic progression, *Am. J. Cardiol.*, 76:34C-39C (1995).

73. M. Aviram, M. Rosenblat, C.L. Bisgaier, R.S. Newton, Atorvastatin and gemfibrozil metabolites, but not the parent drugs, are potent antioxidants against lipoprotein oxidation, *Atherosclerosis*, 138:271-280 (1998).

74. J.A. Kobashigawa, S. Katznelson, H. Laks, et al., Effect of pravastatin on outcomes after cardiac transplantation, *New Engl. J. Med.*, 333:621-627 (1995).

75. K. Wenke, B. Meiser, J. Thiery, et al., Simvastatin reduces graft vessel disease and mortality after heart transplantation, a four year randomized trial Simvastatin reduces graft vessel disease and mortality after heart transplantation - A four-year randomized trial, *Circulation*, 96:1398-1402 (1997).

76. R.S. Rosenson, C.C. Tangney. Antiatherothrombotic properties of statins: implications for cardiovascular event reduction [see comments]. [Review] [160 refs], *JAMA*, 279:1643-1650 (1998).

77. S. Colli, S. Eligini, M. Lalli, M. Camera, R. Paoletti, E. Tremoli. Vastatins inhibit tissue factor in cultured human macrophages - A novel mechanism of protection against atherothrombosis, *Arterioscler. Thromb. Vasc. Biol.*, 17:265-272 (1997).

78. P. Nègre-Aminou, A.K. Van Vliet, M. Van Erck, G.C.F. Van Thiel, R.E.W. Van Leeuwen, L.H. Cohen, Inhibition of proliferation of human smooth muscle cells by various HMG-CoA reductase inhibitors: Comparison with other human cell types, *Biochim. Biophys. Acta Lipids Lipid Metab.*, 1345:259-268 (1997).

79. J. Dimitroulakos, D. Nohynek, K.L. Backway, et al., Increased sensitivity of acute myeloid leukemias to lovastatin- induced apoptosis: A potential therapeutic approach, *Blood*, 93:1308-1318 (1999).

80. W. Feleszko, R. Zagozdzon, J. Golab, M. Jakobisiak, Potentiated antitumour effects of cisplatin and lovastatin against MmB16 melanoma in mice, *Eur. J. Cancer* [A] 1998;34:406-411 (1998).

81. B.A. Masters, M.J. Palmoski, O.P. Flint, R.E. Gregg, D. Wang-Iverson, S.K. Durham, *In vitro* myotoxicity of the 3-hydroxy-3-methylglutaryl coenzyme A reductase inhibitors, pravastatin, lovastatin, and simvastatin, using neonatal rat skeletal myocytes, *Toxicol. Appl. Pharmacol.* 131:163-174 (1995).

82. S. Pierno, A. De Luca, D. Tricarico, et al., Potential risk of myopathy by HMG-CoA reductase inhibitors: A comparison of pravastatin and simvastatin effects on membrane electrical properties of rat skeletal muscle. *J. Pharmacol. Exp. Ther.* 275:1490-1496 (1995).

83. A.P. Gadbut, A.P. Caruso, J.B. Galper, Differential sensitivity of C_2-C_{12} striated muscle cells to lovastatin and pravastatin. *J. Mol. Cell. Cardiol.*, 27:2397-2402 (1995).

84. M. Crisby, G. Fredriksson-Norden, J. Nilsson, Pravastatin treatment decreases lipid content, inflammation and cell death in human carotid plaques. *The Lancet Conference. The Challenge of Stroke*, October (1998).

85. K.S. Hafez, S.R. Inman, N.T. Stowe, A.C. Novick, Renal hemodynamic effects of lovastatin in a renal ablation model. *Urology*, 48:862-867 (1996).

86. G. Mundy, G. Gutierrez, R. Garrett, et al., Identification of a new class of powerful stimulators of new bone formation in vivo, clarification of mechanism of action, and use in animal models of osteoporosis. Second joint meeting Am.Soc.Bone Mineral Res.& Internat. Bone Mineral Soc. San Francisco, Dec.4 (1998).

HOMOCYSTEINE AS A RISK FACTOR IN CARDIOVASCULAR DISEASE

David E. C. Cole, MD PhD FRCPC

Departments of Laboratory Medicine & Pathobiology,
Medicine and Paediatrics (Genetics),
University of Toronto,
Toronto Ontario   M5G 1L5 Canada

INTRODUCTION

Homocysteine is a naturally occurring, sulphur amino acid of established clinical relevance. Excess homocysteine excretion is characteristic of patients with the rare inborn error of metabolism -- homocystinuria -- a connective tissue disorder with spontaneous, early dislocation of the ocular lens, marfanoid habitus, and mental retardation.[13] Homocystinuria is also characterized by early death due to vaso-occlusive disease, and is accompanied by hemostatic changes consistent with a thrombophilic state. Increased plasma homocysteine is associated with histopathologic evidence of vascular endothelial injury, vascular smooth muscle proliferation, and progressive arterial stenosis. After its identification, homocystinuria was studied by investigators hypothesizing that a milder disturbance of homocysteine metabolism might be a significant factor in common cardiovascular conditions and coagulopathies. It is only recently that strong evidence for this hypothesis has emerged.[8;11]

METABOLISM OF HOMOCYSTEINE

Homocysteine is generated by demethylation of the essential amino acid, methionine, but significant amounts of methionine are regenerated by remethylation, a reaction requiring folate and vitamin B_{12}.[18] Nevertheless, the majority of homocysteine is further metabolized to cystathionine in a reaction requiring pyridoxal-5'-phosphate, then converted to cysteine, and finally oxidized to CO_2 and inorganic sulfate.[13]

Homocysteine can bind nitric oxide (NO) to form S-nitrosohomocysteine (Hcy-NO), which may limit the beneficial vasodilating effects of intrinsic nitric oxide production. However, NO production by vascular endothelium may act to limit homocysteine toxicity to the endothelium, and the precise relationship between these two endogenous compounds has not been determined.

The plasma level of homocysteine reflects cellular homocysteine synthesis. Clearance studies in healthy human subjects indicate that about 5-10% of all the homocysteine formed from methionine is exported from cells to plasma every 24 hours [17]. In renal failure,

Diabetes and Cardiovascular Disease: Etiology, Treatment and Outcomes
Edited by Aubie Angel et al., Kluwer Academic/Plenum Publishers, 2001

59

homocysteine clearance is reduced, suggesting an important role of kidney in elimination of homocysteine from plasma.

EPIDEMIOLOGY

Neural tube defects (NTDs), including spina bifida and anencephaly, occur more frequently in the offspring of women with folate deficiency [20]. Prospective trials have proven statistically significant protective effects of folate supplementation [5;12]. The minimum amount of folate required to ensure this protective effect – about 400µg per day – is close to the dose required to correct elevated homocysteine levels in asymptomatic adults. Rosenquist et al. [19] found L-homocysteine teratogenic to both neural tube and to cardiac tissue in avian embryos at concentrations known to occur in humans, and showed that the effect is blocked by folate supplementation. The results of this study give strong experimental support to the hypothesis that NTDs and cardiovascular disease result from elevated homocysteine.

Boushey et al. [3] performed a meta-analysis of 27 studies correlating elevated homocysteine to arteriosclerotic vascular disease. The odds ratio (OR) for coronary artery disease (CAD) of a 5 µmol/L increment in total homocysteine was 1.6 (95% confidence interval [CI], 1.4 to 1.7) for men and 1.8 (95% CI, 1.3 to 1.9) for women. Up to 10% of the overall disease risk appears attributable to homocysteine. The authors concluded that a 5 µmol/L increment in homocysteine increases the risk for atherosclerotic disease to the same extent as a 0.5 mmol/L increase in cholesterol. In a prospective study by Nygård et al. [14] of 587 patients with angiographically confirmed coronary artery disease, homocysteine levels were found to be strong predictors of mortality. In patients with concentrations less than 9 µmol/L as the reference group, the mortality odds ratios were 1.9 for patients with 9.0 - 14.9 µmol/L homocysteine, 2.8 for those with levels of 15.0 - 19.9 µmol/L, and 4.5 for those with levels greater than 20.0 µmol/L. Another study involving 19 centres in 9 European countries [7] found comparable relative risks for atherosclerotic disease.

Elevated homocysteine is also associated with deep vein thrombosis and pulmonary embolism.[2] Ray [16] conducted a similar metanalysis of 9 studies relating elevated homocysteine to deep venous thromboembolic disease and found an odds ratio of 2.95 (CI 2.08 - 4.17) for a homocysteine greater than 15 µmol/L. This ratio climbed to 4.37 (CI 1.94 - 9.84) if when patients older than 60 were excluded .

CLINICAL ASSAY

About 90% of the total plasma homocysteine is bound to plasma proteins. Although measurement of free homocysteine might be more sensitive, it is highly variable and unstable, and is not clinically used. Sample handling is critical. Plasma must be separated within an hour or, if refrigerated, within four hours, because erythrocytes and leukocytes export appreciable amounts of homocysteine into the plasma. Once the plasma is separated, however, homocysteine remains stable up to 24 hours. Most laboratories find that the normal adult range (5th to 95th percentile) for fasting total plasma homocysteine is 5 to 15 µmol/L.[21]

CLINICAL DETERMINANTS OF HOMOCYSTEINE

There are many physiological variables that influence homocysteine concentrations (Table 1). Levels in men are about 25% higher than in premenopausal women, but the differences between men and women decrease after female menopause. Hormone replacement therapy may lower homocysteine, and in pregnancy, homocysteine is decreased because of reduced serum proteins and increased conversion of maternal homocysteine to cysteine, a semi-essential amino acid in the growing fetus.

Food intake affects a plasma homocysteine result. Levels may actually decrease modestly in the first few hours after a single high-carbohydrate meal, but they normally increase substantially by the late afternoon and early evening in proportion to the methionine (i.e., protein) content of daytime meals. To avoid this problem, homocysteine should be measured after overnight fasting.

Vitamin supplements are also associated with lower homocysteine levels. In young adults, vitamin B_{12} has only a minimal influence on levels, whereas folate supplementation usually leads to a substantial decrease in homocysteine.[1] Smoking, high coffee consumption, and lack of exercise are all associated with elevated plasma homocysteine, but the influence of alcohol is less clear.

Pyridoxine status is less important in determining fasting homocysteine but can be evaluated by administering a standardized methionine load. Some authorities suggest that evaluation of homocysteine status is not complete without a methionine load, but this provocative test is not generally available.

Elevated homocysteine is associated with other major contributors to cardiovascular risk, including hypertension and hypercholesterolemia, but the interaction with lipid status is relatively weak. In otherwise healthy populations, homocysteine is higher in individuals not taking vitamin supplements.

Among hematologists, there is general agreement that homocysteine (for B_{12} and folate deficiencies) and methylmalonic acid (for B_{12} deficiency) are clinically useful markers. The degree of elevation of homocysteine depends on the degree of vitamin deficiency; thus, plasma homocysteine levels can range from high normal to more than 100 μmol/L.

Table 1. Determinants of Homocysteine

Physiologic
- age ↑
- male sex ↑
- pregnancy ↓
- dietary protein (methionine) ↑
- dietary vitamins (folate, B_6 and B_{12}) ↓
- menopause ↑

Pathologic
- vitamin deficiency ↑
- renal disease ↑
- transplantation ↑
- hypoalbuminemia ↓
- post-stroke ↓
- psoriasis (severe) ↓
- cancer ↑
- hypothyroidism ↑

Medications
- oral contraceptives/hormone replacement ↓
- corticosteroids, theophylline anticonvulsants ↑
- cyclosporine, methotrexate ↑
- smoking ↑
- penicillamine, N-acetylcysteine ↓

Table 2. Guidelines for determination of total homocysteine [11]

Group 1. Homocystinurics and high risk groups
- cystathionine β-synthase deficiency, MTHFR deficiency
- renal failure, transplantation
- patients with lupus erythematosis or rheumatoid arthritis

Group 2. Vitamin deficiency
- clinical signs of B_{12} or folate deficiency with normal serum vitamin levels
- aberrant serum vitamin levels but normal clinical status

Group 3. Deep vein thrombosis
- family history, without other risk factors, of:
    - recurrent pulmonary embolism
    - other deep vein thromboemboli
- personal history of these conditions in patients < 45 yr

Group 4. Cardiovascular disease
- family history, without other risk factors, of:
    - myocardial infarction
    - peripheral arterial disease
    - stroke
- personal history of these conditions in patients < 45 yr

GUIDELINES FOR HOMOCYSTEINE TESTING

There are four patient groups who may benefit from homocysteine testing (Table 2). The first group includes those rare patients, many of them paediatric, with inborn errors of metabolism causing homocystinuria. For them, homocysteine measurements are an important part of continuing care. The second group comprises patients with some indication of folate or vitamin B_{12} deficiency, such as unexplained megaloblastic anemia or sub-acute combined degeneration. In these individuals, a plasma total homocysteine may confirm the diagnosis, if the vitamin levels are not diagnostic. Alternatively, homocysteine testing may help delineate the extent of the cobalamin deficiency, which can be difficult in older patients with borderline serum levels. In the third group, which includes patients with unexplained or recurrent deep vein thrombosis or pulmonary embolism, homocysteine is an important analyte in the panel of tests that should be used to assess the risk of recurrence and the need for prophylaxis.[6]

It is the fourth and last group – healthy adults seeking to establish their cardiovascular risk – that constitutes the largest and most complex public health concern. Should homocysteine testing be considered in risk assessment for atherosclerotic disease? The American Heart Association has suggested that maintenance of a homocysteine of less than 10 μmol/L is a reasonable goal,[9] but implementing this recommendation may impose a substantial new burden on our health care system.

MANAGEMENT

Regardless of homocysteine level, all women should be prescribed 0.4 mg (400 μg) supplement of folic acid daily either pre- or peri-conceptually, to prevent homocysteine-associated neural tube defects in their offspring.[22] Otherwise, healthy adults with no other contributing risk factors should be encouraged to maintain a healthy diet rich in folates to achieve the recommended daily intake of 400 μg. There is no strong evidence yet that homocysteine testing is warranted in healthy children or adolescents. In other patients, efforts should be made to ensure that the blood sample is processed appropriately and the assay performed by a reliable laboratory before embarking on intensive or long-term treatment. Patients with levels below 15 μmol/L will generally respond to dietary advice aimed at increasing folate intake, and repeat measurements would not normally be indicated for this group, providing no other risk factors are present. In this regard, the move to by legislators in the United States and Canada to mandate higher fortification of flour and its products seems entirely appropriate.[15] Homocysteine levels are significantly decreased by consumption of folate-fortified breakfast cereals, even though the folate intake is increased by less than 150 μg per day.[10]

Where there is a positive family history for vaso-occlusive disease, it may be worthwhile measuring homocysteine in the affected family member to ascertain whether homocysteine is contributing to familial risk. When the affected family member is a close relative of the patient, there is a valid perception of higher personal risk and prophylactic vitamin supplements may be appropriate, at least until their benefit is disproven.

Folate supplementation has been advocated for homocysteine levels between 10 and 15 μmol/L, if diet is not effective, but most of the risk from hyperhomocysteinemia accrues to those with higher levels. Both diet and supplementation may be considered in patients a homocysteine between 15 and 20 μmol/L, even in the absence of other risk factors. Patients with a history of unexplained, early onset thrombo-embolic diseases or those with a strong family history may be advised that long-term folate supplements could be protective, with the caveat that prospective trials proving medical effectiveness have not yet been completed. If other risk factors such as hypercholesterolemia or hypertension are present, efforts should remain focussed on their effective management, until clinical interactions with hyperhomocysteinemia are clarified. Emphasis on additional theoretical risk factors might distract the patient from compliance with primary proven therapy, and should be avoided.

The unusual patient with a homocysteine above 20 μmol/L should be retested and folate, B_{12}, and creatinine should be measured at the same time. In patients with unexplained homocysteine concentrations that persist above 20 μmol/L, in-depth workup is indicated.

CONCLUSION

Homocysteine is a natural amino acid that may promote heart disease, stroke, and other vascular diseases if present in excess amounts. Regulation of homocysteine is dependent on vitamin status, specifically folate, B_6 and B_{12}. Homocysteine is now firmly established as a risk factor for neural tube defects -- prevented in large part by folate supplementation during pregnancy. Plasma homocysteine levels are influenced by many pre-existing medical conditions and/or treatment with many pharmacological agents, so that some of the increased risks for vaso-occlusive diseases in these patient groups may be amenable to similar preventive measures.

Plasma total homocysteine concentrations should be interpreted with regard to clinical context. Determination of homocysteine should probably be limited to centres with the necessary expertise.

Management of mild hyperhomocysteinemia should start with enhancement of dietary folate intake. Folate supplements should be prescribed as part of routine prenatal care, but may be considered for other patients with positive risk factors -- personal or familial. Patients with unexplained, persistent homocysteine levels greater than 20 μmol/L need further investigation.

The mandated increase in folate fortification of flour-based foods (bread, cereal) is already leading to a decreased plasma homocysteine in the general population. If this public health measure is coupled with judicious use of homocysteine testing and folate supplementation for the truly high-risk patient groups, we can expect to see a substantial overall reduction in this risk factor for vaso-occlusive disease. However, ongoing trials should tell us how much of an improvement in outcome can be achieved.

REFERENCES

1. Homocysteine Lowering Trialists' Collaboration. Lowering blood homocysteine with folic acid based supplements: meta- analysis of randomised trials. Br Med J. 1998;316:894-898.
2. Bos GM, den Heijer M: Hyperhomocysteinemia and venous thrombosis. Semin.Thromb.Hemost. 1998;24:387-391.
3. Boushey CJ, Beresford SA, Omenn GS, Motulsky AG: A quantitative assessment of plasma homocysteine as a risk factor for vascular disease. Probable benefits of increasing folic acid intakes. J Am Med Assoc 1995;274:1049-1057.
4. Cole DE, Ross HJ, Evrovski J, Langman LJ, Miner SE, Daly PA, Wong PY: Correlation between total homocysteine and cyclosporine concentrations in cardiac transplant recipients. Clin Chem 1998;44:2307-2312.
5. Czeizel AE, Dudas I: Prevention of the first occurence of neural-tube defects by periconceptional vitamin supplementation. N.Engl.J.Med. 1992;327:1832-1835.
6. Francis JL: Laboratory investigation of hypercoagulability. Semin. Thromb.Hemost. 1998;24:111-126.
7. Graham IM, Daly LE, Refsum HM, Robinson K, Brattstrom LE, Ueland PM, et al.: Plasma homocysteine as a risk factor for vascular disease: The European concerted action project. J Am Med Assoc 1997;277:1775-1781.
8. Langman LJ and Cole DEC. Homocysteine: Cholesterol of the 90s? Clin.Chim.Acta . 1999; 286:63-80.
9. Malinow MR, Bostom AG, Krauss RM: Homocyst(e)ine, diet, and cardiovascular diseases: a statement for healthcare professionals from the Nutrition Committee, American Heart Association. Circulation 1999;99:178-182.
10. Malinow MR, Duell PB, Hess DL, Anderson PH, Kruger WD, Phillipson BE, Gluckman RA, Block PC, Upson BM: Reduction of plasma homocyst(e)ine levels by breakfast cereal fortified with folic acid in patients with coronary heart disease. N.Engl.J.Med. 1998;338:1009-1015.
11. Miner SES, Evrovski J, Cole DEC: Clinical chemistry and molecular biology of homocysteine metabolism: An update. Clin.Biochem. 1997;30:189-201.
12. MRC Vitamin Study Research Group: Prevention of neural tube defects: Results of the Medical Research Council vitamin study. Lancet 1991;338:131-137.
13. Mudd SH, Levy HL, Skovby F: *Disorders of transsulfuration*; in: Scriver CR, Beaudet AL, Sly WS, Valle D (eds): In: The molecular and metabolic bases of inherited disease.(5th ed) New York, McGraw Hill Inc., vol. I, 1995, pp 1279-1327.
14. Nygard O, Nordrehaug JE, Refsum H, Ueland PM, Farstad M, Vollset SE: Plasma homocysteine levels and mortality in patients with coronary artery disease. N.Engl.J.Med. 1997;337:230-236.
15. Oakley GPJ: Eat right and take a multivitamin. N.Engl.J.Med. 1998;338:1060-1061.
16. Ray JG: Meta-analysis of hyperhomocysteinemia as a risk factor for venous thromboembolic disease. Arch.Intern.Med. 1998;158:2101-2106.
17. Refsum H, Guttormsen AB, Fiskerstrand T, Ueland PM: Hyperhomocysteinemia in terms of steady-state kinetics. Eur.J.Pediatr. 1998;157 Suppl 2:S45-9:S45-S49.
18. Rosenblatt DS: *Inherited disorders of folate transport and metabolism*; in: Scriver CR, Beaudet AL, Sly WS, Valle D (eds): The molecular and metabolic bases of inherited disease.(5th ed.) New York, McGraw Hill, 1995, vol. II, pp 3111-3128.
19. Rosenquist TH, Ratashak SA, Selhub J: Homocysteine induces congenital defects of the heart and neural tube: Effect of folic acid. Proc Nat Acad Sci USA 1996;93:15227-15232.
20. Smithells RW, Seller MJ, Harris R, Fielding DW, Schorah CJ, Nevin NC, Sheppard S, Read AP, Walker S, Wild J: Further experience of vitamin supplementation for prevention of neural tube defect recurrences. Lancet 1983;1:1027-1031.
21. Ueland PM, Refsum H, Stabler SP, Malinow MR, Andersson A, Allen RH: Total homocysteine in plasma or serum: methods and clinical applications.. Clin.Chem. 1993;39:1764-1779.
22. Wilson RD, Van Allen MI: SOGC Genetics Committee: Recomendations on the use of folic acid for the prevention of neural tube defects. J Soc Obs Gynecol Can 1993;March Suppl.:41-46.

ENDOTHELIAL INTEGRITY AND REPAIR

Tsu-Yee Joseph Lee, Sabrena Noria, Joanne Lee, Avrum I. Gotlieb

Toronto General Hospital
200 Elizabeth Street
CCRW 1-857
Toronto, Ontario   M5G 2C4

INTRODUCTION

Large artery endothelial integrity and repair is an important area of investigation in atherosclerosis research.   The development of an atherosclerotic plaque (fibrofatty plaque) is a dynamic and complex process that is closely associated with the structure and dysfunction of endothelial cells. Although the sequence of events that lead to the initiation and growth of fibrofatty atherosclerotic plaques is not well understood, there is much experimental and clinical support for the concept that disruption of structural and functional endothelial integrity plays an important role in atherogenesis.

In addition to acting as a thromboresistant surface and a macromolecular barrier, endothelial cells are very active metabolically. The endothelium plays a dynamic biological role in the regulation of normal vascular function, in the regulation of coagulation and fibrinolysis, in platelet and leukocyte activation and in the repair of the arterial wall following injury.   Both endothelial integrity and repair are associated with dynamic remodeling of the endothelial cytoskeleton, including actin microfilaments and centrosomes/microtubules, which appear to be regulated by intracellular signal transduction pathways some of which involve small GTPases. Proteins associated with transduction pathways some of which involve small GTPases. Proteins associated with cell-cell and cell-substratum adhesion sites are important regulators of endothelial integrity. Endothelial cells act as signal transducers by regulating a variety of smooth muscle cell functions via paracrine pathways, including vasomotion, cell proliferation, and matrix secretion. Many endothelial functions are inducible and may become dysfunctional. Important interactions that regulate these endothelial activities occur at the vessel wall-blood interface and at the endothelial-subendothelial matrix interface.   Thus there may be two endothelial phenotypes, one regulating integrity at rest and one modulating endothelial repair following injury.

Diabetes and Cardiovascular Disease: Etiology, Treatment and Outcomes
Edited by Aubie Angel et al., Kluwer Academic/Plenum Publishers, 2001

ENDOTHELIAL STRUCTURAL INTEGRITY

The wall of large and medium sized arteries such as the aorta and its branches, the coronary arteries and the cerebral and peripheral vascular arteries consist of an intima, media and adventitia. The intima is bounded on its inner surface by the endothelium and its outer surface by the internal elastic lamina[1].The area just beneath the endothelium is referred to as the subendothelium. The intima also contains some smooth muscle cells and the occasional macrophage. The smooth muscle cells are likely to be the source of intimal hyperplasia in the response to injury in human arteries. These smooth muscle cells may proliferate over time to produce mild eccentric or diffuse intimal thickening, especially at branch points. Endothelial cells of normal arteries form a continuous single layer of flattened cells orientated in areas of uncomplicated laminar flow with the long axis of the cell in the direction of blood flow. There is normally very little proliferation of endothelial cells in the aorta except at a few specific sites that are predisposed to atherosclerotic plaque formation[2,3]. Thus endothelial integrity is maintained in the normal resting state by quiescent endothelial cells. In areas of turbulent flow or fluctuating shear stress, the cells are altered in shape[4,5]. High shear stress causes cells to elongate, and in low shear conditons they are polygonal in shape. Cell shape is maintained by the endothelial cytoskeleton consisting of actin microfilaments and microtubules. Cell-cell interactions are mediated by adherens junctions, tight junctions, gap junctions, and junctions formed by PECAM-1[6]. Tight junctions regulate permeability[7,8], across the monlayer and adherens junctions are essential in preventing gap formation between cells. Cell to cell contact between endothelial cells is initiated and maintained via calcium-dependent adjesion molecules of the cadherin family found in adherens junctions[9]. N (neural) and VE (vascular endothelial) cadherin are found in endothelial cells with the latter being specific to the endothelium. VE cadherin forms complexes and α-catenin, β-catenin, and plakoglobin (catenin). β binding α-catenin which directly associates with F-actin[10]. These proteins undergo changes in distribution when endothelial cells undergo shape changes in response to alterations in hemodynamic shear stress[11] (Figure 1). Vinculin is also colocalized with peripheral F-actin microfilament bundles at sites of cell to cell contact. The role of microtubules at these sites is not yet understood.

Adhesion plaques containing vinculin are important sites for the anchoring of endothelial cells to the subendothelium at focal adhesion sites[12]. These sites contain many proteins including talin, ezrin, focal adhesion kinase, and α actinin. These sites also associate matrix proteins such as fibronectin, and vitronectin with the cell membrane through integrins and other transmembrance proteins which may become part of the focal adhesion complex. Dysfunction and/or disruption of these junctions or adhesion plaques results in loss of endothelial integrity due to subtle changes in intercellular adhesion, or retraction of adjacent cells leaving small interendothelial gaps, or frank loss of endothelial cells. In preliminary studies, we have shown that endothelial monolayers treated with colchicine, which disrupts the microtubules, show a redistribution of vinculin, talin, and focal adhesion kinase toward the periphery of the cell, possibly to enhance or stabilize remaining cell-substratum contacts (Figure 2).

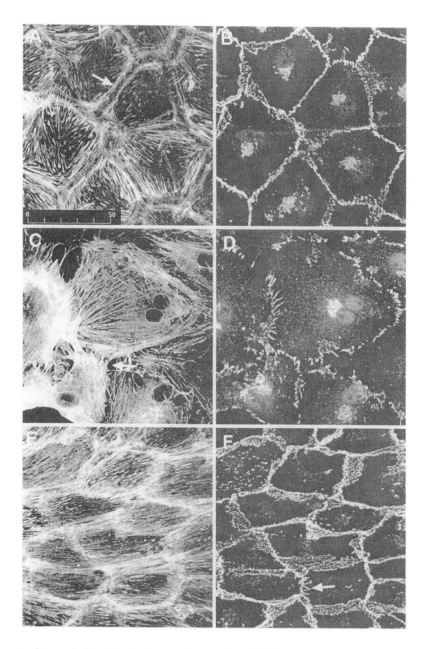

Figure 1. β-catenin localization in porcine aortic endothelial cells exposed to 15 dynes/cm^2 laminar shear stress. Cells were double stained for β-catenin (B, D and F) and F-actin (A, C, and E). Under static conditions, confluent endothelial cells were cuboidal and F-actin was distributed primarily around the periphery of cells, in the dense peripheral band (A, arrow). Under these conditons, staining for β-catenin was continuous, linear and distributed around the entire periphery of the cell. After 8.5 hours of shear stress, gaps were formed between cells (C, arrow). The dense peripheral band was less prominent and F-actin stress fibers were distributed randomly throughout the cell ©. Staining for β-catenin (D) was discontinuous and occurred only at sites of cell-cell contact. After adaptation to shear stress (48 hours exposure), endothelial cells were elongated and aligned in the direction of flow (E, direction of flow is left to right). The cells were continuously apposed to each other and F-actin formed long thick stress fibers that ran the length of the cell. β-catenin was distributed around the entire periphery of the cell as small dashes (F, arrow) that colocalized with the ends of stress fibers that inserted into the lateral plasma membraine. Bar=50 μm.

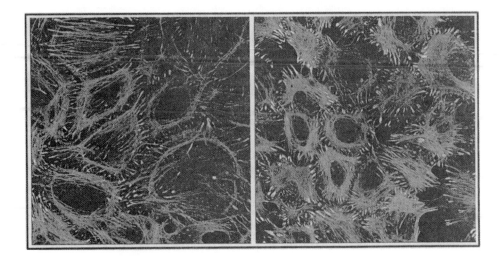

Figure 2. Porcine aortic endothelial cells double-stained to localize actin and vinculin using rhodamine phalloidin and mouse monoclonal anti-vinculin antibody. A) Normal confluent monolayer; B) Confluent monolayer after sic hours of incubation with 10^{-1} μg/ml colchicine.

CYTOSKELETAL FIBER SYSTEMS AND IN VITRO REPAIR

Once endothelial integrity is disrupted, dynamic cytoskeletal fiber systems are essential in regulating endothelial repair[13,14]. Actin microfilaments play a role in force-generation needed for migration[15] and in cell-substratum and cell-cell adhesion[16,17] while the centrosomes and associated microtubules play an essential role in directional cell migration[14,18,19,20]. In endothelial cells in normal confluent monolayers, the actin cytoskeleton is organized as a peripheral dense peripheral band (DPB) of actin microfilament bundles and as central microfilament bundles[21]. The DPB is most prominent in vivo in areas of low shear stress, while the central microfilaments are most prominent in areas of elevated shear stress, especially at sites of vascular branching. The centrosomes are normally found randomly distributed around the nucleus of the endothelial cell with no specific orientation[18,19].

In vitro models of small and large endothelial wounds made in a confluent monolayer show a specific sequence of cellular events[13,14,19,22,23,24]. Adjacent endothelial cells repair a denuded area by rapidly extruding lamellipodia into this area, a process that depends on the presence of intact actin microfilaments. For small wounds, surrounding cells rapidly repair the denuded area by lamellipodia extrusion. In larger wounds, repair cannot be accomplished by lamellipodia alone so a second set of events occur that lead to cell migration and eventual proliferation. This is characterized by the redistribution of the centrosome toward the front of the cell between the nucleus and the leading lamellipodia, and elongation of the endothelial cell in preparation for translocation into the wound. The ensuing breakdown of the dense peripheral band (DPB) results in decreased cell-cell adhesion, followed by directed migration, continuing the process of reendothelialization. In large wounds, cell proliferation is necessary and is dependent on cell migration[6].

THREE STAGES OF EARLY IN VITRO REPAIR

Following denuding endothelial injury, the endothelial cell must undergo a transition from resting, with a cytoskeleton organized to optimize endothelial integrity, to active in which cell spreading and translocation are promoted. Since we had shown that actin microfilaments are critical for both maintaining the integrity of the resting monolayer and for optimum reendothelialization, we carried out a detailed study of the organization of actin microfilaments during the phenotypic transition from resting to active[25]. A linear wound was made with a spatula in the middle of a confluent monolayer of porcine aortic endothelial cells. The complex reorganization of actin microfilament bundles following injury was studied in cells at the wound edge using immunofluorescence staining, laser scanning confocal microscopy, and time-lapse videomicroscopy. As noted above, in the resting confluent monolayer, microfilaments were present as dense peripheral bands (DPB) and central microfilament bundles. three distinct stages of microfilament reorganization occurred sequentially during early repair. Stage I followed wounding and involved the reduction of the DPBs of microfilaments. This was associated with rapid forward actin-based lamellipodia extrusions and cell elongation. Stage II occurred by two hours after wounding and was characterized by central microfilaments located behind the lamellipodia and distributed parallel to the wound edge with vinculin plaques at their tips. This was associated with prominent spreading at the front of the cell which enhanced the extent of coverage of the denuded wound area. Stage III occurring from 4 to 8 hours after wounding, was characterized by the perpendicular orientation of central microfilaments to the wound edge with vinculin plaques and paxillin at their tips (Figure 3). This was also associated with the initiation of cell translocation. Thus, the sequential appearance of the three patterns of microfilament distribution define the cytoskeletal events that regulate the reestablishment of endothelial integrity following denuding endothelial injury[25]. The molecular mechanisms that regulate these cytoskeletal changes are not well understood. However protrusion of lamellipodia and filopodia have been shown to be signaled by the small G proteins rac and cdc42 respectively, while assembly of stress fibers and focal contacts is signaled by rho[26].

We found that the persistence and directionality of migration of the endothelial cells are dependent on an intact microtubule system and centrosomes oriented in the direction of migration[18,24,27]. Centrosome redistribution to the front of the cell at the wound edge occurs within 1 to 3 hours after wounding. The redistribution is independent of migration and occurs well before migration. Centrosome redistribution is dependent on intact microtubules and on the presence of FGF-2 in the medium[28]. Disruption of microfilaments with cytochalasin did not inhibit centrosome redistribution but did delay it by a few hours[24].

ORGANIZATION OF ACTIN MICROFILAMENT IN VIVO IN ENDOTHELIAL CELLS

In vivo endothelial actin microfilaments are organized into central and peripheral bundles[5], similar to that seen in vitro[19,29]. The distribution of microfilaments is important since central microfilaments and peripheral microfilaments are thought to have different functions. The former are considered to be essential in cell-substratum adhesion[23] and the latter in cell-

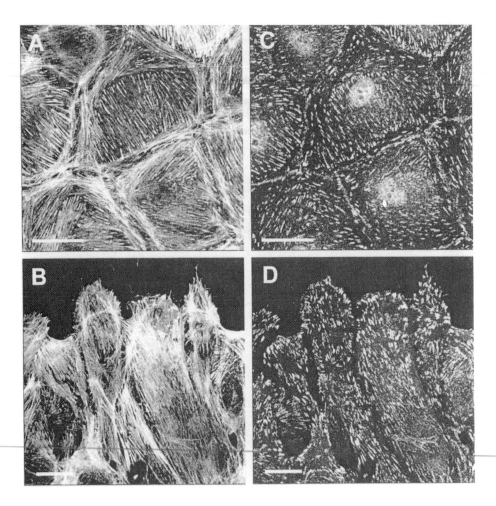

Figure 3. Fluorescence photomicrographs of endothelial cells at confluency (A, C) and at the wound edge 6 hours after wounding (B, D) double stained for actin and phosphotyrosine (A, C) or actin and paxillin (B, D). At confluency phosphotyrosine was localezed at the ends of central microfilaments and within the Dense Peripheral Band (DPB) in a punctuate fashion (A, C). Six hours after wounding, central microfilaments were redistribued perpendicular to the wound (B) with paxillin localized at their ends. Bars, 25μm.

cell adhesion[14,30,31]. The distribution and organization of endothelial microfilaments in the rabbit aorta are a function of the location of cells[32] and the hemodynamic stress exerted on them[5]. Profound variations in the extent of peripheral actin at the cell boundries and the amount, length, and thickness of central microfilaments were seen. An elongated cell shape and prominent central microfilament bundles characterized cells exposed to elevated hemodynamic shear stress, while a cobblestone morphology and prominent peripheral actin bundles are characteristic of cells exposed to static flow conditions or low shear stress[33].

We have carried out a detailed study of the distribution of microfilaments in the immediate vicinity of aortic branches. Branches are of major interest because there is a predilection for atherosclerotic lesions near branch ostia. We made an extensive, systemic examination of branches of the aorta and iliac arteries using in situ staining of perfusion-fixed arteries.

Microfilaments were localized using rhodamine phalloidin. Three patterns of staining were observed by fluorescence microscopy. Some endothelial cells showed prominent central stress fibers. Others had few central stress fibers but prominent peripheral fibers. Major differences can occur over very small distances, so adjacent cells may show strikingly different patters of microfilament distribution. These patterns appear to reflect the geometry of the flow divider and local variations in hemodynamic shear stress. The differences in microfilament distribution may reflect differences in endothelial functions which are essential in maintaining endothelial integrity.

We showed that hypercholesterolemia influences the distribution of endothelial cell microfilaments during the initiation and growth of fatty streak type lesions[34]. We classified the lesions occurring over a twenty week period into four types based on the location and extent of macrophage infiltration observed microscopically. The earliest lesion was characterized by macrophages adherent to the endothelial surface while minimal lesions were characterized by a few cells in the subendothelium. Intermediate and advance fatty streak lesions were elevated with several layers of macrophages. The organization of the dense peripheral band and of central actin microfilament bundles was studied in each of these lesions using fluorescent microscopy. In the aorta away from branch sites and in areas away from lesions, the central microfilament distribution was unaffected by hypercholesterolemia. During the accumulation of subendothelial macrophages in minimal and intermediate lesions, stress fibers were initially increased in comparison to lesion-free areas. In raised advanced lesions however, the central microfilaments became thinner and disappeared. However, at flow dividers, where intermediate lesions showed a reduction in central fibers and peripheral bands became prominent. This was associated with changes in cell shape from elongated to cobblestone cells. Thus actin microfilament bundles in endothelial cells underwent dysfunctional changes in distribution during the accumulation of subendothelial macrophages forming hypercholesterolemia induced fatty streak type lesions. Studies on microtubules were not carried out, however understanding their role in hypercholesterolemic setting awaits future studies.

DYSFUNCTIONAL IN VIVO ENDOTHELIAL WOUND REPAIR

Reduced shear has been identified as a risk factor for atherogenesis. We tested the hypothesis that reduced shear induces dysfunctional endothelial repair. Blood flow rates and shear stresses was decreased in common carotid arteries of rabbits by ligating the ipsilateral external carotid artery. After 24 hours of decreased flow, endothelial cells were less elongated, contained fewer central microfilament bundles, and showed less polarity of the centrosome toward the heart when compared to endothelial cells in carotid arteries with normal flow. To test endothelial repair, we made narrow longitudinal intimal wounds at the time of flow reduction using a nylon monofilament device. In arteries with normal blood flow, endothelial cells at the edge of the wound spread and elongated in the direction of the wound. The dense peripheral band of actin (DPB) was attenuated and central microfilaments became more prominent. Endothelial cells remained in close contact with their neighbors in the monolayer. The centrosome of cells adjacent to the wound was redistributed toward the wound side of the nucleus at 6 and 12 hours. Complete closure occurred by 24 hours, at which time the elongated endothelial cells covering the wound were organized in a herringbone pattern with their downstream ends at the center of the wound. In arteries with decreased flow and shear stress, repair was dysfunctional. The cells at the wound edge spread less than those in normal vessels at 12h after wounding and were randomly oriented and polygonal in shape. Reendothelialization proceeded more slowly and there was a marked reduction of central microfilaments in cells at the wound edge so that at 24 hours, the wounds were still open. The endothelial cells covering the central portion of the wound did not maintain intimate contact with their neighbors and reorientation of the centrosome toward the wound was markedly reduced. We hypothesize that repair at low flow rates and low shear stress disrupts intercellular communication and results in disruption of cytoskeletal reorganization thereby slowing the repair process[35].

REGULATION OF ENDOTHELIAL WOUND REPAIR

There are numerous soluble factors that promote or inhibit repair in addition to the hemodynamic shear stress we described above. We hypothesized that increased susceptibility to atherosclerosis in diabetes mellitus may be due, in part, to delayed reendothelialization following endothelial injury. To test this, the effects of high insulin concentrations on the reendothelialization of small wounds was examined using an in vitro porcine aortic endothelial cell wound model. Elevated concentrations of insulin did not disrupt the confluent endothelial monolayer or alter endothelial cell shape. Insulin also did not induce detectable alterations in the distribution of microtubules and microfilaments in the confluent monolayer. High insulin did not reduce the extent of reendothelialization of the wound. Centrosomal reorientation was similar to that of control wounded cultures as was the reorganization of the microfilaments and microtubules. The data suggests that the atherogenic effects of hyperinsulinemia may not be due to disruption of endothelial repair[36].

Matrix composition is also an important regulator of large vessel endothelial migration. Fibronectin reduces the rate of wound repair while collagen I and III promote it[37]. Exogenous FGF-2 has been shown to enhance migration and repair as well[38,39].

Directed cell migration, an early essential event in the repair is thought to be initiated by centrosome redistribution towards the front of the cell prior to the onset of migration. We have shown that transient inhibition of translation and transcription at the time of wounding disrupts rapid repair by reducing centrosome redistribution to the front of the cell[27]. One of the signals that promotes transcription of unknown factors that regulates redistribution is the release of FGF2 from the cells at the time of wounding[28]. FGF-2 also promotes rapid appearance of long microfilament bundles distributed along the long axis of the cells at the wound edge[40].

Prednisolone[41], TGFβ and oxidized LDL delay in vitro endothelial repair[42]. Thrombin inhibited human iliac artery endothelial cell monolayer repair and proliferation after in vitro denuding mechanical injury[43].

We showed that genistein, a tyrosine kinase inhibitor, and sodium orthovandate, a tyrosine phosphatase inhibitor, inhibited both cell elongation and progression of endothelial cells through the early three stages of endothelial repair described above. Genistein did not have an effect on endothelial cell progression through stage I or II, but had dramatic inhibitory effects on the formation of central microfilaments perpendicular to the wound edge during Stage III[44]. Sodium orthovanadate resulted in inhibiting early endothelial repair by disrupting proper actin central microfilament formation in each of the early stages (unpublished date).   Thus tyrosine kinase and phosphatase activity is critical in the regulation and progression of early endothelial would repair.

Our studies have shown the endothelial integrity and repair require complex dynamic processes which are closely associated with the cytoskeleton and are regulated by soluble extracellular factors and subendothelial matrix, and undergoes dysfunction in response to known risk factors such as low shear stress and hypercholesterolemia.

REFERENCES

1. Stary, HC, Blankenhorn, D, Chandler, AB, Glagov, S, Insull, W Jr, Richardson, M, Rosenfeld, ME, Schaffer, SA, Schwartz, CJ, Wagner, WD, Wissler, RW. A definition of the intima of human arteries and its atherosclerotic-prone regions. Circulation 1992;85:391-405.
2. Lin S-J, Jan K-M, Weinbaum S, Chien S. Transendothelial transport of low density lipoprotein in association with cell mitosis in rat aorta. Arteriosclerosis 1989;9:203-236.
3. Caplan BA, Schwartz CJ. Increase endothelial turnover in areas of in vivo Evans blue uptake in the pig aorta. Atherosclerosis 1973;17:401-417.
4. Langille BL, Adamson SL. Relationship between blood flow direction and endothelial cell orientation at arterial branch sites in rabbits and mice, Circ Res 1981;48:481-488.
5. Kim DW, Gotlieb AI, Langille BL. In vivo modulation of endothelial F-actin microfilaments by experimental alterations in shear stress. Arteriosclerosis 1989a;9:439-445.
6. Dejana E, Corada M, Lampugnani MG. Endothelial cell-to-cell junctions. FASEB Jr. 1995;9:910-918.
7. Hüttner I, Boutet M, More RH. Studies on protein passage through arterial endothelium: II. Regional differences in permeability to fine structural protein tracers in arterial endothelium of normotensive rat,. Lab Invest 1973;28:678-685.
8. Hinsbergh VWM. Endothelial permeability for macromolecules. Arterioscler Thromb Vasc Biol 1997;17:1018-1023.
9. Kemler R. From cadherins to catenins: cytoplasmic protein interactions and regulation of cell adhesion. Trends Gent 1993;9:317-321.
10. Noria S, Cown D, Gotlieb AI, Langille BL. Transient and steady state effects of shear stress on endothelial cell adherens junction. Circ Res 1999;85:504-514.
11. Albelda SM, Buck CA. Integrins and other cell adhesion molecules, FASEB j 1990;4:2868-2880.
12. Wong MKK, Gotlieb AI. In vitro reendothelialization of a single cell wound: Role of microfilament bundles in rapid lamellipodia mediated would close. Lab Invest 1984;51:75-81.
13. Wong MKK, Gotlieb AI. The reorganization of microfilaments, centrosomes, and microtubules during the in vitro small wound reendothelialization. J Cell Biol 1988;107:1777-1783.
14. Kreis TE, Birchmeier W. Stress fibre sarcomeres of fibroblasts are contractile. Cell 1980;22:555-561.
15. Singer I. Association of fibronectin and vinculin with focal contacts and stress fibers in vascular endothelial cells in vivo. J Cell Biol 1982;92:398-408.
16. Wong AJ, Pollard TD, Herman IM. Actin filament stress fibers in vascular endothelial cells in vivo. Science 1983;219:867-869.
17. Gotlieb AI, McBurnie-May LM, Subrahmanyan L, Kalnins VI. Distribution of microtubule organizing centeres in migrating sheets of endothelial cells. J Cell Biol 1981;91:589-594.
18. Gotlieb AI, Spector W, Wong MKK, Lacey C. In vitro reendothelialization: microfilament bundle redistribution in migrating sheet of porcine endothelial cells. Arteriosclerosis 1984;4:91-96.
19. Kupfer A, Louvard D, Singer SJ. Polarization of the Golgi apparatus and the microtubule-organizing center in cultured fibroblasts at the edge of an experimental wound. Proc Natl Acad Sci USA 1982;79:2603-2607.

20. Wong MKK, Gotlieb AI. Endothelial cell monolayer integrity I. Characterization of dense peripheral band of microfilaments. Arteriosclerosis 1986;6:212-219.
21. Coomber BL, Gotlieb AI. In vitro endothelial wound repair: interaction of cell migration and proliferation. Arteriosclerosis 1990;10:215-222.
22. Gotlieb AI, Langille BL, Wong MKK, Kim DW. Structure and function of the endothelial cytoskeleton. Lab Invest 1991;65:123-127.
23. Gotlieb AI, Subrahmanyan L, Kalnins VI. Microtubule organizing centers and cell migration: Effects of inhibition of migration and microtubule disruption in endothelial cells. J Cell Biol 1983;96:1266-1272.
24. Lee TYJ, Rosenthal A, Gotlieb AI. The transition of aortic endothelial cells from resting to migrating cells is associated with three sequential patterns of micrfilament organization. J Vasc Res 1996;33:13-24.
25. Chrzanowska-Wodnicka M, Burridge K. Rho-stimulated contractility drives the formation of stress fibers and focal adhesions. J Cell Biol 1996;133:1403-1415.
26. Ettenson D, Gotlieb AI. In vitro large-wound re-endothelialization. Arteriosclerosis and Thrombosis 1993;13:1270-1281.
27. Ettenson D, Gotlieb AI. Basic fibroblast growth factor is a signal for the initiation of centrosome redistribution to the front of migrating endothelial cells at the edge of an in vitro wound. Arterioscler Thromb Vasc Viol 1995;15:515-521.
28. Colangelo S, Langille BL, Gotlieb AI. Endothelial microfilament distribution in the immediate vicinity of arterial branch sites. Cell Tissue Res 1994;278:235-242.
29. Shasby DM, Shasby SS, Sullivan JM, Peach MJ. Role of endothelial cell cytoskeleton in control of endothelial permeability. Circ Res 1982;51:657-661.
30. Wong MKK, Gotlieb AI. Endothelial monolayer integrity: perturbation of F-actin filaments and DPB vinculin network. Arteriosclerosis 1990;10:76-84.
31. Kim DW, Langille BL, Wong MKK, Gotlie AI. Patterns of endothelial microfilament distribution in the rabbit aorta in situ. Circ Res 1989;64:21-31.
32. Walpola PL, Gotlieb AI, Langille BL. Monocyte adhesion and changes in endothelial cell number, morphology and F-actin distribution elicited by low shear stress in vivo. Am J Pathol 1993;142:1392-1400.
33. Cogangelo S, Langille BL, Steiner G, Gotlieb AI. Alterations in endothelial F-actin microfilaments in rabbit aorta in hypercholesterolemia. Arterioscler Thromb Vasc Biol 1998;18:52-56.
34. Vyalov S, Langille BL, and Gotlieb AI. Low shear stress disrupts repair processes and slows in vivo reendothelialization: effects of shear stress. Am J Pathol 1996;149:2107-2118.
35. Eshraghi S, Gotlieb AI. Insulin does not disrupt actin microfilaments, microtubules in in vitro aortic endothelia wound repair. Biochem Cell Biol J 1995;73:507-514.
36. Madri JA, Bell L, Marx M, Mervin JR, Basson C, Prinz C. Effects of soluble factors and extracellular matrix components on vaxular cell behaviou in vitro and in vivo: models of de-endothelialization and repair. J Cell Biochem 1991;45:123-130.
37. Biro S, YuZ-X, Fu Y-M, Smale G, Sasse J, Sanchez J, Ferrans VJ, Casscells W. Expression of subcellular distribution of basic fibroblast growth factor are regulated during migration of endothelial cells. Circulation Res. 1994;74:485-494.
38. Sato Y, Rafkin DB. Autocrine activities of basic fibrobast grwoth factor: regulation of endothelial cell movement, plasminogen, activator synthesis, and DNA synthesis. J Cell Biol 1988;107:1199-1205.
39. Wang D, Gotlieb AI. Effect of FGF-2 on the early stages of in vitro endothelial repair. Exp Mol Pathol 1999;66:179-190.
40. Fyfe AI, Rosenthal A, Gotlieb AI. Immunosuppresive agents and endothelial repair: prednisolone delays migration and cytoskeletal rearrangement in wounded porcine aortic monolayers. Arterioscler Thromb Vasc Biol 1995;15:1166-1171.
41. Heimark RL, Twardzki DR, Schwartz S. Inhibition of endothelial regeneration by type-beta transforming growth factor from platelet. Science 1986;233:1078-1080.
42. DiMuzio PJ, Pratt KJ, Park PK, Carabasi RA. Role of thrombin in endothelial cell monolayer repair in vitro. J Vasc Surg 1994;20:621-628.
43. Lee T-Y J, Gotleib AI. Genistein inhibits cell elongation during the initiation of endothelial wound repair. FASEB J 1996;10:A1001 (abstract).

MOLECULAR MECHANISMS OF ENDOTHELIAL DYSFUNCTION IN THE DIABETIC HEART

Peter Rösen, Xueliang Du, Guang Zhi Sui

Diabetes Research Institute
Department of Clinical Biochemstry
40225 Düsseldorf, Germany

INTRODUCTION

Healthy endothelium is thromboresistent, tight and supports vasodilatation by the release of various mediators such as nitric oxide and prostacyclin[1-3]. In addition, endothelium inhibits the proliferation of smooth muscle cells and migration of leukocytes across the vessel wall[4]. Taken together, all these properties of healthy endothelium are necessary to maintain an intact circulation and a blood flow sufficient to supply tissues and organs not directly exposed to the blood stream with oxygen and nutrients[1-6]. Disturbances of these processes are often summarised as endothelial dysfunction and have been proposed to play a most important role for the development of vascular complications either in the form of micro- or macroangiopathy[4-6].

It has become clear in the last years that early changes in the function and structure of endothelium are closely associated with the development of various vascular diseases determining the quality and expectancy of life in patients with hypertension, atherosclerosis and diabetes mellitus. Typical alterations such as deposition of lipids, enhanced vasoconstriction, release of growth factors and proliferation of smooth muscle cells, endothelial cells and others, an reinforced adhesion of leukocytes at the vessel wall and changes in the permeability of the vessel wall are typically observed not only in diabetes, but mostly in all these disease states. That the endothelium is affected by diabetes and which changes specifically occur in endothelium of the heart in diabetes has previously described in detail[7,8,9].

What are the molecular mechanisms which cause this thrombogenic transformation of endothelium in diabetes mellitus. What is the link between hyperglycaemia and endothelial dysfunction? These questions cannot be answered at present and are a matter of discussion. In the following, we try to summarise our observations and to draw a concept about the molecular mechanisms which may be responsible to the increased susceptibility of diabetic patients to develop or vascular disease processes and thereby to increase the cardiac risk.

Diabetes and Cardiovascular Disease: Etiology, Treatment and Outcomes
Edited by Aubie Angel et al., Kluwer Academic/Plenum Publishers, 2001

To study the molecular basis of endothelial dysfunction in diabetes we used human umbilical vein endothelial cells (HUVEC) exposed to high glucose to mimic hyperglycaemic conditions and rat heart endothelial cells which can be isolated from healthy and diabetic rats (RHEC). We hypothesise that the formation of reactive oxygen intermediates (ROI) represents a key event for the initiation of endothelial dysfunction leading to a reduced bioavailability of nitric oxide and to a disturbed synthesis of prostacyclin. The activation of redox sensitive transcription factors such as nuclear transcription factor κB and AP-1 may transform the endothelium from an anticoagulant to a procoagulant state[10,11]. The induction of the programmed cell death (apoptosis) can be taken as an indicator of endothelial damage and loss of functional endothelium[12-14].

GENERATION OF NO: INFLUENCE OF HIGH GLUCOSE AND DIABETES

We and others[7,8] have previously shown that the endothelium (NO)-dependent vasodilatation is impaired in the diabetic heart. A diminished production of NO might be one cause for the disturbed vascular reactivity. However such an assumption is not in line with other observations:

- Incubation with high glucose (up to 30 mM) leads to an activation of NO-synthase as shown in human and porcine endothelial cells[15-17].
- After long term incubation with high glucose (22mM, 24 hrs) the amount of mRNA encoding endothelial NO-synthase was elevated, an effect which was clearly prevented by α-lipoic acid suggesting that redox dependent mechanisms are involved. Endothelial cells isolated from diabetic hearts seem to be more sensitive for hyperglycaemia than those from control hearts[18].
- More recently we have provided evidence that the expression of both types of NO-synthases (the endothelial (ecNOS) and the inducible isoform (iNOS)) are increased in diabetic hearts. Not only the amount of protein, but also the amounts of mRNA encoding ec-and iNOS were elevated in the heart of streptozotocin diabetic rats after a diabetes duration of 3-8 weeks. In this model a reduced NO-synthase activity was only observed after a diabetes duration longer than 25 weeks and was associated with an irreversible loss of functional endothelium[18,19].

Thus we have to face the situation that the NO dependent vasodilatation is impaired in heart of diabetic rats, but that the NO-synthase activity and its expression is increased at least temporarily. Therefore, other mechanisms than changes in NO-synthase activity have to be responsible for the impaired NO-dependent vasodilatation in the diabetic heart (for review 20).

GENERATION OF ROI BY ENDOTHELIAL CELLS

To analyse the generation of reactive oxygen intermediates (ROI), HUVEC or RHEC were stained with 2',7'-dichlordihydrofluorescein ester (H$_2$DCF, 21,22) which is oxidised by ROI to an intensive fluorescent dye.

High glucose caused a dramatic increase in the fluorescence intensity of HUVEC which was time and concentration dependent. In contrast to high concentrations of D-glucose L-glucose or D-mannitol (25 mM) did not cause an increase in fluorescence intensity suggesting that the generation of ROI is a process mediated specifically by D-

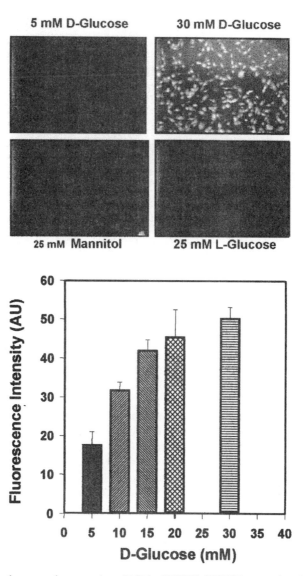

Figure 1. Influence of high glucose on the generation of ROI by HUVEC. HUVEC were cultured in 24-well plates coated with gelatine. After removing the medium and washing, the cells were preincubated with 1 µM H_2DCF ester and 10 µM H_2DCF (dissolved in ethanol) for 45 min. After washing the cells were incubated with medium containing glucose (5 to 30 mM, 15 min). Thereafter the cells were observed under the fluorescent microscope.

a: light microscopic picture with L-glucose and D-mannitol (25 mM) as controls b: concentration dependency

glucose. A similar increase in fluorescence intensity was also observed when RHEC were incubated with high glucose (22 mM). There was no significant difference in fluorescence intensity if RHEC isolated from control or diabetic rats were compared. That high glucose induces the formation of ROI has also been shown in other types of endothelial cells[17]. Of note, Yan et al[23] have reported that advanced glycation endproducts (AGE) are also able to cause the generation of ROI by a receptor-mediated process in endothelial cells.

Table 1. The generation of ROI by endothelial cells is inhibited by:

Compound	Properties
α-Tocopherol	Antioxidant
Lipoic Acid	Antioxidants
BAPTA	Calcium Chelator
N-nitro-L-arginine	Inhibition of NO-synthase
SOD mimetic	Degradation of superoxide anions
Superoxide dismutase	Degradation of superoxide anions
Diphenyleneiodonium	Inhibition of NAD(P)H-Oxidase

Furthermore, it has been shown that the intracellular formation of AGE is completely inhibited if the generation of ROI as measured by the synthesis of lipid peroxides is suppressed, suggesting that the production of ROI is a necessary step during the formation of AGE[24]. These observations suggest that both "glucose spikes" seen often even in well treated patients as well as long term hyperglycaemia expose the endothelium to an oxidative stress.

The underlying mechanisms are not yet fully understood. The observations that the generation of ROI is not only inhibited by antioxidants (α-tocopherol, α-lipoic acid) and superoxide dismutase, but also by BAPTA (1,2-bis(aminophenoxy)ethane-N,N,N,`N`-tetraacetic acid), N-nitro-L-arginine and diphenyleneiodonium suggest that the production of ROI is depending on the presence of NO-synthase and NADPH-oxidase activities (Table 1).

If both superoxide anions and NO are synthesised simultaneously, the formation of peroxynitrite is likely[25]. It has been already shown that peroxynitrite leads to tyrosine nitration of various proteins which can be taken as marker of oxidative stress[25]. To test this hypothesis we determined the amount of tyrosine nitrated proteins by Western blot in endothelial cells incubated at high glucose.

After incubation of HUVEC with the NO-donor sodium nitroprusside (as positive control) or high glucose (20, 30, 40mM), but not with low glucose (5mM) various tyrosine nitrated proteins were detected in the Western-blot with a molecular weight in the range from 18 to 180kD (Figure 2). The high glucose mediated o-tyrosine nitration was inhibited by antioxidants (α-tocopherol, α-lipoic acid) and N-nitro-L-arginine (100 µM, 1 hr preincubation). In addition, in monocytes from diabetic patients with a blood glucose higher than 150 mg % for one month at least the amount of o-nitrated proteins was elevated, too, and strongly associated with the amount of HbA1 (data not shown). These findings suggest that hyperglycaemia leads to an enhanced formation of peroxynitrite and that o-nitration of tyrosine may be a useful marker of oxidative stress in diabetes.

Taking into account
- the results of the pharmacological interventions (Table 1),
- the activation of NO-synthase by high glucose,
- the increased expression of NO-synthases in the diabetic heart, and
- the evidence for the formation of peroxynitrite in human endothelial cells incubated with high glucose and in monocytes of diabetic patients,

we propose the following tentative scheme (Figure 3).

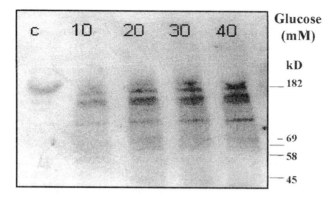

Figure 2. The formation of nitrotyrosine as marker of oxidative stress and specifically peroxynitrite is dependent on the concentration of glucose.

The formation of nitrotyrosine was studied in HUVEC incubated with glucose (5 to 40 mM, 6 hrs). After lysis the proteins were collected and loaded on a gradient gel. After electrophoresis and blotting the membranes were stained with an anti-human-nitrotyrosine antibody. The signals were detected after addition of the second antibody with the ECL system.

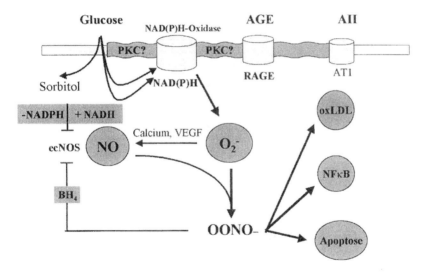

Figure 3. Proposed mechanism for the formation of peroxynitrite by endothelial cells grown in high glucose or in the presence of AGE.

We assume that in diabetes the generation of superoxide anions is stimulated either by high glucose or advanced glycation endproducts (AGE), presumably by activation of a specific NAD(P)H-oxidase as it has been suggested in hypercholesterolemia or by an activation of the AT1 receptor in endothelial cells incubated with angiotensin II (AII). Superoxide anions may a have double function: a further activation of NO-synthase, a process in which the vascular endothelial growth factor (VEGF) and the mobilisation of intracellular calcium might be of importance[26]. On the other hand, it is well known that the simultaneous production of NO and superoxide anions enables the generation of peroxynitrite[25]. This may reduce the bioavailability of NO resulting in an impaired vasodilatation. Other consequences are the observed o-nitration of tyrosine residues in various proteins and the inactivation of tetrahydrobiopterin (BH$_4$), a necessary cofactor of NO-synthase. The reduction of glucose by the "sorbitol"-pathway would diminish NADPH in vivo, another important cofactor of NO-synthase. Thus in vivo, peroxynitrite would effect NO-synthase activity by several mechanisms which would not be seen in the in vitro enzyme test, which is performed under optimised conditions of cofactors and substrates. The in diabetes observed increased expression of NO-synthase could be understood as an adaptation process to compensate the in vivo reduced bioavailability of NO.

It is not yet clear if the NAD(P)H-oxidase activity responsible for the synthesis of superoxide anions is a specific entity. We cannot exclude that the NO-synthase itself is the source of superoxide anions, since it is known that NO-synthase presents NAD(P)H-oxidase activity if the electron flux in the enzyme complex is disturbed. It is furthermore not yet clear in which way the receptors for AGE (RAGE) and AII are coupled to NAD(P)H-oxidase activity. Preliminary data suggest that an isoform of protein kinase C is involved.

WHAT ARE THE CONSEQUENCES FOR THE HEART IN DIABETES?

Impairment of endothelium dependent vasodilatation

A rapid inactivation by superoxide anions diminishes the biological availability of NO. As consequence a shift in the dose-response curve to the right is to be expected as it has been observed in isolated perfused hearts of streptozotocin- and BB-diabetic rats[8,20]. In line with this assumption, we could normalise the impaired endothelium-dependent vasodilatation by treatment of the diabetic rats with high doses of α-tocopherol, but also by perfusion of the isolated hearts with SOD which destroys superoxide anions released in the vascular lumen[8]. The enhanced release of NO and the increased expression of ecNOS can be understood as an adaptive process to compensate for the reduced bioavailability of NO. Of note, a similar mechanism has been suggested to be effective in hypertension[27].

Peroxynitrite mediates the activation of the transcription factor κB

We assume that it is the peroxynitrite which largely promotes the transition of the intact endothelium into a procoagulant state by activation of the transcription factor κB (NFκB). It has been shown by others that peroxynitrite is able to activate NFκB[28].

We have already shown that high glucose and AGE activate NFκB in human umbilical vein endothelial cells[21] and that the activation of this transcription factor is inhibited under the same conditions as the formation of ROI (Table 1) suggesting a role of peroxynitrite. To test if a similar mechanism as in large vessels is working in cells from resistance vessels and capillaries we used rat heart endothelial cells (RHEC).

Incubation of RHEC with high glucose (22 mM) led to an activation of NFκB which reached a maximum after an incubation time of 4 to 6 hrs (Figure 4). The glucose stimulated increase in ROI as well as the activation of NFκB were both inhibited by the antioxidants vitamin C (1 mM) and thioctic acid (1 μM, data not shown). Thus, macro- and microvascular endothelial cells and specifically endothelial cells from the heart do not differ in their responses to activate NFκB by high glucose and AGE (not shown).

To get additional evidence we used a histochemical assay as described in detail by

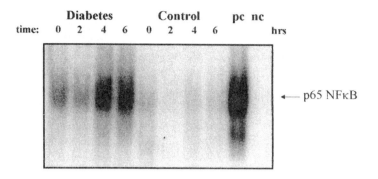

Fig. 4: Activation of NFκB high concentrations of D-glucose in RHEC

RHEC were isolated from collagenase-perfused hearts as described by Linssen et al.[29]. The endothelial cells were identified by the uptake of acetylated low density lipoproteins (Dil-LDL) as described by Voyta et al.[30] and by positive staining for factor VIII[31,32]. Electrophoretic mobile shift assay (EMSA); the EMSAs were performed as described by Bierhaus et al.[29]. The nuclear proteins were collected and incubated with the NFκB-oligonucleotide labelled with γ-32p-ATP. As negative control (nc), 3.5 pmol non-labelled NFκB consensus oligonucleotide was added to block the binding of the labelled probe, as positive control (pc), cultured rat heart endothelial cells were incubated with interleukin 1β and rat γ–interferon. After electrophoresis the signals were detected and quantified using a phophoimager (Fuji-Bas 1000). For further details see[18].

Xie[33,34]: after treatment with DNAse the cells were incubated with HEPES buffer containing 0.25% bovine serum albumin, 1 μg/ml poly [dl-dC], 100 ng/ml poly dC, and 1 ng/ml 3`-rhodamine-labelled oligodeoxynucleotides coding for the NFκB binding site[27,28]. After an incubation for 6 hrs with 22 mM glucose an strong increase in red fluorescence was observed indicating an activation of NFκB which could largely be prevented by preincubation of the cells with vitamin C (1 mM) and α-lipoic acid (1 μM).

As already outlined, the activation of NFκB is one of the necessary steps for the transformation of endothelium into a procoagulant state as indicated for example by an increased expression of the adhesion molecule VCAM-1 or ICAM-1. That there exists a causal relationship between the activation of NFκB and the expression of VCAM-1 follows from experiments using antisense oligodeoxynucleotides against the binding sites of NFκB and/or the RAGE receptor. In both cases, activation of NFκB by AGE, but also the increased expression of VCAM-1 were largely prevented[21,36]. Interestingly and in line with our observations, Nishio et al.[37] have recently reported that the activities of several transcription factors and related genes is altered in whole cardiac tissue of streptozotocin-diabetic rats.

NFκB has been demonstrated to mediate not only expression of VCAM-1, but also a variety of additional important reactions which contribute to the thrombogenic transformation of endothelium[10,11,38,39]: the expression of other adhesion molecules such as the intercellular cell adhesion molecule (ICAM-1) and E-selectin, the release of tumor necrosis factor α and interleukin 1β (proinflammatory), release of growth factors such as the monocyte-colony stimulating factor (M-CSF) and the granulocyte-monocyte-colony stimulating factor (GM-CSF), activation of the monocyte chemoattractant factor (MCP-1), expression of tissue factor which is important for the thrombogenesis.

Induction of apoptosis by peroxynitrite

An accumulation of partly damaged and dysfunctional cells has to be expected in diabetic conditions in the vasculature as consequence of oxidative stress, which could rapidly lead to severe vascular defects in the regulation of vasomotion and thromboresistance. Slowly proliferating cells such as endothelial cells may particularly be affected by these pathophysiological alterations. Induction of apoptosis or the programmed cell death[40] could represent one mechanism to eliminate the damaged cells, to prevent the fixation of vascular defect in these cells and to delay the development of vascular complications in diabetes. On the other hand, endothelial cell death and loss of functional endothelium is associated with a reduced thromboresistance of the vessel wall and may be one important factor to enhance the thrombogenic risk of diabetic patients.

That ROI can induce apoptosis has already been shown very clearly[41]. Furthermore we and others have very recently shown that incubation of endothelial cells in high glucose causes an substantial increase in the number of apoptotic cells[14], however, the molecular mechanism is not yet understood. If we assume that in most cells apoptosis is a process which requires energy as well as de novo gene transcription and protein synthesis[42,43], it is intriguing to suggest that the necessary changes in gene expression mediated by activation of transcription factors such as a NFκB are also of importance for induction of apoptosis. Since AGE products have also been shown to increase the generation of ROI and lead to an activation NFκB, it has to be expected that not only an incubation of endothelial cells with high glucose, but also with AGE is able to induce apoptosis and that this process can be inhibited by interventions which block the activation of NFκB. In addition, if peroxynitrite is involved, it should also be possible to inhibit the induction of the apoptotic process by inhibitors of NO-synthase.

As can be seen, a typical pattern of fragmented low molecular weight (internucleosomal) DNA is obtained from cells incubated either with AGE-BSA or high glucose, but not from those cultivated in the presence of BSA or low glucose (5 mM). Induction of apoptosis was not only prevented by preincubation of the cells with the antioxidants α- tocopherol (10 µg/ml) and thioctic acid (0.5 µM), but also with N-nitro-L-arginine. Similarly, the sharp increase in caspase 3 activity - an early marker for induction of apoptosis - by high glucose (30 mM, 24 hrs) was prevented by incubation with α-tocopherol (10 µg/ml), lipoic acid (0.5 µM) and N-nitro-L-arginine (100 µM, data not shown). Both observations clearly suggest that the induction of apoptosis is dependent on the generation of ROI and specifically of peroxynitrite. That peroxynitrite is able to induce apoptosis in various types of cells has already been shown by others[45,46]

The role of NFκB is controversial discussed and opposite effects have been described dependent on the type of cells[47]. For HUVEC, we can show that the p65 NFκB antisense deoxynucleotide, but not the sense one inhibits the induction of apoptosis by high glucose and AGE. This observation strongly indicates a role of NFκB for the shift of endothelial cells from the cell cycle to apoptosis.

Taken together, our observations indicate that diabetogenic conditions as hyperglycaemic concentration of glucose and AGE are able to induce apoptosis in endothelial cells (HUVEC and similarly in RHEC, data not shown) and that this process is strictly dependent on the formation of peroxynitrite followed by activation of NFκB. The induction of apoptosis might represent a surviving mechanism for vascular cells in diabetes, to eliminate severely damaged cells and to remain the functional integrity of the

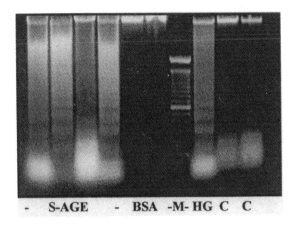

Figure 5. Influence of high glucose and AGE on the apoptosis in HUVEC
HUVEC were incubated with glycated bovine serum albumin (AGE-BSA, 72 hrs, 100 µg/ml) and high glucose (HG, 30 mM, 72 hrs). The low molecular weight DNA was isolated by chloroform/methanol extraction and analysed by agarose gel-electrophoresis after staining with ethidium bromide (44). M = molecular weight standards, C = controls (5 mM glucose)

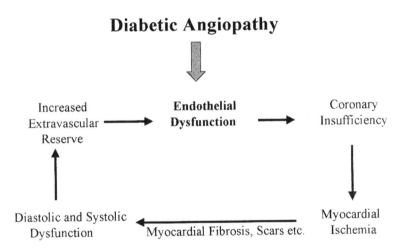

Figure 6. Proposed vicious circle leading from endothelial dysfunction to cardiac dysfunction and remodelling of the heart in diabetes.

vascular wall for some time and to delay the development of vascular complications which is a long time consuming process. Thus, induction of apoptosis may contribute to limit the damage of the vasculature by peroxynitrite generated in excess in diabetes.

SUMMARY

Our observations show that long term hyperglycaemia by the formation of AGE, but also short term hyperglycaemic periods ("glucose spikes") damage the endothelium of the heart in diabetes. The endothelium is exposed to oxidative stress. The simultaneous generation of NO and superoxide anions enables the reaction of both species to form peroxynitrite which has been identified as an important mediator for the transformation of endothelium from an anticoagulant to a procoagulant state. Together with a functional loss of endothelium these processes are assumed to impair the coronary perfusion and to provoke adaptive processes which finally lead to cardiac dysfunction and remodelling of cardiac structure (Figure 6) as it has been described for the heart in diabetes[8,9].

Acknowledgements

This work was supported by the Ministerium für Frauen, Familie und Gesundheit der Bundesrepublik Deutschland and the Wissenschaftsministerium des Landes NRW, the Deutsche Forschungsgemeinschaft, Bonn, and the "Klinische Zellbiologie und Biophysik" e.V., Düsseldorf.

REFERENCES

1. S. Moncada, R.M.J. Palmer, E.A. Higgs, Nitric oxide: physiology, pathophysiology, and pharmacology, Pharmacol. Rev. 43:109-142 (1991).

2. E. Nava, T.F. Lüscher, Endothelium and hypertension, in: The Endothelial Cell in Health and Disease, J.R. Vane, G.V.R. Born, E. Weizel, eds,. Schattauer, Stuttgart (1995).

3. J.P. Cooke, V.J. Dzau, Nitric oxide synthase: role in the genesis of vascular disease, Ann. Rev. Med. 48: 489-509 (1997).

4. P. Kubes, M. Suzuki, D.N. Granger, Nitric oxide: an endogenous modulator of leukocyte adhesion, Proc. Natl. Acad. Sci. USA 88:4651-4655 (1991).

5. M. Lorenzi, E. Cagliero E, Pathobiology of endothelial and other vascular cells in diabetes mellitus, Diabetes 40: 653-659 (1991).

6. R.A. Cohen, Dysfunction of vascular endothelium in diabetes mellitus, Circ. 87 (Suppl. V): V-67-V-76 (1993).

7. A. Nitenberg, P. Valensi, R. Sachs, M. Dali, E. Aptecar, J.R. Attali, Impairment of coronary vascular reserve and Ach-induced coronary vasodilatation in diabetic patients with angiographically normal coronary arteries and normal left ventricular systolic function, Diabetes 42: 1017-1025 (1993).

8. P. Rösen, Th. Ballhausen, W. Bloch, K. Addicks, Endothelial relaxation is disturbed in the diabetic rat by oxidative stress: The influence of tocopherol as antioxidant, Diabetologia 38: 1157-1168 (1995).

9. P. Rösen, U. Kiesel, H. Reinauer, C. Boy, K. Addicks, Cardiopathy in the spontaneously diabetic BB rats: evidence for microangiopathy and autonomic neuropathy in the diabetic heart, in: The Diabetic Heart, M. Nagano, N.S. Dhalla , eds, Raven Press, New York (1991).

10. P.A. Baeuerle, T. Henkel, Function and activation of NF-κB in the immune system, Ann. Rev. Immunol. 12: 141-179 (1994).

11. K. Brand, S. Page, G. Rogler, A. Bartch, R. Brandl, R. Knuechel, M. Page, P.A. Kaltschmidt, P.A. Baeuerle, D. Neumeier, Activated transcription factor-kappa B is present in the atherosclerotic lesion, J. Clin. Invest. 97: 1715-1722 (1996).

12. S.M. Baumgartner-Parzer, L. Wagner, M. Pettermann,, J. Grillari, A. Gessl, W. Waldhäusl, High-glucose-triggered apoptosis in cultured endothelial cells, Diabetes 44: 1323-1327 (1995).

13. S. Dimmeler, A.M. Zeiher, Nitric oxide and apoptosis: another paradigm for the double-edged role of nitric oxide, Nitric Oxide 1: 275-281 (1997).

14. X.L. Du, G.Z. Sui, K. Stockklauser, J. Weiß, S. Zink, B. Schwippert, Q.X Wu, D. Tschöpe, P. Rösen, Induction of apoptosis by high proinsulin and glucose in cultured human umbilical vein endothelial cells is mediated by reactive oxygen species. Diabetologia 41: 249-256 (1998).

15. P. Rösen, X.L. Du, G.Z. Sui, Oxidative stress in diabetes. Why does hyperglycemia induce the formation of reactive oxygen species? in: Oxidative Stress in Diabetes and Its Complications, P. Rösen, G. King, A. Azzi, H. Tritschler, L. Packer, eds, Marcel Dekker, New York, 17-32 (2000).

16. F. Cosentino, K. Hishikawa, Z.S. Katusic, T.F. Lüscher, High glucose increases nitric oxide synthase expression and superoxide anion generation in human aortic endothelial cells, Circ. 96: 25-28 (1997).

17. W.F. Graier, S. Simecek, W.R. Kukovetz, D.M., High D-glucose-induced changes in endothelial Ca^{2+}/EDRF signalling are due to generation of superoxide anions, Diabetes 45: 1386-1396 (1996).

18. K. Stockklauser-Färber, Th. Ballhausen, T. Lauffer, P. Rösen, Influence of diabetes on myocardial nitric oxide synthase expression and activity, submitted

19. P. Rösen, Th. Ballhausen, K. Stockklauser, Impairment of endothelium dependent relaxation in the diabetic rat heart: mechanisms and implications. Diabetes Res. Clin. Pract. 31 (Suppl): S143-S155 (1996).

20. G.M. Pieper, A review of alterations in endothelial nitric oxide production in diabetes. Protective role of arginine on endothelial dysfunction, Hypertension; 31: 1047-1060 (1998)

21. X.L. Du, K. Stockklauer-Färber, P. Rösen, Generation of reactive oxygen intermediates, activation of NF-kB, and induction of apoptosis in human endothelial cells by glucose: role of nitric oxide synthase? Free Rad Biol Med 27:752-763 (1999).

22. J.P. Crow, Dichlorodihydroflurescein and dihydrorhodamine 123 are sensitive indicators of peroxynitrite in vitro: implications for intracellular measurement of reactive and oxygen species, Nitric Oxide 1: 145-157 (1997).

23. S.D. Yan, A.M. Schmidt, G.M. Anderson, J. Zhang, J. Brett, Y.S. Zhou, D. Pinsky, D. Stern, Enhanced cellular oxidant stress by the interaction of advanced glycation end products with their receptors/binding proteins, J. Biol. Chem. 269: 9889-9897 (1994).

24. I. Giardino, D. Edelstein, M. Brownlee, BCL-2 expression or antioxidants prevent hyperglycaemia-induced formation of intracellular advanced glycation end-products in bovine endothelial cells, J. Clin. Invest. 94: 110-117 (1996).

25. J. Beckmann, W.H. Koppenol, Nitric oxide, superoxide, and peroxynitrite: the good, the bad, and the ugly, Am. J. Physiol. 271: C1424-1437 (1996).

26. R.G. Tilton, T. Kawamura, K.C. Chang, Y. Ido, R.J. Bjercke, C.C. Stephan, T.A. Brock, J.R. Williamson, Vascular dysfunction induced by elevated glucose levels in rats is mediated by vascular endothelial growth factor, J. Clin. Invest. 99: 2192-2202 (1997).

27. A. Bouloumie, J. Bauersachs, W. Linz, B.A. Schölkens, G. Wiemer, I. Fleming, R. Busse R, Endothelial dysfunction coincides with an enhanced nitric oxide synthase expression and superoxide anion production, Hypertension 30: 934-941 (1997).

28. A. Rodriguez-Ariza, A. Paine, Rapid induction of NF-kappaB binding during liver cell isolation and culture: inhibition by L-NAME indicates a role for nitric oxide synthase, Biochem. Biophys. Res. Commun. 257: 145-8 (1999).

29. M.C.J.G. Linssen, P.H.M. Willemsen, V.V.Th. Heijnen, G.L. van de Vusse, Arachidonic acid incorporation in cardiomyocytes, endothelial cells and fibroblast-like cells isolated from adult rat heart, Biochim. Biophys. Acta 1268: 88-96 (1995).

30. J.C. Voyta, D.P. Via, C.E. Butterfield, B.R. Zetter, Identification and isolation of endothelial cells based on their increased uptake of acetylated low density lipoproteins, J. Cell Biol. 99: 2034-2040 (1984).

31. F.A. Jaffe, L.W. Hoyer, R.L. Nachman, Synthesis of antihemophilic factor antigen by cultures human endothelial cells, J. Clin. Invest. 52: 2757-2764 (1973).

32. J. Thomas, M. Linssen, G.J. van de Vusse, B. Hirsch, P. Rösen, H. Kammermeier, Y. Fischer, Acute stimulation of glucose transport by histamine in cardiac microvascular endothelial cells, Biochim. Biophys. Acta 1268, 88-96 (1995).

33. Q.W. Xie, Y. Kashiwabara, C. Nathan, Role of transcription factor NF–κB/rel in induction of nitric oxide synthase, J. Biol. Chem. 269: 4705-4708 (1994).

34. Q.W. Xie, R. Whisnant, C. Nathan, Promotor of the mouse gene encoding calcium independent nitric oxide synthase confers inducibility by interferon and bacterial lipopolysaccaride, J. Exp. Med. 177: 1779-1784 (1993).

35. A. Bierhaus, S. Chevion, M: Chevion; M. Hofmann, P. Quehenberger, T. Illmer, T. Luther, E. Berentshtein, H. Tritschler, M. Müller, P. Wahl, R. Ziegler, P. Nawroth, Advanced glycation end product-induced activation of NF–κB is suppressed by α-thioctic acid in cultured endothelial cells, Diabetes 46: 1481-1490 (1997).

36. P. Rösen, G.Z. Sui, X.L: DU, C. Bünting, Th. Koschinsky, AGE, but not glucose stimulate the expression of VCAM-1 in human endothelial cells, Diabetes 48 (Suppl. 1): A32 (1999).

37. Y. Nishio, A. Kashiwagi, H. Taki, K. Shinozaki, Y. Maeno, H. Kojima, H. Maegawa, M. Haneda, H. Hidaka, H. Yasuda, K. Horiike, R. Kikkawa, Altered activities of transcription factors and their related gene expression in cardiac tissues of diabetic rats, Diabetes 47: 1318-1325 (1998).

38. M. Morigi, S. Angioletti, B. Imberti, R. Donadelli, G. Micheletti,, M. Figliuzzi, A. Remuzzi, C. Zoja, G. Renuzzi, Leukocyte-endothelial interaction is augmented by high glucose concentrations and hyperglycemia in a NF–κB-dependent fashion, J. Clin. Invest. 101: 1905-1915 (1998).

39. T. Marumo, V.B. Schini-Kerth, R. Busse, Vascular endothelial growth factor activates nuclear factor-κB and induces monocyte chemoattractant protein-1 in bovine endothelial cells, Diabetes 48: 1131-1137 (1998).

40. J.F.R. Kerr, A.H. Wyllie, A.R. Currie, Apoptosis: a basic biological phenomenon with wide-ranging implications in tissue kinetics, Br. J. Cancer 26: 239-257 (1972).

41. G. Powis, J.R. Gasdaska, A. Baker, Redox signaling and the control of cell growth and death, in: Antioxidants in Disease: Mechanisms and Therapy, H. Sies, ed., Academic Press, New York (1997).

42. K.S. Sellins, J.J. Cohen, Gene induction by gamma-irradiation leads to DNA fragmentation in lymphocytes, J. Immunol. 139: 3199-3206 (1987).

43. A.H. Wyllie, Glucocorticoid-induced thymocytes apoptosis is associated with endogenous endonuclease activation, Nature 284: 555-556 (1980).

44. R.C. Fabio RC, Inhibition of anchorage-dependent cell spreading triggers apoptosis in cultured human endothelial cells, J. Cell Biol. 127: 537-546 (1994).

45. C. Szabo, H. Ohshima, DNA damage induced by peroxynitrite: subsequent biological effects, Nitric Oxide 1: 373-385 (1997).

46. K.T. Lin, J.Y. Xue, P.Y. Wong, Peroxynitrite. An apoptotic agent in HL-60 cells, Adv. Exp. Med. Biol. 407: 413-419 (1997).

47. V.R. Baichwal, P.A. Baeuerle, Activate NF-kappa B or die? Curr. Biol. 1: R94-R96 (1997).

A STUDY OF VASCULAR WOUND HEALING
IN A RABBIT MODEL OF TYPE I DIABETES

Natalie K. Schiller, Donald L. Akers, Brian Burke,
Alvin M. Timothy, Brenda Bedi and Dennis B. McNamara

Departments of Pharmacology and Surgery
Tulane University School of Medicine
New Orleans, Louisiana 70112

INTRODUCTION

The pathophysiology of restenosis following balloon catheterization involves a sequence of events similar to wound healing (1). Mechanical stress and mitogens released by cells at the site of injury activate quiescent vascular smooth muscle cells (VSMC) of the contractile phenotype to dedifferentiate to the synthetic phenotype and, subsequently, divide. Activated VSMC of the synthetic phenotype migrate through breaks in the internal elastic lamina to the intima where they continue to proliferate and synthesize abundant extracellular matrix (ECM), resulting in an increased neointimal mass. This intimal hyperplasia has been suggested to contribute to a decrease in lumen diameter and patency of the vessel resulting in ischemic symptoms. It should be noted, however, that the contribution of intimal thickening to the pathophysiology of restenosis has recently been questioned.

In vitro studies suggest that growth factors modulate the events following balloon catheter-induced arterial injury. Platelet-derived growth factor (PDGF), insulin-like growth factor-1 (IGF-1), basic fibroblastic growth factor (bFGF), epidermal growth factor (EGF), and transforming growth factor-β (TGF-β) all increase cellular proliferation (1). It is recognized that no one growth factor is responsible for VSMC activation and proliferation following balloon catheterization, rather they operate through a network of complex cellular interactions. Growth factors, such as bFGF and PDGF, regulate the initial event in the mitogenic response by allowing G_0-arrested VSMC to enter the G_1 phase of the cell cycle. Competent cells then proceed through the cell cycle into the S phase under the influence of progression factors, such as IGF-1. To keep the cell progressing through the G_1 phase, simultaneous stimulation by both competence and progression factors is necessary (2).

The mitogen activated protein kinase (MAPK) signaling cascade plays a role in the response to balloon catheter injury. It has been shown that catheter-induced arterial injury causes an increase in medial VSMC proliferation, which is associated with an up-regulation of MAPK phosphorylation and activation (3). MAPK relays cytoplasmic signals to the nucleus and phosphorylates transcription factors required for the expression of genes involved in cell growth and proliferation. Many of the growth factors involved in the events following arterial injury are also known to activate MAPK. MAPK has been shown to be present in both

Diabetes and Cardiovascular Disease: Etiology, Treatment and Outcomes
Edited by Aubie Angel *et al.*, Kluwer Academic/Plenum Publishers, 2001

87

contractile and proliferative phenotypes of VSMC, however, the role of MAPK in highly differentiated, non-proliferating tissues, such as muscle, is poorly defined. It has been postulated that in proliferating cells activation of MAPK results in phosphorylation of specific cytoplasmic and nuclear proteins need for passage through certain checkpoints in the cell cycle (i.e., G_1/S) (4).

This study provides evidence for attenuated neointimal thickening and VSMC proliferation in the diabetic rabbit compared to euglycemic control. This study also documents for the first time evidence for the early phase of VSMC activation following catheter injury in the diabetic animals as being associated with increased MAPK activity.

MATERIALS AND METHODS

Male New England White rabbits (3.0-3.5 kg) were treated with alloxan monohydrate (125-175 mg/kg i.v.) to induce the diabetic state, and glucose levels were checked routinely using an Accu-chek III blood glucose monitor. Alloxan-treated animals exhibited a spectrum of blood glucose levels and were grouped accordingly: non-responders (glucose ≤ 170 mg/dL), low hyperglycemic (171-285 mg/dL), high hyperglycemic (286-399 mg/dL), and diabetic (≥ 400 mg/dL) (Table 1). It was found that the mean glucose levels of rabbits prior to alloxan treatment was 139 ± 3 mg/dL. One standard deviation from that mean was equal to a glucose of 170 mg/dL. Thus, animals with glucose levels over 170 mg/dL but less than 400 mg/dL were classified as hyperglycemic. Animals which received alloxan and did not exhibit an increase in blood glucose were grouped as non-responders. This definition of diabetes (glucose ≥ 400 mg/dL) is consistent with the literature of diabetic animals models (5). Serum IGF-1 (Diagnostic Systems Laboratories, Webster, TX) and insulin levels (Diagnostic Products Corporation, Los Angeles, CA) were measured using radioimmunoassay kits.

Vascular injury was produced using a 4 Fr embolectomy catheter. Rabbits were anesthetized using a mixture of ketamine and xylazine i.m. (50 mg/kg ketamine; 10 mg/kg xylazine). Nitrous oxide was used as an inhalational anesthetic and sodium pentobarbital was given i.v. (25 mg/kg). The superficial femoral artery was isolated through a short incision in the right groin. Through an arteriotomy, the catheter was inserted and passed to the level estimated to be the ascending aorta. The balloon was inflated with saline and withdrawn to the level of the abdominal aorta. This was repeated three times. Because the response to injury is directly proportional to the degree of injury induced (6), the catheter was attached to a force gauge in order to consistently and reproducibly maintain a constant pressure (approximately 300 g) transmitted to the vessel wall. Sham-operated animals underwent simple ligation of the femoral artery. These procedures were conducted under sterile conditions in a vivarial operating room. Following surgery, the rabbits were housed in the vivarium and given water and standard rabbit diet ad libitum until time of sacrifice.

Table 1. Serum insulin and IGF-1 levels of alloxan-treated and untreated rabbits grouped according to glycemic classifications prior to catheter injury.

	Glucose (mg/dL)	Insulin (μIU/mL)
Euglycemic	139 ± 3	33 ± 8
Non-responder	≤ 170	27 ± 4
Low hyperglycemic	171-285	$14 \pm 3^{*\dagger}$
High hyperglycemic	286-399	$9.2 \pm 2^{*\dagger}$
Diabetic	≥ 400	$9.3 \pm 3^{*\dagger}$

Values are mean ± SE. n = 6-10 animals; *P <0.005 vs. euglycemic; †P <0.05 vs. non-responder.

Animals were given a lethal dose of sodium pentobarbital (250 mg/kg i.v.) and thoracic aortas were removed. After harvest aorta were placed in ice-cold Krebs buffer solution containing (in mM): 118 NaCl, 4.7 KCl, 5.6 glucose, 25 NaHCO$_3$, 1.5 CaCl$_2$, 1.2 KH$_2$PO$_4$, 1.2 MgSO$_4$, pH 7.4 at which time fat and loose adventitia were dissected from the vessels. Vessels were cut into 3-mm rings for fixation.

To obtain a semiquantitative measurement of intimal thickening, specimens were prepared for light microscopy via fixation in 10% neutral buffered formalin and embedded in paraffin. The tissues were sectioned (5 μm) and stained with Verhoeff-Van Gieson stain for elastic tissue. These slides were examined morphometrically using videomicroscopy and a computerized digital image analysis system. The data were reported as the I/M ratio or the absolute mean of the intima divided by the absolute area of the media multiplied by 100. Medial areas were not affected by catheter injury. Therefore, any increase in the I/M ratio was indicative of increased intimal area.

Harvested thoracic aortas were fixed in 10% neutral buffered formalin. Rings of tissue were embedded in paraffin, sectioned at approximately 6 μm, and mounted on positive-charge glass slides. Slides were de-paraffinized in xylene and rehydrated in a descending ethanol series. Endogenous peroxidase activity was quenched by incubating in 0.3% hydrogen peroxide in methanol for 30 min at room temperature. Proliferating cell nuclear antigen (PCNA) was unmasked by microwaving just short of boiling in 10 mM citric acid (pH 6.0). Nonspecific binding was blocked by incubating tissue in 5% normal goat serum in 1% bovine serum albumin (BSA)-PBS for 30 min at room temperature. Anti-PCNA antibody (PC10; Dako, Carpintera, CA) was diluted in 1% BSA-PBS 1:70 and allowed to incubate at room temperature for 1 hr. Control sections were incubated in normal mouse IgG in place of the primary antibody and as a positive control, a section of intestine was included. Biotin goat anti-mouse IgG diluted 1:3500 in 1% BSA-PBS followed by streptavidin-horseradish peroxidase (SA-HRP) diluted 1:2000 were incubated each for 1 hr at room temperature. The antibody-antigen complex was visualized by reacting 0.02% diaminobenzidine (DAB) containing 0.006% hydrogen peroxide. Sections were counter stained with Gill's Hematoxylin #3 dehydrated in ethanol to xylene and coverslips mounted with permount.

Color video images were captured (x430 magnification) and digitized with a Panasonic color CCTV camera (WV-CP410). Images were analyzed using IP Lab Spectrum software package (Signal Analytics Corp.) The digital color images wee split into their red and blue components to determine cells staining blue (hemotoxylin-positive) and red (DAB-positive). Positive and negative staining cells were differentiated according to cell size and threshold values. The analysis was validated by doing manual counts of positively staining cells. An average of four consecutive cross-sections of the thoracic aorta harvested from each animal was stained and analyzed by a blinded observer. Cells of three random regions of each of the cross-sections were counted. The proliferative index (number of positively-labeled cells divided by the total number of cells x 100) in each region was averaged for each cross-section examined. The individual data points used in the statistical analysis represent the vessel means for percent of proliferating cells at each time point.

Sections of harvested thoracic aortas were snap-frozen in liquid nitrogen. The tissue was homogenized in Triton X-100 Lysis buffer (50 mM Tris-HCl, pH 7.3, 150 mM NaCl, 1% Triton X-100, 5 mM EDTA, 1 mM phenylmethylsulfonyl fluoride, 50 U/ml aprotinin, 1 mM DTT, 1 mM sodium vanadate, 25 mM NaF, 10 mM Na-pyrophosphate, 25 mM beta-glycerophosphate) using a polytron apparatus. Protein homogenate was then centrifuged at 12,000 g for 10 min at 4°C to remove tissue debris. The supernatant was used to determine MAPK activity.

Serine/threonine kinase activity was measured by examining tyrosine phosphorylation of MAPK by immunoprecipitation using myelin basic protein as a substrate. Samples containing equal amounts of protein were incubated with anti-rat MAPK antibody (Upstate Biotechnology, erk 1-CT) for 1 hr at 4°C. Immunoprecipitates were recovered by incubating in 50% protein G-Sepharose for 1 hr at 4°C. Immunoprecipitates were spun down, washed, and incubated at 30°C for 10 min in a final volume of 44 μl with 20 μg of myelin basic protein and 2 μCi [γ-32P]-ATP in kinase reaction buffer containing 18 mM HEPES (pH 7.5) and 10 mM Mg acetate. The reaction was stopped by the addition of 0.1 M EDTA. This reaction mixture was blotted on a P-81 phosphocellulose filter and washed 5 times in 180 mM phosphoric acid and then once in 95% ethanol for 5 min each. The filters were dried and prepared for scintillation counting. Results were expressed as cpm released per μg of protein.

The data obtained within an experimental group were averaged and reported as mean ± SEM. These data were then analyzed using Statview SE+ statistics package using ANOVA and the Scheffe's F test to determine differences between the groups. P <0.05 was considered significant. The n refers to the number of animals per experiment.

RESULTS

Measurement of Neointimal Thickening

Neointimal thickening reported as the absolute area of the intima divided by the absolute area of the media multiplied by 100 (I/M ratio) was measured at 1, 2, 4, and 8 weeks following catheterization (Fig. 1). One week after injury neointimal formation was detectable only in euglycemic animals. Two weeks after injury neointimal formation was present in both diabetic and euglycemic rabbits, though approximately 50% less in the diabetics (P <0.05). I/M ratios for diabetic rabbits remained attenuated by approximately 40% by 8 weeks which was the maximum time-period studied to date (P <0.001). The I/M ratios of alloxan-treated rabbits grouped according to the classifications described in Table 1 were measured 2 weeks following catheterization. It was found that animals in the non-responder and low hyperglycemic groups showed a normal response to injury in a manner similar to the euglycemic group. The I/M ratio of the rabbits in the high hyperglycemic group, however, was attenuated to the degree seen in the diabetic rabbits (P <0.001) (Fig. 2).

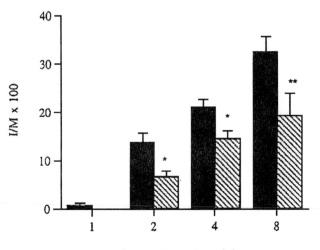

Figure 1. I/M ratios for euglycemic and diabetic rabbits at 1, 2, 4, and 8 weeks following catheter injury. I/M ratio is defined as the absolute area of the intimal divided by the absolute area of the media multiplied by 100. I/M ratios were significantly attenuated 2, 4, and 8 weeks following catheter injury in the diabetic animals (hatched bars) compared to euglycemic animals (black bars). n=5-8 animals, excluding weeks 1 and 8 where n=3 animals. *indicates P <0.05 vs. euglycemic; ** indicates P <0.001 vs. euglycemic.

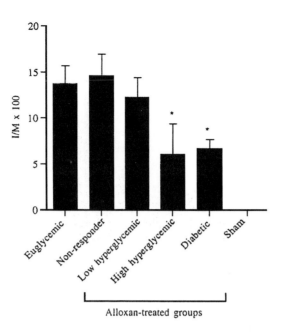

Alloxan-treated groups

Figure 2. I/M ratios for euglycemic and alloxan-treated rabbits 2 weeks after catheter injury. Sham-operated animals underwent simple ligation of the femoral artery. n=6-10 animals. *indicates P <0.05 vs. euglycemic animals.

VSMC Proliferation in Response to Injury

The characterization of neointimal formation following vascular injury was extended by determining VSMC proliferation immunohistochemically using PCNA (a marker of cell cycle protein present during the S-phase of cycling cells). Medial and neointimal cellular proliferation was measured at 1, 3, 5, 7, and 14 days after catheter injury. Figure 3 is a graphical representation of the percent of positively stained VSMC within the media and neointima combined. The proliferative index, defined as the number of VSMC staining for PCNA divided by the total number of VSMC multiplied by 100, was calculated to demonstrate differences in proliferative activity between specimens from euglycemic and diabetic animals. Neither euglycemic nor diabetic animals showed staining for PCNA prior to injury, indicating that VSMC are maintained in a quiescent state and do not undergo proliferation. Upon catheter injury, aortic specimens from both euglycemic and diabetic animals exhibited staining within the media as early as day 1. Medial staining at day 5 was significantly increased (P <0.001) in diabetic animals (10.6% ± 3) compared to euglycemic animals (3.2% ± 1). However, medial staining in diabetic animals by day 14 returned to control, whereas euglycemic animals maintained elevated medial staining through day 14. VSMC were first present within the neointima by day 7 in both euglycemic and diabetic animals at which point neointimal cell number and percent positive were comparable (Table 2). Between days 7 and 14, euglycemic animals underwent a significant increase in neointimal cell number, as well as a 50% increase in PCNA staining (% positive: 22 ± 10 vs. 32 ± 9). During the same time-frame, neointimal cell number in diabetic animals also increased, however, the PCNA staining decreased by 50% (% positive: 29 ± 6 vs. 15 ± 4).

Activation of MAPK following vascular injury has been suggested to mediate growth factor-stimulated VSMC proliferation. MAPK (p42/p44) activity in the thoracic aorta of both euglycemic and diabetic rabbits increased approximately 1.3-fold by day 1 after injury and plateaued at 2.4-fold above baseline by day 5. There was no significant difference between the two experimental groups (Fig. 4).

91

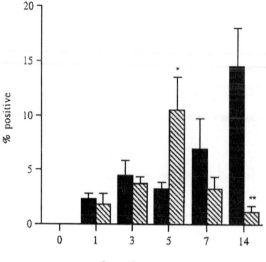

Days after catheter injury

Figure3. Proliferative index of total VSMC (medial and neointimal) following catheter injury in euglycemic (black bars) and diabetic (hatched bars) animals. The proliferative index equals the number of VSMC stained for PCNA divided by the total number of VSMC multiplied by 100 (% positive). n=4-7 animals. *indicates P <0.005 vs. euglycemic at the same time point; **indicates P <0.0001 vs. euglycemic at the same time point.

Table 2. Comparison of PCNA proliferative indices (% positive) and VSMC number within the neointima and media of diabetic and euglycemic animals days 7 and 14 after injury.

	Neointima	Media
Day 7:		
Euglycemic		
Positives	6.8 ± 3	9.9 ± 4
Total VSMC	25 ± 5	220 ± 14
% positive	22 ± 10	5.2 ± 3
Diabetic		
Positives	6.8 ± 2	5.1 ± 3
Total VSMC	23 ± 2	260 ± 9
% positive	29 ± 6	3.1 ± 2
Day 14:		
Euglycemic		
Positives	18 ± 9	12 ± 5
Total VSMC	52 ± 12	200 ± 1
% positive	32 ± 9	5.8 ± 2
Diabetic		
Positives	4.4 ± 1**	0 ± 0*
Total VSMC	32 ± 5**	250 ± 22
% positive	15 ± 4*	0 ± 0*

Values are mean ± SE. Proliferative index equals the number of medial or neointimal VSMC stained for PCNA divided by the total number of medial or neointimal VSMC multiplied by 100 (% positive). n=4-7 animals. *P <0.05 vs. euglycemic; **P <0.005 vs. euglycemic.

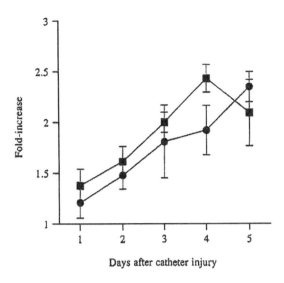

Figure 4. Increase in aortic MAPK enzymatic activity following catheter injury in euglycemic (squares) and diabetic (circles) animals. The data are expressed as fold-increase from basal enzymatic activity. $n=3$ animals.

DISCUSSION

An analogy can be made between the events following balloon catheter-induced vascular injury and any other wound healing response. It has been reported that impaired wound-healing in diabetes is due, in part, to a deficiency in growth factor activity or glucose-induced resistance to growth factors within the wound environment (7). Thus, the attenuated response to injury in the diabetic rabbit may also be a function of the degree of hyperglycemia. Growth factor resistance induced by hyperglycemic states is clinically significant in non-insulin-dependent diabetes mellitus (NIDDM), as well as in IDDM. The attenuated neointimal thickening seen in the diabetic animals could be a function of the hyperglycemia-induced resistance to IGF-1 and may explain why diabetic and euglycemic rabbits have significantly different I/M ratios, yet the increase in IGF-1 shown immunohistochemically following injury in this model is similar (8). If this were the case, then these animals would essentially lack a functional progression factor and have decreased IGF-1 activity, although IGF-1 staining within the vessel was the same. It would be of interest to measure IGF-1 receptor expression and binding activity in the VSMC of these animals. Improving the hyperglycemic state with troglitazone or vanadate might also help in further characterizing the contribution of these factors in the response to injury. Troglitazone and other thiazolidinediones are novel insulin-sensitizing agents that have been shown to significantly reduce hyperglycemia in diabetic animal models, as well as humans (9).

In this study VSMC proliferation was hypothesized to be reduced in diabetic animals compared to euglycemic animals, thus, contributing to the attenuation in neointimal thickening that was observed. It was found that diabetic animals had a significant decrease in actively proliferating cells within the neointima, as well as a significant reduction in neointimal cell number, compared to euglycemic animals. It was noted that, although the number of cells within the neointima was increased from control at day 7 and day 14 in both euglycemic and diabetic animals, the total number of VSMC within the aortic specimen did not change. These results suggest that the degree or rate of cellular migration may be critical in the decreased neointimal thickening present in the diabetic animals. IGF-1 has been shown to be a potent stimulator of directed migration (chemotaxis) or VSMC mediated primarily through the IGF-1 receptor (10). Therefore, it could be that a decrease in circulating IGF-1 levels or hyperglycemia-induced desensitization of IGF-1 receptors may affect VSMC migration and decrease neointimal thickening upon vascular injury.

The response to arterial injury is also accompanied by an acute medial cell loss (minutes) due to apoptotic cell death (11). Apoptosis within the adventitia, media, and neointima has been shown to peak at 6 hr, 18 hr, and 7 days, respectively, following porcine coronary angioplasty (12). Chronic diabetes has also been shown to cause a 6-fold increase in TUNEL (terminal uridine nick-end labeling) staining within the media of the rat aorta (13). Increased apoptosis may be one mechanism by which the diabetic rabbits have a decreased I/M ratio. Increased cell death would contribute to a lower cellular content of vascular lesions following balloon catheter injury in the diabetic rabbits. Reactive oxygen species have also been shown to promote apoptotic cell death in rat VSMC and could also account for increased apoptosis in diabetes (14).

MAPK (p42/p44) activity was measured over the first 5 days after injury prior to the arrival of VSMC within the neointima. There occurred a comparable increase in enzymatic activity through day 5 in diabetic and euglycemic animals. The increase in VSMC proliferation in the diabetic and euglycemic animals upon catheter injury was shown to have a similar time-course as MAPK activity. This signaling cascade, therefore, could be suggested to be a mechanism by which VSMC proliferation occurs in response to balloon catheter injury. MAPK enzymatic activity has been suggested to mediate growth factor-stimulated proliferation (15). The increase in immunoreactive vascular IGF-1, VSMC proliferation, and MAPK activity following catheter injury parallel one another (8). These data suggest for the first time an association between growth factor-induced MAPK activity and VSMC proliferation following injury in diabetic animals (8), as previously reported in euglycemic animals (3). It is of interest to note that 5 days after catheter injury there is a significant difference between diabetic and euglycemic animals in medial VSMC proliferation, yet MAPK activity is similar. This suggests that, although MAPK enzymatic activity is increased by catheter injury, it may not be the only signaling cascade involved in VSMC proliferation upon catheter injury. Studies have shown that IGF-1 and PDGF activate distinct signaling cascades which result in their synergistic effect on VSMC proliferation (16). Moreover, it has been suggested that the differential activation of phosphatidylinositol (PI) 3-kinase and MAPK by IGF-1 and PDGF, respectively, may explain their synergistic effect on proliferation (17).

Alterations in proliferation may partly explain the difference between the neointimal areas of diabetic and euglycemic animals. VSMC proliferation is not alone in its contribution to the formation of the neointima following vascular injury. Cellular migration and the accumulation of ECM are important factors in the expansion of the neointima. Accumulating evidence has shown that remodeling of ECM is necessary to permit migration and proliferation of VSMC (18). The fact that in this study the total cell number is unaltered in the 2 weeks following injury, yet the number of cells within the intima increases significantly from control, provides evidence that cell migration is an important factor in the reduced neointimal thickening seen in the diabetic rabbit. In normal vessels VSMC are surrounded by ECM and basement membrane components, such as proteoglycans, laminin, and collagen. These matrix components exert biochemical and mechanical barriers to cell movement. One of the primary enzymes responsible for the degradation of basement membrane-type collagen (collagen IV) is matrix metalloproteinase-2 (MMP-2). It has been shown that MMP-2 expression and activity are up-regulated upon vascular injury (19). MMP-2 degrades basement membranes surrounding VSMC and allows for VSMC migration following injury. A decreased level of expression or activation of MMP-2 within the vasculature of the diabetic rabbit may decrease VSMC migration following injury and, thus, account in part for their decreased neointimal thickening. Therefore, it would be of interest to measure the enzymatic activity of the metalloproteinases in the catheterized vessels of diabetic rabbits.

It has also been suggested that VSMC proliferation in response to injury may be beneficial and, in some cases, required for arterial repair and, therefore, inhibiting their replication may result in a weakening of the fibrous skeleton of the target lesion (20). In humans, acute coronary events are often due to plaque rupture and thrombus formation. Plaque stability depends upon the presence of a thick fibrous cap made up in part by VSMC. A stable plaque with a thick fibrous cap rarely ruptures or precipitates life-threatening events. Accumulating evidence suggests that intimal VSMC protect plaque from rupturing and stabilize the lesion and, therefore, are part of essential reparative processes whose inhibition would not necessarily be desirable (20). Regardless of whether proliferation upon vascular injury is suggested to be beneficial or detrimental, more studies are required to elucidate our understanding of the factors involved in the modulation of VSMC proliferation.

In another study we addressed the role of the endothelium in the attenuated hyperplastic response to catheter injury in this animal model (21). It was hypothesized that endothelial cell regrowth, morphology, and endothelium-dependent vasoreactivity after catheter injury are improved in the diabetic rabbit (glucose ≥ 400 mg/dL) compared with the euglycemic rabbit. Two weeks after catheter injury, the percent endothelial regrowth was significantly increased in diabetic animals compared with euglycemic animals (32.1 ± 2 and 15.6 ± 1, respectively; $P < 0.05$). The endothelial cell morphology analyzed by scanning electron microscopy was also restored 2 weeks after catheter injury in thoracic aortas from the diabetic animals compared with vessels from euglycemic animals. Endothelium-dependent relaxation to acetylcholine in vessels from diabetic and euglycemic rabbits was attenuated 2 weeks after injury, and, although improved by 4 and 8 weeks, relaxation remained significantly depressed. These results suggest that endothelial cell regrowth and morphology in diabetic animals was improved compared with euglycemic animals; however, endothelium-dependent vasoreactivity remained impaired. Thus, the attenuated neointimal thickening seen in the diabetic rabbit may be a function of the rate and degree of regrowth rather than the normalization of acetylcholine-induced relaxation.

In conclusion, this study shows a reduction in neointimal thickening and VSMC proliferation following vascular injury in chemically-induced diabetic rabbits. Evidence published elsewhere supports the argument against a direct effect of circulating IGF-1 levels in mediating these events; and the immunohistochemical data suggest that local aortic IGF-1 content does not differ between euglycemic and diabetic rabbits following catheter injury (8). This study further shows for the first time an association between vascular growth factor-induced MAPK activity and medial VSMC proliferation in response to injury in the diabetic, as well as confirming the previously reported association of the euglycemic animal. Thus, we suggest that factors, such as hyperglycemia-induced growth factor resistance, alterations in cellular migration, or matrix accumulation may have a critical role in the attenuation of neointimal thickening in the diabetic rabbit.

Acknowledgments

Tables 1 and 2 and Figures 1, 2, 4 and 6 are reproduced or adapted with permission from citation 8; support was from HL 46737.

REFERENCES

1. Dangas G., Fuster B. Management of restenosis after coronary intervention. Prog Cardiol 1996;132:428-436
2. Yarden T, Ullrich A. Growth factor receptor tyrosine kinases. Ann Rev Biochem 1995;57:443-450
3. Lai K, Wang H, Lee W, Jain MK, Lee M, Haber E. Mitogen-activated protein kinase phosphatase-1 in rat arterial smooth muscle cell proliferation. J Clin Invest 1996;98:1560-1567
4. Pyles JM, March KL, Franklin M, Mehdi K, Wilensky RL, Adam LP. Activation of MAP kinase in vivo follows balloon overstretch injury of porcine coronary and carotid arteries. Circ Res 1997;81:904-910
5. Bornfeldt KE, Arnqvist JH, Capron L. In vivo proliferation of rat vascular smooth muscle in relation to diabetes mellitus insulin-like growth factor 1 and insulin. Diabetologia 1992;35:104-108

6. Indolfi C, Esposito G, Di Lorenzo E, Rapacciuolo A, Feliciello A, Porcellini A, Avvedimento VE, Condorelli M, Chiariello M. Smooth muscle cell proliferation is proportional to the degree of balloon injury in a rat model of angioplasty. Circulation 1995;92:1230-1235

7. Bitar MS, Labbad ZN. Transforming growth factor-β and insulin-like growth factor-1 in relation to diabetes-induced impairment of wound healing. J Surg Res 1996;61:113-119

8. Schiller NK, McNamara DB. Balloon catheter vascular injury of the alloxan-induced diabetic rabbit: the role of insulin-like growth factor-1. Mol Cell Biochem 1999;accepted

9. Law RE, Meehan WP, Xi X-P, Graf K, Wuthrich DA, Coats W, Faxon D, Hsueh WA, Troglitazone inhibits vascular smooth muscle cell growth and intimal hyperplasia. J Clin Invest 1996;98:1897-1905

10. Bornfeldt KE, Raines EW, Nakano T, Graves LM, Krebs EG, Ross R. Insulin-like growth factor-1 and platelet-derived growth factor-BB induce directed migration of human arterial smooth muscle cells via signaling pathways that are distinct from those of proliferation. J Clin Invest 1994;93:1266-1274

11. Pollman MJ, Hall JL, Gibbons GH. Determinants of vascular smooth muscle cell apoptosis after balloon angioplasty injury. Influence of redox state and cell phenotype. Circ Res 1999;84:113-121

12. Malik N, Francis SE, Holt CM, Gunn J, Thomas GL, Shepherd L, Chamberlain J, Newman CM, Cumberland DC, Crossman DC. Apoptosis and cell proliferation after porcine coronary angioplasty. Circulation 1998;98:1657-1665

13. Chu Y, Faraci FM, Ooboshi H, Heistad DD. Increase in TUNEL positive cells in aorta from diabetic rats. Endothelium 1997;5:241-250

14. Li PF, Dietz R, von Harsdorf R. Reactive oxygen species induce apoptosis of vascular smooth muscle cell. FEBS Lett 1997;404:249-252

15. Hu Y, Cheng L, Hochleitner BW, Xu Q. Activation of mitogen-activated protein kinases (ERK/JNK) and AP-1 transcription factor in rat carotid arteries after balloon injury. Arterioscler Thromb 1997;17:2808-2816

16. Thommes KB, Hoppe J, Vetter H, Sachinidis A. The synergistic effect of PFGF-AA and IGF-1 on VSMC proliferation might be explained by the differential activation of their intracellular signaling pathways. Exp Cell Res 1996;226:59-66

17. Karenberg T-A, Fenn A, Sachinidis A, Hoppe J. The differential activation of phosphatidylinosil-3 kinase and mitogen-activated protein kinases by PDGF-AA and IGF-1 might explain the synergistic effect of the two growth factors on the proliferation of AKR-2B fibroblasts. Exp Cell Res 1994;213:266-274

18. Bendeck MP, Irvin C, Reidy MA. Inhibition of matrix metalloproteinase activity inhibits smooth muscle cell migration but not neotintimal thickening after arterial injury. Circ Res 1996;78:38-43

19. Zempo N, Kenagy RD, Au YPT, Bendeck M, Clowes MM, Reidy MA, Clowes AW. Matrix metalloproteinases of vascular wall cells are increased in balloon-injured rat carotid artery. J Vasc Surg 1994;20:209-217

20. Libby P. Gene therapy of restenosis: promise and perils. Circ Res 1998;82:404-406

21. Schiller NK, Timothy AM, Chen I-L, Rice JC, Akers DL, Kadowitz PJ, McNamara DB. Endothelial cell regrowth and morphology after balloon catheter injury of alloxan-induced diabetic rabbits. Am J Physiol 1999; in press

ENDOTHELINS IN THE MICROVASCULATURE AND HEART IN DIABETES

Subrata Chakrabarti,[1] Shali Chen,[1] Terry Evans,[1] and Morris Karmazyn[2]

[1]Department of Pathology
[2]Department of Pharmacology and Toxicology
The University of Western Ontario
London, Ontario, Canada, N6A 5C1

INTRODUCTION

Diabetes and its complications impose a global health problem of enormous proportion[1]. One of the most challenging problems during the last few decades has involved the elucidation of the pathogenetic mechanisms responsible for chronic diabetic complications, in an attempt to develop targeted treatment strategies. The establishment of hyperglycemia as the key initiating factor for the development of chronic diabetic complications is a milestone in diabetes research[2]. However the mechanisms, at the cellular level, by which hyperglycemia affects tissue structures and functions leading to diabetic complications remain poorly understood. Exploration of these mechanisms are challenging due to their complex nature and are of vital importance as they will form the backbone for the development of adjuvant treatment strategies. Chronic complications affects multiple organ systems in diabetes. In this article we will address some of the pathogenetic mechanisms of diabetic heart disease as well as diabetic retinopathy where microvascular affection is of major pathogenetic importance.

Diabetic Retinopathy: Brief Overview

Diabetic retinopathy is the leading cause of blindness in the 25-74 years age group[3]. Untreated diabetic retinopathy manifests itself in progressive stages, starting from preretinopathy to non-proliferative retinopathy and ultimately to proliferative retinopathy. Macular edema in the non-proliferative stage and hemorrhage and traction retinal detachment in the proliferative stage are the major lesions leading to blindness. Several interactive mechanisms have been implicated in the development of diabetic retinopathy including biochemical, hemodynamic and rheological factors, all of which may be of importance[4]. These biochemical alterations in hyperglycemia may influence expression of several growth factors and extracellular matrix protein genes[4-8] and in turn affect structural components of retinal microvasculature producing characteristic lesions namely, capillary basement membrane (BM) thickening, pericyte loss etc.[4-8]. Subsequently, secondary effects develop as a result of structural alteration, leading to clinical retinopathy. In the later stages of retinopathy, neovascular proliferation develop secondary to retinal ischemia. Neovascularization may lead

Diabetes and Cardiovascular Disease: Etiology, Treatment and Outcomes
Edited by Aubie Angel et al., Kluwer Academic/Plenum Publishers, 2001

to hemorrhage or tractional retinal detachment.

Diabetic Heart Disease: Brief Overview

Cardiac complications are a major cause of morbidity and mortality in the diabetic population. Diabetic people are 2 to 4 times more likely to have heart disease compared to the normal population and 75% of diabetes related deaths are due to heart disease[9]. Cardiac involvement in diabetes may include coronary atherosclerosis, diabetic cardiomyopathy and autonomic neuropathy[10-12]. The presence of accelerated atherosclerosis and occurrence of microvascular lesions in both type I and type II diabetes have been well documented[13-16]. In addition, for poorly understood reasons, diabetic patients develop congestive cardiac failure more readily and have significantly worse prognosis than their non-diabetic counterparts once they develop coronary disease[17-19]. Several mechanisms may be involved in the generation of diabetic heart diseases[10-12]. The list includes metabolic abnormalities such as defective glucose transport, cellular overload of fatty acid metabolites, altered calcium metabolism in cardiomyocytes and structural alterations in the form of microangiopathy, interstitial and perivascular fibrosis[10-12]. Clinically 40 to 50% of diabetics without known cardiac disease manifest abnormalities of left ventricular mechanical function primarily affecting diastolic properties. These changes manifest clinically as failure of left ventricular contractile function and prolonged relaxation[10-12]. Pathological findings include cardiomegaly and myocardial fibrosis. Myocardial hypertrophy, interstitial and perivascular fibrosis, myocyte necrosis as well as thickening of the capillary basement membrane are some other abnormal structural findings in diabetic hearts[10-12].

PATHOGENESIS OF CHRONIC DIABETIC COMPLICATIONS

Hyperglycemia is the most important factor leading to generation of almost all chronic diabetic complications[2,4,20]. Major clinical trials have shown that better glycemic control can definitely improve trends in cardiovascular complications along with prevention of retinopathy, nephropathy and neuropathy[2]. Both in micro and macro vessels hyperglycemia can cause several metabolic defects. Hyperglycemia leads to increased non-enzymatic glycation[5], sorbitol-myoinositol mediated changes[6], redox potential alteration[4,6,7] and diacylglycerol (DAG) mediated PKC activation[7,8]. Although at first glance, these mechanisms appear isolated, there are several interrelationships among them. For example, fructose generated as an end product of polyol-pathway activation can glycate structural proteins[4,21]. Hyperglycemia causes an increase in DAG level by promoting its direct synthesis in diabetes[7,8,22]. Increased DAG level in the diabetic heart and other organs is directly related to PKC activation[22,23,25]. Augmented DAG mediated PKC activation, especially of the PKC-β isoform has been demonstrated in several target organs of diabetic complications including the heart and retina[7,8,22-24]. An altered NADH/NAD$^+$ ratio formed due to augmented polyol pathway further favours PKC activation[4].

PKC activation exerts extensive effects on cellular functions. PKC can activate calcium sensitive phospholipase A$_2$ (cPLA$_2$) leading to increased PGE$_2$ and reduced Na$^+$-K$^+$-ATPase activity[25]. Loss of Na$^+$-K$^+$-ATPase activity will perturb membrane integrity leading to increased intracellular Na$^+$ and defective contractile properties of the myocardium[26]. Alteration of several growth factors, cytokines, vasoactive molecules, extracellular matrix proteins have been demonstrated in diabetes. The list includes plasminogen activator 1, endothelins (ET), fibronectin, c-fos and vascular endothelial growth factor (VEGF)[4,7,22]. All of these factors have been reported to be regulated by PKC and it has been hypothesized that these alterations are mediated through hyperglycemia induced PKC activation[27-31]. An increased PKC activity has been demonstrated in several target organs of diabetic complications including the heart and retina in diabetes[7,8,22,31-33]. PKC activation may affect many vascular functions including vascular tone, hemodynamics and cellular proliferation[23].

PKC Activation In Diabetes and The Interrelationship With Vasoactive Factors

PKC is a known upregulator of ET-1 and ET receptor production[4,7,8,34-38]. ET-1, in turn, causes phospholipase C activation, formation of inositol trisphosphate (IP3) and DAG, the latter producing PKC activation[34-38]. ETs are a family of potent vasoactive substances[34]. The ET family consists of 4 distinct isoforms each containing 21 amino acid residues, known as ET-1, ET-2, ET-3 and the vasoactive intestinal contractor. These peptides interact with three populations of receptors, ET_A, ET_B and ET_C[35-39]. In addition to acting as important autocrine and paracrine growth factors, ETs appear to function as neuromodulators and neurotransmitters[37,40,41]. ETs further have crucial roles in morphogenesis, smooth muscle contraction and steroidogenesis[35-41]. ET-1 knockout mice show elevation of blood pressure and extensive cardiovascular abnormalities including ventricular septal defects with abnormalities of the outflow tract[39,42].

In the endothelin (ET) system, ET-1 is the most widely studied peptide. ET-1 has several important cardiovascular functions[43]. Intravenous injection of ET-1 causes initial transient pressor response followed by a sustained increase in blood pressure[37]. In the heart ET-1 is produced by both myocytes and endothelial cells[44,45]. High affinity ET-1 binding sites are present in the cardiac myocytes. ET-1 evokes positive inotrophic and chronotrophic effects and prolongation of action potential[37,46,47]. In addition, ET-1 can affect cardiac function by its effect on coronary circulation[37]. In the hearts of diabetic rats, increased ET-1 binding sites have been demonstrated suggesting receptor upregulation may be an additional factor along with peptide upregulation[48]. ET-1 mRNA is elevated in the rat heart within 2 weeks of diabetes, which can be prevented by insulin treatment[49]. In addition a duration-dependant alteration of ET-1 responsiveness has been seen in the diabetic hearts[50]. Hypoxia and ischemia are two important up-regulators of ET-1 expression in the heart[43]. Several changes seen in diabetes are similar to the changes seen in hypoxia[4]. Hence it is possible that the duration of sustained hyperglycemia has modulating effects on ETs and/or their receptor expression.

The long-term effects of upregulation of ET-peptides involve cellular changes requiring differential gene expression[40,42]. Altered extracellular matrix protein synthesis and subsequent structural alteration such as BM thickening are hallmarks of diabetic microangiopathy[4,5,7]. It has been demonstrated, that diabetes-induced increased expression of glomerular $\alpha1(I)$, $\alpha1(III)$, $\alpha1(IV)$ collagen, laminin B1 and B2, can be completely blocked by treatment with an ET_A receptor antagonist[51]. Although similar matrix protein changes have been demonstrated in diabetic heart a possible role of ET in such alteration has not been characterized[14-16].

ETs interact with other potent vasoactive substances such as NO[35,36,43,55]. ET-1 possesses a positive feedback regulatory action on NO-synthesis[34]. NO in turn has an inhibitory effect on ET-1 synthesis[34,35]. ET-1 further acts through distinct receptors and stimulates DAG activity via a G protein-dependent process, which in turn activates PKC[34-38]. It has been demonstrated that in the aorta ET-1 stimulates Na^+-K^+-ATPase activity by a PKC dependent pathway[53]. In kidneys from diabetic animals PKC has been shown to increase ET-1 synthesis concomitantly with a downregulation of ET receptors[54]. Moreover, it has been demonstrated that down regulation of ET receptors in the kidneys of diabetic animals can be prevented by PKC inhibitors[54]. It is of further interest to note that treatment of diabetic animals with α-tocopherol (a PKC inhibitor) has been shown to prevent diabetes induced endothelial relaxation (mediated by NO) in the rat heart[55]. PKC is further an important regulator of VEGF production in the target organs of diabetic complications and inhibition of the specific β isoform of PKC has been shown to prevent VEGF expression as well as functional alteration in the retina[33,56]. VEGF also increases endothelin converting enzyme expression in heart[57]. It has further recently been shown that in the endothelial cells, both ET-1 and ET-3, via a PKC dependant mechanism, are stimulators of VEGF production[58].

ENDOTHELINS AND CHRONIC DIABETIC COMPLICATIONS

Table 1. Resistivity index of the retinal blood flow

	1 Month	6 Months
Control	0.42 ± 0.04 (9)	0.57 ± 0.03 (7)
Diabetic	0.54 ± 0.03 (8)[*]	0.52 ± 0.02 (8)
Galactose-fed	0.55 ± 0.03 (5)[*]	0.54 ± 0.04 (8)
Diabetic & Bosentan	0.46 ± 0.02 (6)[**]	0.55 ± 0.04 (8)
Galactose-fed & Bosentan	0.46 ± 0.04 (6)[***]	0.49 ± 0.02 (8)[*]

[*] significantly different from control group.
[**] significantly different from diabetic group.
[***] significantly different from galactose-fed group.

Functional Disturbances in The Microvasulature in Diabetes:

Abnormalities of several and partly interrelated metabolic pathways in diabetes affect vascular tone and blood flow in early diabetes. These changes have particularly been investigated in early diabetic retinopathy[3,4,7]. Loss of autoregulation is a characteristic feature of diabetic retinopathy. In early human diabetes, retinal blood flow is decreased, which increases later with background retinopathy[7,8]. Although there are some conflicting reports, the majority of studies have shown that in early diabetes retinal blood flow is decreased in animals[4,7,8,59,60]. Using non-invasive ultrasound laser-Doppler method, we have demonstrated an increased resistivity index in the central retinal artery after 1 month of diabetes and galactosemia[61,62,Table 1].

Resistivity index of the central retinal artery, calculated from the blood flow data obtained from color Doppler ultrasound, indicates obstruction in the distal vascular bed, i.e., retinal capillary vasoconstriction. This blood flow alteration is preventable by treatment with a general ET receptor blocker, blocking both ET_A and ET_B suggesting that alteration of the ET-system is an early phenomenon in the retina secondary to hyperhexosemia which works via both ET-receptor subtypes[61,62]. After 6 months of follow-up increased resistivity index was no longer demonstrable in diabetes or galactosemia. These may be due to age related changes such as thickening of basement membrane which may cause loss of distensibility of the vasculature. It is of interest to note that in the non-diabetic animal there is an age related increase in the resistivity index of retinal blood flow. In these experiments as galactose fed animals were simultaneously investigated and showed identical results as those of diabetic rats, the alterations demonstrated appear to be due secondary to hyperhexosemia and not due to insulin or other hormonal alterations in diabetes. Data from these studies indicates that ET mediated blood flow alteration is of significant importance in the pathogenesis of blood flow alteration in early diabetes.

Alteration of Components of ET System in the Heart and Retina in Hyperhexosemia

We have investigated two target organs of diabetic complications at various time points after onset of diabetes and following feeding the animals with galactose. In the retina both ET-1 and ET-3 are present with no evidence for the presence of ET-2. In addition in the retina both ET_A and ET_B receptors are present reflecting local synthesis[63-69]. In the rat retina ET-1 and ET-3 immunoreactivity is localized in the microvasculature and in the neuronal and glial components (Fig. 1).

The peptides were present in the endothelial cells, but not in the pericytes[69]. In the heart, only ET-1 was immunocytochemically demonstrable, which was seen both in the endothelial cells and in the cardiomyocytes (Fig. 1). ET-1 and ET-3 immunoreactivity is increased in the retina of diabetic animals[69]. These changes reflect local synthesis as increases were

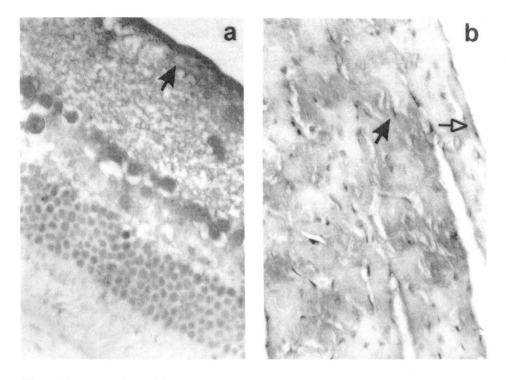

Figure 1: Immunocytochemical localization of ET-1 in the rat a) retina and b) heart. In the retina positive immunoreactivity was present in the neuronal and glial components as well as in the microvasculature (arrow). Cardiomyocytes (large arrow) and endothelium (small arrow) in the heart showed positive immunoreactivity.

associated with increases in retinal ET-1 and ET-3 mRNA by semiquantitative RT-PCR from the RNA isolated from the retina of rats[61,62,67]. Investigation of the ET receptor mRNAs showed that after 1 month of diabetes or galactosemia only ET_A receptor mRNA is upregulated whereas after 6 months of follow-up both ET_A and ET_B receptor mRNAs are upregulated[61,62,67,Fig. 2].

The altered receptor synthesis were further confirmed by receptor autoradiography which showed increased ET receptor concentration in the retina without any alteration of cellular distribution. It is of great interest that different components of ET system were altered at various time points after onset of diabetes. It is possible that ET_B receptor upregulation in long term diabetes may produce vasodilatation, counteracting vasoconstricting effects of ET-1. Such time dependent alteration of blood flow have further been demonstrated in human diabetes[7,70]. Investigation of the mRNA from the heart of chronically diabetic animals, using similar semiquantitative RT-PCR showed that ET-1 mRNA is similarly upregulated in diabetes. Assessment of the ET-receptor mRNAs showed that both ET_A and ET_B mRNA upregulation after long term diabetes (Fig. 3).

The long-term consequences of ETs may involve cellular changes requiring differential gene expression contributing to long term nuclear signaling[35-39,70-74]. Increased extracellular matrix protein synthesis and subsequent structural alteration such as BM thickening are hallmarks of diabetic microangiopathy[4-7,75]. It has been demonstrated, that diabetes-induced increased expression of glomerular $\alpha 1(I)$, $\alpha 1(III)$, $\alpha 1(IV)$ collagen, laminin B1 and B2, tumor necrosis factor α, platelet derived growth factor, transforming growth factor β, and basic FGF can be completely blocked by treatment with an ET_A receptor antagonist[51].

Both in the heart and retina of the diabetic rats after 6 months of follow-up we have found increased mRNA expression for two extracellular matrix proteins, collagen $\alpha 1(IV)$ and fibronectin, by semiquantitative RT-PCR. The increased extracellular matrix protein mRNAs, were completely prevented by treatment of the animals with Bosentan (Fig 4).

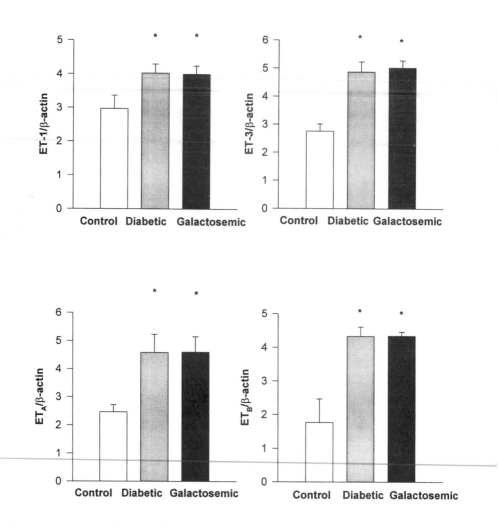

Figure 2. Increased ET-1, ET-3, ET_A and ET_B mRNA in the retina after 6 months of diabetes (* = significantly different from controls).

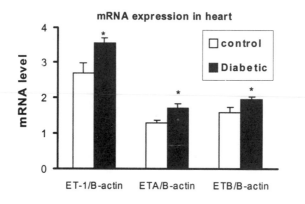

Figure 3. Increased ET-1, ET_A and ET_B mRNA in the heart after 6 months of diabetes.(* = significantly different from controls).

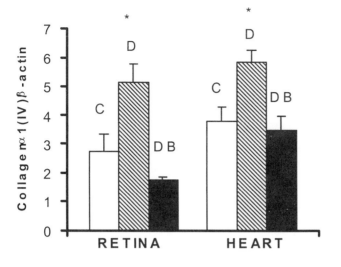

Collagen α1(IV) mRNA Expression

Figure 4.   Semiquantitative RT-PCR from retina and heart from control(C), Diabetic (D) and diabetic rats treated with Bosentan (DB). (*significantly different from controls).

Regulation of ET-1 synthesis via PKC and other vasoactive factors in hyperglycemia

ETs interact with other potent vasoactive substances such as NO and VEGF[78,34-38,44,57]. ET-1 possesses a positive feedback regulatory action on NO-synthesis[34-38,44]. NO in turn has an inhibitory effect on ET-1 synthesis[34-38,44]. Of relevance to this paper, in diabetes, activation of the polyol-pathway limits NO synthesis, hence limiting the inhibitory effect of NO on ET-1, resulting in increased ET-1 production[4]. Among the specific isoforms of NO synthase (NOS), both constitutively expressed endothelial NOS (ecNOS) and inducible NOS (iNOS) are of importance for this phenomenon[79-81].

VEGF acts both as a permeability factor and as an angiogenesis factor in the retina[56,82,83,84]. VEGF is a 35-45 KD homodimeric protein which is highly conserved with several isoforms resulting from alternative RNA splicing. VEGF is 20 times more potent than histamine as a permeability factor[85,86]. Two types of VEGF receptors, high and low affinity, are localized primarily in the endothelial cells[87]. ET-1 and ET-3 have been demonstrated to upregulate VEGF production in endothelial cells leading to endothelial proliferation[57,78]. On the other hand VEGF increases preproET-1 mRNA and protein expression in the endothelial cells[78].

We investigated high glucose induced ET-1 expression regulation in the endothelial cells as well as in cardiomyocytes. Both Human Umbilical Vein Endothelial Cells, fetal and adult cardiomyocytes   show increased ET-1 immunoreactive protein expression and mRNA expression when incubated with 25mM glucose for 48 hours compared to the incubation in the media containing 5mM glucose (Fig. 5).

The increased ET-1 expression is associated with increased permeability across the HUVEC cell confluent monolayer.   To assess the interaction with various vasoactive substances HUVEC cells in both high and low glucose were incubated with various compounds. Incubation of the cells at normal glucose (5mM) with L-NAME and VEGF showed increased ET-1 expression. Increased ET-1 expression in high glucose was completely prevented by general PKC inhibitors, H7 and Chelerythrene, a specific PKC β inhibitor and a VEGF neutralizing antibody but not by a VEGF non-neutralizing antibody or ET-receptor

Effect of glucose level on ET-1 mRNA expression in HUVECs

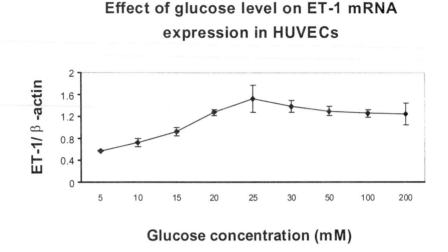

Glucose concentration (mM)

Figure 5: Effect of glucose levels on ET-1 mRNA expression as measured by semiquantitative RT-PCR.

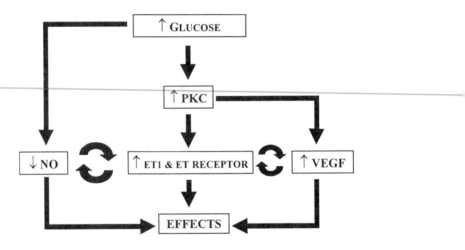

Figure 6. A simplified putative outline of interaction of PKC and vasoactive factors in diabetes.

blocker .

These interactions probably represent regulatory mechanisms controlling availability of these peptides. In the context of diabetic complications, as VEGF induces endothelial cell proliferation and ET-1 causes smooth muscle cell proliferation, together they may have important roles in diabetic micro- and macroangiopathy[57,58]. PKC is further an important regulators of VEGF production in the target organs of diabetic complications and inhibition of specific β isoform of PKC has been shown to prevent VEGF expression and diabetes induced increased permeability in the retina[56]. VEGF on the other hand increases preproET mRNA[78]. It has further been shown that in the endothelial cells, both ET-1 and ET-3, stimulate VEGF production via a PKC dependant mechanism[57]. It appears that the interplay between the endothelium derived factors such as NO and ET may ultimately determine the net effects of these peptides.

CONCLUDING REMARKS

Data presented herein indicate that alteration of ET system is of importance in the pathogenesis of diabetes induced changes in several target organs of diabetic complications. ET system alteration may lead to a variety of functional and structural alterations. However, the components of the ET system may be differentially activated and may have temporal variation. The functional effects of ETs may vary depending on the structure and function of the particular organ involved. ET-1 expression is modulated by several other vasoactive factors and PKC in diabetes. The nature of PKC involvement is undoubtedly complex. PKC activation in diabetes may effect vascular endothelium derived factors such as ETs, VEGF and NO[4,5,7,55,88]. Figure 6 shows a simplified putative outline of possible complex interactions among the vasoactive factors and PKC in diabetes. A detailed delineation of such interactions will help us understand the pathogenesis of diabetic complications which will be pivotal in the development of adjuvant treatment strategies.

Acknowledgement

Authors acknowledge grant support from Canadian Diabetes Association in honour of Florence Langille and Heart and Stroke Foundation of Ontario.

REFERENCES

1. International Diabetes Federation Triennial Report 1991-1994, IDF, Brussels, 1994
2. The Diabetes Control and Complications Trial Research Group, The effect of intensive treatment of diabetes on the development and progression of long-term complications in insulin-dependent diabetes ellitus, *N Engl J Med,* 329:977 (1993).
3. National Society to prevent blindness; Vision problems in US. New York, 1980
4. J.R. Williamson, K. Chang, M. Frangos, K.S. Hasan, Y. Ido, T. Kawamura, J.R. Nyengaard, M. van den Enden, C. Kilo, R.G. Tilton, Hyperglycemic pseudohypoxia and diabetic complications. *Diabetes.* 42:801 (1993).
5. M. Brownlee, A. Cerami, and H. Vlassara, Advanced products of nonenzymatic glycosylation and the pathogenesis of diabetic vascular disease. *Diabetes Metab Rev.* 4:437 (1988).
6. D.A. Greene, S.A. Lattimer, A.A. Sima, Sorbitol, phosphoinositides, and sodium-potassium-ATPase in the pathogenesis of diabetic complications. *N Engl J Med.* 316:599 (1987).
7. G.L. King, F.J. Oliver, T. Inoguchi, T. Shiba, N.K. Banskota, Abnormalities of vascular endothelium in diabetes, in: Diabetes Annual, S.M. Marshall, P.D. Home, K.G.M.M. Alberti, L.P. Krall, eds., Elsevier Publication, Amsterdam pp107 (1993).
8. D. Koya, G.L. King, Protein kinase C activation and the development of diabetic complications. *Diabetes.* 47:859 (1998).
9. NIH Publication # 96: 3926 (1995).
10. A. Shehadeh, T.J. Regan, Cardiac consequences of diabetes mellitus. *Clin Cardiol.* 18:301 (1995).
11. D.S. Bell, Diabetic cardiomyopathy. A unique entity or a complication of coronary artery disease? *Diabetes Care.* 18:708 (1995).
12. M.M. LeWinter, Diabetic cardiomyopathy: an overview. *Coron Artery Dis.* 7:95 (1996).
13. C.D. Furberg, H.P. Adams Jr, W.B. Applegate, R.P. Byington, M.A. Espeland, T. Hartwell, D.B. Hunninghake, D.S. Lefkowitz, J. Probstfield, W.A. Riley, B. Young, Effect of lovastatin on early carotid atherosclerosis and cardiovascular events. Asymptomatic Carotid Artery Progression Study (ACAPS) Research Group. *Circulation.* 90:1679 (1994).
14. K. Pyorala, M. Laakso, M. Uusitupa, Diabetes and atherosclerosis: an epidemiologic view. *Diabetes Metab Rev.* 3:463 (1987).
15. J. Stamler, O. Vaccaro, J.D. Neaton, D. Wentworth, Diabetes, other risk factors, and 12-yr cardiovascular mortality for men screened in the Multiple Risk Factor Intervention Trial. *Diabetes Care.* 16:434 (1993).
16. M. Laakso, T. Ronnemaa, S. Lehto, P. Puukka, V. Kallio, K. Pyorala, Does NIDDM increase the risk for coronary heart disease similarly in both low- and high-risk populations? *Diabetologia.* 38:487

(1995).

17. M.P. Savage, A.S. Krolewski, G.G. Kenien, M.P. Lebeis, A.R. Christlieb, S.M. Lewis, Acute myocardial infarction in diabetes mellitus and significance of congestive heart failure as a prognostic factor. *Am J Cardiol.* 62:665 (1988).

18. A.S. Jaffe, J.J. Spadaro, K. Schechtman, R. Roberts, E.M. Geltman, B.E. Sobel, Increased congestive heart failure after myocardial infarction of modest extent in patients with diabetes mellitus. *Am Heart J.* 108:31 (1984).

19. J.W. Smith, F.I. Marcus, R. Serokman, Prognosis of patients with diabetes mellitus after acute myocardial infarction. *Am J Cardiol.* 54:718 (1984).

20. J. Pirart, Diabetes mellitus and its degenerative complications. A prospective study of 4400 patients observed between 1947 and 1973. *Diabetes Care.* 1:168 (1978).

21. G. Suarez, Nonenzymatic browning of proteins and the sorbitol pathway. *Prog Clin Biol Res.* 304:141 (1989).

22. G.L. King, M. Kunisaki, Y. Nishio, T. Inoguchi, T. Shiba, P. Xia, Biochemical and molecular mechanisms in the development of diabetic vascular complications. *Diabetes*, 45 Suppl. 3:S105 (1996).

23. T. Inoguchi, R. Battan, E. Handler, J.R. Sportsman, W. Heath, G.L. King, Preferential elevation of protein kinase C isoform beta II and diacylglycerol levels in the aorta and heart of diabetic rats: differential reversibility to glycemic control by islet cell transplantation, *Proc Natl Acad Sci USA*, 89:11059 (1992).

24. Y. Tanaka, A. Kashiwagi, T. Ogawa, N. Abe, T. Asahina, M. Ikebuchi, Y. Takagi, Y. Shigeta, Effect of verapamil on cardiac protein kinase C activity in diabetic rats, *Eur J Pharmacol.* 200:353 (1991).

25. N. Kaiser, S. Sasson. E.P. Feener, N. Boukobza-Vardi, S. Higashi, D.E. Moller, S. Davidheiser, R.J. Przybylski, G.L. King, Differential regulation of glucose transport and transporters by glucose in vascular endothelial and smooth muscle cells. Diabetes, 42:80 (1993).

26. L.A. Vasilets, W. Schwarz, Structure-function relationships of cation binding in the Na$^+$K$^+$-ATPase, *Biochim Biophys Acta.* 1154:201 (1993).

27. Y. Nishio, C.E. Warren, J.A. Buczek-Thomas, J. Rulfs, D. Koya, L.P. Aiello, E.P. Feener, T.B. Miller Jr, J.W. Dennis, G.L. King, Identification and characterization of a gene regulating enzymatic glycosylation which is induced by diabetes and hyperglycemia specifically in rat cardiac tissue, *J Clin Invest.* 96:1759 (1995).

28. Y. Nishio, L.P. Aiello, G.L. King, Glucose induced genes in bovine aortic smooth muscle cells identified by mRNA differential display, *FASEB J.* 8:103 (1994).

29. L.P. Aiello, G.S. Robinson, Y.W. Lin, Y. Nishio, G.L. King, Identification of multiple genes in bovine retinal pericytes altered by exposure to elevated levels of glucose by using mRNA differential display, *Proc Natl Acad Sci USA.* 91:6231 (1994).

30. Y. Nishizuka, Intracellular signaling by hydrolysis of phospholipids and activation of protein kinase C, *Science.* 258:607 (1992).

31. T. Shiba, T. Inoguchi, J.R. Sportsman, W.F. Heath, S. Bursell, G.L. King, Correlation of diacylglycerol level and protein kinase C activity in rat retina to retinal circulation, *Am J Physiol.* 265:E783 (1993).

32. P.A. Craven, F.R. DeRubertis, Protein kinase C is activated in glomeruli from streptozotocin diabetic rats. Possible mediation by glucose, *J Clin Invest.* 83:1667 (1989).

33. H. Ishii, M.R. Jirousek, D. Koya, C. Takagi, P. Xia, A. Clermont, S.E. Bursell, T.S. Kern, L.M. Ballas, W.F. Heath, L.E. Stramm, E.P. Feener, G.L. King, Amelioration of vascular dysfunctions in diabetic rats by an oral PKC beta inhibitor, *Science.* 272:728 (1996).

34. P.M. Vanhoutte, Endothelin-1. A matter of life and breath, *Nature.* 368:693 (1994).

35. M.S. Simonson, Endothelins: multifunctional renal peptides, *Physiol Rev.* 73:375 (1993).

36. E.L. Schiffrin, The endothelium and control of blood vessel function in health and disease, *Clin Invest Med*, 17:602 (1994).

37. G.M. Rubanyi, M.A. Polokoff, Endothelins: molecular biology, biochemistry, pharmacology, physiology, and pathophysiology, *Pharmacol Rev*, 46:325 (1994).

38. J.P. Huggins, J.T. Pelton, R.C. Miller, The structure and specificity of endothelin receptors: their importance in physiology and medicine, *Pharmacol Ther.* 59:55 (1993).

39. Y. Kurihara, H. Kurihara, H. Suzuki, T. Kodama, K. Maemura, R. Nagai, H. Oda, T. Kuwaki, W.H. Cao, N. Kamada, K. Jishage, Y. Ouchi, S. Azuma, Y. Toyoda, T. Ishikawa, M. Kumada, Y. Yazaki, Elevated blood pressure and craniofacial abnormalities in mice deficient in endothelin-1, *Nature.* 368:703 (1994).

40. A. Peri, G.B. Vannelli, G. Fantoni, S. Giannini, T. Barni, C. Orlando, M. Serio, M. Maggi, Endothelin in rabbit uterus during pregnancy, *Am J Physiol*, 263:E158 (1992).

41. E.A. Woodcock, J.K. Tanner, L.M. Caroccia, P.J. Little, Mechanisms involved in the stimulation of aldosterone production by angiotensin II, vasopressin and endothelin, *Clin Exp Pharmacol Physiol.* 17:263 (1990).

42. Y. Kurihara, H. Kurihara, H. Oda, K. Maemura, R. Nagai, T. Ishikawa, Y. Yazaki, Aortic arch malformations and ventricular septal defect in mice deficient in endothelin-1, J Clin Invest, 96:293 (1995).

43. E.R. Levin, Endothelins as cardiovascular peptides, *Am J Nephrol*, 16:246 (1996).

44. B.H.L. Chua, C.C. Chua, C.A. Diglio, B.B. Siu, Regulation of endothelin-1 mRNA by angiotensin II in rat heart endothelial cells, *Biochim Biophys Acta*, 1178:201 (1993).
45. T. Suzuki, T. Kumazaki, Y. Mitsui, Endothelin-1 is produced and secreted by neonatal rat cardiac myocytes in vitro, *Biochem Biophys Res Commun*, 191:823 (1993).
46. J.R. Hu, R. Von Harsdorf, R.E. Lang, Endothelin has potent inotropic effects in rat atria, *Eur J Pharmacol*, 158:275 (1988).
47. T. Ishikawa, M. Yanagisawa, S. Kimura, K. Goto, T. Masaki, Positive chronotropic effects of endothelin, a novel endothelium-derived vasoconstrictor peptide, *Pflugers Arch*, 413:108 (1988).
48. L. Vesci, G.G. Mattera, P. Tobia, N. Corsico, M. Calvani, Cardiac and renal endothelin-1 binding sites in streptozotocin-induced diabetic rats, *Pharmacol Res*, 32:363 (1995).
49. Y.W. Lin, E. Duh, Z. Jiang, Expression of preproEndothelin-1 mRNA in Streptozotocin-induced diabetic rats, *Diabetes*, 45(suppl. 2) 48A (1996).
50. A.T. Lieu, J.J. Reid, Changes in the responsiveness to endothelin-1 in isolated atria from diabetic rats, *Eur J Pharmacol*, 261:33 (1994).
51. T. Nakamura, I. Ebihara, M. Fukui, Y. Tomino, H. Koide, Effect of a specific endothelin receptor A antagonist on mRNA levels for extracellular matrix components and growth factors in diabetic glomeruli, *Diabetes*, 44:895 (1995).
52. T.F. Luscher, C. Boulanger, Z. Yang, Y. Dohi, Interaction between endothelin and endothelial derived relaxing factors, in: Endothelin, G.M. Rubanyi, ed., Oxford University Press, New York (1992).
53. S. Gupta, N.B. Ruderman, E.J. Cragoe Jr, I. Sussman, Endothelin stimulates Na^+/K^+-ATPase activity by a protein kinase C-dependent pathway in rabbit aorta, *Am J Physiol*, 261:H38 (1991).
54. M. Awazu, R.E. Parker, B.R. Harvie, I. Ichikawa, V. Kon, Down-regulation of endothelin-1 receptors by protein kinase C in streptozotocin diabetic rats, *J Cardiovasc Pharmacol*, 17:S500 (1991).
55. P. Rosen, T. Ballhausen, W. Bloch, K. Addicks, Endothelial relaxation is disturbed by oxidative stress in the diabetic rat heart: influence of tocopherol as antioxidant, *Diabetologia*, 38:1157 (1995).
56. L.P. Aiello, S.E. Bursell, A. Clermont, E. Duh, H. Ishii, C. Takagi, F. Mori, T.A. Ciulla, K. Ways, M. Jirousek, L.E. Smith, G.L. King, Vascular endothelial growth factor-induced retinal permeability is mediated by protein kinase C in vivo and suppressed by an orally effective beta-isoform-selective inhibitor, *Diabetes*, 46:1473 (1997).
57. A. Pedram, M. Razandi, R.M. Hu, E.R. Levin, Vasoactive peptides modulate vascular endothelial cell growth factor production and endothelial cell proliferation and invasion, *J Biol Chem*, 272:17097 (1997).
58. A. Ladoux, C. Frelin, Hypoxia is a strong inducer of vascular endothelial growth factor mRNA expression in the heart, *Biochem Biophys Res Commun*, 195:1005 (1993).
59. E.M. Kohner, V. Patel, S.M. Rassam, Role of blood flow and impaired autoregulation in the pathogenesis of diabetic retinopathy, Diabetes, 44:603 (1995).
60. R.G. Tilton, K. Chang, K.S. Hasan, S.R. Smith, J.M. Petrash, T.P. Misko, W.M. Moore, M.G. Currie, J.A. Corbett, M.J. McDaniel, J.R. Williamson, Prevention of diabetic vascular dysfunction by guanidines. Inhibition of nitric oxide synthase versus advanced glycation end-product formation, *Diabetes*, 42:221 (1993).
61. D.X. Deng, T. Evans, K. Mukherjee, D. Downey, S. Chakrabarti, Diabetes induced vascular dysfunction in the retina: role of endothelins, *Diabetologia*, 42:1228 (1999).
62. T. Evans, D.X. Deng, D. Downey, S. Chakrabarti, Endothelins, their receptors, and retinal vascular dysfunction in galactose-fed rats, *Diabetes Res Clin Pract Canad*, 48:75(2000).
63. K. Takahashi, R.A. Brooks, S.M. Kanse, M.A. Ghatei, E.M. Kohner, S.R. Bloom, Production of endothelin 1 by cultured bovine retinal endothelial cells and presence of endothelin receptors on associated pericytes, *Diabetes*, 38:1200 (1989).
64. M.W. MacCumber, H.D. Jampel, S.H. Snyder, Ocular effects of the endothelins. Abundant peptides in the eye, *Arch Ophthalmol*, 109:705 (1991).
65. M.W. MacCumber, C.A. Ross, B.M. Glaser, S.H. Snyder, Endothelin: visualization of mRNAs by in situ hybridization provides evidence for local action, Proc *Natl Acad Sci USA*, 86:7285 (1989).
66. D. McDonald, J. Bailie, D. Archer, U. Chakravarthy, Molecular characterization of endothelin receptors and the effect of insulin on their expression in retinal microvascular pericytes, *J Cardiovasc Pharmacol*, 26 Suppl 3:S287 (1995).
67. S. Chakrabarti, X.T. Gan, A. Merry, M. Karmazyn, A.A. Sima, Augmented retinal endothelin-1, endothelin-3, endothelinA and endothelinB gene expression in chronic diabetes, *Curr Eye Res*, 17:301 (1998).
68. U. Chakravarthy, A.J. Douglas, J.R. Bailie, B. McKibben, D.B. Archer, Immunoreactive endothelin distribution in ocular tissues, *Invest Ophthalmol Vis Sci*, 35:2448 (1994).
69. S. Chakrabarti, A.A. Sima, Endothelin-1 and endothelin-3-like immunoreactivity in the eyes of diabetic and non-diabetic BB/W rats, *Diabetes Res Clin Pract*, 37:109 (1997).
70. G.L. King, M. Brownlee, The cellular and molecular mechanisms of diabetic complications, *Endocrinol Metab Clin North Am*, 25:255 (1996).
71. D. Pribnow, L.L. Muldoon, M. Fajardo, L. Theodor, L.Y. Chen, B.E. Magun, Endothelin induces transcription of fos/jun family genes: a prominent role for calcium ion, *Mol Endocrinol*, 6:1003 (1992).

72. L.L. Muldoon, D. Pribnow, K.D. Rodland, B.E. Magun, Endothelin-1 stimulates DNA synthesis and anchorage-independent growth of Rat-1 fibroblasts through a protein kinase C-dependent mechanism, *Cell Regul*, 1:379 (1990).
73. L.L. Muldoon, K.D. Rodland, M.L. Forsythe, B.E. Magun, Stimulation of phosphatidylinositol hydrolysis, diacylglycerol release, and gene expression in response to endothelin, a potent new agonist for fibroblasts and smooth muscle cells, *J Biol Chem*, 264:8529 (1989).
74. M.S. Simonson, J.M. Jones, M.I. Dunn, Differential regulation of fos and jun gene expression and AP-1 cis-element activity by endothelin isopeptides. Possible implications for mitogenic signaling by endothelin, *J Biol Chem*, 267:8643 (1992).
75. S. Chakrabarti, N. Ma, A.A. Sima, Anionic sites in diabetic basement membranes and their possible role in diffusion barrier abnormalities in the BB-rat, *Diabetologia,*. 34:301 (1991).
76. S. Roy, M. Lorenzi, Early biosynthetic changes in the diabetic-like retinopathy of galactose-fed rats, *Diabetologia*, 39:735 (1996).
77. T. Evans, D.X. Deng, S. Chen, S. Chakrabarti, Hyperhexosemia induced extracellular matrix protein gene expression and basement membrane thickening in the retinal microvasculature are mediated via augmented endothelin production, *Canad. J. Diab. Care,* 23(Suppl. 1):A177 (1999).
78. A. Matsuura, S. Kawashima, W. Yamochi, K. Hirata, T. Yamaguchi, N. Emoto, M. Yokoyama, Vascular endothelial growth factor increases endothelin-converting enzyme expression in vascular endothelial cells, *Biochem Biophys Res Commun,* 235:713 (1997).
79. Y. Oyama, H. Kawasaki, Y. Hattori, M. Kanno, Attenuation of endothelium-dependent relaxation in aorta from diabetic rats, *Eur J Pharmacol*, 132:75 (1986).
80. P. Rosen, T. Ballhausen, K. Stockklauser, Impairment of endothelium dependent relaxation in the diabetic rat heart: mechanisms and implications, *Diabetes Res Clin Pract*, 31 Suppl:S143 (1996).
81. J. Nadler, L. Winer, Free radicals, nitric oxide and diabetic complications, in: Diabetes Mellitus, D. LeRoith, et al. (eds), Lippincott-Raven, Philadelphia (1996).
82. H.P. Hammes, J. Lin, R.G. Bretzel, M. Brownlee, G. Breier, Upregulation of the vascular endothelial growth factor/vascular endothelial growth factor receptor system in experimental background diabetic retinopathy of the rat, *Diabetes*, 47:401 (1998).
83. L.P. Aiello, R.L. Avery, P.G. Arrigg, B.A. Keyt, H.D. Jampel, S.T. Shah, L.R. Pasquale, H. Thieme, M.A. Iwamoto, J.E. Park, et al, Vascular endothelial growth factor in ocular fluid of patients with diabetic retinopathy and other retinal disorders, *N Engl J Med*, 331:1480 (1994).
84. J.W. Miller, A.P. Adamis, L.P. Aiello, Vascular endothelial growth factor in ocular neovascularization and proliferative diabetic retinopathy, *Diabetes Metab Rev*, 13:37 (1997).
85. K. Cullinan-Bove, R.D. Koos, Vascular endothelial growth factor/vascular permeability factor expression in the rat uterus: rapid stimulation by estrogen correlates with estrogen-induced increases in uterine capillary permeability and growth, *Endocrinology*, 133:829 (1993).
86. T. Murata, K. Nakagawa, A. Khalil, T. Ishibashi, H. Inomata, K. Sueishi, The relation between expression of vascular endothelial growth factor and breakdown of the blood-retinal barrier in diabetic rat retinas, *Lab Invest*, 74:819 (1996).
87. L.B. Jakeman, J. Winer, G.L. Bennett, C.A. Altar, N. Ferrara, Binding sites for vascular endothelial growth factor are localized on endothelial cells in adult rat tissues, *J Clin Invest*, 89:244 (1992).
88. J.P. Liu, Protein kinase C and its substrates, *Mol Cell Endocrinol*, 116:1 (1996).

DIABETES AND ENDOTHELIAL FUNCTION: IMPLICATIONS FOR CORONARY ANGIOPLASTY

Todd J. Anderson

University of Calgary
Calgary AB T2N 2T9

DIABETES AND CORONARY INTERVENTION

Clinical Trials

Complications from coronary artery disease remain the leading cause of mortality in subjects with diabetes mellitus. As such, coronary revascularization is frequently performed in patients with diabetes. Percutaneous coronary intervention has been widely applied to patients with coronary disease including those with diabetes. [1] Whereas success rates remain high it is clear that outcomes in patients with diabetes are worse than those without diabetes. Kip et al. reported on the 9 year follow-up from the 1985-86 NHLBI angioplasty registry. [2] Patients with diabetes tended to be older, were more likely to be female, have more extensive coronary disease and have greater comorbidity. Despite this, acute success and the degree of revascularization were the same, but in-hospital events were higher. The 9 year mortality was almost twice as high in those with diabetes (35.9 vs 17.9%). Similarly, there was an excess of non-fatal myocardial infarctions, coronary bypass surgery and repeat angioplasty. Diabetes remained a significant independent risk factor in multivariate analysis. Similar long-term registry data has been reported by others. [3; 4]

Over the last 5 years percutaneous interventional procedures have changed from mainly balloon angioplasty to coronary stenting. This has resulted in lower restenosis and repeat revascularization rates. [5] Van Belle and colleagues demonstrated that angiographic restenosis rates were significantly higher in diabetics (63 vs 36 %) undergoing balloon angioplasty. [6] However, in those diabetics that were stented, restenosis was not increased compared with non-diabetics. Elizi recently reported a large series of patients (2839 non-diabetes, 715 diabetics) from a single interventional site who had undergone coronary stenting. [7] One year event free survival was worse in those with diabetes (73.1 vs 78.8%) as were major adverse cardiac events (6.7 vs 3.8%). Intravascular ultrasound studies have demonstrated that subjects with diabetes have exaggerated intimal hyperplasia following both balloon angioplasty and coronary stenting leading to increased restenosis rates. [8] Thus

Diabetes and Cardiovascular Disease: Etiology, Treatment and Outcomes
Edited by Aubie Angel et al., Kluwer Academic/Plenum Publishers, 2001

stenting is effective in those with diabetes, but has not eliminated the adverse effects of diabetes including restenosis.

Diabetes also remains a signficant risk factor for patients undergoing coronary bypass grafting. [3] It was recently reported in the Bypass Angioplasty Revascularization Investigation (BARI) trial, that 5 year survival amongst treated diabetics was significantly worse for patients treated by angioplasty compared with bypass surgery (35 vs 19%). [9] While this was not confirmed in the BARI registry [10], it is a general belief that angioplasty is not the revascularization procedure of choice for diabetics with multivessel disease. [11]

Mechanisms for Increased Risk

There are a multitude of reasons why risk is increased in diabetics following coronary intervention. An increase in acute in-hospital complications is consistently seen. [2,7] This is felt to be due to patient demographics and angiographic factors. These patients are often older, more often female, have smaller arteries, more extensive coronary disease and decreased LV function. Despite this, diabetes remains an independent risk factor in multivariate analysis for acute complications. This may in part be the result of the vascular abnormalities associated with diabetes that create an abnormal leukocyte, platelet and endothelial interaction. [12] Recent evidence from a large multicenter trial has demonstrated that the platelet glycoprotein IIb/IIIa receptor blocker abciximab may reduce acute complications of angioplasty in diabetics. [13]

Intermediate term results following percutaneous intervention are dominated by restenosis. A detailed discussion of restenosis is beyond the scope of this review. Increased smooth muscle cell (VSMC) proliferation in diabetics may result from mitogens such as platelet derived growth factor and insulin that stimulate cell growth and excessive extracellular matrix production. [14] Although, insulin stimulates endothelial cell production of nitric oxide, it also promotes vascular smooth muscle cell growth [15], can stimulate PAI-1 production in VSMC, and it stimulates extracellular matrix production. [16] Although a number of pathways may be involved, the mitogen-activated protein kinase (MAPK) pathway may play a prominent role. [17] Insulin resistance likely disturbs the balance between potential vasoprotective effects of insulin which are mediated by NO, and the atherogenic effects of insulin which involve VSMC proliferation.

The long-term detrimental effects of diabetes are due in large part to the progression of atherosclerosis following angioplasty. [18] It is well known that patients with insulin-resistance or type II diabetes often have associated risk factors that make up metabolic syndrome X. [19] These include hypertension, central obesity, and hyperlipidemia. Recent data from Framingham demonstrated that an astounding 48% of coronary events in women can be attributed to clusters of metabolically related risk factors that include diabetes. [20] Overt diabetes is well known to increase cardiovascular risk [21] and this may occur at only mildly increased levels of glucose and insulin. [22] Even though there is significant data to suggest that secondary prevention strategies, such as lipid lowering are beneficial in these patients, we are undertreating to a great degree. [23] Diabetes imposes metabolic disturbances that have adverse vascular effects. Endothelial dysfunction plays an important role in the vascular complications of diabetes, including those post coronary intervention. Endothelial cell biology as it applies to diabetes will be reviewed below.

ENDOTHELIAL FUNCTION

The endothelium controls a number of processes that maintain vascular integrity. [24] Local vascular control depends on a balance between dilators and constrictors, with endothelium-dependent nitric oxide (NO) being the best characterized and probably the most important. [25] NO is stimulated by a variety of stimuli which serve as the basis for the assessment of endothelium-dependent vasodilation. Opposing NO are vasoconstrictors such as endothelin and angiotensin II. In health, the endothelium is vasodilatory, but is also anti-atherogenic as a result of other properties (Table 1).

Table 1. Functions of the Healthy Endothelium

Vasodilation	Inhibits leukocyte adhesion
Inhibits platelet aggregation	Inhibits smooth muscle cell proliferation
Selective permeability	Fibrinolysis

Table 2. Mechanisms of Endothelial Dysfunction in Diabetes

Hyperglycemia	Increased tumor necrosis factor
Oxidation of LDL	Increased endothelin-1
Protein glycosylation	Sympathetic nervous system activation
Advanced glycosylation end-products	Leukocyte adhesion
Protein Kinase C activation	Concomitant risk factors (hypertension)
Insulin resistance	

There is extensive evidence that insulin-mediated vasodilation in humans is NO dependent and this may be important in insulin's effect on glucose uptake. [26] In conditions of insulin-resistance, insulin-mediated vasodilation is markedly blunted.

Endothelial Dysfunction And Diabetes

Observational Studies There is a wealth of information in animals and humans that diabetes impairs endothelium-dependent vasodilation. The data in humans is somewhat more consistent for states of insulin-resistant such as type II diabetes. Williams et al. demonstrated attenuated increases in forearm blood flow to acetylcholine and sodium nitroprusside in type II diabetics compared with controls. [27] However, the same group demonstrated impaired endothelial function in type I diabetics as well, [28] although others have not confirmed this in type I diabetics. [29] Baron has done extensive work in this area, and has also been able to demonstrate that subjects with insulin resistance and no evidence of diabetes have impaired vasodilator function as well. [30] The acute induction of insulin resistance by increasing free fatty acids also impairs endothelial function. [31] Diabetes results in other manifestations of endothelial dysfunction including leukocyte adhesion and platelet activation. [32]

Mechanisms of Dysfunction There are several important mechanisms whereby diabetes impairs vascular regulation. Central to the metabolic abnormality of diabetes is an increase in oxidative stress. Hyperglycemia induces superoxide formation in vitro, [33] and acutely impairs endothelium-dependent vasodilation. [34] A recent study demonstrated that increased level of F_2-isoprostanes in diabetic patients, a measure of lipid peroxidation, correlated with glycemic control. [35] Oxidative stress impairs NO mediated vasodilation in part by inactivating NO. In addition the chronic hyperglycemia leads to glycosylation of proteins including hemoglobin. Advanced glycosylation end-products (AGE's) have been shown to adversely affect endothelial cell function. [36] Other metabolic derangements affecting endothelial function are listed below. These ongoing abnormalities are certainly associated with the increased risk of atherosclerosis progression in patients who have undergone percutaneous interventions.

Endothelial Dysfunction and Angioplasty

Balloon injury of an atherosclerotic coronary artery results in severe trauma to the vessel wall and the endothelium. The result is deep arterial injury and platelet and leukocyte adhesion, an increase in oxidative stress, and serotonin and endothelin release, leading to attenuated endothelial function early after intervention. The effect that this process has on coronary blood flow had not been well studied. We recently studied coronary blood flow responses to acetylcholine in 30 subjects immediately following coronary stenting. [37] Marked attenuation of ACh-induced increases in CBF was noted compared with atherosclerotic control subjects, despite excellent angiographic results and normal appearing flow by angiography. In addition, animal studies have demonstrated enhanced platelet and leukocyte adhesion particularly following stenting. [38] This likely accounts for the increased incidence of myocardial infarctions following stenting. The fact that the glycoprotein IIb/IIIa receptor blocker abciximab markedly decreases events following stenting would support an important role for endothelial dysfunction. [39] The effect of diabetes per se on endothelial dysfunction post intervention has not been specifically studied, but work is ongoing in this area.

CONCLUSION

Diabetes presents a major challenge to interventional cardiologists. The metabolic derangement present in these subjects, along with the concomitant diseases increase the acute and long-term events following intervention. Similar statements apply to bypass surgery as well. Acute complications may in part be mediated by abnormalities of coronary blood flow induced by endothelial dysfunction following intervention. Accelerated atherosclerosis in the long-term certainly contributes to the increased event rates in these individuals. Endothelial dysfunction plays a predominant role here. We need to be more aggressive in our treatment of diabetes, the lipid abnormalities and hypertension in these patients. There is good evidence that lowering cholesterol and using angiotensin-converting enzyme inhibition improves endothelial function in diabetics. The effect of tight glucose control on endothelial function is not clear, but it is probable that macrovascular complications are reduced with more aggressive diabetes control. Whether this will have specific benefit in lowering complications post coronary intervention needs to be studied, but this should be the goal in our high risk diabetic patients who do undergo coronary revascularization.

REFERENCES

1. Topol EJ, Serruys PW: Frontiers in interventional cardiology. *Circulation* 1998;98:1802-1820
2. Kip KE, Faxon DP, Detre KM, Yeh W, Kelsey SF, Currier JW: Coronary angioplasty in diabetic patients. The National Heart, Lung, and Blood Institute Percutaneous Transluminal Coronary Angioplasty Registry. *Circulation* 1996;94:1818-1825
3. Barsness GW, Peterson ED, Ohman EM, Nelson CL, DeLong ER, Reves JG, Smith PK, Anderson RD, Jones RH, Mark DB, Califf RM: Relationship between diabetes mellitus and long-term survival after coronary bypass and angioplasty. *Circulation* 1997;96:2551-2556
4. Stein B, Weintraub WS, Gebhart SP, Cohen-Bernstein CL, Grosswald R, Liberman HA, Douglas JSJ, Morris DC, King SB: Influence of diabetes mellitus on early and late outcome after percutaneous transluminal coronary angioplasty. *Circulation* 1995;91:979-989
5. Serruys PW, de Jaegere P, Kiemeneij F, Macaya C, Rutsch W, Heyndrickx GR, Emanuelsson H, Marco J, Legrand V, Materne P, Belardi J, Sigwart U, Colombo A, Goy JJ, van den Heuvel P, Delcan J, Morel MA, for the BENESTENT Study Group: A comparison of balloon-expandable-stent implantation with balloon angioplasty in patients with coronary artery disease. *N Engl J Med* 1994;331:489-495
6. Van Belle E, Bauters C, Hubert E, Bodart JC, Abolmaali K, Meurice T, McFadden EP, Lablanche JM, Bertrand ME: Restenosis rates in diabetic patients: a comparison of coronary stenting and balloon angioplasty in native coronary vessels. *Circulation* 1997;96:1454-1460
7. Elezi S, Kastrati A, Pache J, Wehinger A, Hadamitzky M, Dirschinger J, Neumann FJ, Schomig A: Diabetes mellitus and the clinical and angiographic outcome after coronary stent placement. *J Am Coll Cardiol* 1998;32:1866-1873

8. Kornowski R, Mintz GS, Kent KM, Pichard AD, Satler LF, Bucher TA, Hong MK, Popma JJ, Leon MB: Increased restenosis in diabetes mellitus after coronary interventions is due to exaggerated intimal hyperplasia. A serial intravascular ultrasound study. *Circulation* 1997;95:1366-1369

9. The BARI Investigators: Influence of diabetes on 5-year mortality and morbidity in a randomized trial comparing CABG and PTCA in patients with multivessel disease: the Bypass Angioplasty Revascularization Investigation (BARI). *Circulation* 1997;96:1761-1769

10. Detre KM, Guo P, Holubkov R, Califf RM, Sopko G, Bach R, Brooks MM, Bourassa MG, Shemin RJ, Rosen AD, Krone RJ, Frye RL, Feit F: Coronary revascularization in diabetic patients : A comparison of the randomized and observational components of the bypass angioplasty revascularization investigation (BARI). *Circulation* 1999;99:633-640

11. Weintraub WS, Stein B, Kosinski AS, Douglas JS, Jr., Ghazzal ZMD, Jones EL, Morris DC, Guyton RA, Craver JS, King SB, III: Outcome of coronary bypass surgery versus coronary angioplasty in diabetic patients with multivessel coronary artery disease. *J Am Coll Cardiol* 1998;31:10-19

12. Keaney JFJ, Loscalzo J: Diabetes, oxidative stress, and platelet activation [In Process Citation]. *Circulation* 1999;99:189-191

13. Kleiman NS, Lincoff AM, Kereiakes DJ, Miller DP, Aguirre FV, Anderson KM, Weisman HF, Califf RM, Topol EJ: Diabetes mellitus, glycoprotein IIb/IIIa blockade, and heparin: evidence for a complex interaction in a multicenter trial. EPILOG Investigators. *Circulation* 1998;97:1912-1920

14. Aronson D, Bloomgarden Z, Rayfield EJ: Potential mechanisms promoting restenosis in diabetic patients. *J Am Coll Cardiol* 1996;27:528-535

15. Banskota NK, Taub R, Zellner K, King GL: Insulin, insulin-like growth factor I and platelet-derived growth factor interact additively in the induction of the protoncogene c-myc and cellular proliferation in cultured bovine aortic smooth muscle cells. *Mol Endocrinol* 1989;3:1183-1190

16. Tamaroglio TA, Lo GS: Regulation of fibronectin by insulin-like growth factor-1 in cultured rat thoracic aortic smooth muscle cells and glomerular mesangial cells. *Exp Cell Res* 1994;215:338-346

17. Xi XP, Graf K, Goetze S, Fleck E, Hsueh WA, Law RE: Central role of the MAPK pathway in ang II-mediated DNA synthesis and migration in rat vascular smooth muscle cells. *Arteriosclerosis, Thrombosis & Vascular Biology.* 1999;19:73-82

18. Mick MJ, Piedmonte MR, Arnold AM, Simpfendorfer C: Risk stratificication for long-term outcome after elective coronary angioplasty: a multivariate analysis of 5000 patients. *J Am Coll Cardiol* 1994;24:74-80

19. Reaven GM: Role of insulin resistance in human disease. *Diabetes* 1988;37:1595-1607

20. Wilson PWF, Kannel WB, Silbershatz H, D'Agostino RB: Clustering of metabolic factors and coronary heart disease. *Archives of Internal Medicine* 1999;159:1104-1109

21. Kannel WB, McGee DL: Diabetes and glucose tolerance as risk factors for cardiovascular disease:the Framingham Study. *Diabetes Care* 1979;2:120-126

22. Gerstein HC, Pais P, Pogue J, Yusuf S: Relationship of glucose and insulin levels to the risk of myocardial infarction:A case-control study. *J Am Coll Cardiol* 1999;33:612-619

23. Pyorala K, Pedersen TR, Kjekshus J, Faergeman O, Olsson AG, Thorgeirsson G: Cholesterol lowering with simvastatin improves prognosis of diabetic patients with coronary heart disease. A subgroup analysis of the Scandinavian Simvastatin Survival Study (4S) [see comments] [published erratum appears in Diabetes Care 1997 Jun; 20(6):1048]. *Diabetes Care* 1997;20:614-620

24. Moncada S, Higgs A: The l-arginine-NO pathway. *N Engl J Med* 1993;329:2002-2012

25. Furchgott RF, Zawadski JV: The obligatory role of endothelial cells in the relaxation of arterial smooth muscle by acetylcholine. *Nature* 1980;288:373-376

26. Steinberg HO, Brechtel G, Johnson A, Fineberg N, Baron AD: Insulin-mediated skeletal muscle vasodilation is nitric oxide dependent. A novel action of insulin to increase nitric oxide release. *Journal of Clinical Investigation* 1994;94:1172-1179

27. Williams SB, Cusco JA, Roddy M-A, Johnstone M, Creager MA: Impaired nitric oxide-mediated vasodilation in humans with non-insulin-dependent diabetes mellitus. *JACC* 1996;27:567-574

28. Johnstone M, Creager SJ, Scales K, Cusco JA, Lee B, Creager MA: Impaired endothelium-dependent vasodilation in patients with insulin-dependent diabetes mellitus. *Circulation* 1993;88:2510-1516

29. Smits P, Kapma J-A, Jacobs M-C, Lutterman J, Thien T: Endothelium-dependent vascular relaxation in patients with type I diabetes. *Diabetes* 1993;42:148-153

30. Steinberg HO, Chaker H, Leaming R, Johnson A, Brechtel G, Baron AD: Obesity/insulin resistance is associated with endothelial dysfunction. Implications for the syndrome of insulin resistance. *Journal of Clinical Investigation* 1996;97:2601-2610

31. Steinberg HO, Tarshoby M, Monestel R, Hook G, Cronin J, Johnson A, Bayazeed B, Baron AD: Elevated circulating free fatty acid levels impair endothelium-dependent vasodilation. *Journal of Clinical Investigation* 1997;100:1230-1239

32. Tsao PS, Niebauer J, Buitrago R, Lin PS, Wang B, Cooke JP, Chen Y, Reaven GM: Interaction of diabetes and hypertension on determinants of endothelial adhesiveness. *Arterioscler Thromb Vasc Biol* 1998;18:947-953

33. Cosentino F, Hishikawa K, Katusic ZS, Luscher TF: High glucose increases nitric oxide synthase expression and superoxide anion generation in human aortic endothelial cells. *Circulation* 1997;96:25-28

34. Williams SB, Goldfine AB, Timimi FK, Ting HH, Roddy M-A, Simonson DC, Creager MA: Acute hyperglycemia attenuates endothelium-dependent vasodilation in humans in vivo. *Circ* 1998;97:1695-1701

35. Davi G, Ciabattoni G, Consoli A, Mezzetti A, Falco A, Santarone S, Pennese E, Vitacolonna E, Bucciarelli T, Costantini F, Capani F, Patrono C: In vivo formation of 8-iso-prostaglandin f2alpha and platelet activation in diabetes mellitus : effects of improved metabolic control and vitamin E supplementation [In Process Citation]. *Circulation* 1999;99:224-229

36. Vlassara H, Fuh H, Makita Z, Krungkrai S, Cerami A, Bucala R: Exogenous advanced glycosylation end products induce complex vascular dysfunction in normal animals: a model for diabetic and aging complications. *Proc Natl Acad Sci USA* 1992;89:12043-12047

37. Anderson TJ, Shewchuk L, Buller CE, Carere R, Teefy P: Endothelium-dependent resistance vessel function is impaired immediately following coronary intervention. *Can J Cardiol* 1998;188F(Abstract)

38. Merhi Y, Provost P, Guidoin R, Latour JG: Importance of platelets in neutrophil adhesion and vasoconstriction after deep carotid arterial injury by angioplasty in pigs. *Arterioscler Thromb Vasc Biol* 1997;17:1185-1191

39. The EPISTENT Investigators: Randomised placebo-controlled and balloon-angioplasty-controlled trial to assess safety of coronary stenting with use of platelet glycoprotein-IIb/IIIa blockade. *Lancet* 1998;352:87-92

THE EFFECT OF HYPERTENSION IN DIABETES

Ellen D. Burgess

Faculty of Medicine
University of Calgary
Calgary, Alberta, Canada

The Hypertension in Diabetes Study (HDS) reported the prevalence of hypertension in newly-diagnosed type2 diabetics was 39%, using the criteria of a blood pressure >160/90 or taking medication for hypertension[1]. If the criterion of 140/90 is used instead, the prevalence could be as high as 90%. In the HDS the newly-diagnosed diabetic patients had already had an increased event-rate compared to the normo-tensive diabetic patients, and a follow-up study demonstrated that hypertensive diabetic patients had about twice the rate of fatal and non-fatal diabetic outcomes[2]. Since diabetic persons have a risk of events about twice that of non-diabetic persons, then the hypertensive diabetic person has a risk about 4-times that of a normo-tensive non-diabetic individual.

Hypertension in diabetes affects the outcome of microvascular and macrovascular outcomes, including death. This is most clearly proven by intervention trials including the United Kingdom Prospective Diabetes Study Group[3,4] that have demonstrated that the treatment of hypertension in diabetes reduces the risk of death related to diabetes (32% reduction), and the risk of microvascular end-points including retinopathy. Although the reduction of blood pressure is beneficial, the use of a specific class of anti-hypertensives, the ACE inhibitors, may be particularly useful; this has been clearly demonstrated in diabetic nephropathy in type 1 diabetes[5], and other studies are ongoing evaluating renal, retinal, and other outcomes.

HYPERTENSION IN DIABETES

Why should there be such a high prevalence of hypertension in diabetes? Studies have demonstrated that there is an elevation in total body exchangeable sodium in both normotensive and hypertensive diabetic patients. Other studies have demonstrated an increased sensitivity to infused vasopressor substances, including angiotensin II and norepinephrine, in all diabetic patients compared to that in essential hypertensive or normotensive individuals. Insulin is normally a vasodilating substance; in diabetic subjects, there is attenuated vasodilation from insulin. Therefore, the enhanced sensitivity to vasopressors and blunted response to vasodilators is a set up for the development of hypertension, particularly when there may be volume expansion or an increase in intracellular sodium and other ion imbalances.

Diabetes and Cardiovascular Disease: Etiology, Treatment and Outcomes
Edited by Aubie Angel et al., Kluwer Academic/Plenum Publishers, 2001

DIABETIC NEPHROPATHY

Diabetes is the leading cause for patients requiring renal replacement therapy (dialysis or transplantation). There is a predictable natural history of type 1 diabetic nephropathy with microalbuminuria coming on about 5-7 years after diagnosis, macro-proteinuria at 10-12 years, with decreasing renal function thereafter until renal replacement is needed at about year 15. Only about 30-40% of all diabetic patients develop nephropathy. The risk factors for type 1 diabetic nephropathy are a) poor glycemic control/lack of insulin secretion, b) family history of hypertension, and c) cigarette smoking. Since the onset of type 2 diabetes is not always clear, the natural history of the development of type 2 diabetic nephropathy is not as clear. These diabetic patients may have nephropathy at the time they are diagnosed with diabetes. Therefore it is not possible to discuss risk factors, but we can discuss promotors of nephropathy. These include a) hypertension, b) poor glycemic control, and c) cigarette smoking. Although blood sugar control is probably more important in preventing the initiation of diabetic nephropathy, control of the blood pressure is more important in slowing the progression of established nephropathy. A recent study has shown that the probability of deterioration of renal function is much less if the diastolic blood pressure is < 85 mmHg than if it is ≥85mmHg[6].

The role of intraglomerular hypertension was presented in the mid-1980's by Dr Brenner. It would appear that the afferent arteriole has a decreased resistance due to poor overall tone, thus exposing the glomerulus to systemic blood pressure. To make matters worse, the efferent arteriolar resistance is not as reduced relative to the afferent arteriole, and so there is an increase in intraglomerular pressure. This is an adaptive means to maintain glomerular filtration when there is a reduction in overall renal function. However, this adaptation results in longterm deterioration of the glomeruli. The reduction in systemic blood pressure, by any anti-hypertensive agents, results in a decrease of intra-glomerular pressure relevent to the transmission of pressure from the systemic vasculature. However, the efferent arteriole is predominantly under the control of angiotensin II, and therefore agents which will interfere with angiotensin II must be used to specifically decrease efferent arteriolar resistance. This has been the reason for using ACE inhibitors, and more recently Angiotensin II type 1 receptor blockers. The use of ACE inhibitors results in an initial reduction in filtration due to reduction in intraglomerular pressure[6]. This is a temporary phenomenon, reversible with discontinuation of ACE inhibitor therapy. This initial phenomenon may contribute to a significant reduction in proteinuria. This reduction in protein excretion predicts the long-term response of the patient; that is, a patient who reduces proteinuria by >50% is likely to have a good long-term result with a significant slowing of the rate of deterioration of renal function. This is due in part to the harmful effects on the proximal tubular cells as they reabsorb the filtered protein. In addition, the long-term slowing of renal deterioration has been hypothesized to be primarily related to the blocking of the angiotensin II effect of stimulating transforming growth factor-beta (TGF-b) and other cytokines which promote scarring within the interstitium of the kidney and other organs.

ENDOTHELIAL DYSFUNCTION

The presence of microalbuminuria has been shown to predict cardiovascular outcome in diabetic and non-diabetic groups. Microalbuminuria is a marker for small vessel damage, likely related to endothelial dysfunction. Endothelial dysfunction from diabetes appears to include enhanced NO turnover, advanced glycosylation end-products, increased oxidative stress, altered mechanical forces, and increased angiotensin II formation and effect[7]. Hypertension affects endothelial function through shear stress, circumferential stress and pressure, decreased endothelial NO synthetase, and increased VEGF mRNA expression. This results in increased permeability and access to subendothelial areas, both required for arteriolosclerosis. The renin-angiotensin system has been implicated in the generation of superoxide anions, regulating a membrane-bound flavin which produces oxygen radicals, and upregulating VEGF mRNA expression (which is blocked by AT1 receptor blockers). ACE inhibition has been demonstrated to restore endotheial function, and animal studies have shown that it can prevent the development of diabetic vasculopathy.

TREATING FOR IMPROVED DIABETIC OUTCOMES

Diabetic retinopathy may, in part, be related to hyperperfusion and increased vascular permeability. Treatment with ACE inhibition has been demonstrated to decrease the progression of diabetic retinopathy in patients receiving lisinopril for microalbuminuria. Vascular factors appear to be important in the development of diabetic neuropathy also. In a small study, trandolapril was given for 12 months, and was shown to improve motor nerve conduction velocity, although there was no change in patient symptoms.

There is conclusive proof that the treatment of hypertension, particularly with ACE inhibitors which disrupt the angiotensin II system, is beneficial for diabetic nephropathy and cardiovascular endpoints. ACE inhibitor therapy may be particularly important for nephropathy, retinopathy, vasculopathy, and neuropathy. The target blood pressure should be <130/80 mmHg, perhaps as low as 125/75 if there is more than 1 gm protein per day in the urine. Treatment should include an ACE inhibitor, used at close to the maximum dose so as to maximize the potential effect on the tissue level where angiotensin II interacts with growth factors and cytokines. Without outcome study results, it is not yet appropriate to recommend substituting or adding angiotensin II type 1 receptor blockers to the therapeutic plan. However, combining ACE inhibitors with diuretics and/or calcium channel blockers will likely be necessary in order to attain the target blood pressure.

REFERENCES

1. The Hypertension in Diabetes Study Group.Hypertension in Diabetes Study (HDS): I. Prevalence of hypertension in newly presenting type 2 diabetic patients and the association with risk factors for cardiovascular and diabetic complications. J Hypertens 1993;11:309-317.
2. The Hypertension in Diabetes Study Group.Hypertension in Diabetes Study (HDS): II. Increased risk of cardiovascular complications in hypertensive typpe 2 diabetic patients. J Hypertens 1993;11:319-325.
3. UK Prospective Diabetes Study Group. Tight blood pressure control and risk of macrovascular and microvascular complications in type 2 diabetes: UKPDS 38. BMJ 1998;317:703-13.
4. UK Prospective Diabetes Study Group. Efficacy of atenolol and captopril in reducing risk of macrovascular and microvascular complications in type 2 diabetes: UKPDS 39. BMJ 1998;317:713-20.
5. Lewis EJ, Hunsicker LG, Bain RP, Rohde RD. The effect of angiotensin-converting-enzyme inhibition on diabetic nephropathy. New Engl J Med 1993;329:1456-1462.
6. Bjork S. Clinical trials in overt diabetic nephropathy. in.The Kidney and Hypertension in Diabetes Mellitus. CE Mogensen (ed). Kluwer Academic Publishers, Boston. 1998 pp409-418.
7. Cooper ME, Cao Z, Rumble JR, Jandeleit K, Allen TJ, Gilbert RE. Attenuation of diabetes-associated mesenteric vascular hypertrophy with perindopril: morphological and molecular biological studies. Metabolism 1998;47(Suppl1):24-27.

THE DIABETIC HYPERTENSIVE (OR HYPERTENSIVE DIABETIC) - A COMPELLING NEED TO OPTIMIZE BLOOD PRESSURE

S. George Carruthers

London Health Sciences Centre
The University of Western Ontario
London, Ontario

INTRODUCTION

In North America and other parts of the developed world, obesity is increasingly common and is associated with the pathophysiology of both hypertension and diabetes. Both the prevalence of Type 2 diabetes mellitus and the prevalence of hypertension are expected to increase substantially in the first two decades of the next century as aging Baby Boomers enter the ranks of senior citizens. Worldwide, the demographic trends of increasing urbanization, weight gain, increasing blood pressure and increasing prevalence of diabetes mellitus that mimic current Western cardiovascular risk profiles will also create a major public health problem of unprecedented proportions in developing countries. The preeminence of cardiovascular diseases as the leading international cause of mortality that was anticipated in the early years of the third millennium is already a reality at the end of the 1990s.

Overlap of diabetes and hypertension is common, with 8 to 10% of hypertensives over the age of 60 years exhibiting diabetes and some 50% of diabetics in this age group experiencing elevated blood pressure. Undetected and unmanaged diabetes and hypertension are both common in older persons. In a cohort of older persons with hypertension, Johnson and his colleagues found that 11.6% had undiagnosed NIDDM and many more had impaired glucose tolerance[1]. The combination of hypertension and diabetes greatly aggravates the progressive cardiovascular morbidity and mortality associated with aging[2,3]. Diabetics typically demonstrate dyslipidemia with increased triglyceridemia and reduced HDL - cholesterolemia.

As discussed elsewhere in this book, cardiovascular diseases including myocardial infarction, stroke and heart failure as the major cause of morbidity and mortality in both Type 1 and 2 diabetes, and are increased two-to four-fold compared to age-and sex-matched individuals in the nondiabetic population. Premenopausal women who become diabetic assume the cardiovascular risk of age-matched men and lose the benefits asiociated with normal ovarian function. Silent ischemia and myocardial infarction (MI) are more common and the outcome of an MI is worse than in people who are not diabetic.

Diabetes and Cardiovascular Disease: Etiology, Treatment and Outcomes
Edited by Aubie Angel *et al.*, Kluwer Academic/Plenum Publishers, 2001

In Type 1 diabetes, blood pressure is usually "normal" at presentation. Hypertension typically develops with the onset of nephropathy, and is characterized by systolic and diastolic blood pressure elevation. About half of Type 1 diabetics with 30 or more years of diabetes have hypertension. People with Type 2 diabetes are generally older and are often hypertensive at the time of diagnosis. The increase in blood pressure is generally correlated with obesity, decreased physical activity and older age. Isolated systolic hypertension (usually defined as systolic BP of 160 mmHg or greater in association with diastolic BP less than 90 mmHg) is particularly common in Type 2 diabetes.

Because hypertension is a major contributor to the dramatically increased morbidity and mortality in both Type 1 and 2 diabetes, it seems entirely reasonable to argue that high blood pressure should be diagnosed and treated early and aggressively. Despite the lack of rigorous scientific evidence to support this approach until recently, most international guidelines have urged that diabetics with hypertension be treated to lower blood pressures than non-diabetics, especially if they show renal involvement with microalbuminuria[4]. Both non-pharmacological and pharmacological treatments are recommended to achieve the goal of near-normal or ideal blood pressure.

PROSPECTIVE CLINICAL TRIALS OF HYPERTENSION AND DIABETES

Major clinical trials published during the past few years provide ample evidence that aggressive lowering of blood pressure can indeed result in marked reduction of cardiovascular morbidity and mortality in hypertensive diabetics. This will be the major focus of this chapter. Some earlier trials have conducted *post hoc* subgroup analyses of diabetic patients, e.g. SHEP[5] and Syst-Eur[6]; more recent studies have prospectively stratified for specific risk factors including the presence of diabetes in a major trial of hypertension outcomes (HOT)[7] and a study of hypertensives within a trial designed initially to investigate the benefits of strict euglycemic control (UKPDS)[8]. The latter trials are the most convincing by virtue of their prospective hypotheses and their designs which included sufficient patients over an adequate period of time to be methodologically robust.

HOT - The Hypertension Optimal Treatment Study

The Hypertension Optimal Treatment (HOT)[7] investigated the effects of targeting blood pressure to <90, <85 and <80 mmHg blood pressure among 18,780 patients in 26 countries followed for almost 4 years. Within this entire HOT Study population, 1501 patient (8%) were diabetic. At study entry, diabetic patients in HOT were approximately 63 years of age, a little older than the study-wide average of 61.5 years. While average diastolic BP at entry was similar between diabetic and non-diabetic participants at 105 mmHg, systolic BP was higher in diabetics, 175 vs. 170 mmHg. Patients were treated with a 5-step regimen consisting of the dihydropyridine vasoselective calcium blocker felodipine 5 mg, followed as needed by an ACE inhibitor, a beta-blocker and/or a low dose thiazide diuretic.

The overall HOT study results showed no difference by intention to treat between the <90, <85 and <80 mmHg treatment groups, with approximately 10 major cardiovascular events per 1000 patient-years in each study group. However, major cardiovascular events (fatal and nonfatal myocardial infarctions, fatal and nonfatal strokes and all other cardiovascular deaths) were reduced from 24.4 events per 1000 patient-years in the 501 patients in the <90 mmHg group to 11.9 events per 1000 patient-years in the 499 diabetic patients in the <80 mmHg group, p-value for trend 0.005. Cardiovascular mortality dropped from 11.1 per 1000 patient-years to 3.7 per 1000 patient-years, p-value for trend 0.016, while total mortality was 15.9 per 1000 patient-years in the <90 group versus 9.0 in the <80 mmHg group, p-value for trend 0.068. Consequently, HOT was the first prospective, randomised trial of rigorous BP control in a diabetes population to show that the anticipated benefits of lower BP do indeed occur, with reduced macrovascular morbidity and mortality.

UKPDS - The United Kingdom Prospective Diabetes Study

The United Kingdom Prospective Diabetes Study (UKPDS)[8] investigated tight blood pressure control and risk of macrovascular and microvascular complications in Type 2 diabetes. UKPDS was designed with the major objective of determining the impact of tight glycemic control in middle-aged diabetic patients. At study entry patients were 56 years of age on average and 1,544 (38%) were hypertensive. Of these, a total of 1,148 patients entered the hypertension in diabetes substudy. Patients were randomized to less tight control of blood pressure (n=390) or to tight control of blood pressure (target <150/85 mmHg, n=758), of whom 400 were further randomized to treatment with an ACE inhibitor based treatment and 358 to control with a regimen that started with beta-blockade.

The salient findings in UKPDS were an approximately 10/5 mmHg greater reduction in blood pressure and an average achieved blood pressure of 144/82 in the patients treated with the tight blood pressure control policy. There was a reduction in any diabetes-related endpoint by 24%, p=0.0046; a decrease in diabetes-related death by 32%, p=0.019; a reduction in stroke by 44%, p=0.013; a reduction in microvascular disease by 37%, p=0.0092; a reduction by heart failure by 56%, p=0.0043; a delay in retinopathy progression by 34%, p=0.0038 and less deterioration of vision by 47%, p=0.0036. There was no difference in BP lowering or clinical outcomes between the ACE inhibitor and beta-blocker based protocols. UKPDS confirmed the benefits of better blood presssure control on macrovascular events and on mortality and was the first study to demonstrate prospectively the benefits of BP control on microvascular disease in the eye and the kidney. The treatment of middle-aged and older hypertensives is very cost-effective[9]. In UKPDS only 11 (6 to 29) patients needed to be treated (NNT) more aggressively over the 8.4 years duration of the study to prevent any diabetes-related clinical end point and the NNT to avoid a diabetes-related death was only 20.

RETROSPECTIVE ANALYSES OF TRIALS WITH DIABETIC POPULATIONS

While HOT and UKPDS have independently demonstrated the merits of BP control in a scientifically robust manner, we should also respect the lessons learned from other major studies in which there have been sufficient hypertensive patients with diabetes for adequate substudies to be undertaken. The most important of these have been SHEP[5] and Syst-Eur[6].

SHEP - The Systolic Hypertension in the Elderly Program

Cardiovascular outcomes in a subgroup of 583 non-insulin-dependent diabetic patients in the Systolic Hypertension in the Elderly Program (SHEP)[5] were compared retrospectively with outcomes in 4,149 nondiabetic patients. The SHEP antihypertensive drug regimen of chlorthalidone 12.5-25 mg daily with a step-up to atenolol 25-50 mg daily or reserpine 0.05-0.1 mg daily lowered systolic BP effectively in both diabetic and nondiabetic patients and was well tolerated. All outcome rates were lower for participants randomized to the active treatment group than for those randomized to the placebo group. Five year major cardiovascular disease rate was lowered by 34% for active treatment compared with placebo for both diabetic patients and nondiabetic patients. Absolute risk reduction with active treatment compared with placebo was twice as great for diabetic versus nondiabetic patients (101/1000 versus 51/1000 randomized participants at the five year follow-up), presumably reflecting the higher baseline risk of diabetic patients.

Syst-Eur - The Systolic Hypertension in Europe Trial

Likewise, in the Systolic Hypertension Europe Study (Syst-Eur)[6] antihypertensive therapy beginning with the calcium channel blocker nitrendipine was at least as effective in patients with diabetes as in those without diabetes at entry. A detailed comparison of SHEP and Syst-Eur concludes that there may be advantages of the calcium channel blocker based regimen in the European study over the diuretic based regimen employed in the North American study[10].

RECENT CARDIOVASCULAR STUDIES

There are other lessons to be learned from three more recent studies in which results from subgroups of diabetics have been examined to determine the benefits of BP control or of specific medications. These are CAPPP[11], STOP Hypertension-2[12], and HOPE[13], all of which will be discussed in more detail below. Data on diabetic patients are presently incomplete and will likely be described in greater detail in later publications.

CAPPP - The Capopril Prevention Project

The Captopril Prevention Project (CAPPP)[11] was a prospective, randomised intervention trial to compare the effects of ACE inhibition and conventional therapy on cardiovascular morbidity and mortality in patients with hypertension. 10,985 patients aged 25-66 years with a diastolic blood pressure of 100 mmHg or more were enrolled in Sweden and Finland. Patients were randomly assigned the ACE inhibitor captopril or "conventional" antihypertensive treatment (diuretics, beta-blockers). Primary endpoint events occurred at rate of 11.1 per 1000 patient-years in the captopril group and 10.2 per 1000 patient-years in the conventional-treatment group (relative risk 1.05 [95% CI 0.90- 1.22], p=0.52). Cardiovascular mortality was lower with captopril than with conventional treatment (76 vs 95 events; relative risk 0.77 [0.57- 1.04], p=0.092). The rate of fatal and non-fatal myocardial infarction was similar (162 vs 161), but fatal and non-fatal stroke was more common with captopril (189 vs 148; RR1.25 [1.01-1.55]. p=0.044). Captopril and conventional treatment did not differ in efficacy in preventing cardiovascular morbidity and mortality. The difference in stroke risk was thought to be due to the lower levels of blood pressure obtained initially in previously treated patients randomised to conventional therapy.

There were 572 patients with diabetes mellitus Type 2 in CAPPP. In this group the ACE inhibitor captopril was superior to the diuretic/beta-blocker regimen in preventing cardiovascular complications. This conclusion conflicts, therefore, with that of UKPDS in which no difference was found between beta-blocker based treatment and a regimen based on an ACE inhibitor.

STOP Hypertension-2 - The Swedish Treatment of Old Patients with Hypertension-2 Study

The second Swedish Treatment of Older Persons with Hypertension 2 (STOP Hypertension-2)[12] compared the efffiacy of "newer" antihypertensive drugs with the effects of "conventional" antihypertensive drugs on cardiovascular mortality and morbidity in elderly patients. This was a prospective, randomised trial involving 6614 patients aged 70-84 years with hypertension (blood pressure of 180 mmHg systolic or greater, 105 mm Hg diastolic or greater, or both). Patients were randomly assigned "conventional" antihypertensive drugs (atenolol 50 mg, metoprolol 100 mg, pindolol 5 mg, hydrochlorothiazide 25 mg plus amiloride 2.5 mg daily) or "newer" drugs (enalapril 10 mg or lisinopril 10 mg, or felodipine 2.5 mg or isradipine 2.5 mg daily). Primary outcome included fatal stroke, fatal myocardial infarction and other fatal cardiovascular disease.

Blood pressure was decreased to a similar extent in all treatment groups. The primary combined endpoint of fatal stroke, fatal myocardial infarction, and other fatal cardiovascular disease occurred in both drugs group at a rate of 19.8 events per 1000 patient-years. Decrease in blood pressure was of major importance for the prevention of cardiovascular event. Among the 719 diabetic patients randomised to either conventional or newer antihypertensive treatment, neither treatment was found to be superior to the other.

HOPE - The Heart Outcomes Prevention Evaluation Study

The Heart Outcomes Prevention Evaluation (HOPE)[13] study was not really an investigation of hypertension or diabetes but its conclusions are relevant to this discussion. HOPE investigated the possible benefits of the ACE inhibitor ramipril, Vitamin E, or their combination in a double-blind, placebo controlled randomised study of individuals at higher risk of cardiovascular events because of their age, and the presence of diabetes, hypertension or other known risk factors. Greatest absolute benefit of ramipril was observed within the group of subjects with both diabetes and hypertension, but blood pressure reduction with ramipril was only 2 mmHg greater than in the control group. To date Vitamin E has shown no protective benefit, even in higher risk patients with diabetes and hypertension.

IS THERE A PREFERRED DRUG OR DRUGS TO LOWER BP?

The studies discussed have used a variety of antihypertensive regimens. Benefits observed in all of these studies, irrespective of the initial antihypertensive medication chosen, suggest that blood pressure reduction itself is more important than the choice of a particular treatment. The results confirm earlier recommendations that systolic BP should be targeted to <130 and diastolic blood pressure should be targeted to <80 mmHg.

Aggressive blood pressure control in the hypertensive with diabetes is associated with absolute risk reduction approximating 30-50% compared with more conventionally managed patients. Benefits are observed with very small numbers of patients needed to be treated and treatment is extremely cost-effective[9]In any case, most patients will require two or more antihypertensive drugs to achieve optimal blood pressure lowering [7,8]. Although ACE inhibitors have generally been preferred because of their proven benefits in delaying progression of end stage renal disease[14,15,16], UKPDS suggests that beta-blocker based treatment is equally effective and well tolerated. Although there have been concerns about the use of thiazide diuretics in Type 2 diabetic patients, the results of SHEP indicate that a diuretic-based regimen is not only effective but well tolerated in older diabetics with isolated systolic hypertension. The debate about the use of calcium channel blockers will likely continue given the observations that some may increase CV risk relative to ACE inhibitors[17,18,19]. However, results from HOT, a retrospective analysis of Syst-Eur and STOP Hypertension-2 add needed balance to this discussion. There appear to be equal benefits from the older diuretics and beta-blockers and the newer ACE inhibitors and calcium blockers.

Whether or not the latest antihypertensive medication class, the Angiotensin II AT1 receptor antagonists/blockers (ARAs, ARBs), will be as effective in reducing the morbidity and mortality associated with hypertension in the diabetic remains unknown. Given the similarity of their pharmacological action to ACE inhibitors on the endothelium, kidney and myocardium, one would be hard pressed to argue that ARBs will be any less effective in "hard" clinical outcomes. The excellent tolerability of ARBs augurs well for long term concordance with treatment. They are useful in combination with diuretics and other classes of antihypertensives and are not associated with any important kinetic or dynamic interactions with other medications likely to be ingested by patients with hypertension and diabetes. Longterm studies with clinical outcomes are awaited with interest. They should be used in patients intolerant of ACE inhibitors.

NON-PHARMACOLOGIC TREATMENT

A brief word on non-pharmacologic intervention is needed. Weight loss, reduced alcohol consumption and limited salt intake are recommended and must be strongly encouraged. A recent study demonstrates the utility of weight loss or aerobic exercise in improving blood pressure in diabetic hypertensives[20]. Remarkably, the combination of exercise and weight loss was not better than either intervention alone. However, longterm clinical outcomes might be improved by combining exercise and weight loss.

SUMMARY

In summary, the present information on treating hypertension in the diabetic overwhelmingly indicates a compelling need to lower BP to target diastolic BP of 80 mmHg or less[21], to be less concerned about the types of drugs used than the blood pressures achieved and the concordance with therapy and to rely on two or more antihypertensive drugs in the majority of cases. Management of the hypertensive diabetic is very cost-effective. It is clear that we must engage in total cardiovascular risk management if we are to prevent the microvascular and macrovascular complications in the hypertensive diabetic (or the diabetic hypertensive).

REFERENCES

1. Johnson KC, Graney MJ, Applegate WB et al Prevalence of undiagnosed non-insulin dependent diabetes mellitus and impaired glucose tolerance in a cohort of older persons with hypertension. J Am Geriatr Soc 1997; 45:695-700.
2. Kannel WB, McGee DL. Diabetes and cardiovascular disease: the Framingham study. JAMA 1979;241:2035-939.
3. Wang SL, Head J, Stevens L, Fuller JH. Excess mortality and its relation to hypertension and proteinuria in diabetic patients. The WHO Multinational Study of Vascular Disease in Diabetes. Diabetes Care 1996;19:305-12.
4. The sixth report of the Joint National Committee on prevention, detection, evaluation, and treatment of high blood pressure. Arch Intern Med 1997; 157:2413-46. [Erratum, Arch Intern Med 1998;158:573.]
5. Curb JD, Pressel SL, Cutler JA et al Effective diuretic-based antihypertensive treatment on cardiovascular disease risk in older diabetic patients with isolated systolic hypertensive. Systolic Hypertension in the Elderly Program Cooperative Research Group JAMA 1996; 276:1886-1892 Comment in ACP J Club 1997 126 (3):57.
6. Staessen JA, Thijs L,Gasowski J et al. Treatment of isolated systolic hypertension in the elderly: Further evidence from the systolic hypertension in Europe (SYST-EUR) trial. Am J Cardiol 1998; 82(9B): 20R-22R.
7. Hansson L, Zanchetti A, Carruthers SG, et al. Effects of intensive blood pressure lowering and low dose aspirin in patients with hypertension: Principal results of the Hypertension Optimal Treatment (HOT) randomized trial. HOT Study Group. Lancet 1998; 351: 1755-62.
8. UK Prospective Diabetes Study Group. Tight blood pressure control and risk of macrovascular and microvascular complications in Type 2 diabetes: UKPDS 38. BMJ 1998; 317: 703-713.
9. UK Prospective Diabetes Study Group. Cost effectiveness analysis of improved blood pressure control in hypertensive patients with type 2 diabetes: UKPDS 40. BMJ 1998;317:720-6
10. Tuomilehto J, Rastenyte D, Birkenhager WH et al. Effects of calcium-channel blockade in older patients with diabetes and systolic hypertension. NEJM 1999; 340:677-84.
11. Hansson L, Lindholm LH, Niskanen L, Lanke J et al. Effect of angiotension-converting-enzyme inhibition compared with conventional therapy on cardiovascular morbidity and mortality in hypertension: the Captopril Prevention Project (CAPPP) randomised trial. Lancet 1999;353:611-6.
12. Hansson L, Lindholm LH, Ekbom T, Dahlof B et al. Randomised trial of old and new antihypertensive drugs in elderly patients: cardiovascular mortality and morbidity the Swedish Trial in Old Patients with Hypertension-2 study. Lancet 1999;354:1751-6
13. The Heart Outcomes Prevention Evaluation Study Investigators. Effects of an angiotensin-converting-

enzyme inhibitor, ramipril, on death from cardiovascular causes, myocardial infarction, and stroke in high risk patients. NEJM 2000; (to be published January 20, 2000)

14. Mathiesen ER, Hommel E, Giese J, Parving HH. Efficacy of captopril in postponing nephropathy in normotensive insulin dependent diabetic patients with microalbuminuria. BMJ 1991;303:81-7.

15. Bjorck S, Mulec H, Johnsen SA, Norden G et al. Renal protective effect of enalapril in diabetic nephropathy. BMJ 1992;304:339-43.

16. Lewis EJ, Hunsicker LG, Bain RP, Rohde RD. The effect of angiotension-converting-enzyme inhibition on diabetic nephropathy. N Engl J Med 1993;329:1456-62.

17. Tatti P, Pahor M, Byington RB et al. Outcome results of the Fosinopril Versus Amlodipine Cardiovascular Events Randomized Trial (FACET) in patients with hypertension and NIDDM. Diabetes Care 1998; 21:597-603.

18. Estacio RO, Jeffers BW, Hiatt WR et al. The effect of nisoldipine as compared with enalapril on cardiovascular outcomes inpatients with non-insulin-dependent diabetes and hypertension. NEJM 1998; 338:645-52.

19. Malmberg K, Ryden L, Wedel H. Calcium antagonists, appropriate therapy for diabetic patients with hypertension? Eur Heart J 1998; 19:1269-72.

20. Dengel DR, Galecki AT, Hagberg JM et al. The independent and combined effects of weight loss and aerobic exercise on blood pressure and oral glucose tolerance in older men. Am J Hypertens 1998; 11;1405-12.

21. Feldman RD, Campbell N, Larochelle P Bolli et al. 1999 Canadian recommendations for the management of hypertension. CMAJ 1999;161:S1-S17.

LEFT VENTRICULAR DIASTOLIC DYSFUNCTION IN DIABETIC OR HYPERTENSIVE SUBJECTS: ROLE OF COLLAGEN ALTERATIONS

T. J. Regan, G. N. Jyothirmayi, C. Laham and A. Jain

Department of Medicine, UMDNJ-NJ Medical School
185 South Orange Avenue, Newark, NJ 07103

INTRODUCTION

Diabetes and hypertension may be associated with myocardial rather than coronary diseases as the preventing clinical abnormality[1,2]. An early functional alteration of the left ventricle in these states is often diastolic rather than systolic. In addition abnormalities of glucose and insulin metabolism that are less than seen in frank diabetes have recently been described for the hypertensive state[3]. In view of the observation that glucose intolerance in a normotensive canine model has been associated with diastolic dysfunction and interstitial fibrosis of the ventricle,[4] a potential role of the metabolic abnormality in the myocardial response to hypertension has been raised.

Since moderate obesity is often present in patients with these disease states and may itself affect diastolic function,[5] as well as insulin and glucose metabolism,[3] the influence of associated obesity has been examined. Left ventricular diastolic and systolic function, as well as mass, have been assessed in the absence of significant coronary occlusive disease.

In addition patients with normal or elevated arterial pressure who were either lean or obese constituted 4 groups that were compared for hemodynamic and metabolic alterations. Two groups of normotensive diabetics were studied to determine if the left ventricular abnormalities of chronic hyperglycemia differed in lean and obese subjects.

METHODS

Subjects undergoing catheterization for chest pain were included in the study when significant coronary disease was not present. There were two groups of diabetics, the lean and the obese. For the non-diabetic study groups 1 (lean) and 2 (obese) were normotensive and groups 3 (lean) and 4 (obese) were hypertensive. Intraventricular pressures and angiographic volumes of the left ventricle were determined. Fasting plasma glucose, insulin, hemoglobin$_{A1c}$ and glucose tolerance were assessed[6] in each group.

RESULTS

Diabetes and Cardiovascular Disease: Etiology, Treatment and Outcomes
Edited by Aubie Angel *et al.*, Kluwer Academic/Plenum Publishers, 2001

127

Table 1 Clinical Characteristics of Diabetic Groups

	Diabetic/Lean (n=8)	Diabetic/Obese (n=7)
Age (Y)	59.4 ± 2.1	54.0 ± 2.8
Sex (M/F)	3/5	4/3
BMI (kg/m^2)	25.1 ± 0.86	30.9 ± 0.86*
Heart rate (bpm)	77.1 ± 4.0	83.5 ± 11.3
Arterial pressure (mmHg)		
Systolic	131.6 ± 6.3	132.0 ± 8.7
Diastolic	73.0 ± 4.4	70.3 ± 4.2

bpm indicates beats per minute.
*-Significant difference.

Table 2 Left Ventricular Parameters

	Diabetic/Lean (n=8)	Diabetic/Obese (n=7)
Diastolic Parameter		
LVDP (end) (mmHg)	12.0 ± 1.7	22.1 ± 2.1*
LVDP (early) (mmHg)	1.20 ± 0.5	1.30 ± 0.6
EDVI (mL/kg)	77.06 ± 9.13	89.90 ± 7.4
H$_{80}$ (cm)	0.96 ± 0.02	0.99 ± 0.06
LVMI (g/m)	139.0 ± 18.19	166.0 ± 16.71
KP (mmH .m^2.mL^{-1})	0.86 ± 0.26	1.44 ± 0.26*
KPV (mmH .m^2.mL^{-1})	56.96 ± 14.04	120.6 ± 12.92*
K*EDWS (g/cm^2)	1.80 ± 0.55	3.01 ± 0.5
Systolic Parameter		
Ejection fraction (%)	61.6 ± 4.2	58.6 ± 3.8
ESWS (g/cm^2)	77.2 ± 14.5	91.4 ± 18.1

LVDP-left ventricular diastolic pressure; EDVI-end diastolic volume index; H$_{80}$-left ventricular end-diastolic wall thickness; LVMI-left ventricular mass index; KP-chamber stiffness; KPV-chamber stiffness normalized for volume; EDWS-end-diastolic wall stress; ESWS-end-systolic wall stress.
*-Significant difference.

Diabetics

The lean and obese diabetics had similar clinical characteristics except for the adiposity parameters (Table 1). Arterial pressure was normal in both groups. Fasting blood glucose and hemoglobin$_{A1c}$ were 154 ± 22 mg% and 6.9 ± 0.85% respectively, in the lean subjects while the obese diabetics had values of 175 ± 36.7 mg% (NS) and 10.9 ± 1.4% (P<0.05).

Ejection fraction was normal in both groups. Left ventricular end-diastolic pressure, and chamber stiffness (KPV) were significantly greater in the obese group whereas K*EDWS was just outside this range (Table 2).

Table 3 Clinical Characteristics of Nonhypertensive and Hypertensive Groups

	Nonhypertensive		Hypertensive	
	Group 1 (n=8)	Group 2 (n=7)	Group 3 (n=17)	Group 4 (n=15)
Age (Y)	53 ± 3.1	46 ± 4.63*	59.4 ± 1.95	57 ± 2.49
Sex (M/F)	3/5	4/3	8/9	6/9
BMI (kg/m²)	23.8 ± 0.89	30.0 ± 1.1*	24.7 ± 0.51	32.2 ± 0.75*
Heart rate (bpm)	70.9 ± 4.3	73.7 ± 2.6	77.2 ± 3.9	75.6 ± 3.9
Systolic blood pressure (mmHg)	118 ± 3.9	129 ± 3.2*	150 ± 4.3*	157 ± 4.2*
Diastolic blood pressure (mmHg)	69 ± 3.7	75 ± 3.9	79 ± 1.8*	83 ± 1.9*

bpm – beats per minute.
* - Significantly different vs. group 1.

Hypertensives

Ages were comparable in the four subgroups of the hypertensive study (Table 3). Groups 2 and 4 had a mean BMI that was significantly higher than that of groups 1 and 3. Heart rate was similar in the four groups, and arterial pressure was normal in groups 1 and 2. Systolic blood pressure was significantly higher in both hypertensive groups.

Systolic function did not differ in the four groups (Table 4). Left ventricular end-diastolic pressure was significantly higher in lean and obese hypertensives than in either normotensive group; the initial diastolic pressure did not differ. End-diastolic volume index was comparable in the four groups. The nonindexed volume was 165 ± 13 mL in group 1, 195 ± 11 mL in group 2 (P<0.02), 151 ± 7.4 mL in group 3, and 189 ± 14 mL in group 4 (P<0.03).

Chamber stiffness values, KPV and K*EDWS were significantly higher in lean and obese hypertensives than in the control subjects of group 1. The association of obesity with hypertension revealed a significantly higher KPV and K*EDWS than in group 3. LVMI was significantly higher in lean and obese hypertensives than in the respective normotensives, but the difference between the hypertensive groups was not significant.

Fasting blood sugar and insulin levels were significantly higher in groups 2 through 4 than in group 1 (Table 5). Group 4 was considered glucose intolerant rather than diabetic because fasting glucose was 116 ± 4.6 mg%, below the 140 mg% threshold for the diagnosis of diabetes. Moreover, hemoglobin$_{A1c}$ and glucose tolerance did not differ significantly from groups 2 and 3. The planimetered area for plasma glucose during the glucose tolerance test was increased in each group compared with group 1 but did not reach significance. Only the obese of group 2 showed a significant insulin response to the oral feeding, 64.8 ± 18.2 mU h/L versus 37 ± 5.3 in group 1.

The parameters of diastolic function in the four groups were compared with metabolic variables by univariate analysis. Fasting glucose correlated with KPV (P<0.006). LVMI was not significantly related to fasting glucose, insulin or KPV. When comparing lean hypertensives with lean diabetics, only KP was significantly higher in the latter. Obese diabetics, however, had significantly higher KP, KPV and LVMI than did obese hypertensives.

Table 4 Left Ventricular Characteristics

| | Nonhypertensive | | Hypertensive | |
	Group 1 (n=8)	Group 2 (n=7)	Group 3 (n=17)	Group 4 (n=15)
Diastolic Parameter				
LVDP (end) (mmHg)	9.1 ± 0.79	12.6 ± 2.25	15.0±1.41*	22.7±0.94*†‡
LVDP (early) (mmHg)	1.7 ± 0.48	2.3 ± 0.60	2.3 ± 0.63	2.7 ± 0.89
EDVI (mL/kg)	80.19 ± 6.61	83.7 ± 4.93	75.6 ± 4.17	84.1± 6.42
H_{80} (cm)	0.83 ± 0.04	0.97 ± 0.06	1.03 ± 0.04*	1.08± 0.06*
LVMI (g/m)	95.63 ± 4.20	129.8 ± 9.42*	126.5 ± 7.41*	141.0±13.3*
KP (mmH .m².mL⁻¹)	0.14 ± 0.002	0.16 ± 0.03	0.32 ± 0.04*†	0.39±0.06*†
KPV (mmH .m².mL⁻¹)	23.56 ± 3.26	32.4 ± 6.9	49.3 ± 9.5*	72.1± 7.7*†‡
K*EDWS (g/cm²)	0.73 ± 0.14	1.43 ± 0.48	1.08 ± 0.25*	2.2± 38*†
Systolic Parameter				
Ejection fraction (%)	70.3 ± 3.14	72.1 ± 2.8	68.8 ± 2.1	72.0 ± 2.7
ESWS (g/cm²)	78.5 ± 10.3	69.4 ± 16.4	72.9 ± 9.6	83.7 ± 4.0

*-Significant difference vs. group 1; †-vs. group 2; ‡- vs. group 3.
Abbreviations as for Table 2.

Table 5 Basal Plasma Glucose and Insulin

	Group 1	Group 2	Group 3	Group 4
Glucose (mg%)	83 ± 2.8	101 ± 6.2*	103 ± 5.4*	116 ± 4.6*†
Hemoglobin$_{A1c}$ (%)	5.64 ± 0.65	5.52 ± 0.8	5.80 ± 0.37	6.50 ± 0.28
Plasma Insulin (μU/mL)	8.8 ± 1.2	17.9 ± 3.2*	14.9 ± 2.2*	15.3 ± 2.7*

*-Significant difference vs. group 1.
†- Significant difference vs. groups 2 and 3.

DISCUSSION

Diabetes

Prior hemodynamic descriptions in diabetics have not distinguished between the lean and obese states[1]. When moderate obesity was associated with diabetes in this study, there was a greater abnormality of end-diastolic function, which is assumed to be related to further alterations in myocardial interstitium, but a contribution of hypertrophy in diabetics with the larger ventricular mass is an important consideration.

Hemoglobin$_{A1c}$ levels were significantly higher in the obese diabetics, which is consistent with a greater degree of glycation in proteins that have a relatively slow turnover. Such a process affecting myocardial collagen may result in further interstitial accumulation and thus affect end-diastolic stiffness. Morphological evidence for collagen accumulation has been reported in human diabetes [1,7,8,9].

Hypertension

Diastolic stiffness was increased in lean hypertensives compared with lean control subjects, associated with an increase in basal fasting plasma glucose and insulin. The modest extent of the diastolic abnormality in the lean hypertensives suggests that the development of heart failure may be less likely in the absence of obesity.
Diastolic abnormalities observed in the lean hypertensives were generally greater in group 4. In the obese hypertensives, further alterations that promote myocardial stiffness are suggested, which may be related to the higher fasting plasma glucose, as discussed below.
Left ventricular hypertrophy, as a potential contributor, did not significantly correlate with KPV in the hypertensive groups. A clear dissociation of these phenomena has been achieved in the spontaneously hypertensive rat with use of a therapeutic intervention that normalized myocardial fibrosis without affecting hypertrophy[10]. Nevertheless, left ventricular stiffness was also normalized. A myocyte contribution to stiffness has been described in cell cultures and has been attributed to proteins of the cytoskeleton,[11] but the role in hypertensive hypertrophy is not known.

Pathogenesis

The pathophysiology of the diastolic abnormality in the obese hypertensive may be related to alterations in glucose and insulin metabolism. Although plasma insulin increments have been associated with hypertrophy in moderately obese subjects[12] and hypertensives,[3] the hypertrophy of obese hypertensives was not associated with additional insulin increments. A prior observation indicated that experimental glucose intolerance associated with enhanced diastolic stiffness was not related to plasma insulin [13]. The influence of other hormones and cytokines on this process is not yet defined.

The observation that the degree of fasting hyperglycemia in the hypertensives correlated with myocardial stiffness abnormality may provide a clue to pathogenesis. In the glucose intolerant canine model, fasting glucose was in the high normal range and apparently was sufficient to elicit an increase in diastolic stiffness and interstitial collagen in the absence of hypertension. That hyperglycemia may have a major role in pathogenesis is supported by observations in cultured mesangial[14] and neural cells[15] in which collagen synthesis as enhanced when the media contained elevated glucose concentrations.   A more complex situation has been suggested from preliminary observations in the canine model with chronic glucose intolerance[16]. Insoluble collagen was increased in myocardium. This appeared to be attributable to the formation of advanced glycosylation products, presumed to result in increased collagen cross-links.

An increase of left ventricular diastolic stiffness without systolic dysfunction characterized this canine model of impaired glucose tolerance compared to normal controls[16]. Diastolic dysfunction was associated with an increased concentration of collagen in myocardium in the absence of left ventricular hypertrophy. On morphologic study interstitial fibrosis was observed in diabetic animals without evidence of replacement fibrosis. Although a change in collagen phenotypes may occur during cardiac remodeling, a disproportionate increase of Type I collagen, which may enhance stiffness, compared to Types III and V has not been found in the myocardium of the glucose intolerant model[16].

Aminoguanidine has been used to modify the glucose derived cross-link formation in diabetes without affecting enzymatically derived collagen cross-links[17]. Persistence of collagen accumulation after pharmacologic intervention suggested that concentration increases were unrelated to advanced glycosylation. Improved diastolic function occurred despite increased myocardial collagen concentrations. Of interest is the observation that diminished collagenase gene expression in diabetic kidney may be a basis for collagen accumulation[18] and has recently been observed in myocardium[19].

PERMISSIONS

American Heart Association has approved Publication of the tables.

REFERENCES

1. T.J. Regan, M.M. Lyons, S.S. Ahmed, G.E. Levinson, H.A. Oldewortel, M.R. Ahmad, and B. Haider, Evidence for cardiomyopathy in familial diabetes mellitus, *J. Clin. Invest.* **60**, 885-899 (1977).
2. E. Frohlich, Coordinating Committee Working Group of the National High Blood Pressure Education Program: the heart in hypertension, *New Engl. J. Med.* **327**, 998-1007 (1992).
3. A.L.M. Swislocki, B.B. Hoffman, and G.M. Reaven, Insulin resistance, glucose intolerance and hyperinsulinemia in patients with hypertension, *Am. J. Hypertens.* **2**, 419-423 (1989).
4. G.F. Avendano, R.K. Agarwal, R.I. Bashey, M.M. Lyons, B.J. Soni, G.N. Jyothirmayi, and T.J. Regan, Effects of glucose intolerance on myocardial function and collagen-linked glycation, *Diabetes.* **48** 1443-1447 (1999).
5. B.A. Carabello and L. Gitten, Cardiac mechanics and function in obese normotensive persons with normal coronary arteries, *Am. J. Cardiol.* **59**, 469-473 (1987).
6. A. Jain, G. Avendano, S. Dharamsey, A. Dasmahapatra, R. Agarwal, A. Reddi, and T. Regan, Left ventricular diastolic function in hypertension and role of plasma glucose and insulin: comparison with diabetic heart, *Circulation.* **93**, 1396-1402 (1996).
7. E.K. Shirey, W.L. Proudfit, and W.A. Hawk, Primary myocardial disease: correction with clinical findings, angiographic and biopsy diagnosis: follow-up of 139 patients. *Am. Heart. J.* **99**, 198-207 (1980).
8. U. Baandrup and E.G.J. Olsen, Critical analysis of endomyocardial biopsies from patients suspected of having cardiomyopathy. I: morphological and morphometric aspects, *Br. Heart J.* **45**, 475-486 (1981).
9. K.H. Van Hoeven and S.M. Factor, A comparison of the pathological spectrum of hypertensive, diabetic and hypertensive-diabetic heart disease, *Circulation.* **82**, 848-855 (1990).
10. C.G. Brilla , J.S. Janicki, and K.T. Weber, Impaired diastolic function and coronary reserve in genetic hypertension, *Circ. Res.* **69**, 108-114 (1991).
11. A.J. Brady, Mechanical properties of isolated cardiac myocytes, *Physiol. Rev.* **71**, 413-428 (1991).
12. Z. Sasson, Y. Rasolly, T. Bhesania, and I. Rasolly, Insulin resistance is an important determinant of left ventricular mass in the obese, *Circulation.* **88**, 1431-1436 (1993).
13. T.J. Regan, C.F. Wu, C.K. Yeh, H.A. Oldewurtle, and B. Haider, Myocardial composition and function in diabetes: the effect of chronic insulin use, *Circ. Res.* **49**, 1268-1277 (1981).
14. T. Danne, M.J. Spiro, and R.G. Spiro, Effect of high glucose on type IV collagen production by cultured glomerular epithelial, endothelial and mesangial cells, *Diabetes.* **42**, 170-177 (1993).
15. P. Muona, J. Peltonen, S. Jaakkola, and J. Uitto, Increased matrix gene expression by glucose in rat neural connective tissue cell in culture, *Diabetes.* **40**, 605-611 (1991).
16. G. Avendano, R. Agrawal, R. Bashey, and P. Rameshwar, and T.J. Regan, Role of TGF-β_1 in the collagen accumulation of diabetic myocardium, *J. Invest. Med.* **44**, 292A (1996).
17. M. Brownlee, Glycation and diabetic complications, *Diabetes.* **43**, 836-841 (1994).
18. T. Nakamura, T. Takahashi, M. Fukul, I. Eblhara, S. Osada, Y. Tomino, and H. Koide, Enalapril attenuates increased gene expression of extracellular matrix components in diabetic rats, *J. Am. Soc. Nephrol.* **5**, 1492-1497 (1995).
19. T.J. Regan, B.J. Soni, M. Masurekar, and G.N. Jyothirmayi, Role of matrix metalloproteinases (MMPs) and advanced glycation (AGE) in interstitial fibrosis of diabetic heart (Abstract), *FASEB.* **13**, A508 (1999).

ALTERATIONS IN THE VASCULAR ACTIONS OF INSULIN IN THE PATHOGENESIS OF INSULIN RESISTANCE AND HYPERTENSION

Subodh Verma[1] and John H. McNeill[2]

[1] The Division of Cardiology
Faculty of Medicine
University of Calgary, Canada

[2] The Division of Pharmacology and Toxicology
Faculty of Pharmaceutical Sciences
The University of British Columbia, Canada

INTRODUCTION

Resistance to the metabolic effects of insulin (insulin resistance) and hyperinsulinemia have been suggested to contribute to a cluster of abnormalities including diabetes, hypertension, obesity, hyperlipidemia, atherosclerosis, coronary artery disease and polycystic ovary syndrome.[1-5] One of our primary interests has been the role of insulin resistance and hyperinsulinemia in the pathogenesis of hypertension independent of obesity and diabetes. In a series of studies we have demonstrated that drugs that specifically improve insulin sensitivity (counter insulin resistance) and decrease plasma insulin levels both prevent and reverse hypertension in experimental models of high blood pressure (BP).[3,4,6-12] These data lend credence to the notion that insulin resistance and hyperinsulinemia may play an important role in the final expression of high BP. Following these observations, we focussed our efforts towards elucidating the mechanisms through which insulin resistance and hyperinsulinemia lead to hypertension in these models. Our studies have focussed on the interaction of insulin with endothelium derived relaxing and contracting factors. A growing body of evidence suggests that insulin exerts direct effects on vascular tone through stimulation of endothelium derived nitric oxide (NO). This has led to the suggestion that changes in the actions of insulin (in states of insulin resistance) may be important in modulating the expression of both cardiovascular and metabolic endpoints. For example, resistance to the vasodilatory action of insulin (vascular insulin resistance) has been documented in the insulin resistant states of diabetes, obesity and hypertension.[13-16] Vascular insulin resistance may sensitize/predispose the vasculature to the effects of pressors and lead to an increased vascular smooth muscle (VSM) tone and reactivity. As the vasodilatory actions of insulin contribute significantly to whole body glucose disposal, vasoconstriction (secondary to vascular insulin resistance) may play a role in the development and/or reinforcement of skeletal muscle/whole body insulin resistance. In this paper, we briefly discuss the relationship between insulin resistance and

Diabetes and Cardiovascular Disease: Etiology, Treatment and Outcomes
Edited by Aubie Angel et al., Kluwer Academic/Plenum Publishers, 2001

133

hypertension from a pharmacological and mechanistic standpoint. We then present some data from our laboratory that suggest that the vascular actions of insulin are altered in insulin resistant hypertensive rats and that these effects may antedate the development of high BP. For a general discussion of insulin resistance in cardiovascular regulation, the reader is referred to several comprehensive reviews.[1,3,4,17]

HEMODYNAMIC EFFECTS OF INSULIN

BP control and hypertension reflect forces governing systemic hemodynamic variables, specifically blood flow (cardiac output) and peripheral vascular resistance.[18] Arterial pressure is determined by the diverse combination of factors that affect either (or both) of these variables. Hypertension therefore results from a relative imbalance of cardiac output and systemic vascular resistance.[18] The kidney contributes to the maintenance of BP by regulating the volume of intravascular fluid. Baroreflexes, mediated by sympathetic nerves, act in combination with humoral mechanisms, including the renin-angiotensin system (RAS) to coordinate function at each level of control. One of the key observations in the field of hypertension has been the observation that insulin may have a "physiological role" in modulating the function of each of these parameters.[3,4,13] This has led to the hypothesis that that in states of insulin resistance and hyperinsulinemia, alterations in insulin's cardiovascular actions may be important in the development and/or reinforcement of high BP. The section to follow discusses some of the emerging data on insulin and vascular tone.

Effects of Insulin on Endothelial Function and Vascular Tone

The current literature supports a vasodilatory role of insulin in humans.[13-15,19-25] Insulin has specific and physiologically relevant effects to increase skeletal muscle blood flow. In recent years, results have repeatedly shown that intravenous insulin, independent of glucose changes, increases blood flow in the leg.[22-25] By combining the euglycemic clamp with the leg balance technique, these investigators also demonstrated that insulin-induced vasodilation was specific for skeletal muscle.[22-25] This effect was dose-dependent and occurred at physiological insulin concentrations with an apparent ED_{50} of 35-40 μU/ml in lean insulin-sensitive subjects. The vasodilating action of insulin has been confirmed by several groups over a range of physiological insulin concentrations and by using different techniques.[26-31]

Much current attention has focused on the interaction between insulin and the endothelium-derived nitric oxide (NO) system in mediating vasodilation, key evidence for which comes from Baron's group.[13-15,19-25,32-36] There is now compelling evidence that insulin-mediated vasodilation in humans is NO dependent. Studies by Steinberg *et al.*[36] have provided evidence for this mechanism. In their studies, intrafemoral artery infusion of the specific inhibitor of endothelium-derived NO synthesis, N^{ω}-monomethyl-L-arginine (L-NMMA), were performed under basal conditions in healthy volunteers and leg blood flow was measured by thermodilution. In a separate group, L-NMMA infusions were performed after 3 h of hyperinsulinemia during a euglycemic clamp designed to increase leg blood flow approximately two fold. At baseline, L-NMMA caused ≈25% fall in leg blood flow. During hyperinsulinemia, leg blood flow increased approximately two fold, and in contrast to baseline, L-NMMA caused a ≈50% fall in leg blood flow indicating that insulin-mediated vasodilation was NO dependent. Although the exact mechanism/s through which insulin interacts with the NO pathway in humans are unclear, studies indicate that this may involve synthesis/release of NO, but not NO action on VSM.[36] In a recent study, we examined the proposition that insulin mediated vasodilation may be mediated via tetrahydrobiopterin, an absolute cofactor requirement for NOS activation.

Our data indicate that pharmacological blockade of tetrahydrobiopterin synthesis significantly attenuates insulin's vasodepressor effects in rat femoral arteries.[35] This suggests that the effects of insulin on the L-arginine NO system may be mediated via increasing cofactor (tetrahydrobiopterin) availability.[35]

The vasodilating action of insulin raises a number of questions regarding the physiological significance of this effect. Two areas of intense research are (a) the contribution of insulin-mediated vasodilation towards glucose metabolism and (b) the role of the insulin-mediated vasodilation in the maintenance of vascular tone. In regard to the first question, Baron et al.[24] examined the contribution of insulin-mediated vasodilation to insulin's overall effect to stimulate glucose uptake in skeletal muscle. Steady state euglycemia alone caused ≈15% increase in leg glucose extraction and a two-fold increase in leg blood flow. When insulin-mediated vasodilation was inhibited, leg blood flow returned to baseline rates and the glucose extraction decreased by 50% with a net effect to reduce leg glucose uptake by ≈25%. Thus, it has been suggested that vasodilation *per se* may account for approximately one-fourth of insulin's overall effect to stimulate glucose uptake.

The role of insulin in the maintenance of vascular tone in humans has been a subject of much discussion and debate. Studies demonstrating that the vasodilatory actions of insulin are blunted in insulin resistant states of obesity and diabetes[14,15] have been extrapolated to imply that insulin-mediated vasodilation is an important determinant of vascular tone and BP. However, acute systemic or local infusions of insulin produce no change or a small change in mean arterial pressure. Studies by Anderson et al.[31] have elegantly demonstrated that although insulin causes marked reductions in forearm vascular resistance (due to vasodilation), the reason why insulin does not alter blood pressure is because it simultaneously activates the sympathetic nervous system (SNS). Thus, the effects of vasodilation are offset by an increase in SNS activity. Notwithstanding the above discussion, it is possible that in states of insulin resistance, a loss of vasodilation associated with insulin resistance could diminish vasodilatory reserve and thus "sensitize" the vasculature to the pressor forces.

A brief discussion about the effects of insulin on vascular tone in experimental animals merits attention. Studies in intact blood vessels *in-vitro* have reported both constrictory and dilatory effects of insulin.[37-44] Insulin (in pharmacological concentrations) has been shown to attenuate pressor responses in aortae from control rats.[39-42] Similar observations were made in rabbit femoral arteries and veins, where supraphysiological concentrations of insulin inhibited the vasoconstrictor effect of angiotensin II (A II).[43] Studies examining the effects of insulin on the mesenteric vasculature (MVB) have reported conflicting results. Studies have shown that physiological insulin concentrations attenuate vasoconstriction by norepinephrine (NE), serotonin and potassium chloride in mesenteric arterioles.[41,44] However, when the effects of similar concentrations of insulin are examined in the entire perfused mesenteric vascular bed (MVB), insulin consistently exaggerates the pressor responses to vasoactive agents.[39,40] We have consistently observed that at pharmacological concentrations (100 mU/ml), insulin attenuates the vasoconstrictor responses in aortae and femoral arteries. By contrast, at lower concentrations (100 μU/ml) insulin exaggerates the pressor responses of MVB to NE. These data are discussed in the sections to follow.

In contrast to the effects on NO, reports indicate that physiological concentrations of insulin stimulate the synthesis, secretion and gene expression of the potent vasoconstrictor agent endothelin (ET)-1.[45-48] Studies have demonstrated elevated ET-1 levels in insulin-treated diabetic patients and in experimental models of diabetes during insulin treatment.[47,49] Although the exact mechanism through which insulin increases ET-1 production is not known, reports indicate that this effect may be mediated through the tyrosine kinase action of insulin and probably results from the stimulation of a nuclear protein which acts in trans on cis elements of the ET-1 promoter.[45,47]

In summary, accumulating evidence from experimental and clinical studies indicate that insulin, in addition to its well-known effects on carbohydrate, lipid and protein metabolism, exhibits important hemodynamic effects. At the level of the vasculature, physiological insulin concentrations appear to cause vasodilation in humans. This, in turn, may be part of insulin's overall action to enhance glucose uptake. Studies examining the effects of insulin on reactivity of blood vessels in rats have yielded inconsistent results. This is, in part, due to the pharmacological concentrations of insulin employed and the apparent species differences in the effects of insulin in rats vs. humans. Insulin may activate completely divergent pathways, for example insulin may stimulate the L-arginine-NO system while activating the synthesis and release of the potent vasoconstrictor ET-1. Although the question as to what role insulin plays in regulating vascular tone *in-vivo* remains far from being resolved, the observation that insulin exhibits vascular effects poses the intriguing question: *are changes in insulin's cardiovascular effects in states of hyperinsulinemia and insulin resistance important in the development and/or reinforcement of hypertension?*

PHARMACOLOGICAL AND MECHANISTIC STUDIES: OUR EXPERIENCE AND INTERPRETATION

Pharmacological Modulation of Insulin Resistance and Hyperinsulinemia in Hypertension

In a series of experiments, we have recently examined the proposition that insulin resistance and hyperinsulinemia contribute causally to the development of high BP.[1,4] Essentially, if these defects were pathogenic in the development of hypertension, then drugs that counter these defects should decrease BP. We, therefore, examined the effects of multiple agents (that were known to improve insulin sensitivity; metformin, vanadium, pioglitazone) on BP in rodent models of hypertension. We found that chemically diverse drugs that had the common property of attenuating hyperinsulinemia also lowered BP in both the spontaneously hypertensive rat (SHR) and the fructose-induced hypertensive (FH) rat.[4,6-12] All of these drugs not only caused sustained reductions in plasma insulin concentrations and BP, but the antihypertensive effects of these drugs could be reversed by simply restoring the plasma insulin levels in the drug-treated rats to those that existed before drug treatment. These data indicated that insulin resistance and hyperinsulinemia were closely associated with the final expression of high BP in these models. Following these observations, our research was geared to determining the mechanisms linking these defects to hypertension with emphasis on the alteration in insulin's vascular actions in states of insulin resistance and hyperinsulinemia. Most of the studies were conducted in the FH rat. The FH rat is an acquired form of hypertension, where feeding normal male Sprague Dawley rats a fructose-enriched diet (60% fructose) results in hyperinsulinemia, insulin resistance and hypertension without changes in body weight. By employing the euglycemic hyperinsulinemic clamp technique in conscious rats, we recently demonstrated that these rats are extremely insulin resistant and hyperinsulinemic as compared to their controls.[10]

Direct Vascular Effects of Insulin in Control and Insulin Resistant and Hypertensive Rats

In a series of studies we examined the direct *in-vitro* effects of insulin on the reactivity of aortae and MVB from insulin resistant and hypertensive FH rats.[4,16,51] These studies were aimed at examining whether the vascular actions of insulin are altered in states of insulin resistance. Two key observations emanated from these studies. First, insulin's vascular effects are vessel-specific and dose-dependent. In control rat aortae, insulin at concentrations of 100 mU/ml attenuated the contractile responses to NE (Figure 1)[51] and A II, while in the MVB, insulin at concentrations of 100 µU/ml exaggerated the pressor responses to NE (not shown).[4]   Similar vessel-specific effects of insulin have been previously reported.   Second, in arteries from FH rats, insulin's vascular effects were altered in both arterial beds studied. In aortae from FH rats, insulin (100 mU/ml) failed to attenuate NE- or A II-induced contractile responses (Figure 1).[51]   By contrast, insulin-induced potentiation of MVB NE responses was further augmented in arteries from FH rats (not shown).[4] Thus, the direct vascular effects of insulin are altered in hyperinsulinemic, insulin resistant FH rats in favor of increased peripheral vascular resistance. It is important to note that the effects of insulin on aortic reactivity were observed at pharmacological insulin concentrations (100 mU/ml vs. 100 µU/ml in the MVB). As the plasma insulin levels of hyperinsulinemic rats in the post-prandial state are $\approx$ 80-100 µU/ml, it is reasonable to conclude that the effects of insulin on MVB reactivity are more relevant to altered hemodynamics in FH rats than a loss of insulin-mediated vasodilation in aortae. This factor assumes greater significance given the contribution of the MVB towards global systemic vascular resistance. Thus, based on these observations, we suggest that in FH rats, chronic hyperinsulinemia may serve to increase peripheral vascular resistance (via exaggeration of MVB responses) which, in turn, may play an important role in the development or maintenance of elevated BP in these rats.

Do Alterations in Insulin's Vascular Effects Precede the Development of FH?

A critical point to clarify is whether these changes in MVB reactivity precede the development of high BP. To this aim, we examined the effects of physiological insulin concentrations (100 µU/ml) on MVB reactivity in FH rats after one week of fructose

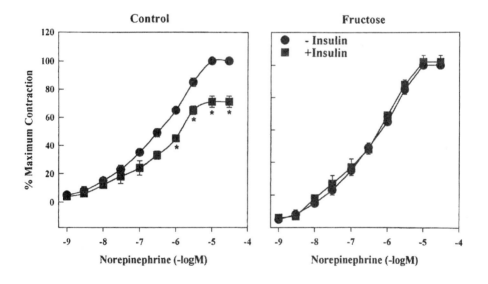

Figure 1. Reactivity of isolated aortae from control (n=8, left panel) and fructose-hypertensive rats (n=8, right panel) to norepinephrine (NE) in the absence ● and presence ■ of insulin (100mU/ml for 2 hours). Absolute tension values corresponding to 100% in g/mm²: control 2.7±0.2, control+insulin 1.49±0.3, fructose 2.6±0.2, fructose+insulin 2.8±0.3. Insulin caused vasodepressor effects in control rat aortae; in the presence of pharmacological insulin concentrations both the percent maximum contraction and the sensitivity were attenuated (percent maximum attenuation by insulin 30±3, pD2 values: 7.35±0.07 vs. control+insulin 8.4±0.05, P<0.05). Insulin induced attenuation of NE responses was absent in aortae from fructose-hypertensive rats indicating the presence of vascular insulin resistance. See text for details. From 51.

Table 1. General Characteristics of the Rats in the Pre-Hypertensive Study

	Control (n=10)	Fructose (n=10)
Systolic BP (mmHg)	126±3	124±5
Plasma Insulin (ng/ml)	2.1±0.3	3.1±0.1*
Plasma Glucose (mM)	4.7±0.6	5.3±0.5
Body Weight (g)	205±4	210±9

*P<0.05, different from control.

Male Sprague Dawley rats were assigned to two groups, control and fructose. The fructose group received a 60% fructose diet for one week. Following one week of treatment, the rats in the fructose group were hyperinsulinemic, normoglycemic and normotensive. We used this time point to represent the pre-hypertensive state. MVB were isolated from these rats at this time point and MVB responses to NE were studied in the presence and absence of insulin as shown below (Figure 2).

feeding.[51]   We chose the one-week post-fructose time point to represent the pre-hypertensive state.   After one week of fructose feeding the rats in the F group were hyperinsulinemic yet normotensive (Table 1).[51] Results from our study in pre-hypertensive FH rats demonstrate that altered MVB responses to insulin were evident prior to the development of hypertension in these rats.[51] MVB from pre-hypertensive FH rats exhibited a greater potentiation of NE reactivity when compared to C rats (Figure 2). Thus, it is reasonable to suggest that hyperinsulinemia in FH rats may serve to exaggerate MVB responses and increase BP through increasing systemic vascular resistance and that this effect is evident prior to the development of hypertension.

In-vitro and In-vivo Studies Examining the Role of ET-1 in the Development of FH

As discussed earlier, studies indicate that insulin may stimulate the production of the potent vasoconstrictor ET-1. We hypothesized that hyperinsulinemia in FH rats may serve as a continual stimulus for ET-1 release, which could increase BP via increases in vascular tone and reactivity. To this aim, we examined (a) the effects of acute ET receptor blockade (with bosentan) on insulin-induced changes in MVB reactivity[4,51] and (b) effects of chronic ET receptor blockade on plasma insulin levels, systolic BP and total MVB ET-1 content[52,53]. ET receptor blockade (with bosentan) did not affect in-vitro insulin-mediated MVB potentiation of NE responses in control rats. By contrast, indomethacin completely prevented the insulin response in MVB from control rats.[4] The marked inhibition by indomethacin of insulin potentiation of NE responses in the MVB of control rats suggests that a cyclooxygenase metabolite from the endothelium may be involved in this response. In FH rats, as observed earlier, insulin potentiated MVB to a significantly greater degree than control rats.[4] Although indomethacin attenuated the pressor responses in FH rats (to a similar degree to that seen in control rats), in the presence of both indomethacin and bosentan, the effects of insulin were completely abrogated. As bosentan is a potent inhibitor of ET_A and ET_B receptors it is reasonable to speculate that the component of hyper-reactivity observed in MVB's from FH rats in response to insulin may be mediated via ET-1. Analysis of the total ET-1 content in MVB's revealed that FH rats had an almost two fold higher mesenteric ET content compared to control rats.[52] More importantly, chronic bosentan treatment completely prevented the development of hypertension in FH rats.[52] Taken together, these data indicate that hyperinsulinemia in FH rats may serve to exaggerate MVB responses (possibly through increases in ET-1 production) which in turn may lead to increases in vascular tone, reactivity and BP.

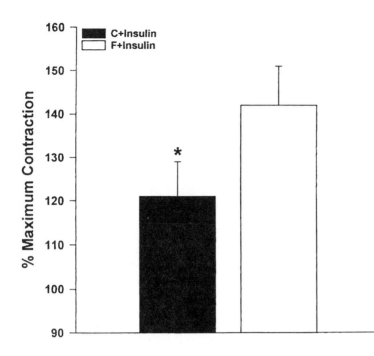

Figure 2. Insulin-induced potentiation of MVB responses in pre-hypertensive FH rats. MVB were isolated from control rats and fructose rats following one week of fructose feeding (pre-hypertensive). The graph depicts the percent maximum potentiation by insulin (100 μU/ml for 2 hours) in control and pre-hypertensive FH rats. 100% corresponds to the %maximum contraction in the absence of insulin. *P<0.05 different from fructose+insulin. The data show that in the pre-hypertensive fructose rat the MVB responses to insulin are exaggerated when compared to control.

Effects of Calcium Channel Blockade in FH Rats

As highlighted in the introduction section, perfusion per se is as an independent determinant of glucose uptake into skeletal muscle. Basically, if increased peripheral vascular tone plays a role in the development and/or maintenance of the insulin resistant state, then vasodilator-antihypertensive agents should attenuate these defects in FH rats. To this aim, we studied the long-term effects of two vasodilator calcium antagonists (mibefradil, pioglitazone) on the development of hyperinsulinemia and hypertension in FH and Spontaneously Hypertensive rats respectively.[53,54] Data from these studies indicated that the antihypertensive effects of chronic mibefradil treatment are associated with sustained and marked reductions in plasma insulin levels.[54] Although insulin sensitivity was not directly measured, analysis of the 5-hour fasted insulin/glucose ratios (an index of insulin sensitivity) revealed an improvement in insulin sensitivity after mibefradil treatment.[54] These data provide indirect evidence that vasodilation may play a role in modulating insulin resistance/hyperinsulinemia in experimental models of rodent hypertension. Similar observations were made using pioglitazone, which in addition to enhancing the effects of insulin is also a calcium antagonist, in SHR.[55]

CONCLUDING REMARKS

Several lines of evidence suggest that insulin resistance and hyperinsulinemia may play a pathogenic role in the development of high BP in rodent models of hypertension.

We have examined this relationship from both a pharmacological and mechanistic standpoint. Our data indicate that drugs, that specifically counter insulin resistance and decrease plasma insulin levels lower BP in experimental hypertension. The link between insulin resistance/hyperinsulinemia in the pathogenesis of hypertension may be due to an alteration in the vascular actions of insulin. Indeed, data from our studies reveal that insulin's vascular effects are altered in favor of increased vascular tone and reactivity in states of whole body insulin resistance. Importantly, these defects may antedate the development of high BP. Our studies also serve to uncover the differences in the vascular effects of insulin between humans and rats. In humans, insulin has a physiological role to vasodilate skeletal muscle vasculature. In contrast in rats, insulin concentrations within the physiological range serve to exaggerate resistance vessel function. This exaggeration may be due to an increased ET-1 production (secondary to hyperinsulinemia). The observation that vasodilator antihypertensive agents (mibefradil/pioglitazone and others) improve insulin sensitivity and decrease plasma insulin levels suggests that increases in vascular tone may be linked to insulin resistance and hyperinsulinemia.

Although the exact contribution of hyperinsulinemia and insulin resistance towards the pathogenesis and clinical course of essential hypertension in humans is still debatable, the evidence that these defects are associated with an atherogenic risk profile and other cardiovascular diseases stands strong. There is compelling evidence that insulin resistance and hyperinsulinemia assume an early and integral role in the development and natural history of a wide spectrum of cardiovascular and metabolic diseases such as diabetes, hypertension, atherosclerosis, hyperlipidemia, endothelial dysfunction, polycystic ovary syndrome, obesity and increased risk for coronary artery disease. Thus it is logical to propose that treating insulin resistance in hypertension may serve to prevent or improve other insulin resistant disorders and may be beneficial in countering global cardiovascular risk.

Acknowledgements

The grant support of the following organizations is acknowledged (JHMcN): Heart and Stroke Foundation of BC and Yukon, Medical Research Council of Canada, Canadian Diabetes Association. Studies outlined in this paper were conducted by Dr. Subodh Verma, Dr. Sanjay Bhanot, Dr. Linfu Yao, and Ms. Emi Arikawa in my laboratory and Dr. Ismail Laher in the Faculty of Medicine University of BC. Dr. Subodh Verma is an MRC Fellow. We thank Ms. Mary Battell and Ms. Sylvia Chan for technical and secretarial assistance respectively. The gift of bosentan from Dr.M.Clozel, Actelion Ltd, Switzerland is kindly acknowledged.

REFERENCES

1. Reaven GM. Role of insulin resistance in human disease. Diabetes. 1988; 37:1595-1607.
2. DeFronzo RA. Insulin resistance, hyperinsulinemia and coronary artery disease: a complex metabolic web. J Cardiovasc Pharmacol. 1992; 20:S1-S16.
3. Bhanot S and McNeill JH. Insulin and hypertension: a causal relationship? Cardiovasc. Res. 1996; 31:212-221.
4. Verma S and McNeill JH. Insulin resistance and hypertension: pharmacological and mechanistic studies. Can J Diab Care (in press).
5. Verma S, MatherK, Dumont A and Anderson TJ. Pharmacological modulation of insulin resistance and hyperinsulinemia in polycystic ovary syndrome: the emerging role. The Endocrinologist 1998; 8: 418-424.
6. Bhanot S, McNeill JH. Vanadyl sulfate lowers plasma insulin levels and blood pressure in spontaneously hypertensive rats. Hypertension. 1994; 24:625-632.
7. Bhanot S, Bryer-Ash M, Cheung A, McNeill JH. Bis(maltolato)oxovanadium(IV) attenuates hyperinsulinemia and hypertension in spontaneously hypertensive rats. Diabetes. 1994; 43:857-861.

8. Bhanot S, Bryer-Ash M, Nichoulas A, McNeill JH. Pioglitazone attenuates hyperinsulinemia and lowers systolic blood pressure in spontaneously hypertensive rats.(abstract) Can. J. Physiol. Pharmacol. 1994; 72(Suppl. 1):P1.9.29.

9. Verma S, Bhanot S and McNeill, JH. Metformin decreases plasma insulin levels and blood pressure in spontaneously hypertensive rats. Am. J. Physiol. 1994; 36:H1250-H1253.

10. Bhanot S, McNeill H and Bryer-Ash M. Vanadyl sulfate prevents fructose induced hyperinsulinemia and hypertension in rats. Hypertension. 1994; 23:308-12.

11. Bhanot S, Verma S, Michoulas A, McNeill JH. Drugs that attenuate hyperinsulinemia in spontaneously hypertensive rats cause concurrent decreases in systolic blood pressure (abstract). Diabetes 1994; 43(Suppl 1):40A.

12. Verma S, Bhanot S and McNeill JH. Antihypertensive effects of metformin in fructose-fed hyperinsulinemic, hypertensive rats. J. Pharmacol. Exp. Therap. 1994; 271:1334-1337.

13. Baron AD. Cardiovascular actions of insulin in humans. Implications for insulin sensitivity and vascular tone. Baillere's Clin Endocrinol Metab 1993; 7: 961-987.

14. Laakso M, Edelman SV, Brechtel G and Baron AD. Impaired insulin-mediated skeletal muscle blood flow in patients with NIDDM. Diabetes 1992; 41: 1076-1083.

15. Laakso M, Edelman SV, Brechtel G and Baron AD. Decreased effect of insulin to stimulate skeletal muscle blood flow in obese men. J Clin Invest 1990; 85: 1844-1852.

16. Verma S, Bhanot S, Yao L and McNeill JH. Vascular insulin resistance in fructose hypertensive rats. Eur J Pharmacol 1997; 322:R1-R2.

17. Reaven GM. Syndrome X: 6 years later. J. Intern Med. 1994; 236(Suppl 736): 13-22.

18. Textor SC. Pathogenesis of hypertension. In: Primer on Kidney Diseases (Ed Greenberg A) 2nd edition, National Kidney Foundation, Academic Press, 1998; pp491-495.

19. Brands MW, Mizelle HL, Gaillard CA, Hildebrandt DA, Hall JE. The hemodynamic response to chronic hyperinsulinemia in conscious dogs. Am. J. Hypertens. 1991; 4:164-168.

20. Dela F, Larsen JJ, Mikines KJ and Galbo H. Normal effect of insulin to stimulate leg blood flow in NIDDM. Diabetes. 1995; 44:221-226.

21. Egan BM and Stepnaikowski K. Compensatory hyperinsulinemia and the forearm vasodilator response during an oral glucose tolerance test in obese hypertensives. J. Hypertens. 1994; 12:1061-1067.

22. Baron AD, Brechtel G. Insulin differentially regulates systemic and skeletal muscle vascular resistance. Am. J. Physiol. 1993; 265:E61-E67.

23. Baron AD. Hemodynamic actions of insulin. Am. J. Physiol. 1994; 267:E187-E202.

24. Baron AD, Steinberg HO, Chaker I., Leaming R, Johnson A and Brechtel G. Insulin-mediated skeletal muscle vasodilation contributes to both insulin sensitivity and responsiveness in lean humans. J. Clin. Invest. 1995; 96:786-792.

25. Baron AD, Laakso M, Brechtel G and Edelman SV. Mechanism of insulin resistance in insulin-dependent diabetes mellitus: a major role for reduced skeletal muscle blood flow. J. Clin. Endo. Metab. 1991; 73:637-643.

26. Richter EA, Mikines KG, Galbo H and Kiens B. Effect of exercise on insulin action in human skeletal muscle. J. Appl. Physiol. 1989; 66:876-885.

27. Bennett WM, Connacher AA, Scrimgeour CM, Jung RT and Rennie MJ. Euglycemic hyperinsulinemia augments amino acid uptake by human leg tissue during hyperaminoacidemia. Am. J. Physiol. 1990; 259:E185-E194.

28. Edelman SV, Marco M, Wallace P, Buchtel J, Olefsky JL and Baron AD. Kinetics of insulin-mediated and non-insulin mediated glucose uptake in humans. Diabetes. 1990; 39:955-964.

29. Vollenweider P, Tappy L, Randin D, Schneiter P, Jequier E, Nicod P and Scherrer U. Differential effects of hyperinsulinemia and carbohydrate metabolism on sympathetic nerve activity and muscle blood flow in humans. J. Clin. Invest. 1993; 92:147-154.

30. Boden G, De Santis R, Chen X, Morris M and Badoza F. Glucose metabolism and leg blood flow after pancreas/kidney transplantation. J. Clin. Endocrinol. Metabol. 1993; 76:1229-1233.

31. Anderson EA, Hoffmann RP, Balon TW, Sinkey CA and Mark AL. Hyperinsulinemia produces both sympathetic neural activation and vasodilation in normal humans. J. Clin. Invest. 1991; 87:2246-2252.

32. Baron AD and Steinberg HO. Vascular actions of insulin in health and disease. In: Endocrinology of the vasculature, Sowers JR Editor, Humana Press, Totowa, New Jersey. 1996; pp95-107.

33. Baron AD. The coupling of glucose metabolism and perfusion in human skeletal muscle. The potential role of endothelium-derived nitric oxide. Diabetes. 1996; 45 (Suppl. 1):S105-S109.

34. Baron AD, Brechtel G, Johnson A, Fineberg N, Henry DP, Steinberg HO. Interactions between insulin and norepinephrine on blood pressure and insulin sensitivity: studies in lean and obese men. J. Clin. Invest. 1994; 93:2453-2462.

35. Verma S, Arikawa E, Yao L, Laher I and McNeill JH. Insulin induced vasodilation is dependent upon tetrahydrobiopterin synthesis. Metabolism. 1998; 47: 1037-1039.

36. Steinberg HO, Brechtel G, Johnson A, Fineberg N and Baron AD. Insulin-mediated skeletal muscle blood flow is nitric oxide dependent. J. Clin. Invest. 1994; 94:1172-1179.

37. Juncos LA and Hito S. Disparate effect of insulin on isolated rabbit afferent and efferent arterioles. J. Clin. Invest. 1993; 92:1981-1985.
38. Yanagisawa-Miwa A, Ito H and Sugimot T. Effects of insulin on vasoconstriction induced by thromboxane A2 in porcine coronay artery. Circulation. 1990; 81:1654-1659.
39. Wu H, Jeng YY, Yue C, Chye KY, Hsueh WA and Chan TM. Endothelium derived vascular effects of insulin and insulin-like growth factor 1 in the perfused mesenteric artery and aortic ring. Diabetes. 1994; 43:1027-1032.
40. Townsend RR, Yamamoto R, Nickols M, Dipette DJ and Nickols GA. Insulin enhances pressor responses to norepinephrine in rat mesenteric vasculature. Hypertension. 1992; 19 (Suppl. II):II-105-II-110.
41. Walker AB, Savage MW, Dores J and Williams G. Insulin-induced attenuation of noradrenaline-mediated vasoconstriction in resistance arteries from Wistar rats is nitric oxide dependent. Clin. Sci. 1997; 92:147-152.
42. Alexander WE and Oake RJ. The effect of insulin on vascular reactivity to norepinephrine. Diabetes. 1977; 26:611-614.
43. Yagi S, Takata S, Kiyokawa H, Yamamoto M, Noto Y, Ikeda T and Hattori N. Effects of insulin on vasoconstrictive responses to norepinephrine and angiotensin II in rabbit femoral artery and vein. Diabetes. 1988; 37:1064-1067.
44. Wambach GK and Liu D. Insulin attenuates vasoconstriction by noradrenaline, serotonin and potassium chloride in rat mesenteric arterioles. Clin. Exp. Hyper. 1992; A14(4):733-740.
45. Oliver FJ, De la Rubia G, Feener EP et al. Stimulation of endothelin-1 gene expression by insulin in endothelial cells. J. Biol. Chem. 1991; 266:23251-23526.
46. Frank HJL, Levin ER, Hu RM and Pedram A. Insulin stimulates endothelin binding and action on cultured vascular smooth muscle cells. Endocrinology. 1993; 133:1092-1097.
47. Hu R-M, Levin ER, Pedram A and Frank HJL. Insulin stimulates production and secretion of endothelin from bovine endothelial cells. Diabetes. 1993; 42:351-358.
48. Hattori Y, Kasai K, Nakamura T, Emoto T, Shimoda S-I. Effect of glucose and insulin on immunoreactive endothelin-1 release from cultured porcine aortic endothelial cells. Metabolism 1991; 40:165-169.
49. Takahashi K, Gathei MA, Lam HC, O'Halloran DJ and Bloom SR. Elevated plasma endothelin in patients with diabetes mellitus. Diabetologia. 1990; 33:306-310.
50. Hopfner RL, Misurski D, Wilson TW, McNeill JR and Gopalakrishnan V. Insulin and vanadate restore decreased plasma endothelin concentrations and exaggerated vascular responses to normal in the streptozotocin diabetic rat. Diabetologia. 1998; 41:1233-1240.
51. Verma S. Mechanisms of hypertension in hyperinsulinemic and insulin resistant fructose hypertensive rats. PhD Thesis. 1997; The University of British Columbia, Canada.
52. Verma S, Bhanot S and McNeill JH. Effect of chronic endothelin blockade in hyperinsulinemic hypertensive rats. Am. J. Physiol. 1995; 269:H2017-H2021.
53. Verma S, Skarsgard P, Bhanot S, Yao L, Laher I and McNeill JH. Reactivity of mesenteric arteries from fructose-hypertensive rats to endothelin-1. Am. J. Hypertens. 1997; 10: 1010-1019.
54. Verma S, Bhanot S, Hicke A and McNeill JH. Chronic T-type calcium channel blockade in hyperinsulinemic, hypertensive rats. Cardiovasc. Res. 1997; 34:121-128.
55. Verma S, Bhanot S, Arikawa E, Yao L and McNeill JH. Direct vasodepressor effects of pioglitazone in spontaneously hypertension rats. Pharmacol. 1998; 56:7-16.

CARDIAC HYPERTROPHY IN DIABETES PATIENTS WITH AND WITHOUT HYPERTENSION: EFFECTS OF TROGLITAZONE, A NOVEL ANTIDIABETIC DRUG, ON DIASTOLIC FUNCTION

Naoki Makino, Hiroyoshi Hirayama, Hidetoshi Yonemochi*, Ken-ichi Yano, Nobuyuki Abe**.

Dep. of Bioclimatology & Med. Medical Inst. of Bioregulation,
Kyushu University, Beppu,
*Department of Clinical Laboratory, Oita Medical University, Hasamachou,
**Abe Medical Clinic, Oita,
JAPAN

INTRODUCTION

Patients with non-insulin-dependent- (type 2) diabetes mellitus (NIDDM) have excessive cardiovascular morbidity and mortality even in the absence of albminuria and hypertension[1]. Left ventricular hypertrophy (LVH), which is an ominous prognostic sign and an independent risk factor for cardiac events, is often present in NIDDM patients[2,3]. It is also demonstrated that reversal of LVH reduced the increased cardiovascular risk in patients with essential hypertension and LVH[4,5]. Possible contributions of hyperinsulinemia and insulin resistance to LV mass have also been suggested in normotensive NIDDM patients but the results reported are not consistent[6,7]. Thus, LVH in diabetes patients is associated with hyperinsulinemia in the regardless of the presence or absence of albminuria and hypertension. Those patients also show the early diastolic dysfunction of the left ventricle rather than systolic dysfunction[8]. There are several literatures in which calcium antagonists or angiotensin converting enzyme (ACE) inhibitors could reduce left ventricular mass in hypertensive NIDDM patients[9,10], but ACE inhibitors seemed to offer a reduction beyond that explained by their blood pressure-lowering properties as reviewed by Schmieder et al.[11]. Troglitazone, a novel member of the insulin-sensitizing thiazolidinediones, has been widely used to treat patients with NIDDM. The treatment with Troglitazone reduced hyperglycemia, plasma trigycerides, and blood pressure[12-15]. In addition, recent studies show that Troglitazone attenuate high glucose-induced abnormalities in relaxation and intracellular calcium in rat ventricular myocytes[16] and may improve cardiac function in diabetic patients[17]. Thus, the beneficial effects of Troglitazone on heart have described but not been clearly established in the diastolic function of NIDDM patients. The present study were therefore undertaken to assess that whether or not Troglitazone affects the diastolic dysfunction of the left ventricle in diabetes patients with LVH.

Diabetes and Cardiovascular Disease: Etiology, Treatment and Outcomes
Edited by Aubie Angel et al., Kluwer Academic/Plenum Publishers, 2001

Table 1. Clinical data in NIDDM patients with or without hypertension and in control subjects

	NIDDM Patients with Hypertension	NIDDM Patients with Normotension	Control Subjects
Sex (M / F)	36 / 16	28 / 14	29 / 18
AGE (y)	64 ± 3	59 ± 6	56 ± 8
Body mass index. (kg/m2)	24.5 ± 5	23.6 ± 7	22.9 ±10
Fasting glucose (mmol/L)	6.3 ± 0.5*	6.4 ± 0.5*	5.4 ± 0.4
insulin -90 (pmol)	354 ± 125	2 43 ± 167=	-
HbA1c (%)	7.3 ±1.7*	7.2 ± 1.4*	5.2 ± 0.4
Urinary albumin excretion rate (mg 24-1)	1012(260-7620)	11(3-27)=	9(2-28)=
Serum creatine (mmol-1)	82 (57-246)	68 (54-120)=	58 (51-118)
Systolic-BP (mmHg)	168 ± 6*	134 ± 4=	126 ± 3=
Diastolic-BP (mmHg)	94± 5*	81 ± 4=	74 ± 3=

Data are mean ± SD or median (range), * p< vs control subjects. = p<0.01 vs NIDDM with hypetension.

METHODS

Patients

All NIDDM patients with hypertensive (n=52) and normotensive (n=42) patients attending the out patient clinic were identified. Diabetes mellitus was diagnosed by the criteria of the WHO[18]. Subjective who had a fasting glucose level of 7.8 mmol /L or higher and /or a 2-hour postload glucose level of 11.1 mmol/L or higher were diagnosed as having diabetes mellitus by 75-g OGTT. Hypertension was diagnosed as repeated arterial blood pressure>160/90 mmHg and normotension was <140/90 mmHg. We measure BP in the subject's right arm using the first and fifth phases of Korotkoff sounds by mercury sphygmomanometer after at least 5 minutes of rest in the sitting position. Measurements were repeated three times and average of the two lower values was used for analysis. BMI (body weight divided by squared height) was used as a marker of obesity. Normotensive NIDDM subjects was not previous antihypertensive treatment and nonalbumiuric (urinary albumin excretionrate <100 mg/24hr) as seen in Table 1. Hypertensive subjects have previous antihypertensive treatment and albumiuric (urinary albumin excretionrate >100 mg/24hr). Both subjects were without any history of cardiovascular disease and no significant Q waves in more than one ECG reading. Healthy normal subjects (n=47) were recruited as a control.

Echocardiography

To evaluate LV mass and LV geometry, echocardiography (two-dimensional targeted M mode) was performed with an ultrasound imager (SSA-160A. Toshiba Medical Co Ltd) with either a 2.5- or 3.75-MHZ transducer by expert physicians. Patients were examined in the left lateral decubitus position. End-diastolic and endsystolic LV diameters and thickness of the interventricular septum and LV posterior wall were obtained according to the Pen convention. LV mass was calculated by use of the formula of Devereux and Reichek[19]. LV mass index was obtained by dividing LV mass by body surface area. Relative wall thickness was calculated as the ratio of two times posterior wall thickness to end-diastolic LV diameter[20]. The mean value from at least three cardiac cycles was used for data analysis, which had been measured by one physician blinded to the patient's information. In the apical four chamber view, the Doppler sample volume was placed in the middle of the LV inflow tract ~1 cm below the plane of the mitral annulus between the mitral leaflet tips, where maximal flow velocity in early diastole was recorded[21]. From Doppler spectra of 3 to 5 consecutive cardiac cycles, average values were calculated for the following diastolic variables: the maximal early flow velocity, and the deceleration time of early filling[22]. The isovolumetric relaxation time was measured as the time interval between the aortic valve closure and the onset of the mitral valve inflow.

Study Protocol

We assessed effects of Triglitazone (400 mg/day), a novel member of the insulin-sensitizing thiazolidinediones on the diastolic function in NIDDM patients with hypertension and normotension. Twelve and fourteen patients in NIDDM with hypertension and normotension, respectively, accepted participation in the present randomized, double-blind parallel group 6-month study. Two patients in each group did not complete the study. Before and after Triglitazone treatment (mean interval; 5.2 0. 8 month), we compared glucose levels, HbA1c and arterial blood pressure (BP) measured by noninvasive ambulatory BP monitoring (ABPM-630, Nippon Colin Co). The accuracy of this device was previously validated[23]. Reexamination was performed in the three-hypertensive patients whose BP data were not available due to the presence of artifacts in more than 10 % of the total measurements. Using echocardiography, diastolic function was examined the peak E/A wave velocity ratio, the deceleration time and the isovolumetric relaxation time pre- and post-treatment with Triglitazone.
Statistical analysis:

Data are expressed as, mean ± SD. Statistical analysis was performed with the use of SAS version 6.07 (SAS Inc). Differences between groups were assessed by ANOVA with the multiple comparison test (Scheffe's test). A value of p<0.05 was regarded as statistically significant.

RESULTS

Table 1 shows pertinent clinical data in three groups. The groups were well-matched with regard to sex, age, and body mass index. The 24-h systolic blood pressure was higher in NIDDM patients with nephropathy as compared with normoalbuminuric

Table 2. Echocardiographic Profiles in NIDDM patients with or without hypertension and in control subjects

	NIDDM Patients with Hypertension	NIDDM Patients with Normotension	Control Subjects
LV Mass (g)	261 ± 37*	231 ± 36*=	182 ± 25
LVM index (g/m2)	166 ± 21*	145 ± 17*=	112 ±13
LV diastolic dimension (mm)	47.2 ± 3.0*	45.6 ± 2.6*	31.3 ± 2.2
LV systolic dimension (mm)	36.2 ± 2.4*	35.2 ±2.0*	41.3 ±2.0
Interventricular septum thickness (mm)	13.1 ±1.3*	11.8 ±1.0*=	9.6 ±0.9
Posterior wall thickness (mm)	11.4 ±1.0*	10.8 ±0.9*	8.4 ±0.7
Relative posterior wall thickness (mm)	0.46 ± 0.06*	0.40 ±0.04=	0.36 ±0.03
LV shortening fraction, %	23.3± 4.2	22.8 ± 3.5	24.2±2.9

Data are mean ± SD. *p< vs control subjects. = p<0.01 vs NIDDM with hypetension.
LV mass was calculated by use of the formula of Devereur and Reichek

Table 3. Effects of Troglitazone on clinical and echocardiographic data in NIDDM patients with or without hypertension

	NIDDM Patients with Hypertension (n=10)		NIDDM Patients with Normotension (n=12)	
	pre	post	pre	post
Fasting glucose(mmol/L)	6.2 ± 0.7	$5.7 \pm 0.5*$	6.4 ± 0.5	$5.6 \pm 0.4*$
HbA1c (%)	7.7 ± 1.1	$6.8 \pm 1.8*$	7.5 ± 1.2	$6.7 \pm 1.0*$
24-h s-BP (mmHg)	146 ± 23	138 ± 23	123 ± 16	121 ± 153
24-h d-BP (mmHg)	78 ± 11	74 ± 12	73 ± 11	72 ± 10
LVM index, g/m2	172 ± 22	166 ± 18	152 ± 17	$136 \pm 15*$
LV shortening fraction (%)	32.7 ± 4.8	33.8 ± 4.0	33.4 ± 3.9	35.1 ± 3.5

Data are mean $\pm$ SD, *$p < 0.01$ vs data before the treatment with Troglitazone (400 mg/day)

patients and control subjects. The latte two groups had almost identical values. Compared to normotensive patients, insulin levels at 90 min in 75g-OGTT study and serum creatine values increased in hypertensive patients. There was no difference in the fasting glucose and HbA1c levels between hypertensive and normotensive patients. Table 2 shows echocardiographic profiles in both groups of NIDDM patients and in control subjects. All ehocardiographic data were more increased in NIDDM patients than in normal control subjects, except for the LV shortening fraction, which was not different between two NIDDM groups. LV mass as well as LV mass index were significantly greater in hypertensive patients than in normotensive NIDDM patients. LV hypertrophy in NIDDM patients was explained for the increased thickness in the both of interventricular septum and relative posterior wall. In diastolic function of NIDDM patients, maximal early flow velocity was reduced, while both of deceleration time and Isovolumic relaxation time were prolonged in comparison to control subjects. Compared with normotensive NIDDM patients, maximal early flow velocity was significantly reduced in hypertensive patients, and the both of deceleration time and Isovolumic relaxation time were significantly increased.

Table 3 shows results clinical and echocardiographic data in normotensive or hypertensive NIDDM patients pre- and post-Troglitazone treatment. Diabetic state (fasting glucose and HbA1c levels) in both groups were significantly improved after the treatment with Troglitazone. However, 24-h systolic and diastolic BP as well as LV shortening fraction was not changed in both groups by the treatment.

LV mass index decreased in normotensive patients, but not in hypertensive patients by Troglitazone treatment. Diastolic dysfunction was also assessed in the present study. In normotensive patients treated with Troglitazone, the maximal early flow velocity was larger, while both of the deceleration time and the isovolumic relaxation time were less than those of the pre-treatment. On the other hand, in hypertensive patients both of the deceleration time and the isovolumic relaxation time were not changed although the maximal early flow velocity was larger by Troglitazone treatment.

DISCUSSION

The present study demonstrates that Troglitazone causes regression of LVH in normotensive, nonalbuminuric NIDDM patients as compared with pre-treatment. This effect was independent of systemic BP. However, this antidiabetic agent did not affect LVH in hypertensive NIDDM patients although hyperglycemic state was improved. All patients included in our study fulfilled established criteria of LVH (LVM index >130 g/m2 in men and >100 g/m2 in women)[19] at baseline even though the other mean values of the echocardiogarphic measurements were within normal limits. Troglitazone, a novel member of the insulin-sensitizing thiazolidinediones, has been widely used to treat patients with NIDDM and reduced hyperglycemia, plasma trigycerides, and BP[12-15]. However, by this agent 24-h systolic BP did not significantly decrease in both of hypertensive and normotensive patients. This indicates that the pathogenesis of hypertension in NIDDM patients is not only contributed to a high insulin resistance, but also may be due to renal dysfunction (albuminuria). The present study also showed the diastolic dysfunction in normotensive patients to be improved after the treatment with Troglitazone. Thus, abnormalities in LV diastolic dysfunction often precede systolic dysfunction in cardiac hypertrophy[8]. Troglitazone has also an action to attenuate high glucose-induced abnormalities in relaxation and intracellular calcium in rat ventricular myocytes[16]. These findings may explain for the improved diastolic function in diabetic patients studied here[17].

Epidemiological data indicate that LVH represents a serious risk factor for cardiovascular events and congestive heart failure[2,3]. ACE inhibitors and calcium-channel antagonists are effective both in controlling blood pressure and in reversing LVH[9,10]. Hypertension occurs about twice as often in individuals with diabetes as it dose in the nondiabetic population[24]. Up to 50% of diabetic individuals ultimately become hypertensive[25]. The pathogenesis of this association is complex, involving familiar trait for essential hypertension, hyperinsulinemia, dyslipidemia, obesity, and Na-exchange alterations[26,27]. The results of the present study show that the 6-month Troglitazone therapy is as effective as ACE inhibitors in reducing LVH in nonhypertensive diabetic patients as well as hypertensive patients. LV mass index was no significance differences in hypertensive subjects between the pre- and the post Troglitazone treatment. LV end-diastolic volume and ejection fraction did not change significantly during the follow -up period. Considerable efforts have been recently directed toward the development of noninvasive techniques capable of accurate and serial assessment of LV diastolic properties. As expected,b o th the isovolumetric relaxation time and early deceleration times were prolonged and the maximal early flow velocity reduced in LV hypertrophy of NIDDM patients when compared with age-matched control subjects, reflecting impaired LV relaxation and compliance[28]. Our data also confirm that Troglitazone could improve those three parameters in the diastolic dysfunction in NIDDM patients without hypertension, but not in NIDDM patients with hypertension except for the maximal early flow velocity. These results suggest that this antidiabetic therapy for reducing insulin resistance is useful in NIDDM patients.

REFERENCES

1. Gall M-A, Borch-Jhonsen K, Hougaard P, Nielsen FS, Parving H-H: Albiminemia and poor glycemic control predicts mortality in NIDDM. Diabetes   44:1303-1309, 1995.
2. Sampson MJ, Denver E, Foyle WJ ,Dawson D, Pinkney J, Yudkin JS: Association between left ventricular hypertrophy and erythrocyte sodiun-lithium exchange in normotensive subjects with and without NIDDM. Diabetologia 38:454-460,1995.
3. Nielsen FS, Ali S, Rossing P, Bang LE, Svendsen TL, Gall M-A, Smidt UM, Kastrup J, Parving H-H. Left ventricular hypertrophy in non-insulin dependent diabetic patoents with and without diabetic nephropathy. Diabet Med 14:538-46,1997.
4. Yurenv AP, Dyakonova HG, Novikov ID, Viols A, Pahl L, Haynemann G, Wallrabe D, Tsifkova R, Romanovska L, Niderle P, Tsiskarishvili DL, Davarashvili T, GelovaniK, Kochachidze T, Balash A: Management of essential hypertension in patients with different degrees of left ventricular hypertrophy. Am J Hypertens 5:S182-S189,1992.
5. Lorenza Muiesan M, Salvetti M, Rizzoni D, Castellano M, Donato F. Agabiti-Rosie E: Association of change in left ventricular mass with prognosis during long-term antihypertensive treatment. J Hypertens 13:1091-1095, 1995.
6. Shrap SD, Williams RR. Fasting insulin and left ventricular mass in hypertensives and normotensive

controls. Cardiollogy. 81:207-212,1992.

7. Swislocki ALM, Hoffman BB, Reaven GM. Insulin resistance glucose intolerance and hyperinsulinemia in patients with hypertension. Am J Hypertens. 2:419-4231989.

8 Topol EJ, Traill TA, Fortuin NJ. Hypertensive hypertrophic cardiomyopathy of the elderly. New Engl J Med. 312:277-283,1985.

9. Nielsen FS, Smidt UM, Sato A, Kastrup J, Ali S, Parving H-H, Tarnow L. Beneficial impact of ramipril on left ventricular hypertrophy in normotensive   nonalbuminuric NIDDM patients. Diabetic Care 21:804-809,1998.

10. Clement DL, DeBuyzere M, Duprez D: left ventricular hypertrophy in essential hypertension. Am J Hypertens 6:14S-19S,1993.

11. Schmieder RE, Martus P, Klingbeil A: Reversal of left ventricular hypertrophy in essential hypertension: a meta-analysis of randomized double -blind studies.   JAMA 275:1507-1513,1996.

12. Suter SL, Nolan JJ, Wallance P, Gumbiner B, Olefsky M. Metabolic eddects of new oral hypoglycemic agent CS-045 in NIDDM subjects. Diabetic Care. ;15:193-203,1992.

13. Nolan JJ, Ludvik B, Beerdsen P, Joyce M, Olefsky J. Improvement in glucose telerance and insulin resistance in obese subjects treated with troglitazone. N Eng J Med. 331:1188-1193,1994

14. Schwartz S, Raskin P, Fonseca V, Graveline JF. Effects of Troglitazone in insulin-treated patients with type II diabetes mellitus. N Eng J Med. 338:861-866,1998.

15. Inzucchi SE, Maggs DG, Spollett GR, Page SL, Rife FS, Walton V, Shulman GI. Effecacy and metabolic effects of metformin and troglytazone in type II diabets mellitus. N Eng J Med. ;338:867-872,1998.

16. Ren J, Dominguez LJ, Sowers JR, Davidoff AJ. Triglitazone attenuates high-glucose-induced abnormalities in relaxation and intracellular calcium in rat ventricular myocytes. Diabetes, 45:1922-1825,1996.

17. Ghazzi MN, perez JE, Antonucci TK, Driscoll JH, Huang SM, Faja BW, Whitcomb RW, the Troglytazone Study Group. Cardiac and glycemic benefits of triglitazone treatment in NIDDM. Diabetes.46:433-439,1997.

18. World Health Organization. Impaired glucose telerance and diabetes: WHO criteria. Br Med J. 6:45-86,1985.

19. Devereux RB, Reichek N: Echocardiographic determinationof left ventricular mass in man : anatomic validation of the method. Circulation 55:613-618, 1977.

20. Devereux RBLutas EM, Casale PN, Kligfield P, Eisenberg RR, Hammond IW, Miller DH, Ries G, Alderman MH, Laragh JH; Standardadization of M-mode echocardiographic left ventricular anatomic measurements. J Am Coll Cardiol 4:1222-1230,1984.

21. Appleton CP, Hatle LK, Popp RL. Relation of transmitral flow velocity pattern to left ventricular function: new insight from a combined hemodynamic and Doppler echocardiographic study. J Am Coll Cardiol. 12:426-440,1988.

22. Appleton CP, Hatle LK, Popp RL. Relation of transmitral low velocity patterns to left ventricular diastolic function: new insight from a combined hemodynamic and Doppler ehocardiographic study. J Am Coll Cardiol. 12;426-440,1988.

23. White WB, Lund-Johansen P, McCabe EJ. Clinical evaluation of the Colin BPM 630 at rest and during exercise: an ambulatory blood pressure monitoring with gas-poweredcuff inflation. J Hypertens. 7:477-483,1989.

24. Teusher A Egger M, Hermann JB. Diabetes and nephropathy: blood pressure in clinical diabetic patients and control population. Arch Intern Med 149:1942-1945,1989.

25. Epstein M, Sowers JR; Diabetes mellitus and hypertension. Hypertension 19:403-418,1992.

26. Weidmann P, Ferrari P. Hypertension and the diabetic: central role of sodium. Diabetes Care 14:220-232,1991.

27. Factor SM, Sonnenblick EH. The pathogenesis of clinical and experimental congestive cardimyopahties: recent concepts. Progr Cardiovasc Dis 27:395-420,1985.

28. Myreng Y, Smiseth AO. Assessment of left ventricular relaxation by Doppler echocardiography; compaison of isovolumetric relaxation and transmitral flow velocities with time constant of isovolumic relaxation. 81:260-266,1990.

COST AND BENEFITS OF BLOOD PRESSURE MONITORING AND CONTROL

Arun Chockalingam[1] and Norman R.C. Campbell[2]

1. Centre for Chronic Disease Prevention and Control, Health Canada, Ottawa, Canada.
2. Departments of Medicine and of Pharmacology and Therapeutics, University of Calgary, Calgary, Alberta

INTRODUCTION

In Canada health care costs 127 billions dollars a year (direct costs $ 44 billion, indirect costs $ 83 billion). Of this, cardiovascular diseases (CVD), coronary heart disease (CHD) and stroke combined consume around 29.8 billion (10.9 billion direct & 18.9 billion indirect) dollars and remains as the number one cause of health burden [1]. The direct cost refers to hospitalization (66%), drug costs (21%), Physicians fees (12%) and research (1%). Indirect costs refer to person years of lost life (premature death), disability costs and lost productivity.

Cardiovascular diseases including stroke continue to be the number one cause of death in Canada, like most western countries [2]. It is well established that uncontrolled high blood pressure is a primary risk factor for CVD including stroke [3]. The cost of CVD reflects both on individuals and the society at large. Therefore, early detection and control of cardiovascular risk factors such as high blood pressure, hyperlipidemia, diabetes mellitus, obesity, smoking and alcohol abuse are essential to curb the escalating cost both at the individual and societal level.

Detection, follow-up, treatment and control of high blood pressure are necessary steps to control CVD and its ensuing toll on health care burden [4]. For the purpose of this article, our discussions are limited only to high blood pressure.

In considering the cost to the individuals and the societies, there are four important issues to consider. They are:
Lack of awareness
Diagnostic errors
The decision to intervene and
Lack of comprehensive management.

LACK OF AWARENESS

Diabetes and Cardiovascular Disease: Etiology, Treatment and Outcomes
Edited by Aubie Angel et al., Kluwer Academic/Plenum Publishers, 2001

According to the Canadian Heart Health Survey conducted in all 10 Canadian provinces during the period of 1986-1992 prevalence of high blood pressure was estimated to be at 22% (26% males and 18% females) [5]. This survey included 23,129 randomly selected, non-institutionalized respondents aged 18 to 74 years. High blood pressure was defined as BP ≥ 140/90 mmHg and or on treatment. The interesting and important finding from this survey was that only 58% of the hypertensives were aware of their hypertension status. Of those with hypertension, a mere 16% were treated and controlled, 23% were treated and not controlled while the remaining 19% were neither treated nor controlled. In addition, the remaining 42% (47% men and 35% women) of the hypertensives were completely unaware of their elevated blood pressure status.

Even in a developed country like Canada, with all the medical care available to the population, about 84% of the hypertensives or about 5.5 million adult Canadians are exposed to uncontrolled high blood pressure. It leaves them vulnerable to potential CVD including stroke. In an attempt to address this issue, the Canadian Coalition for High Blood Pressure Prevention and Control and Health Canada have joined forces with a number of non-governmental organizations and public/corporate partners to develop a national strategy for prevention and control of high blood pressure.

DIAGNOSTIC ERRORS

Blood pressure measurement, although a simple procedure, is often not done properly. Improper measurements could lead to either under diagnosis or over diagnosis [6,7]. Under diagnosis will lead to missed opportunities to identify and correct the potential risk for the patient. The patient is left vulnerable and exposed to cardio- cerebro-vascular complication. On the other hand, over diagnosis leads to unnecessary life-long treatment and unwarranted cost of medications and associated adverse drug effects.

McKay and colleagues [8] reported that there are three main factors which contribute to blood pressure measurement errors. They are (i) patient factors, (ii) provider factors and (iii) equipment factors. Their study, conducted in 114 physicians in Newfoundland, reported several important findings. The four key findings include, percentage of physicians who follow the Canadian Hypertension Society recommendations [9] for blood pressure measurement; percentage of physicians who deflated the cuff pressures at the recommended rate of 2-3 mmHg per second; percentage of physicians who were equipped with calibrated sphygmomanometers (either mercury or aneroid); and percentage of physicians who were equipped with various blood pressure cuff sizes.

This study showed that often times patients were not prepared (palpation, two arms, position, rest, etc.) before taking blood pressure measurements. Furthermore, only 15% of physicians deflated the cuff at the recommended deflation rate of 2-3 mmHg while 80% deflated too quickly and the remaining 5% deflated slowly. Only 3.5% of the physicians had calibrated mercury sphygmomanometers and none had calibrated aneroid manometers. Calibration errors of over 4 mmHg were found in 7.7% of mercury and 40.2% aneroid syphgmomanometers while errors of more than 10 mmHg was found to be among 0% of mercury and 10% aneroid syphygomanometers. Very few physicians were possessed with new-born, infant and child size cuffs as well as large and thigh size cuffs. Most physicians used one cuff for patients of all sizes.

As we can see from this report there are multitudes of errors that could contribute to improper blood pressure measurements. A recent study found that over 50% of patients with hypertension changed diagnostic class (normotensive Vs hypertensive) when blood pressure was measured with standardized Vs usual blood pressure measurement technique [10]. In 1994 the Canadian Coalition for High Blood Pressure Prevention and Control through its task force produced a *Guidline for proper blood pressure measurement* [11] and effectively disseminated across Canada. The Coalition also produced a plasticized card, listing 17 important steps for proper blood pressure measurement, that could be carried by the health care professionals.

THE DECISION TO INTERVENE

It is imperative that early detection, treatment and control of high blood pressure not only saves lives but also considerably reduces the health care burden. This is the 'high risk'approach. In other words, identify those at high risk and treat them. Several well controlled clinical trials report the benefit of treating high blood pressure. The well-known meta-analysis of several important clinical trials data by Collins and his colleagues [12] concluded that anti-hypertensive treatment lowering blood pressure by 4-6 mm Hg reduces stroke events by an average of 42% (range 33-50%) and coronary heart disease events by 14%.

In cost-benefit analysis an important parameter is *fraction of benefit* (FOB). The FOB is defined as the actual benefit observed divided by the potential benefit. Bulpitt [13], analysed the findings of Collins et al [12] for cost-benefit and concluded that a 42% 'actual'reduction in stroke could mean an 'observed' reduction of 35-40. Therefore, the FOB obtained for stroke was 100%. Using a similar analysis Bulpitt arrived at a 60% FOB for coronary heart disease.

In addition to a high risk approach, a population-based intervention is highly recommended as a preventive measure by epidemiologists [14]. The population distribution of blood pressure is 'normal' or 'gauzian' with a large percentage of the population falling in the middle of the 'bell' shaped curve and some in both extremities. Shifting the population mean even as low as 2 mmHg could result in significant health gains [15]. Figure 1 shows the population distribution before and after intervention. With a 90 mmHg cut off for high blood pressure, the population at risk of high blood pressure is seen to be at 24% and 20% before and after intervention respectively. Just a mere 2 mmHg shift shows a 4% of the population receiving the benefit.

Figure 1. Effects of a population-based intervention strategy among men and women aged 35 to 65 years of all races combined. (Adopted from Ref. 16)

Cook et al [16] estimated number of coronary heart disease (CHD) events prevented per 100,000 with a reduction of diastolic blood pressure in an untreated population. These authors have shown that a reduction of 2 mmHg (reduction) shift in population distribution through lifestyle intervention only to yield a reduction of 5.6% of CHD events. They have also demonstrated that a reduction of 5-6 mmHg in medical treatment of all those with a diastolic blood pressure greater than or equal to 90 mmHg resulted in 6.7% reduction in CHD events.

Shifting population mean to the left has been demonstrated to be possible over a period of time. The landmark North Karelia study [17] has clearly demonstrated that over a twenty year period (1972-1992), the population mean diastolic blood pressure decreased from 92 down to 85 mmHg (in men) and from 92 down to 80 mmHg (in women). Similar leftward shifts were reported for systolic blood pressures as well. Systolic blood pressure decreased from 149 down to 141 mmHg (in men) and from 153 down to 135 mmHg (in women). Such a favourable trend in hypertension is probably due partly to re-organizing the hypertension care system and partly to the intensive heath education in the community. Heath education has resulted in marked improvements in health behaviours such as smoking [18] and dietary habits [19-21].

When dealing with 'high risk' approach one should be cognizant of the differential distribution of population attributable risk. Referring to Figure 1, percentage of population concentrated in the range of 90-100 mmHg diastolic is higher than that in the range of 105-130. In the MRFIT study [22] people with more than 160 mmHg systolic were reported to be less than 2% of population with all deaths attributable to systolic blood pressure of less than 25%. The corresponding numbers for people in the range of 120-139 and 140-159 mmHg systolic were 33% and 40% respectively. The same study

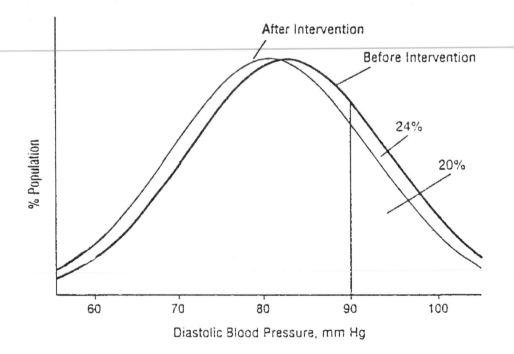

reported that intervention of patients with 105-130 mmHg diastolic resulted in a reduction of 15% excess deaths while those with 80-95 mmHg resulted in a reduction of 57%

excess deaths [23]. Therefore early intervention to reduce hypertension will produce a larger population effect

LACK OF COMPREHENSIVE MANAGEMENT

Studies indicate that lack of patient adherence [24, 25] and health care provider adherence strongly contribute to poor blood pressure control. CVD including stroke is a multifactorial disease. While treating a patient with any one risk factor, it is highly recommended to explore for other co-morbid risk factors such as hyperlipidemia, smoking, obesity, diabetes mellitus and sedentary lifestyle.

CONCLUSIONS

If properly implemented, lifestyle modification can reduce high blood pressure not only at the individual level but also at the population level. This could be highly effective at reducing the incidence and prevalence of high blood pressure and CVD. When lifestyle modification is not feasible or inappropriate one should resort to drug therapy. While doing so, the care giver should keep in mind that high blood pressure is a silent killer and early detection and ongoing treatment to keep it under control is warranted. The caregiver should also be responsible to choosing the right type of medication for the patient concerned since the medication cost is covered by the patient in most instances.

In terms of opportunities to improve cost effectiveness of blood pressure monitoring and control [26], the following issues should be addressed: proper diagnosis of hypertension using well defined guidelines; choice of treatment regimen; counseling patients to improved adherence [24]; step-down of medication dosage as and when the blood pressure is well controlled and at the same time frequently monitoring the patient's blood pressure levels; and the efficiency of the office practice in terms of providing prevention counseling in addition to drug treatment.

In a condition like high blood pressure which requires a lifelong intervention one should pay attention to both cost as well as benefit [27]. In an effort to keep the cost down and at the same time respecting the moral responsibility, the society should engage in both 'high risk' and population approaches. They are not mutually exclusive but are vital complementary.

REFERENCES

1. Heart and Stroke Foundation of Canada. The changing face of heart disease and stroke in Canada 2000. Ottawa, Canada, 1999; pp 61-63.
2. The World Health Report 1997. Conquering suffering, Enriching humanity. Geneva, Switzerland, World Health Organization, 1997.
3. WHO Technical Report Series. No. 862, Hypertension Control. Report of a WHO Expert Committee. Geneva, Switzerland, World Health Organization, 1996.
4. Hypertension Detection and Follow-up Program Co-operative Group. Five-year findings of the Hypertension Detection and Follow-up Program: I. Reduction in mortality of persons with high blood pressure, including mild hypertension. J Am Med Assoc 1979; 242: 2562-2571.
5. Joffres MR, Ghadirian P, Fodor JG, et. al. Awareness, treatment, and control of hypertension in Canada. AJH 1997; 10: 1097-1102.
6. Campbell NRC, McKay DW. Accurate blood pressure measurement, why does it matter? Editorial. CMAJ. 1999;161:277-8.
7. Campbell, NRC, Myers MG, McKay DW Usual measurement of blood pressure. is it meaningful? Blood Pressure Monitoring 1999;4:71-6.
8. McKay DW, Campbell NRC, Parab LS, et. al. Clinical assessment of blood pressure. J Human Hypertens 1990; 4: 639-645.

9. Haynes BR, Lacourciere Y, Rabkin S, et. al. Report of the Canadian Hypertension Society Consensus Conference: 2. Diagnosis of hypertension in adults. Can Med Assoc J 1993; 149(4): 409-418.
10. Campbell, NRC, Myers MG, McKay DW Usual measurement of blood pressure. is it meaningful? Blood Pressure Monitoring 1999;4:71-6.
11. Abbot D, Campbell N, Carruthers-Czyzewski P, et. al. Canadian Coalition for High Blood Pressure Prevention and Control Guidelines for measurement of blood pressure, follow-up, and life-style counselling. Can J Pub Hlth 1994; 85 (Suppl. 2): S29-S35.
12. Collins R, Peto R, MacMahon S, et. al. Blood pressure, stroke, and coronary heart disease. Part 2, short-term reductions in blood pressure: overview of randomised drug trials in their epidemiological context. Lancet 1990; 335: 827-838.
13. Bulpitt CJ. A risk-benefit analysis for treatment of hypertension. Postgrad Med J 1993; 69:764-774.
14. Rose G. Strategy of prevention. Lessons from cardiovascular disease. Br Med J 1981; 282: 1847-1851.
15. Rose G. Strategies of prevention: the individual and the population. In Coronary heart disease epidemiology. From aetiology to public health (eds.) Marmot M and Elliott P. Oxford University Press, Oxford, UK. 1994. Pp 311-324.
16. Cook NR, Cohen J, Hebert P, Taylor JO, Hennekens CH. Implications of small reductions in diastolic blood pressure for primary prevention. Arch Intern Med. 1995;155:701-9.
17. Nissinen A, Tuomilehto J, Salomaa V, Puska P. Hypertension Control. In The North Karelia Project. 20 years results and experiences (eds.) Puska P, Tuomilehto J, Nissinen A, Vartiainen E. The National Piblic Health Institute (KTL), Finland. 1995. Pp 95-105.
18. Salonen JT, Puska P, Kottke TE. Smoking, blood pressure and serum cholesterol as risk factors of acute myocardial infarction and death among men in Eastern Finland. Eur Heart J 1981; 2: 365-373.
19. Tuomilehto J, Puska P, Tanskanen A, et. al. A community-based intervention study on the fesibility and effects of the reduction of salt intake in North Karelia, Finland. Acta Cardiol 1981; 36: 83-104.
20. Tuomilehto J, Puska P, Nissinen A, et. al. Community-based prevention of hypertension in North Karelia, Finland. Ann Clin Res 1984; 16 (Suppl. 43): 18-27.
21. Puska P, Iacono J, Nissinen A, et. al. Controlled, randomized trial of the effect of dietary fat on blood pressure. Lancet 1983; 1: 1-5.
22. Stamler J. Blood pressure and high blood pressure. Aspects of risk. Hypertension . 1991;18(suppl 1): 95-107.
23. Stamler J, Neaton JD, Wentworth DN. Blood pressure (systolic and diastolic) and risk of fatal coronary heart disease. Hypertension 1989;13(suppl I):2-12.
24. Chockalingam A, Bacher M, Campbell NRC, Cutler H, Drover A, Feldman R, Fodor JG, Irving J, Ramsden V, Thivierge R, Tremblay G. Adherence to management of high blood pressure: Recommendations of the Canadian Coalition for High Blood Pressure Prevention and Control. Can J Publ Hlth 1998; 89(Suppl. I): 5-11.
25. Berlowitz DR, Ash AS, Hickey EC, Friedman RH, Glickman M, Kader B, Moskowitz MA. Inadequate management of blood pressure in a hypertensive population. NEJM 1998;339:1957-63.
26. Staeson WB. Opportunities to improve the cost-effectiveness of treatment for hypertension. Hypertension 1991; 18 (Suppl. I): 161-166.
27. Fletcher A. Pressure to treat and pressure to cost: a review of cost-effectiveness analysis. J Hypertens 1991; 9: 193-198.

MALONYL COA CONTROL OF FATTY ACID OXIDATION IN THE DIABETIC RAT HEART

Gary D. Lopaschuk

Cardiovascular Research Group
University of Alberta
Edmonton, Alberta, Canada

INTRODUCTION

Diabetics have a significantly greater incidence and severity of angina, acute myocardial infarctions (AMI), congestive heart failure, and other manifestations of atherosclerosis than non-diabetics [37]. Long-term mortality rates following an AMI are 2-3 times higher in diabetics compared with non-diabetics, while mortality rates following coronary artery bypass grafting are also 2 times as high [9,37,87]. While a high incidence of coronary artery disease is a major contributor to the high prevalence of heart disease in the diabetic, it is also clear that non-coronary factors contribute to the severity of ischemic injury. In particular, diabetes-induced changes within the heart itself are important contributing factors to injury during and following an AMI [6,70,71,84].

Accumulating evidence suggests that an over-reliance of the heart on fatty acid oxidation as a source of energy is an important contributing factor to the severity of ischemic injury in the diabetic [10,17,18,49,68,86,91]. In particular, fatty acid inhibition of myocardial glucose use is an important contributing factor to ischemic injury [10,49,68,91]. Furthermore, it is now clear that a link exists between improving glucose use and overcoming the biochemical changes that occur in the diabetic heart [17,18,34,35,49,68,91]. This review will discuss the subcellular changes that occur in the myocardium of the diabetic that contribute to this abnormal fatty acid metabolism. In particular, the importance in this process of malonyl CoA, a potent inhibitor of fatty acid uptake into the mitochondria, will be discussed.

CARDIAC ENERGY METABOLISM IN THE DIABETIC

Energy Metabolism In The Aerobic Heart

Myocardial ATP production under aerobic conditions arises predominantly from the mitochondrial oxidation of acetyl CoA, derived from carbohydrates (primarily glucose and lactate), free fatty acids and to a lesser extent ketone bodies and amino acids [see reviews 40,64,75]. Glucose is taken up by the cardiomyocytes in an insulin-dependent manner (via GLUT 4 and GLUT 1 transporters) and is then predominantly metabolized through

Diabetes and Cardiovascular Disease: Etiology, Treatment and Outcomes
Edited by Aubie Angel et al., Kluwer Academic/Plenum Publishers, 2001

155

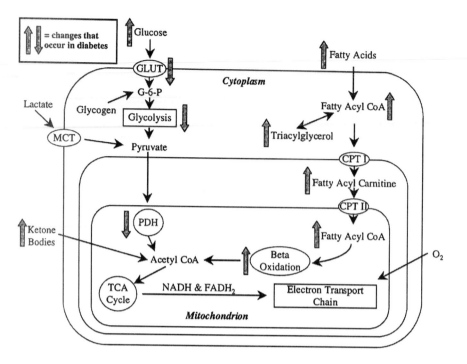

Figure 1. Overview of fatty acid metabolism in the heart

glycolysis to form pyruvate. Pyruvate produced by glycolysis is either converted to acetyl CoA (oxidative metabolism) or is converted to lactate and released from the heart. Pyruvate taken up by the mitochondria is converted to acetyl CoA by the pyruvate dehydrogenase complex (PDC) [Figure 1].

In uncontrolled diabetics, myocardial glucose use is reduced and fatty acid oxidation can account for almost all of the myocardial oxygen consumption [30,74,75,78,91]. This is due in part to a decrease in the number and activity of glucose transporters in the membrane [19]. However, a major reason for the decrease in myocardial glucose metabolism is the elevated levels of plasma fatty acids that can be found in the diabetic [76]. Use of fatty acids for mitochondrial oxidative metabolism results in a marked decrease in both the activty of PDC and

phosphofructose-1 kinase, a key enzyme in the glycolytic pathway [26,67,73,75]. While high circulating levels of fatty acids in the diabetic decrease glucose metabolism, it is clear that other metabolic changes in the heart are also responsible for low glucose oxidation rates. For instance, the decrease in PDC activity seen in diabetic rat hearts exceeds what would be expected if the inhibition occurred solely to a high level of circulating fatty acids [74,75]. This is supported by the observation that glucose oxidation rates are significantly lower in diabetic rat hearts compared to control hearts, even if hearts are perfused with similar concentrations of fatty acids [91,82]. As a result, the combination of high levels of circulating fatty acids and direct alterations in insulin control of fatty acid and glucose oxidation, can result in the diabetic rat heart becoming entirely dependent on fatty acid oxidation for its energy requirements [29,30,50,74,75,78,91,82].

Energy Metabolism During And Following Cardiac Ischemia

During ischemia, when the supply of O_2 becomes limiting for oxidative phosphorylation, both fatty acid and carbohydrate oxidation decrease and ATP production is impaired. Anaerobic glycolytic ATP production and glycogenolysis initially increase in an attempt to compensate for this decrease in ATP supply. As a result, decreased glucose uptake and glycolysis during ischemia in the diabetic heart may increase the sensitivity of the diabetic to myocardial ischemia. However, increasing glycolysis during and following ischemia is a "double-edged sword" since during severe ischemia, high glycolytic rates contribute to cellular acidosis, thereby exacerbating cell injury [see 47,51, and 55 for reviews].

During reperfusion following an episode of ischemia, a rapid recovery of mitochondrial oxidative phosphorylation must occur if contractile function is to recover. During this period, fatty acid oxidation is the predominant source of myocardial ATP production in non-diabetics, providing 80 to 90% of the heart's energy requirements [8,43,50,77]. These high rates of fatty acid oxidation are primarily due to: 1) circulating concentrations of fatty acids that occur following acute myocardial infarction or cardiac bypass surgery [2,48,66,69,85], and 2) a decrease in the intracellular regulation of fatty acid oxidation, especially at the level of mitochondrial fatty acid uptake [40,41,44,45] (see next section). Although circulating fatty acid levels can be elevated in diabetics even in the absence of ischemia, it is not clear what effect ischemia has on the control of mitochondrial fatty acid oxidation in the diabetic.

High rates of fatty acid oxidation during reperfusion of ischemic hearts markedly decreases glucose oxidation rates, contributing to contractile dysfunction during reperfusion [44,45,50,53,54,64]. Recent experimental and clinical studies have shown that stimulating glucose oxidation can both improve cardiac function and cardiac efficiency [see 47,51,55,83 for reviews]. Furthermore, a new class of pharmacological agents that inhibit fatty acid oxidation and stimulate glucose oxidation is now being used clinically to treat ischemic heart disease [5]. For instance, trimetazidine, which stimulates glucose oxidation in the heart secondary to an inhibition of fatty acid oxidation, has recently been licensed in over 80 countries for the treatment of ischemic heart disease [51,52].

Although it is clear that high rates of fatty acid oxidation contribute to cardiac ischemic injury in the non-diabetic, it is not clear what effect high rates of fatty acid oxidation have on ischemic injury in the diabetic rat heart. The issue of whether the diabetic rat heart is more or less sensitive to ischemic injury is controversial, has recently been debated [25,72]. While this issue remains to be resolved, it appears that depressed glycolytic rates in the diabetic rat heart contributes to injury in hypoxic or mildly ischemic hearts, but decreases the potential for acidosis and injury in severely ischemic hearts. However, in both mild and severe ischemia, inhibiting fatty acid oxidation and stimulating glucose oxidation will benefit the diabetic heart [see 47,51,55 and 56 for reviews). Therefore, one approach that has potential in treating myocardial ischemia is to decrease mitochondrial fatty acid uptake in the diabetic rat heart.

CONTROL OF MITOCHONDRIAL FATTY ACID UPTAKE BY THE HEART

Fatty acid oxidation can be regulated at a number of different sites in the heart. These different sites are reviewed in a number of recent articles from our laboratory [47,51,55] and others [42,67,88]. One particularly important site is at the level of mitochondrial uptake of fatty acids. A key enzyme in this process is carnitine palmitoyltransferase (CPT) 1 [Figure 2]. CPT 1 is the first committed step of fatty acid oxidation, and transfers the fatty acid moiety from acyl-CoA to carnitine to form long chain acylcarnitine, which is then transported into the mitochondria [see 59 and 62 for reviews]. Malonyl-CoA, which is produced by acetyl-CoA carboxylase, is a potent inhibitor of CPT 1 [59,60]. Unlike the liver, where a 88 kDa isoform of CPT 1 predominates, hearts predominantly express a 82 kDa isoform of CPT 1 [12,23,96]. The 88 kDa isoform of CPT 1 is expressed in the heart, although it is expressed to a much lesser extent then the 82 kDa isoform [22,24,92]. Because the 82 kDa CPT 1 is more sensitive to inhibition by malonyl CoA [92], the cardiac CPT 1 is 10 to 50 times more sensitive to malonyl CoA inhibition then the liver [16,60,61].

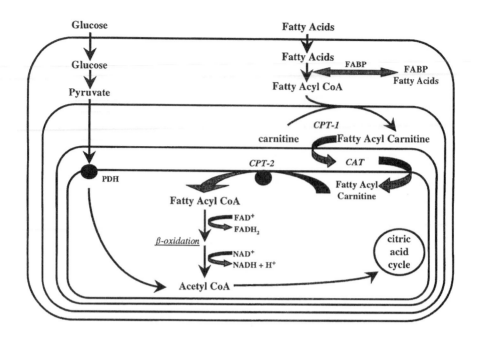

Figure 2: Alterations in malonyl CoA control of cardiac fatty acid oxidation in diabetes.

In liver, the IC_{50} of CPT 1 for malonyl CoA can increase dramatically in diabetes [15,62,80]. As a result, high concentrations of malonyl CoA are required to inhibit fatty acid oxidation and, theoretically, malonyl CoA becomes less important as a regulator of hepatic fatty acid oxidation. In contrast to the liver, previous studies by McGarry's group [59-61] and Cook's group [15,16] have shown that the sensitivity of heart CPT 1 to malonyl CoA inhibition does not change in diabetic animals [16,39,46]. In both newborn hearts and in reperfused ischemic hearts (both of which are conditions in which fatty acid oxidation increase) we have also observed that the sensitivity of CPT 1 to malonyl CoA inhibition does not change [39,46]. Existing evidence suggests that actual changes in malonyl CoA levels appear to be the key factor regulating changes in fatty acid oxidation in the heart, as opposed to changes in sensitivity of CPT 1 to malonyl CoA inhibition.

In light of recent advances in the molecular characterization of CPT 1, the issue of cardiac CPT 1 sensitivity to malonyl CoA inhibition has recently been revisited by the laboratories of Dr. McGarry [12] and Dr. McMillin [63]. In newborn hearts, the expression of 82 kDa isoform of CPT 1 increases and has been suggested to be the major source of CPT 1 activity in the newborn heart [12]. This suggests that in the newborn heart CPT1 is more sensitive to malonyl CoA inhibition. To date, it has not been determined if CPT 1 isoform expression changes in the diabetic heart.

It should be recognized that it is unlikely that all the malonyl CoA present in the heart is accessible to CPT 1. This is because total measured levels of malonyl CoA in the heart range from 5 to 30 nmol/g dry wt [39,76,101,132], which if all cytosolic would roughly translate into a cytoplasmic concentration of 2-15 μM. However, the IC_{50} for cardiac CPT 1 is in the 30-100 nM range [59,60,61,78]. Therefore, malonyl CoA must be compartmentalized in the heart and cannot always be accessible to CPT 1, or the heart would not oxidize fatty acids (which clearly is not the case). A significant amount of malonyl CoA probably exists in the mitochondrial matrix. Unfortunately, it is technically difficult to get an accurate measure of the actual cytoplasmic levels of malonyl CoA accessible to CPT 1. While we have observed a correlation between total tissue levels of malonyl CoA and fatty acid oxidation rates in some of our studies [39,40,46,47,56,57,79], this relationship does not persist under all experimental conditions [27,82].

ACETYL-COENZYME A CARBOXYLASE (ACC) REGULATION OF FATTY ACID OXIDATION IN THE HEART

Cardiac muscle expresses a 280 kDa isoform of ACC that regulates fatty acid oxidation secondary to the production of malonyl CoA. Our studies in isolated working rat hearts have provided direct proof that ACC is an important regulator of fatty acid oxidation [39,40,46,47,56,57,79], an observation that was also confirmed by Awan and Saggerson in isolated myocytes [5]. A role of ACC in regulating skeletal muscle fatty acid oxidation has also recently been shown [65,81,89,93,94]. In pancreatic islet cells ACC may also regulate fatty acid oxidation, and may have a novel and important role in glucose-stimulated insulin secretion secondary to inhibition of fatty acid oxidation [13,14,73], although a recent study did not support this concept [3].

Although very little is known about the transcriptional control of heart ACC, it is clear that ACC activity is regulated both by phosphorylation control and by acetyl CoA supply to the enzyme.

Phosphorylation Control Of ACC

Heart expresses an AMP-activated protein kinase (AMPK) that can phosphorylation and inhibit cardiac ACC activity [39,40]. Research on AMPK in the liver has recently attracted considerable attention, due to its ability to conserve energy by inhibiting anabolic processes when cellular ATP levels are depleted and AMP levels increase [32,33]. We have recently characterized AMPK activity in heart tissue and found that AMPK activity is comparable to the activity observed in liver [39,40]. We have also observed a close correlation between increased AMPK activity, decreased ACC activity and increased fatty acid oxidation in isolated working rat hearts [40,41,57,58].

In liver, AMPK has been termed a "fuel gauge" by Dr. Hardie, and it is thought that during times of metabolic stress AMPK is activated to downregulate anabolic processes in the liver (such as fatty acid and cholesterol biosynthesis). In heart and skeletal muscle AMPK also appears to act as a fuel gauge, but in these tissues AMPK acts to upregulate fatty acid oxidation during times of energy demand. A decrease in AMPK activity also functions to decrease fatty acid oxidation rates in times of low demand (secondary to an increase in ACC activity and malonyl CoA levels). In support of this concept we recently demonstrated that insulin inhibits AMPK activity in the heart [27,57], similar to what has been previously observed in liver [95]. We propose that insulin inhibition of AMPK functions to downregulate fatty acid oxidation in response to the increase in glucose metabolism that occurs following insulin administration. This provides an attractive mechanism by which fatty acid oxidation and glucose metabolism in the heart can be coordinated. To date it has not been determined how insulin inhibits AMPK, although a decreased phosphorylation of AMPK is one possibility.

The effects of diabetes on cardiac AMPK activity depends on the severity and type of diabetes. In severe uncontrolled diabetes (rats administered 100 mg/kg i.v. streptozotocin), AMPK activity increases, while in milder diabetes (rats administered 55 mg/kg i.v.streptozotocin) or in insulin-resistant diabetes (JCR/LA rats), we do not see changes in AMPK activity [56,82].

Substrate Control Of ACC

Our earlier studies demonstrated that cardiac ACC is regulated by acetyl CoA supply and has an important role in ensuring an adequate supply of acetyl CoA for the TCA cycle [79]. During periods of low metabolic demand, intramitochondrial acetyl CoA increases, and the acetyl groups are transferred out of the mitochondria via a carnitine acetyltransferase-translocase pathway [47]. The cytoplasmic acetyl CoA is then used as a substrate by ACC to produce malonyl CoA, resulting in a decrease in fatty acid oxidation rates during periods of low metabolic demand. We also demonstrated that increases in intramitochondrial acetyl CoA supply from glucose oxidation could stimulate this pathway [79]. As a result, this pathway provides an attractive means by which an increase in glucose metabolism can downregulate fatty acid metabolism.

Our previous studies have addressed diabetes-induced changes in ACC expression and activity occur in hearts obtained from streptozotocin diabetic rats [28]. Despite the presence of severe diabetes, neither the levels of mRNA or protein for the cardiac isoforms of ACC are altered. Whether ACC activity is changed depends on the severity and duration of diabetes. In acute diabetes a decrease in ACC activity is observed, which is accompanied by an increase in AMPK activity [28]. We have also recently observed that ACC activity is decreased in hearts obtained from insulin-resistant JCR/LA rats [56]. Accompanying this decrease in ACC activity is an increase in AMPK activity. Combined this data suggests that the change in ACC activity in these hearts occurs due to an alteration in either phosphorylation control or allosteric control, as opposed to an alteration in expression of ACC.

We have also recently demonstrated that insulin can stimulate ACC in heart muscle [27,57]. What is responsible for the increase in ACC activity is not clear, although preliminary evidence suggests that it is due to decreased AMPK phosphorylation of cardiac ACC, resulting in ACC being in a more active dephosphorylated state [28,57].

ISCHEMIA-INDUCED CHANGES IN CARDIAC ACETYL COA CARBOXYLASE

Although ACC expression remains constant under a wide range of fatty acid oxidation rates, we have shown that ACC activity dramatically decreases during reperfusion of previously ischemic hearts [39,40,41]. This is accompanied by a dramatic decrease in malonyl CoA levels [39], and is primarily responsible for the high rates of fatty acid oxidation seen in reperfused ischemic hearts. While a decrease in acetyl CoA supply to ACC may be partly responsible for the ischemia-induced decrease in malonyl CoA levels, a dramatic decrease in ACC activity appears to be responsible for this decrease in malonyl CoA levels and the high fatty acid oxidation rates during reperfusion. The decrease in ACC activity is not due to a degradation of ACC, but rather to a phosphorylation and inhibition of ACC [40,41]. Activation of AMPK during ischemia appears to be primarily responsible for this phosphorylation and inhibition of ACC (Figure 2) [40,41]. This is supported by our recent observation that inhibition of AMPK can increase malonyl CoA levels in the heart, resulting in a decrease fatty acid oxidation rates and an improvement in functional recovery during reperfusion [58].

MALONYL COA DEGRADATION IN THE HEART

Although the importance of malonyl CoA in regulating myocardial fatty acid oxidation has been firmly established, few studies have addressed how malonyl CoA is degraded in the heart. We propose that in heart, malonyl CoA is decarboxylated by a malonyl CoA decarboxylase (MCD). We have recently shown that heart contains an active MCD activity [7,20,21,39,82]. We have also shown that under conditions in which malonyl CoA levels decrease an increase in MCD activity can be observed [7,20]. For instance, in both diabetic or fasted rats (which have high fatty acid oxidation rates), MCD activity is increased [82]. The increase in fatty acid oxidation in the newborn heart is also accompanied by an increase in MCD activity [20].

We recently purified MCD from the rat liver, isolating a protein of approximately 48 kDa [21]. The enzyme exists as a tetramer in viv [36,38]. The activity of this purified

MCD was 1571 times greater than the MCD activity found in the initial 55% ammonium sulphate pellet. Interestingly, like the uropygial gland, MCD also co-purifies with catalase. In collaboration with Dr. Marc Prentki, we were also successful in obtaining the rat islet and liver cDNA sequences for MCD [82,90]. Comparison with the goose uropygial gland cDNA sequence showed only 68% identity with the rat MCD's. Of interest, is that the rat MCD has a potential mitochondrial targeting sequence, and the C terminal part of the enzyme ends with a peroxysomal targeting motif characterized by the SKL signature. The significance of these sequences with regard to the subcellular localization of the enzyme remains to be determined. The uropygial gland of the goose contains two MCD isoforms [36,38], a mitochondria and a cytoplasmic isoform. Whether different isoforms exist in mammalian tissues also remains to be determined.

In both heart and liver, diabetes can induce significant changes in MCD activity. In 6 streptozotocin-diabetic rats, MCD activity is significantly increased in both the heart [82] and liver [21]. This increased activity is due to an increased expression of the enzyme. In fasted rats, MCD activity is also increased, although expression of MCD does not increase. Preliminary experiments sugges that this increase in activity may be due to a decrease in the phosphorylated state of the enzyme. While MCD is inhibited when phosphorylated [20], it has yet to be established which kinases are involved in this process.

Malonyl CoA decarboxylase activity is increased in the diabetic rat heart [82]. Therefore, if malonyl CoA synthesis decreases (such as can occur during reperfusion of hearts following an ischemic insult) then cytoplasmic malonyl CoA levels will decrease to a greater extent then the decrease observed in non-diabetic rat hearts. This will increase fatty acid oxidation to a greater extent in diabetic rat hearts compared to non-diabetic rat hearts. This will result in a further decrease in glucose oxidation during reperfusion of ischemic hearts, thereby decreasing cardiac function and efficiency.

CONTROL OF MALONYL COA LEVELS CONTRIBUTES TO THE SEVERITY OF ISCHEMIC INJURY IN THE DIABETIC RAT HEART

As discussed, experimental data is inconsistent as to whether the diabetic rat heart is more or less sensitive to ischemic injury. However, it is clear that high rates of fatty acid oxidation contribute to ischemic injury in the non-diabetic rat heart [39,40,44,45,49,50] and that myocardial fatty acid oxidation rates can be very high in the diabetic [82,91]. It is also clear that recovery of mechanical function in diabetic rat hearts following an episode low-flow ischemia is depressed compared to control hearts [10,11,25,49]. It has also been shown that if non-diabetic rat hearts are reperfused following ischemia, malonyl CoA levels dramatically drop resulting in high rates of fatty acid oxidation during the critical period of reperfusion [39,40]. This drop in malonyl CoA levels is due to an activation of AMPK during and following ischemia, resulting in an inhibition of ACC during reperfusion. In diabetic rat hearts, we have recently observed that MCD activity is significantly elevated compared to control hearts even in the absence of ischemia [82]. As a result, it is possible that any ischemia induced change in malonyl CoA synthesis could enhance ischemic injury in the diabetic rat heart compared to the control heart.

MALONYL COA CONTROL OF CARNITINE PALMITOYLTRANSFERASE 1 IS ALTERED IN THE DIABETIC HEART

In liver, diabetes results in a significant increase in CPT 1 activity and a decreased sensitivity of CPT1 to malonyl CoA inhibition [15,16,59,60,61,62]. However, unlike the liver, McGarry's group [61] and Cook's group [19] have shown that CPT 1 activity and the sensitivity of CPT 1 to malonyl CoA inhibition does not change in hearts from diabetic rats. However, since these earlier studies were performed it has now been shown that 2 isoforms of CPT 1 exist in the heart (an 82 and 88 kDa) with different affinities for carnitine and different K_i values for malonyl CoA inhibition [22,23,24]. It has also been shown and that a switch in CPT 1 isoform distribution can occur in a number of physiological situations. To date, it is not clear if diabetes results in any changes in CPT 1 isoform expression in the heart.

SUMMARY

Increased fatty acid metabolism can decrease cardiac function and efficiency, and may therefore contribute to the outcome of ischemic injury in the diabetic. Alterations in the control of myocardial malonyl CoA levels is an important contributing factor to these high fatty acid oxidation rates. This includes alterations in AMPK, ACC, and MCD activity in the diabetic rat heart. A further understanding of how malonyl CoA controls fatty acid oxidation in the diabetic heart should help identify new targets for pharmacological intervention which decreases the reliance of the heart on fatty acid oxidation, and ultimately improves heart function.

REFERENCES

1. Abu-Elheiga L, Jayakumar A, Baldini A, Chirala SS. Human acetyl CoA carboxylase: characterization, molecular cloning and evidence for two isoforms. *Proc Natl Acad Sci USA* 1995; **92**:4011-4015.
2. Allison SP, Chamberlain MJ, Hinton P. Intravenous glucose tolerance, insulin, glucose and free fatty acid levels after myocardial infarction. *Br Med J* 1969; **4**:776-778.
3. Antinozzi PA, Segall L, Prentki M, McGarry JD. Molecular or pharmacologic pertubation of the link between glucose and lipid metabolism is without effect on glucose-stimulated insulin secretion. A re-evaluatio n of the long-chain acyl-CoA hypothesis. *J Biol. Chem* 1998; **273**:16146-16154.
4. Asins G, Serra D, Arias G, Hegardt FG. Developmental changes in carnitine palmitoyltransferases I and II gene expression in intestine and liver of suckling rats. *Biochem J* 1995; **306**:379-384.
5. Awan MM, Saggerson ED. Malonyl-CoA metabolism in cardiac myocytes and its relevance to the control of fatty acid oxidation. *Biochem J* 1993; **295**:61-66.
6. Baandrup U, Ledet, T, Rasch, R. Diabetic cardiopathy; quantitative histological studies of diabetic rats in poor and good control. *Lab Invest* 1981; **45**:169-173.
7. Barr RL, Kozak R, Lopaschuk GD. Malonyl CoA degradation in the reperfused ischemic heart. *Circulation* 1996;**64**; I-125.
8. Benzi RH, Lerch R. Dissociation between contractile function and oxidative metabolism in postischemic myocardium. *Circ Res* 1992; **71**:567-576.
9. Bradley RF, Bryfogle JW. Survival of diabetic patients after myocardial infarction. *Am J Med* 1956; **30**:207-216.
10. Broderick T, Barr RL, Quinney A, Lopaschuk GD. Acute insulin withdrawal from diabetic BB rats decreases myocardial glycolysis during low-flow ischemia. *Metabolism* 1992; **41**:33-338.
11. Broderick TL, Quinney HA, Lopaschuk GD. Protection of the ischemic diabetic myocardium by L-carnitine: effects on glycolysis, glucose oxidation and functional recovery. *Cardiovasc Res* 1995;29:373-378.
12. Brown NF, Weis BC, Husti JE, Foster DW, and McGarry JD. Mitochondrial carnitine pPalmitoryltransferase I isoform switching in the developing rat heart. *J Biol Chem* 1995; **270**:8952-8957
13. Brun T, Roche E, Kim K, Prentki M. Glucose regulates acetyl-CoA carboxylase gene expression in a pancreatic ß-cell line (INS-1). *J Biol Chem* 1993; **268**:18905-18911.
14. Chen A, Ogawa A, Ohneda M, Unger RH, Foster DW, McGarry JD. More direct evidence for a Malonyl-CoA-Carnitine palmitoyltransferase I interaction as a key event in pancreatic-cell signaling. *Diabetes* 1994; **43**:87-883.
15. Cook GA, Gamble MS. Regulation of carnitine palmitoyltransferase by insulin results in decreased activity and decreased apparent K_i values for malonyl CoA. *J Biol Chem* 1987; **262**:2050-2055.
16. Cook GA, Lappi MD. Carnitine palmitoyltransferase in the heart is controlled by a different mechanism than the hepatic enzyme. *Mol Cell Biochem* 1992; **116**:39-45.
17. Dillmann WH. Methyl palmoxirate increases Ca^{2+} myosin ATPase activity and changes myosin isoenzyme distribution in the diabetic rat heart. *Am J Physiol* 1985;**248**:E602-E605.
18. Dillmann WH. Myosin isoenzyme distribution and Ca^{2+} activated myosin ATPase activity in the rat heart influenced by fructose feeding and triiodothyronine. *Endocrinology* 1985; **116**:2160-2166.

19. Douen AG, Ramlal T, Rastogi S, Bilan PJ, Cartee GD, Vranic M, Holloszy JO, Klip A. Exercise induces recruitment of the "Insulin-responsive glucose transporter. *J BiolChem* 1990; **265**:13427-13430.
20. Dyck JRB, Barr A, Barr R, Kolattukudy PE, Lopaschuk GD. Characterization of cardiac malonyl-CoA decarboxylase and its putative role in regulating fatty acid oxidation. *Am J Physiol* 1998;**275**:H2122-H2129.
21. Dyck JRB, Berthiuame LG, Kantor PF, Barr AJ, Barr R, Singh D, Hopkins TA, Voilley N, Prentki M, Lopaschuk GD. Isolation and cloning of rat liver malonyl CoA decarboxylkase and characterization of its role in regulating hepatic fatty acid oxidation. (manuscript submitted).
22. Esser V, Britton CH, Weis BC, Foster DW, McGarry JD. Cloning, sequencing, and expression of a cDNA encoding rat liver carnitine palmitoyltransferase I. *J Biol Chem* 1993; **268**:5817-5822.
23. Esser V, Brown NR, Cowan AT, Foster DW, McGarry JD. Expression of a cDNA isolated from rat brown adipose tissue and heart identifies the product as the muscle isoform of predominant CPT I isoform expressed in both white (epididymal) and brown adipocytes. *J Biol Chem* 1996; **271**:6972-77.
24. Esser V, Kuwajima M, Britton CH, Krishnan K, Foster DW, McGarry JD. Inhibitors of mitochondrial carnitine palmitoyltransferase I limit the action of proteases on the enzyme. *J Biol Chem* 1993; **268**:5810-5816.
25. Feuvray D, Lopaschuk GD. Controversies on the sensitivity of the diabetic heart to ischemic injury: the sensitivity of the diabetic heart to ischemic injury is decreased. *Cardiov. Res.* 1997; **34**:113-120.
26. French, TJ, Goode AW, Holness MJ, MacLennan, PA, Sugden MC. The relationship between changes in lipid fuel availability and tissue fructose 2,6-bisphosphateconcentrations and pyruvate dehydrogenase complex activities in the fed state. *Biochem J* 1988; **256**:935-939.
27. Gamble J, Lopaschuk GD. Insulin inhibition of 5' adenosine monophosphate-activated protein kinase in the heart results in activation of acetyl coenzyme A carboxylase and inhibition of fatty acid oxidation. *Metabolism* 1997; **46**: 1270-1274.
28. Gamble J, Witters LA, Makinde O, Lopaschuk GD. Acetyl CoA carboxylase expression in the diabetic rat heart (manuscript submitted).
29. Garland PB, Randle PJ. Regulation of glucose uptake by muscle. X. Effects of alloxan diabetes, starvation, hypophysectomy and adrenalectomy and of fatty acids, ketonebodies and pyruvate on the glycerol output and concentrations of free fatty acids, long-chain fatty acyl coenzyme A, glycerol phosphate and citrate cycle intermediates in rat hearts and diaphragm muscles. *Biochem J* 1970; **93**:678.
30. Goodale WT, Olson RE, Hackel DB. The effects of fasting and diabetes mellitus on myocardial metabolism in man. *Am J Med* 1959; 212-220.
31. Goodwin GW, Taegtmeyer H. Regulation of fatty acid oxidation of the heart by MCD and ACC during contractile stimulation. Am J Physiol 1999;**277**:E772-E777.
32. Hardie DG. An emerging role for protein kinases: the response to nutritional and environmental stress. *Cell Signal* 1994; **6**:813-821.
33. Hardie DG. Regulation of fatty acid and cholesterol metabolism by the AMP-activated protein kinase. *Biochim Biophys Acta* 1992; **1123**:231-238.
34. Hekimian G, Feuvray D. Reduction of ischemia-induced acyl carnitine accumulationby TDGA and its influence on lactate dehydrogenase release in diabetic rat hearts. *Diabetes* 1986; **35**:906-910.
35. Heyliger CE, Rodrigues B, NcNeill JH. Effect of choline and methionine treatment on cardiac dysfunction of diabetic rats. *Diabetes* 1986; **35**:1152-1157.
36. Jang, S-H., Cheesbrough, T.M., Kolattukudy, E. Molecular cloning, nucleotide sequence, and tissue distribution of malonyl-CoA decarboxylase. *J Biol Chem* 1989:**264**, 3500-3505.
37. Kannel WB, McGee DL. Diabetes and cardiovascular risk factors: the Framingham study. *Circulation* 1979; **59**:8-13.
38. Kolattukudy, P. E., Poulose, A. J., Kim, Y-S. (1981) Malonyl-CoA decarboxylase from avian, mammalian, and microbial sources. *Methods-Enzymol* 1981; **71**, 150-163.
39. Kudo N, Barr A, Barr R, Lopaschuk GD. 5'AMP-activated protein kinase inhibition of acetyl CoA carboxylase can explain the high rates of fatty acid oxidation in reperfused ischemic hearts. *J Biol Chem* 1995; 270:17511-17520.
40. Kudo N, Gillespite JG, Kung L, Witters LA, Schulz R, Clanachan AS, Lopaschuk GD. Characterization of 5'AMP-activated protein kinase activity in the heart and its role in inhibiting acetyl-CoA carboxylase during reperfusion following ischemia. *Biochim Biophys Acta* 1996;**1301**:67-75. protein kinase that is involved in the regulation of fatty acid oxidation. *Circulation* 1996; **92**:I-771.
42. Kunau WH, Dommes V, Schulz H. ß-oxidation of fatty acids in mitochondria, peroxisomes, and bacteria: a century of continued progress. *Prog Lipid Res* 1995; **34**:267-342.
43. Liedtke AJ, DeMaison L, Eggleston AL, Cohen LM, Nellis SH. Changes in substrate metabolism and effects of excess fatty acids in reperfused mycoardium. *Circ. Res.* 1988; **62**:535-542.
44. Liu B, Clanachan AS, Schulz R, Lopaschuk GD. Cardiac efficiency is improved after ischemia by altering both the source and fate of protons. *Circ Res* 1996; **79**:940-948.

45. Liu B, El Alaoui-Talibi Z, Clanachan AS, Schulz R, Lopaschuk GD. Uncoupling of contractile function from mitochondrial TCA cycle activity and MV_{O2} during reperfusion of ischemic hearts. *Am J Physiol* 1996; **270**:H72-H80.

46. Lopaschuk G, Witters LA, Itoi T, Barr R, Barr A. Acetyl-CoA carboxylase involvement in the rapid maturation of fatty acid oxidation in the newborn rabbit heart. *J Biol Chem* 1994; **269**:25871-25878.

47. Lopaschuk GD, Belke DD, Gamble J, Itoi T, Schönekess BO. Regulation of fatty acid oxidation in the mammalian heart in health and disease. *Biochim Biophys Acta* 1994; **1213**:263-276.

48. Lopaschuk GD, Collins-Nakai R, Olley PM, Montague,TJ, McNeil G, Gayle, M, Penkoske P, Finegan BA. Plasma fatty acid levels in infants and adults after myocardial ischemia. *Am Heart J* 1994; **128**: 61-67.

49. Lopaschuk GD, Spafford M. Response of isolated working hearts from acutely and chronically diabetic rats to fatty acids and carnitine palmitoyltransferase I inhibition during reduction of coronary flow. *Circ Res* 1989; **65**:378-387.

50. Lopaschuk GD, Spafford MA, Davies NJ, Wall SR. Glucose and palmitate oxidation in isolated working rat hearts reperfused after a period of transient global ischemia. *Circ Res* 1990; **66**:546-553.

51. Lopaschuk GD, Stanley WC. Glucose metabolism in the ischemic heart. *Circulation* 1997; **95**:313-315.

52. Lopaschuk GD, Stanley WC. Manipulation of energy metabolism in the heart. *Science and Medicine* 1997; **4**:2-51.

53. Lopaschuk GD, Wall SR, Olley PM, Davies NJ. Etomoxir, a carnitine palmitoyltranferase I inhibitor, protects hearts from fatty acid-induced ischemic injury independent of changes in long chain acylcarnitine. *Circ Res* 1988; **63**:1036-1043.

54. Lopaschuk GD, Wambolt RB, Barr RL. An imbalance between glycolysis and glucose oxidation is a possible explanation for the detrimental effects of high levels of fatty acids during aerobic reperfusion of ischemic hearts. *J Pharm Exp Ther* 1993; **264**:135-144.

55. Lopaschuk GD. Alterations in fatty acid oxidation during reperfusion of the heart after myocardial ischemia. *Am J Cardiol* 1997; **80**:11A-16A.

56. Lopaschuk GD. Fatty acid metabolism in the heart following diabetes. *Diabetes in the Heart* (in press).

57. Makinde A-O, Gamble J, Lopaschuk GD. Upregulation of 5'-AMP-activated protein kinase is responsible for the increase in myocardial fatty acid oxidation rate following birth in the newborn rabbit. *Circ. Res* 1997; **80**:482-489.

58. Makinde AO, Lopaschuk GD. Evidence that 5' AMP-activated protein kinase regulates fatty acid oxidation in the newborn rabbits hearts. *Circulation* (manuscript submitted).

59. McGarry JD, Foster DW. Regulation of hepatic fatty acid oxidation and ketone body production. *Ann Rev Biochem* 1980; **49**:395-420.

60. McGarry JD, Leatherman GF, Foster DW. Carnitine palmitoyltransferase I. The site of inhibition of hepatic fatty acid oxidation by malonyl-CoA. *J Biol Chem* 1978; **253**,4128-4136.

61. McGarry JD, Mills SE, Long CS, Foster DW. Observations on the affinity for carnitine, and malonyl-CoA sensivity, of carnitine palmitoyltransferase I in animal and human tissues. *Biochem J* 1983; **214**:21-28.

62. McGarry JD, Woeltje KF, Kuwajima M, Foster DW. Regulation of ketogenesis and the renaissance of carnitine palmitoyltransferase *Diabetes* 1989; **5**:271-284.

63. McMillin JB, Wang D, Witters LA, Buja LM. Kinetic properties of carnitine palmitoyltransferase I in cultured neonatal rat cardiac myocytes. *Arch. Biochem. Biophys.* 1994; **312**:375-384.

64. McVeigh JJ, Lopaschuk GD. Dichloroacetate stimulation of glucose oxidation improves recovery of ischemic rat hearts. *Am J Physiol* 1990; **29**:H1079-H1085.

65. Merrill GF, Kurth EJ, Hardie DG, Winder WW. AICA riboside increases AMP-activated protein kinase, fatty acid oxidation, and glucose uptake in rat muscle. *Am J Physiol* 1997; **273**:E1107-E1112.

66. Mueller HS, Ayes ST. Metabolic responses of the heart in acute myocardial infarction in man. *Am J Cardiol* 1978; **42**: 363-371.

67. Neely JR, Morgan HE. Relationship between carbohydrate metabolism and energy balance of heart muscle. *Ann Rev Physiol* 1974; **36**:413-459.

68. Nicholl TA, Lopaschuk GD, McNeill JH. The effects of free fatty acids and dichloroacetate on the isolated working diabetic rat heart. *Am J Physiol* 261:H1053- H1059.

69. Oliver MF, Kurien VA, Greenwood TW. Relation between serum-free-fatty acids and arrythmia and death after myocardial infarction. *Lancet* 1968; **1**: 710-715.

70. Oswald B, Corcovan S, Yudkin JS. Prevalence and risks of hyperglycemia and undiagnosed diabetes in patients with acute myocardial infarction *Lancet* 1984; **1**:1264-1267.

71. Partamian JO, Bradley RF. (Acute myocardial infarction in 258 cases of diabetes. *N Engl J Med* 1965; **273**:455

72. Paulson DJ. The diabetic heart is more sensitive to ischemic injury, *Cardiov. Res.* 1997; **34**:104-112.

73. Prentki M, Vischer S, Glennon MC, Regazzi R, Deeney JT, Corkey BE. Malonyl-CoA and long chain acyl-CoA esters as metabolic coupling factors in nutrient-induced insulin secretion. *J Biol Chem* 1992; **267**:5802-5810.

74. Randle PJ, Hales CN, Garland PB, Newsholme EA. The glucose fatty-acid cycle. Its role in insulin sensitivity and the metabolic disturbances of diabetic mellitus. *Lancet* 1963; **1**:785-789.

75. Randle PJ, Newsholme EA, Garland PB. Regulation of glucose uptake by muscle: effects of fatty acids, ketone bodies and pyruvate and of alloxan-diabetes and starvation, on the uptake and metabolic fate of glucose in rat heart and diaphragm muscles. *Biochem J* ; **93**:652-665.

76. Reaven GM, Hollenbeck C, Jeng CY, Wu MS, Chen YI. Measurements of plasmaglucose, free fatty acid, lactate, and insulin for 24h in patients with NIDDM. *Diabetes* 1988; **37**: 1020-1024.

77. Saddik M, Lopaschuk GD. Myocardial triglyceride turnover during reperfusion of isolated rat hearts subjected to a transient period of global ischemia. *J Biol Chem* 1991; **267**:3825-3831.

78. Saddik M, Lopaschuk GD. Triacylglycerol turnover in isolated working hearts of acutely diabetic rats. *Can J pharmacol* 1994; **72**:1110-1119.

79. Saddik M. Gamble J, Witters LA, Lopaschuk GD. Acetyl-CoA carboxylase regulation of fatty acid oxidation in the heart. *J Biol Chem* 1993;**268**:25836-25845.

80. Saggerson ED, Carpenter CA. Effects of fasting, adrenalectomy and streptozotocin   diabetes on snesitivity of hepatic carnitine acyltransferase to malonyl CoA. *FEBS Lett* 1981; **129**:225-228.

81. Saha AK, Vavvas D, Kurowski TG, Apazidis A, Witters LA, Shafrir E, Ruderman NB. Malonyl-CoA regulation in skeleletal muscle: its link to cell citrate and the glucose-fatty acid cycle. *Am J Physiol* 1997; **272**: E641-E648.

82. Sakamoto J, Barr R, Kavanagh K, Lopaschuk GD. An increase in malonyl-CoA decarboxylase activity contribute to the high fatty acid oxidation rates seen in hearts from diabetic rats. *Am J Physiol* (in press).

83. Stanley WC, Lopaschuk GD, Hall, JL, McCormack JG. Regulation of myocardial carbohydrate metabolism under normal and ischaemic conditions. *Cardiovasc Res* 1997; **33**:243-257.

84. Stone PH, Muller JE, Hartwel T, York BJ, Rutherford JD, Parker CB, Turi ZG, Strauss HW, Willerson JT, Robertson T, Braunwald E, Jaffe AS. The effect of diabetes mellitus on prognosis and serial left ventricular function after acute myocardial infarction: Contribution of both coronary disease and diastolic left ventricular dysfunction to the adverse prognosis. *J Am Coll Cardiol* 1989; **14**:49-57.

85. Svensson S, Svedjeholm R, Ekroth R, Milocco I, Nilsson F, Sabek KG, William-Olsson G. Trauma metabolism and the heart: uptake of substrates and effect of insulin early after cardiac operations. *J Thorac Cardiovasc Surg* 1990; **99**: 1063-1073.

86. Tahiliani AG, McNeill JH. Diabetes-induced abnormalities in the myocardium. *Life Sc* 1986; **38**:959-974.

87. Ulvenstam G, Aberg A, Bergstrand R, Johansson S, Pennert K, Vedin A, Wilhelmsen L, Wilhelmsson C. Long-term prognosis after myocardial infarction in men with diabetes. *Diabetes* 1985; **34**:787-792.

88. Van der Vusse GJ, Glatz JF, Stam HC, Reneman RS. Fatty acid homeostasis in the normoxic and ischemic heart. *Physio. Rev* 1992; **72**: 881-940.

89. Vavvas D, Apazidis A, Saha AK, Gamble J, Patel A, Kemp BE, Witters LA, Ruderman NB. Contraction-induced changes in acetyl-CoA carboxylase and 5'-AMP-activated kinase in skeletal muscle. *J Biol Chem*.1997; **272**: 13255-13261.

90. Voilly N, Roduit R, Vicaretti R, Bonny C, Waeber G, Dyck JRB, Lopaschuk GD, Prentki M. Clongin and expression of rat pancreatic ß-cell malonyl CoA decarboxylase. *Biochem J* 1999;**240**:213-217.

91. Wall SR, Lopaschuk GD. Glucose oxidation rates in fatty acid-perfused isolated working hearts from diabetic rat. *Biochim Biophys Acta* 1989; **1006**:97-103.

92. Weis BC, Esser V, Foster DW, McGarry JD. Rat heart expresses two forms of mitochondrial carnitine palmitoyltransferase I. *J Biol Chem* 1994; **269**:18712-18715.

93. Winder WW, Hardie DG. Inactivation of acetyl-CoA carboxylase and activation of AMP-activated protein kinase in muscle during exercise. *Am J Physiol* 1996;**270**:

94. Winder WW, Wilson HA, Hardie DG, Rasmussen BB, Hutber CA, Call GB, Clayton RD, Conley LM, Yoon S, Zhou B. Phosphorylation of rat muscle acetyl CoA carboxylase by AMP-activated protein kinase and protein kinase A. *J Appl Physiol* 1997; **82**: 219-225.

95. Witters LA, Kemp BE. Insulin activation of acetyl-CoA carboxylase accompanied by inhibition of the 5'-AMP-activated protein kinase. *J Biol Chem* 1992; **267**:854-2867.

96. Xia Y, Buja M, McMillin JB. Change in expression of heart carnitine palmitoyltransferase I isoforms with electrical stimulation of cultured rat neonatal cardiac myocytes. *J. Biol. Chem.* 1996; **271**:12082-12087.

ALTERATIONS IN 1,2-DIACYLGLYCEROLS AND CERAMIDES IN DIABETIC RAT HEART

Kenji Okumura, Kazunori Hayashi, Kichiro Murase, Hideo Matsui, Yukio Toki.

Internal Medicine II
Nagoya University
Nagoya, Japan

INTRODUCTION

Recent evidence has implicated lipid-mediated second messengers such as 1,2-diacylglycerol (DAG)-protein protein kinase C (PKC) pathway as an important mediator underling multiple aspects of myocardial function (1). For example, PKC is involved in Ca^{2+}-induced inotropy, in mediating myocardial preconditioning by diverse stimuli both in animals and humans, and in the signaling processes which lead to the production of proinflammatory mediators. Hyperglycemia and diabetes have been shown to be associated with PKC activities (2). The changes in DAG-PKC pathway are significant in causing cardiovascular dysfunctions and pathologies.

PKC FAMILY

PKC is a ubiquitous Ser-Thr kinase with several isoforms. The PKCs are classified into three groups; conventional PKCs (α,β,γ) which are Ca^{2+} dependent and DAG sensitive, novel PKCs ($\delta,\epsilon,\theta,\eta,\mu$) which are DAG sensitive, and atypical PKCs (ζ,λ) which are Ca^{2+} independent and DAG insensitive. The quantitative immunoblot assay shows that the conventional PKCs are the most abundant, composing approximately 75% of total PKC, in the rabbit heart (3). Multiple isoforms are expressed in each cell. At least six different PKC isoforms have been identified in rat cardiac myocyte (4,5), where PKC regulates a number of functions such as contractility, atrial natriuretic factor secretion, and gene expression. In spite of extensive studies, attribution of a specific function to a specific isoform cannot be consistently established. In the left ventricular sample from failing myocardium, α and β isoforms of PKC are elevated in membrane fractions (6). Several isoforms may mediate a similar range of functions. A physiological activator DAG activates most of PKC isoforms.

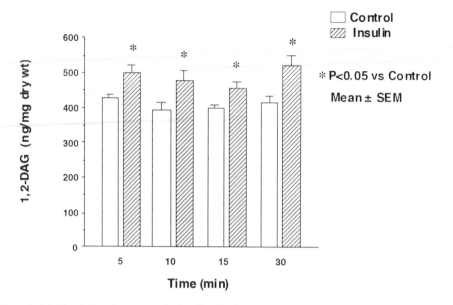

Figure 1. 1,2-Diacylglycerol contents after insulin (25mU/mL) perfusion in the isolated rat heart.

Therefore, the alteration in DAG may well be considered to have a great influence on transmembrane signaling systems.

DAG IN DIABETES

Previously, we demonstrated that the total DAG content is increased in the myocardium from both streptozotocin-induced diabetic rats and insulin-treated diabetic rats. The increases in DAG contents also have been shown in other tissues such as retina, glomeruli, and aorta in diabetic animal models (7). Insulin and a high glucose concentration induced a rapid increase in the formation of DAG. However, we found that the fatty acid profile in the increased DAG in the myocardium differs between diabetic rats and insulin-treated diabetic rats. The fatty acid profiles of DAG in diabetic rats were found to be almost the same as those in control. In contrast, the fatty acid composition of DAG was different in insulin-treated diabetic rat heart from that of either control or diabetic rats. In particular, the percentages of palmitic (16:0) and oleic acids (18:1, n-9) were increased in insulin-treated diabetic rats. These data suggest that the increased DAG contents may be produced from the different sources.

THE EFFECT OF INSULIN AND HIGH GLUCOSE ON DAG CONTENTS IN ISOLATED PERFUSED RAT HEART

Insulin and high glucose concentrations have been shown to increase DAG in cultured cells (8,9). Increases in DAG abundance have been proposed to be mediated by hydrolysis of inositol phospholipids by phospholipase C (10), de novo synthesis, and hydrolysis of phosphatidylcholine by phospholipase D (10). We studied effects of insulin and high glucose on DAG contents using isolated perfused rat hearts (male Wistar rats, 250~350g). In response

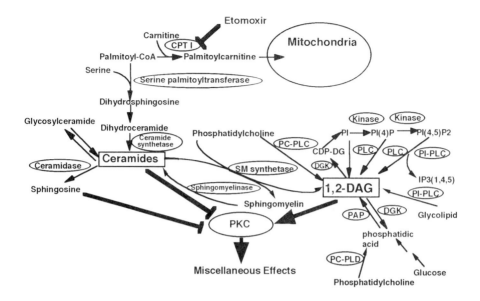

Figure 2. The Scheme of 1,2-diacylglycerol and protein kinase C pathway. CPT: carnitine palmitoyltransferase. PKC: protein kinase C. DAG: diacylglycerol. PC: phosphatidylcholine. PI: phosphtidylinositol. GPI: glycosylphosphatidylinositol. SM: Sphingomyelin. IP3(1,4,5): inositol 1,4,5-trisphosphate. PI(4)P: phosphatidylinositol 4-phosphate. PI(4,5)P2: phosphatidylinositol 4,5-bisphosphate. DGK: DAG kinase. PAP: phophatidate phosphatase. PLC: phospholipase C. PLD: phospholipase D.

to a high concentration (25 mU/ml) of insulin in the presence of 8.6 mmol/L glucose, a decrease in resting tension was accompanied by a significant increase in cardiac muscle contractility and a significant decrease in coronary flow. However, after a 25-minute perfusion in the presence of 3 mmol/L glucose, increasing the concentration to 17 mmol/L had no effect on heart performance (11). Addition of 25 mU/ml insulin to the perfusion medium increased total DAG by 18.2% and 26.4% after 5 and 30 minutes, respectively (Fig. 1). Among the fatty acid molecules involved in DAG, palmitic (16:0), oleic (18:1, n-9), and linoleic (18:2, n-6) acids showed significant increases of 17.2%, 39.8%, and 46.3%, respectively, in the heart after 5 minutes of insulin perfusion when compared with controls. A similar pattern was apparent at 15 and 30 minutes. Other fatty acid species of DAG remained largely unaffected. These results indicated that the distribution of different species of DAG changed in response to insulin perfusion, and that the increased DAG mass contained predominantly 16:0, 18:1 (n-9), and 18:2 (n-6) fatty acids. On the other hand, increasing the glucose concentration of the perfusion medium 3 to 17 mmol/L failed to increase the total mass of DAG or the abundance of specific fatty acids. Thus, we showed that DAG content in the rat hearts is increased by insulin perfusion but not a short exposure to a high glucose concentration. Although palmitic acid and oleic acid are the predominant fatty acids incorporated into DAG via the de novo pathway and the metabolism of PC, the source of increased DAG mass induced by insulin remains to be explored.

CERAMIDE IN DAG-PKC PATHWAY

Sphingolipids are structurally more complex than the glycerophospholipids which are

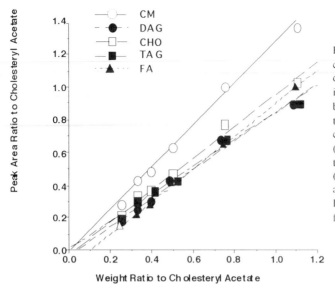

Fig. 3. Calibration curves for ceramide and diacylglycerol determinations. These lines indicate the relationship between the weight ratios and the peak area ratios of ceramides (CM). 1.2-diolein (DAG). cholesterol (CHO). triolein (TAG). and oleic acid (FA) compared to cholesteryl acetate by the FID response. Data represent the mean values from duplicate samples.

precursors of DAG, arachidonate and eicosanoids, and also participate in signal transduction (12). Ceramide and sphingomyelin, derivatives from sphingolipids (Fig.2), are associated with aspects of cell biology such as apoptosis, growth suppression, and stress response. Ceramide generation, resulting chiefly from sphingomyelin hydrolysis, constitutes a signal transduction pathway that mediates cytokines and tumor necrosis factor-α. Ceramide production also has been reported to induce NF-κB, a stress response transcription factor. Sphingolipid metabolites including ceramide inhibit the activity of protein kinase C (13). Therefore, ceramide may oppose the DAG-related action. Recently we developed the simultaneous quantitation of DAG and ceramide from the tissue with the use of the Iatroscan in a study of the significance of the two lipids in the myocardium (14). Figure 3 shows the peak area rations to cholesterol acetate, which is added to the homogenate of tissues as an internal standard, when compared with the weight rations to cholesterol acetate, and the relationship was linear.

CERAMIDE AND DAG CONTENTS IN STREPTOZOTOCIN-INDUCED DIABETIC RATS

We determined the ceramide content as well as DAG content in diabetic rat heart induced by streptozotocin (65mg/kg). Palmitoyl-CoA, an important precursor of sphingolipids synthesized de novo, is a substrate for carnitine palmitoyl transferase I (CPT I). Therefore, the inhibition of CPT I activity enhances sphingolipid synthesis and is associated with the metabolism of ceramide. Moreover, etomoxir, a CPT I inhibitor, has been reported to improve left ventricular performance of pressure-overload rat heart (15), and also may be valuable as a potential anti-diabetic drug (16). We evaluated the effect of etomoxir on ceramide and DAG contents. Left ventricular contractile function estimated by fractional shortening with transthoracic echocardiography was reduced in 6 week diabetic rats. However, one week (-)etomoxir treatment (18 mg/kg) of 5 week diabetic rats prevented the decrease in fractional shortening. Etomoxir itself did not affect left ventricular contractile function. DAG content

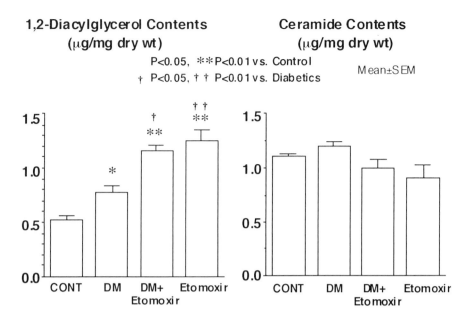

1,2-Diacylglycerol Contents **Ceramide Contents**
(μg/mg dry wt) **(μg/mg dry wt)**

P<0.05, **P<0.01 vs. Control
† P<0.05, † † P<0.01 vs. Diabetics

Mean±SEM

Figure 4. 1,2-Diacylglycerol and cermamide contents from control (CONT), diabetic (DM), etomoxir-treated diabetic (DM+Etomoxir), and etomoxir-treated control (Etomoxir) rats.

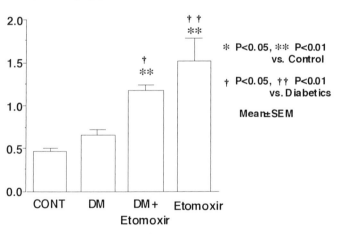

1,2-Diacylglycerol/Ceramide Ratio

* P<0.05, ** P<0.01
vs. Control

† P<0.05, †† P<0.01
vs. Diabetics

Mean±SEM

Figure 5. The ratios of 1,2-diacylglycerol to cermamide contents from control (CONT), diabetic (DM), etomoxir-treated diabetic (DM+Etomoxir), and etomoxir-treated control (Etomoxir) rats.

was increased in diabetic rat hearts more than observed in the previous experiments (7). Etomoxir treatment also elevated the DAG levels in control rats, and further increased those in diabetic rats (Fig. 4). We calculated the ratio of DAG to ceramide, because DAG is an activator and ceramide is an inhibitor of PKC. Therefore, their ratio may well be considered to express the activation of PKC in the tissue. The ratio of DAG to ceramide was increased in diabetic rat hearts (Fig. 5). Etomoxir elevated the ratio twice more than that in diabetic rats. These results suggest that the action of etomoxir is similar to that of insulin regarding lipid-mediated transduction system.

Inhibition of CPT 1 by etomoxir prevents palmitoyl-CoA from entering into mitochondria and leads to its accumulation in the cytoplasm, probably resulting in the augmentation of production of DAG. Ceramide has been shown to incite antiproliferative responses and apoptosis. Sphingomyelin metabolites including ceramide inhibit the activity of PKC. Therefore, elevated DAG levels may oppose this ceramide-related action.

IN CONCLUSION

DAG is elevated in the myocardium of both diabetic and insulin-treated diabetic rats. Insulin also elevates myocardial DAG contents, but the fatty acid profile of DAG in insulin-treated hearts differs from that in diabetic hearts. Etomoxir improves cardiac function of diabetic hearts and increases myocardial DAG. It is very likely that diabetic cardiomyopathy is attributed to the activation of the DAG-PKC pathway. However, the preventive effects of insulin and etomoxir on cardiac dysfunction in diabetic hearts are also via the DAG-PKC pathway. The elevated DAG differs in the fatty acid composition between diabetes and treated diabetes, probably resulting in leading different PKC activation.

REFERENCES

1. P.C. Simpson. β-Protein kinase C and hypertrophic signaling in human heart failure. Circulation. 99:334 (1999).
2. D. Koya. and G.L. King. Perspective in diabetes: Protein kinase C activation and the development of diabetic complications. Diabetes. 47:859 (1998).
3. P. Ping. J. Zhang. Y. Qiu. X.L. Tang. S. Manchikalapudi. X. Cao. and R. Bolli. Ischemic preconditioning induces selective translocation of protein kinase C isoforms ε and η in the heart of conscious rabbits without subcellular redistribution of total protein kinase C activity. Circ Res. 81:404 (1997).
4. V.O. Rybin. and S.F. Steinberg. Protein kinase C isoform expression and regulation in the developing rat heart. Circ Res. 74:299 (1994).
5. M.H. Disatnik. G Buraggi. and D Mochly-Rosen. Localization of protein kinase C isozymes in cardiac myocytes. Exp Cell Res. 210:287 (1994).
6. N. Bowling. R.A. Walsh. G Song. T Estridge. GE Sandusky. RL Fouts. K Mintze. T Pickard. R Roden. MR Bristow. HN Sabbah. JL Mizrahi. G Gromo. GL King. and CJ Vlahos. Increased protein kinase C activity and expression of Ca2+-sensitive isoforms in the failing human heart. Circulation. 98:384 (1998).
7. K.Okumura. N.Akiyama. H. Hashimoto. K. Ogawa. and T. Satake. Alteration of 1,2-diacylglycerol content in the myocardium from diabetic rats. Diabetes. 37:1168(1988).
8. T. Inoguchi. P. Xia. M. Kunisaki. S. Higashi. E.P. Feener. and G.L. King. Insulin's effect on protein kinase C and diacylglycerol induced by diabetes and glucose in vascular tissues. Am J Physiol. 267:E369 (1994).
9. S.H. Ayo. R. Radnik. J.A.Garoni. D.A. Troyer. and J.I. Kreisberg. High glucose increases diacylglycerol mass and activates protein kinase C in mesangial cell cultures. Am J Physiol. 261:F571 (1991).
10. W. Li. W. Wang. and X. Liu. Comparative study of high-glucose effect on phosphatidylcholine hydrolysis of cultured retinal capillary pericytes and endothelial cells. Biochim Biophys Acta. 1222:339 (1994).
11. K. Okumura. H. Matsui. K. Murase. A. Shimauchi. K. Shimizu. Y. Toki. T. Ito. and T. Hayakawa. Insulin increases distinct species of 1,2-diacylglycerol in isolated perfused rat heart. Metabolism. 45:774 (1995).
12. Y.A. Hannun. Functions of ceramide incoordinating cellular responses to stress. Science. 274:1855 (1996).
13. Y.A. Hannun. C.R. Loomis. A.H.Jr. Merrill. and R.M. Bell. Sphingosine inhibition of protein kinase C activity and of phorbol dibutyrate binding in vitro and in human platelets. J Biol Chem. 261:12604 (1986).

14. K. Okumura, K. Hayashi, I. Morishima, K. Murase, H. Matsui, Y. Toki, and T. Ito. Simultaneous quantitation of ceramides and 1,2-diacylglycerol in tissues by Iatroscan thin-layer chromatography-flame-ionization detection. Lipids. 33:529 (1998).
15. M. Turcani, and H. Rupp. Etomoxir improves left ventricular performance of pressure-overloaded rat heart. Circulation. 96:3681 (1997).
16. F.J. Schmitz, P. Rösen, and H. Reinauer. Improvement of myocardial function and metabolism in diabetic rats by the carnitine palmitoyl transferase inhibitor etomoxir. Horm Met Res. 27: 515 (1995).

REGULATION OF MYOCARDIAL PHOSPHOLIPID N-METHYLATION BY INSULIN AND DIABETES

Stephen W. Schaffer and Mahmood Mozaffari

University of South Alabama
School of Medicine
Department of Pharmacology
Mobile, Alabama

INTRODUCTION

Phospholipid N-methylation has been implicated in the actions of several hormones, neurohumoral modulators and pharmaceutical agents in the myocardium (Panagia et al. 1989; Taira et al. 1990; Hamaguchi et al. 1991). During N-methylaltion of phosphatidylethanolamine, the methyl group of S-adenosylmethionine is transferred to the amino head group of the phospholipid, resulting in the ultimate formation of phosphatidylcholine. Although the cytidinediphosphocholine pathway appears to serve as the primary source of phosphatidylcholine in the myocardium (Hatch et al. 1989), the conversion of phosphatidylethanolamine to phosphatidylcholine is considered important because it causes local changes in membrane structure (Post et al. 1995). One of the changes involves the redistribution of phospholipid within the membrane. This occurs because phosphatidylethanolamine, but not phosphatidylcholine, is preferentially located in the inner (cytoplasmic) leaflet of the membrane (Posts et al. 1995). When phosphatidylethanolamine is converted to phosphatidylcholine, a net transfer of phospholipid from the inner (cytoplasmic) leaflet to the outer (extracellular) leaflet of the membrane takes place (Crews 1985).

The other major effect of phospholipid N-methylation is a change in the size of the phospholipid headgroup, causing an alteration in the molecular shape and stable configuration of the phospholipid in aqueous solution. While phosphatidylethanolamine prefers a hexagonal H_{II} structure, phosphatidylcholine assumes a bilayer structure in solution (Cullis et al. 1986). According to the fluid mosaic model, the cell membrane exists as a fluid semipermeable bilayer, which can undergo local, transient departures from the bilayer structure. These transient phase transitions are promoted by hexagonal formers, such as phosphatidylethanolamine, and are thought to regulate several important membrane transport processes.

Among the important transport processes in the heart affected by phospholipid N-methylation and the phospholipid composition of the membrane is calcium transport. Panagia and coworkers (Ganguly et al. 1985; Panagia et al. 1986; Panagia et al. 1987) have reported an inhibition of Na^+-Ca^{2+} exchanger activity and an elevation in sarcolemmal and sarcoplasmic

Diabetes and Cardiovascular Disease: Etiology, Treatment and Outcomes
Edited by Aubie Angel et al., Kluwer Academic/Plenum Publishers, 2001

175

reticular Ca^{2+} activity upon stimulation of phospholipid N-methylation. Therefore, it is not surprising that modulation of phospholipid N-methylation is associated with changes in the contractile state of the heart (Gupta et al. 1988).

Panagia and coworkers (Ganguly et al. 1984; Panagia et al. 1990) have found that defects develop in the N-methylation of various cardiac subcellular membranes in the type I diabetic rat. Since these changes correlated with alterations in calcium transport, it was suggested that these defects may be crucial to the development of cardiac dysfunction in the type I diabetic. However, the mechanism underlying these changes in N-methylation were not investigated. The present study examines the effect of insulin and type II diabetes on phospholipid N-methylation activity.

METHODS

Type II diabetes was induced in 2 day old Wistar rats using the procedure described previously (Schaffer et al. 1985; Allo et al. 1991; Schaffer et al. 1993). As the diabetic animals aged they became markedly glucose intolerant. One hour after an intraperitoneal injection of 2 g/kg glucose, blood glucose levels of the year old diabetic rats rose to values ranging from 500 to 600 mg/dl, compared to levels of 200 to 300 mg/dl in the nondiabetic rats. Fasting blood glucose levels for the nondiabetic and diabetic were 110 ± 4 mg/dl and 139 ± 4 mg/dl, respectively.

Enriched sarcolemma was prepared from diabetic and nondiabetic rat hearts using the method of Pitts (1979) as previously described (Allo et al. 1991). To verify the purity of each preparation, assays of adenylate cyclase, cytochrome c oxidase, Ca^{2+} stimulated ATPase, p-nitrophenylphosphate driven calcium uptake and ATP-dependent calcium uptake in the presence and absence of 2 mM oxalate were performed. Of all reactions examined, diabetes only affected oxalate-independent ATP-dependent calcium uptake, reducing activity from 29.5 ± 2.1 to 23.8 ± 1.4 nmol/mg/min. The purity factor for adenylate cyclase and cytochrome c oxidase in the sarcolemmal preparation relative to the homogenate was about 10 fold and was similar in nondiabetic and diabetic membrane. The purity factor for cytochrome c was 0.5 in both preparations. Based on calcium transport assays, sarcoplasmic reticular contamination was deemed negligible in all preparations.

Phospholipid N-methyltransferase activity was assayed using sarcolemmal membrane prepared from type II diabetic and nondiabetic hearts. Panagia et al. (1987) have shown that the enzyme phospholipid N-methyltransferase contains three catalytic sites, with a site for each of the N-methylation steps in the conversion of phosphatidylethanolamine to phosphatidylcholine. Site I N-methyltransferase activity favoring the formation of phosphatidyl N-monomethylethanolamine, was determined in 50 mM Tris-glycylglycine buffer (pH 8.0) containing 1 mM $MgCl_2$ and 0.1 lM S-adenosyl-L-[^{3}H-methyl[-methionine. When examining the effects of insulin, sarcolemma (0.5 mg) preloaded with buffer containing 1 mM $MgCl_2$, 2 mM ATP and either 0 or 100 lM 5'guanyly imidodiphosphate (GppNHp), was incubated for 10 min at 37°C in the Tris-glycylglycine buffer containing the appropriate concentration of insulin but lacking radioactive S-adenosylmethionine. The assay for site I phospholipid N-methyltransferase (also referred to as PE N-methyltransferase) was initiated by the addition of radioactive S-adenosylmethionine and allowed to proceed for 30 min. The site II reaction favoring the formation of phosphatidyl-N,N-dimethylethanolamine was assayed by a 30 min incubation of 0.5 mg sarcolemmal protein with 50 mM phosphate buffer (pH 7.0) containing 10 lM S-adenosyl-L-[^{3}H-methyl]-methionine. The final reaction favoring phosphatidylcholine formation was assayed in 50 mM glycine buffer (pH 10.0, 37°) containing 150 lM radioactive S-adenosylmethionine. Thirty minutes following the addition of radioactive S-adenosylmethionine, the reaction at each site was terminated by addition of 3 ml chloroform/2N Hcl (6:3:1 by volume). The lipids were extracted according to the procedure of Ganguly et al. (1984) and the radioactive N-methylated phospholipid content was determined.

RESULTS

Prior to examining the effect of insulin on phospholipid N-methyltransferase activity, the effects of ATP and the GTP analog, GppNHp, on phospholipid N-methyltransferase activity were examined. While 2 mM ATP had no effect on site I N-methyltransferase activity, membrane loaded with buffer containing both 100 lM GppNHp and 2 mM ATP exhibited a 21% increase in enzyme activity. The effect of GppNHp was blocked by inclusion of 10 lM staurosporine in the site I incubation buffer. Also capable of reversing the effects of GppNHp was 0.2 U/l insulin (Figure 1). However, the effects of insulin and GppNHp appear to be mutually exclusive since similar insulin-mediated decreases in site I N-methyltransferase activity were observed in the presence and absence of GppNHp. Figure 2 shows the dose-dependent decrease in site I N-methyltransferase activity in the presence of ATP. The EC_{50} of insulin was 0.36 U/l while maximal inhibition of site I N-methyltransferase activity was approximately 50%.

Insulin was also found to inhibit phospholipid N-methyltransferase site III, which preferentially catalyzes the formation of phosphatidylcholine from phosphatidyl N,N dimethylethanolamine. At a concentration of 1.0 U/l, the extent of site III inhibition was 42% (Figure 3). By contrast, 1.0 U/l insulin produced no significant decline in site II phospholipid N-methyltransferase activity.

Despite the effects of insulin on N-methyltransferase activity, membrane isolated from type II diabetic rats contained normal N-methyltransferase activity (Table 1).

Nonetheless, the response to insulin was significantly impaired in the diabetic membrane. At the two concentrations examined (0.2 and 1.0 U/l) insulin mediated nearly a two-fold greater inhibition of site I N-methyltransferase activity with nondiabetic membrane than with diabetic membrane (Figure 4).

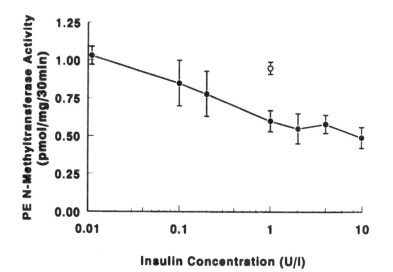

Figure 1. Regulation of phosphatidyletyhanolamine N-methyltransferase.
Enriched sarcolemma from rat heart were loaded with MOPS buffer containing 1 mM $MgCl_2$ and 160 mM NaCl, to which was added either no cofactor (Basal), 2 mM ATP (the ATP groups) or 2 mM ATP plus 100 bM GppNHp (the ATP + GppNHp groups). In some samples, the membranes were incubated for 10 min with 0.2 U/l insulin prior to initiating the N-methylation reaction by addition of radioactive S-adenosylmethionine (0.1 bM). Enzyme activity at site I was expressed as pmol [^{3}H]-methyl groups incorporated/mg protein/30 min. Values shown represent the means ± S.E.M. of four experiments. The asterisks denote significant differences (p < 0.05) between the insulin-treated samples and their corresponding controls lacking insulin. The pound sign denotes a significant difference between the ATP and GppNHp group and the groups lacking GppNHp.

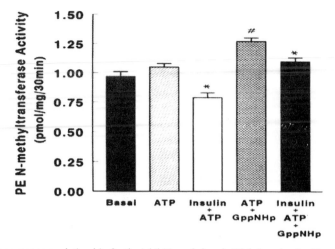

Figure 2. Dose response relationship for the inhibition of phosphatidylethanolamine N-methyltransferase activity by insulin.Enriched sarcolemma from rat heart were loaded with MOPS buffer containing 1 mM MgCl$_2$, 160 mM NaCl and either 0 or 2 mM ATP. After incubation of the preloaded membranes for 10 min with Tris-glycylglycine buffer containing 1 mM MgCl$_2$ and the appropriate concentration of insulin, the N-methyltransferase reaction was initiated by the addition of radioactive S-adenosylmethionine (0.1 bM). Open and closed circles represent phosphatidylethanolamine N-methyltransferase activity in the absence and presence of ATP in the membrane loading buffer. Values shown represent the means ± S.E.M. of 4-5 preparations.

Table 1. Effect of type II diabetes on sarcolemmal phospholipid N-methyltransferase activity.

Catalytic Site	Nondiabetic	Diabetic
I	1.01 ± 0.11	1.17 ± 0.12
II	25.0 ± 2.4	19.8 ± 2.1
III	221 ± 23	287 ± 41

Sarcolemma were prepared form hearts derived from nondiabetic and type II diabetic rats. Phospholipid N-methyltransferase activity at its three catalytic sites was assayed according to the procedure described in the Methods. Values are expressed as [^{3}H]-methyl groups incorporated/mg protein/30 min and represent means ± S.E.M. of 5-7 different membrane preparations.

DISCUSSION

Taira et al. (1990) have previously shown that rats administered isoproterenol i.p. experience an elevation in myocardial site I N-methyltransferase activity, which can be duplicated by exposure of isolated sarcolemma to the catalytic subunit of cAMP dependent protein kinase. It is well established that isoproterenol-mediated activation of cAMP dependent protein kinase involves a cascade of reactions initiated by the coupling of the b adrenergic receptor to a G protein. Thus, our finding that the G protein activator, GppNHp, also stimulates site I N-methyltransferase activity is consistent with the actions of isoproterenol. Similarly, the inhibition of the GppNHp effect by the protein kinase inhibitor, staurosporine, is consistent with the involvement of protein kinases in the signal transduction pathway activated by isoproterenol. By contrast, reversal of the effect by insulin appears unrelated to the signal transduction pathway of the b adrenergic agonist. This conclusion is supported by the observation that insulin (0.2 U/l) mediates a 20% reduction in site I N-methyltransferase activity in both the presence and absence of GppNHp. Also, the EC$_{50}$ of the

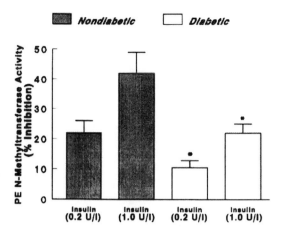

Figure 3. Effect of insulin on sites II and III phospholipid N-methyltransferase activity. Sarcolemma from rat heart were loaded with MOPS buffer containing 1 mM $MgCl_2$, 160 mM NaCl and 2 mM ATP and then incubated with MOPS buffer containing 1 U/l insulin for 10 min prior to assaying site II (closed bars) and site III (open bars) N-methyltransferase activity. Values shown represent the means $\pm$ S.E.M. of 7-8 experiments. The asterisk denotes significant difference ($p < 0.05$) between site III activity with and without insulin.

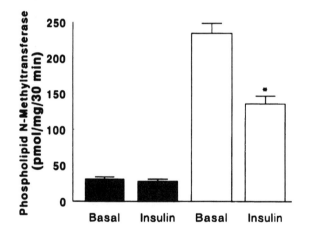

Figure 4. Influence of type II diabetes on insulin-mediated inhibition of site I N-methyltransferase activity. Enriched sarcolemma from diabetic and nondiabetic rat heart were loaded with MOPS buffer as described in Figure 3. After a 10 min incubation with buffer containing 0.2 or 1.0 U/l insulin, the site I N-methyltransferase reaction was initiated. The data are expressed as % inhibition of N-methyltransferase activity by insulin. Values shown represent means $\pm$ S.E.M. of 5-7 different membrane preparations. Asterisks denote significant difference ($p < 0.05$) between the diabetic and nondiabetic preparations.

insulin effect is comparable to the EC_{50} for other insulin-mediated events, such as the stimulation of glucose transport in the isolated rat heart (Schaffer et al. 1993).

In addition to inhibiting site I N-methyltransferase activity, insulin also inhibits site III N-methyltransferase activity, but is without significant influence on site II activity. This differential regulation of the reaction sites of the phospholipid N-methyltransferase has been commonly observed. Panagia et al. (1989) found that quinidine, which presumably alters enzyme activity by changing the structure of the phospholipid bilayer, inhibits site II N-methyltransferase activity without altering sites I and III. On the other hand, phosphorylation of the membrane with cAMP dependent protein kinase stimulates site I activity without affecting sites II and III (Taira et al. 1990). Moreover, activation of site I activity by the reducing agent, dithiothreitol, greatly exceeds the activation of the other two sites (Vetter et al. 1991).

It is noteworthy that sites II and III, but not site I, play a significant role in the modulation of sarcolemmal calcium transport (Panagia et al. 1987; Gupta et al. 1988). This may be related to the characteristics of the phospholipid products of the three N-methylation reactions. While the primary substrate for site I N-methylation, phosphatidylethanolamine, is a nonbilayer former, the products of the site II and III N-methyltransferase reactions, phosphatidylcholine and phosphatidyl-N,N dimethylphosphatidylethanolamine, serve as stabilizers of the bilayer membrane (Cullis et al. 1986). Thus, it is logical to assume that N-methylation-mediated changes in the nonbilayer/bilayer ratio of the membrane can alter the activity of transporters, such as the Na^+,Ca^{2+} exchanger. Indeed, incubation of sarcolemma with medium containing 150 1 M S-adenosylmethionine to promote site III N-methylation, leads to a decrease in Na^+,Ca^{2+} exchanger activity. On the other hand, insulin is known as an activator of the Na^+,Ca^{2+} exchanger. It is possible that insulin stimulates the exchanger in part by inhibiting site III N-methylation.

Panagia et al. (1990) have attributed certain calcium transport defects in the type I diabetic heart to impaired phospholipid N-methyltransferase activity. However, in contrast to the type I diabetic heart, the type II diabetic heart exhibits no significant change in basal phospholipid N-methyltransferase activity. Thus, it is unlikely that the basal calcium transport abnormalities noted in the type II diabetic heart is caused by impaired phospholipid N-methyltransferase activity. Indeed, the primary calcium transport defect found in the type II diabetic, namely, the loss in Na^+,Ca^{2+} exchanger activity, occurs in response to hyperglycemia rather than insulinopenia (Schaffer et al. 1997). However, the activation of the Na^+,Ca^{2+} exchanger by insulin is attenuated in the type II diabetic heart (Schaffer et al. 1997). That observation is consistent with the present study that insulin-mediated activation of site III phospholipid N-methyltransferase activity is impaired in the type II diabetic heart. Thus, the insulin resistance of the type II diabetic heart is reflected in the response of both the Na^+,Ca^{2+} exchanger and phospholipid N-methyltransferase activity to insulin action. Whether the two processes are causatively related remains to be determined.

REFERENCES

Allo SN, Lincoln TM, Wilson GL, Green FJ, Watanabe AM, Schaffer SW. Non-insulin-dependent diabetes-induced defects in cardiac cellular calcium regulation. Am J Physiol 1991;260:C1165-C1171

Crews FT. "Phospholipid methylation and membrane function." In *Phospholipids and cellular regulation*, CRC Press, Boca Raton, pp 131-158, 1986

Cullis PR, Hope MJ, Tilcock CPS. Lipid polymorphism and the roles of lipids in membranes. Chem Physics Lipids 1986;40:127-144

Ganguly PK, Rice KM, Panagia V, Dhalla N. Sarcolemmal phosphatidylethanolamine N-methylation in diabetic cardiomyopathy. Circ Res 1984;55:504-512

Ganguly PK, Panagia V, Okumura K, Dhalla NS. Activation of Ca^{2+}-stimulated ATPase by phospholipid N-methylation in cardiac sarcoplasmic reticulum. Biochem Biophys Res Commun 1985;130:472-478

Gupta MP, Panagia V, Dhalla NS. Phospholipid N-methylation-dependent alterations of cardiac contractile function by L-methionine. J Pharmacol Expt Therap 1988;245:664-672

Hamaguchi T, Azuma J, Schaffer S. Interaction of taurine with methionine: Inhibition of myocardial phospholipid methyltransferase. J Cardiovasc Pharmacol 1991;18:224-230

Hatch GM, Karmin O, Choy PC. Regulation of phosphatidylcholine metabolism in mammalian hearts. Biochem Cell Biol 1989;67:67-77

Panagia V, Okumura K, Makino N, Dhalla NS. Stimulation of Ca^{2+} pump in rat heart sarcolemma by phosphatidylethanolamine N-methylation. Biochim Biophys Acta 1986:856:383-387

Panagia V, Makino N, Ganguly PK, Dhalla NS. Inhibition of Na^+-Ca^{2+} exchange in heart sarcolemmal vesicles by phosphatidylethanolamine N-methylation. Eur J Biochem 1987;166:597-603

Panagia V, Ganguly PK, Gupta MP, Taira Y, Dhalla NS. Alterations of phosphatidylethanolamine N-methylation in rat heart by quinidine. J Cardiovasc Pharmacol 1989;14:763-769

Panagia V, Taira Y, Ganguly PK, Tung S, Dhalla NS. Alterations in phospholipid N-methylation of cardiac subcellular membranes due to experimentally induced diabetes in rats. J Clin Invest 1990;86:777-784

Pitts BJR. Stoichiometry of sodium-calcium exchange in cardiac sarcolemmal vesicles. J Biol Chem 1979;254:6232-6235

Post JA, Verkleij AJ, Langer GA. Organization and function of sarcolemmal phospholipids in control and ischemic/reperfused cardiomyocytes. J Mol Cell Cardiol 1995;27:749-760

Schaffer SW, Ballard-Croft C, Boerth S, Allo SN. Mechanisms underlying depressed Na^+/Ca^{2+} exchanger activity in the diabetic heart. Cardiovasc Res 1997;34:129-136

Schaffer SW, Tan BH, Wilson GL. Development of a cardiomyopathy in a model of noninsulin-dependent diabetes. Am J Physiol 1985;248:H179-H185

Schaffer SW, Warner BA, Wilson GL. Effects of chronic glipizide treatment on the NIDD heart. Horm Metab Res 1993;25:348-352

Taira Y, Panagia V, Shah KR, Beamish RE, Dhalla NS. Stimulation of phospholipid N-methylation by isoproterenol in rat hearts. Circ Res 1990;66:28-36

Vetter R, Dai J, Mesaeli N, Panagia V, Dhalla NS. Role of sulfhydryl groups in phospholipid methylation reactions of cardiac sarcolemma. Mol Cell Biochem 1991;103:85-96

REDUCTION OF PHOSPHATIDYLINOSITOL -4,5-BISPHOSPHATE MASS IN HEART SARCOLEMMA DURING DIABETIC CARDIOMYOPATHY

Paramjit S. Tappia, Song-Yan Liu, Yun Tong, Solomon Ssenyange and Vincenzo Panagia

Institute of Cardiovascular Sciences
St. Boniface Research Centre and
Departments of Human Anatomy & Cell Science and Physiology,
University of Manitoba
Winnipeg, Manitoba, Canada

INTRODUCTION

Phosphatidylinositol 4,5-bisphosphate (PtdIns 4,5-P_2) is an important signaling factor as it is a membrane attachment site for proteins containing PH domains and/or an essential requirement for several proteins, which are associated with the cardiac cell plasma membrane (sarcolemma, SL) for normal cardiac function (1,2). PtdIns 4,5-P_2 is synthesized in the SL membrane by the coordinated and successive action of PtdIns 4-kinase (which catalyses the phosphorylation of PtdIns to PtdIns 4-phosphate) and PtdIns 4-phosphate 5-kinase (which catalyses the phosphorylation of PtdIns 4-phosphate to PtdIns 4,5-P_2) (3). Further, PtdIns 4,5-P_2 can be phosphorylated by phosphatidylinositol 3-kinase to another membrane-delimited messenger, phosphatidylinositol 3,4,5, trisphosphate (PtdIns 3,4,5-P_3) (4). Changes in the membrane phosphoinositide levels due to the activation of the phosphoinositide signaling pathway (5) may be taken into consideration as being part of the receptor-mediated signaling events via this pathway in the heart (3).

Phosphoinositide-phospholipase C (PLC) is a modular monofunctional enzyme which is involved in numerous transmembranal signals (6). Its preferred physiological substrate, PtdIns 4,5-P_2, is converted into two signaling lipid molecules, inositol 1,4,5-trisphosphate (Ins 1,4,5-P_3) and sn-1,2-diacylglycerol (DAG). Ins 1,4,5-P_3 and its phosphorylated derivative inositol 1,3,4,5-tetrakisphosphate (Ins 1,3,4,5-P_4) serve to enhance the sarcoplasmic reticular (SR) Ca^{2+} release and uptake respectively (7,8), and therefore, modulate the cardiac inotropic response to agonists (7,9-11). Immunolocalization of Ins 1,4,5-P_3 receptors at the fascia adherens of the intercalated discs may suggest a possible role in local Ca^{2+} entry or intercellular signaling between cardiomyocytes (12). Amongst the biological functions of DAG, the most important is the activation of protein kinase C family members (9,13). Given the role of PtdIns 4,5-P_2 and its derivatives, it is conceivable

Diabetes and Cardiovascular Disease: Etiology, Treatment and Outcomes
Edited by Aubie Angel et al., Kluwer Academic/Plenum Publishers, 2001

that its synthesis and conversion to Ins 1,4,5-P_3 and DAG or to PtdIns 3,4,5-P_3 are stringently regulated (1).

The molecular events underlying the contractile dysfunction in diabetic cardiomyopathy are incompletely defined. Although abnormal intracellular Ca^{2+} handling is a major factor of myocardial dysfunction in diabetes (14), there is no information available on the SL PtdIns 4,5-P_2 content and enzymes responsible for its synthesis and degradation. Thus, the present study was undertaken to examine possible changes in the SL level of PtdIns 4,5-P_2 and in the function of PtdIns 4 and PtdIns 4-phosphate 5-kinase activities in an experimental model of streptozotocin-induced diabetes, as well as the reversibility of these changes upon treatment of the diabetic animals with insulin. It may be noted that insulin-dependent diabetes mellitus (IDDM, type 1) due to streptozotocin has been shown to result in a cardiomyopathy associated with defects in cardiac ultrastructure, function and metabolism (14,15). The results indicate a reduction in the content of PtdIns 4,5-P_2 during diabetic cardiomyopathy, which seems to be due, at least partially, to its decreased synthesis by defective PtdIns 4 and PtdIns 4-phosphate 5-kinases.

MATERIALS AND METHODS

All experimental protocols for animal studies were approved by the Animal Care Committee of the University of Manitoba, following the guidelines established by the Canadian Council on Animal Care. Male Sprague-Dawley rats weighing approximately 175g each were used in this study. Diabetes was induced by a single tail vein injection of streptozotocin (STZ, 65 mg/kg body weight) dissolved in 0.1 mol/L citrate buffer pH 4.5 (16), while age-matched controls received citrate buffer only. Six weeks after the STZ injection, the diabetic animals were randomly subdivided into two groups. Half of the animals received 3 units Humulin U insulin zinc per day and the other half received a daily injection of saline for 2 weeks.

Animals were killed by decapitation and the hearts were quickly excised and immersed in ice-cold 0.6 mol/L sucrose, 10 mmol/L imidazole, pH 7.0 (buffer A). Three hearts were pooled to prepare the sarcolemmal fraction. After removal of atria, hearts were homogenized in 3.5 ml of buffer A/g tissue with a Polytron homogenizer (6 x 10 s, setting 5). Large particles were removed by centrifugation at 12,000 x g for 30 minutes at 4 °C. The resultant supernatant was diluted with 300 mmol/L KCl-buffer to solubilize weakly associated proteins, and further processed for the preparation of sarcolemmal membranes according to the method used previously (17). As reported recently (17), marker enzyme evaluation indicated an equal degree of enrichment of the SL membrane in control and experimental SL preparations, with only minimal (< 5%) and similar cross-contamination by other subcellular fragments. Protein concentrations were determined by the method of Lowry *et al.* as indicated elsewhere (17).

Isolation of adult rat cardiomyocytes was done essentially as described by Piper *et al.* (18). Male Sprague-Dawley rats, weighing 200-250 g each, were killed by decapitation and the hearts excised, the atria removed, and mounted on the Langendorff apparatus. The heart was initially perfused with calcium-free Krebs solution containing (mmol/L) 110 NaCl, 2.6 KCl, 1.2 KH_2PO_4, 1.2 $MgSO_4$, 25 $NaHCO_3$, and 11 glucose (pH 7.4), and gassed with 95% O_2 and 5% CO_2 mixture. After 10 min of perfusion , the perfusate was switched to 0.1% (w/v) collagenase solution containing 0.1% (w/v) bovine serum albumin, fraction V, (BSA) and 25 μmol/L $CaCl_2$. After a 60 min recirculation period, the heart was removed from the cannula and placed in warm (37 °C) Krebs solution containing 1% (w/v) BSA and 25 μmol/L $CaCl_2$ in a sterile Petri dish. Cells were liberated after gentle pipetting of the tissue. The cell suspension was collected by centrifugation at 6.8 x g for 2 min, the supernatant was removed, the cells resuspended in warm Krebs containing 1% (w/v) BSA and 50 μmol/L $CaCl_2$ and centrifuged again at 1.7 x g for 2 min; the procedure was repeated, resuspending on each occasion in warm Krebs containing 1% BSA (w/v) and increasing $CaCl_2$ concentrations (200-500 μmol/L). Finally the cells were resuspended in warm Krebs solution containing 4% (w/v) BSA and 1 mM $CaCl_2$, and centrifuged at 6.8 x g for 2 min. The cell pellet was then resuspended in medium-199 (M199) containing 0.2% (w/v) BSA and 4% (v/v) fetal calf serum (FCS), and plated out onto laminin-coated 100 mm Petri dishes at about 1x 10^6 cells/plate. After a period of 3 hr, cells were washed with M-199, incubated with 10% FCS-containing M-199 and placed into a 5% CO_2 humidified incubator at 37 °C overnight.

PtdIns 4,5-P_2-PLC activity associated with the sarcolemmal membrane fraction was determined as previously reported (19). The exogenous substrate employed was prepared by mixing an aliquot of [^{3}H]-PtdIns 4,5-P_2 with an aliquot of the nonlabeled substrate. The mixture was dried under N_2 and redissolved in 10% (w/v) Na-Cholate. The assay was performed by incubating 15μg SL protein in 30 mM HEPES-Tris buffer (pH 7.0) at 37^0C for 2.5 min. After terminating the reaction, the mixture was separated in two phases by centrifugation. The upper phase was applied to a microcolumn of Dowex 1 X 8 (formate form, 100-200 mesh); this column was eluted by 5 mmol/L sodium tetraborate in 30 mmol/L sodium formate (to elute inositol) and gradient concentration of ammonium formate (0.2, 0.4 and 1.0 mmol/L) in 0.1mol/L formic acid [to elute inositol 4-phosphate, (Ins 4-P) inositol 1,4-bisphosphate (Ins 1,4-P_2) -and Ins 1,4,5-P_3, respectively]. The radioactivity in each elutant was measured by liquid scintillation counting. As previously reported (20) Ins 1,4,5-P_3 is the primary product of PtdIns 4,5-P_2 hydrolysis by PLC and its alterations reflected those of PLC activity.

Sarcolemmal PtdIns 4,5-P_2 content and myocytal cytosolic concentration of Ins 1,4,5-P_3 were determined using the Biotrak radioimmunoassay kit (Amersham Life Science Inc., Canada). The manufacturer's instructions modified according to the method of Chilvers et al. (21) were followed. In the case of PtdIns 4,5-P_2, the SL mass of PtdIns 4,5-P_2 was quantified by conversion of PtdIns 4,5-P_2 in lipid extracts into Ins 1,4,5-P_3 by alkaline hydrolysis. Extracts were then neutralized and assayed for Ins 1,4,5-P_3 (21).

The activities of PtdIns 4 kinase and PtdIns 4-phosphate 5-kinase were assayed as described previously (22). Thirty μg of SL proteins were preincubated in a solution mixture containing 40 mmol/L HEPES-Tris (pH 7.4), 5 mmol/L $MgCl_2$, 2 mmol/L EGTA, 1 mmol/L dithiothreitol and 30 μg alamethicin for 30 min at 30 °C. PtdIns 4-P kinase was assayed in the presence of 25 μmol/L PtdIns 4-P. The phosphorylation was started by adding [γ-^{32}P]-ATP in a final concentration of 1 mmol/L (0.16 Ci/mmol). The reaction was terminated after 1 min incubation by adding methanol: 10 N HCl (100:1 v/v) followed by the addition of 2.5 N HCl and chloroform. After centrifugation, the aqueous phase was discarded and the organic phase was washed once with chloroform: methanol: 0.6 N HCl (3: 48: 47 v/v). Aliquots of the combined organic phases were used for the analysis of phosphoinositides by thin layer chromatography. The mobile phase for the separation of phosphoinositide species contained chloroform: acetone: methanol: glacial acetic acid: water (40: 15: 13:12: 8 v/v). The ^{32}P-labeled phospholipid spots were visualized by overnight autoradiography using X-Omat-R X-ray film. PtdIns 4-P and PtdIns 4,5-P_2 were scraped from the plates and the radioactivity in each fraction was determined by liquid scintillation counting.

All values are expressed as mean ± SEM. The differences between two groups were evaluated by Student's t-test. The data from more than two groups were evaluated by one-way analysis of variance (ANOVA) followed by Duncan's multiple comparison test. A probability of 95% or more was considered significant.

RESULTS

SL activity of both PtdIns 4 and PtdIns 4-phosphate 5-kinases, which are responsible for the synthesis of the membrane PtdIns 4,5-P$_2$, were found to be significantly depressed in diabetic hearts, as compared to control values (Table 1). The absolute SL level of PtdIns 4,5-P$_2$, was significantly decreased in diabetic hearts *vs* controls (Table 1). Two weeks insulin treatment resulted in a partial recovery of PtdIns 4-kinase activity, whereas, PtdIns 4-P 5-kinase activity was completely normalized. However, no recovery of the SL PtdIns 4,5-P$_2$ mass was observed (Table 1). Analysis of the inositol phosphates revealed diminished Ins 1,4,5-P$_3$ formation in diabetes as a consequence of depressed PLC activity, which was completely normalized with insulin treatment (Table 2).

Ins 1,4,5-P$_3$ is a downstream signal molecule generated by PLC activity, and its concentration was measured in the cytosolic compartment of isolated cardiomyocytes. Ins 1,4,5-P$_3$ concentration was markedly decreased in cytosol from diabetic cardiomyocytes, which was only partially corrected by insulin treatment (Figure 1).

Table 1. Sarcolemmal phosphatidylinositol 4,5-bisphosphate mass and phosphoinositide kinases activity in diabetic hearts.

	PtdIns 4,5-P$_2$	Kinases	
		PtdIns 4	PtdIns 4-P 5
	nmol/mg SL rotein	pmol/min/mg SL protein	
Control	8.0 ± 0.5	2113 ± 12	228 ± 19
Diabetic	2.6 ± 0.2*	1313 ± 67*	164 ± 10*
Diabetic insulin-treated	2.1 ± 0.3*	1856 ± 70*	212 ± 10

Values are means ± SEM of three experiments. Assays were performed in triplicate.
Abbreviations: PtdIns 4,5-P$_2$ = phosphatidylinositol 4,5-bisphosphate, PtdIns = phosphatidylinositol, PtdIns 4-P = phosphatidylinositol 4-phosphate.
* Significantly different (p<0.05) *vs.* corresponding control values.

Table 2. *In vitro* formation of the different inositol phosphate species by sarcolemmal phospholipase C in diabetic cardiomyopathy.

	Inositol phosphate species (nmol/min/mg protein)		
	Ins 4-P	Ins 1,4-P$_2$	Ins 1,4,5-P$_3$
Control	0.02 ± 0.01	1.18 ± 0.04	6.69 ± 0.09
Diabetic	0.02 ± 0.02	0.58 ± 0.04*	5.64 ± 0.14*
Diabetic insulin-treated	0.02 ± 0.02	0.98 ± 0.05	7.45 ± 0.44

Sarcolemmal PLC activity was assayed under standard conditions, in the presence of 20 μmol/L [^{3}H]-PtdIns 4,5-P$_2$, as already described (19). Values are means ± SEM of inositol phosphate formation in three experiments. Assays were performed in triplicate.
Abbreviations: Ins 4-P = inositol 4-phosphate, Ins 1,4- P$_2$ = inositol 1,4-bisphosphate, Ins 1,4,5-P$_3$= inositol 1,4,5-trisphosphate.
* Significantly different (p<0.05) *vs.* corresponding control values.

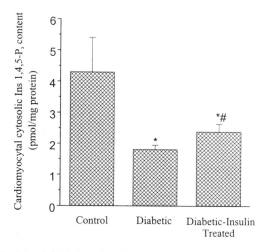

Figure 1. Cytosolic levels of inositol 1,4,5-trisphosphate in isolated diabetic cardiomyocytes. Values are means ± SEM of three experiments. Assays were performed in duplicate.
Abbreviations: Ins 1,4,5-P_3 = inositol 1,4,5-trisphosphate.
*Significantly different (P<0.05) *vs.* corresponding control values.
Significantly different (P<0.05) *vs.* corresponding diabetic values.

DISCUSSION

PtdIns 4,5-P_2 is a versatile phospholipid, not only because it is an important signaling molecule in its own right but because, through the activities of phospholipases, phosphatases and phosphoinositide kinases, it generates several messenger molecules which influence the cellular function. The present study was conducted to examine the SL level of PtdIns 4,5-P_2 as well as the activities of the phosphoinositide kinases responsible for its synthesis and phosphoinositide-specific PLC responsible for its hydrolysis in chronic diabetes.

A significant decrease in the cardiac total SL phosphoinositide-PLC activity was found in the STZ-induced diabetic rats under the *in vitro* assay conditions employed, as indicated by the lower production of Ins 1,4,5-P_3. It is therefore conceivable that a decreased basal PLC activity *in vivo* may also exist in diabetic cardiomyopathy. In support of this contention, additional experiments conducted on isolated cardiomyocytes showed a reduced concentration of basal cytosolic Ins 1,4,5-P_3 in diabetic rats. The regulation of phosphoinositide-PLC activity occurs at several levels, including the receptor, substrate and membrane physico-chemical properties (6,23,24). In this regard, a number of possible mechanisms can be proposed to explain the depression in PLC activity observed in STZ-cardiomyopathic hearts: **1.** Phosphatidic acid (PtdOH) has been shown to stimulate PLC activities *in vitro* (25,26). Since there is a 67% decrease in SL phospholipase D-derived PtdOH concentration, it is possible that the depressed PLC activity *in vivo* may be partially due to the attenuated PtdOH stimulation. **2.** In our past study, IDDM resulted in enhancement of the SL phosphatidate phosphohydrolase activity compared to phospholipase D, with augmented DAG production (17). Increase in total myocardial DAG level has been reported in STZ-injected diabetic rats and in spontaneous autoimmune diabetic BB rats (27,28). Increase in membrane DAG content has been shown to destabilize the membrane and cause structural transitions (29,30), and this may have an inhibitory effect on PLC activity (31). **3.** Diabetes could induce structural modifications of the catalytic domain of PLC (XY domain, 23), resulting in a defective enzyme activity. **4.** An increased oxidative stress has been shown to occur during diabetic cardiomyopathy (14). We have previously reported that SL PLC is inhibited by oxidants through reversible modification of associated thiol groups, which are critical for the enzyme activity (20). Therefore the depressed SL PLC activity seen in diabetes could in part be explained by the oxidant-induced alteration of the enzyme thiol groups.

The sequential phosphorylation of PtdIns on the 4th and 5th positions of the inositol ring by PtdIns 4-kinase and PtdIns 4-P 5-kinase gives rise to the PLC substrate, PtdIns 4,5-P_2 (2). Local substrate availability determines the hydrolytic activity of PLC (32). The reduced synthesis and diminished SL content of PtdIns 4,5-P_2 could contribute, in part, to the observed decrease of the basal PLC activity *in vivo*. In addition, a contributory factor to the reduction in SL PtdIns 4,5-P_2 mass could be PtdIns 3-kinase, which also employs PtdIns 4,5-P_2 as substrate to produce PtdIns 3,4,5-P_3 and has been shown to be activated in vascular smooth muscle cells during diabetes (33). It is not unlikely that a similar situation may exist at the cardiac SL level.

The sarcolemmal mass of PtdIns 4,5-P_2 and the activity of its synthesizing enzymes were diminished in diabetes. Although two weeks insulin treatment was able to normalize the SL PLC activity, its substrate, PtdIns 4,5-P_2, remained depressed to the level seen in the diabetic heart. In order to replenish the membrane PtdIns 4,5-P_2 pool, the precursors for PtdIns 4,5-P_2, PtdIns 4-P and PtdIns have to be maintained at a certain level. In this regard, it is worth noting that the SL level of the PtdIns 4-kinase substrate, PtdIns, is unchanged during diabetes without or with insulin therapy (34), which may also indicate that the cytosolic PtdIns-transfer protein translocates normaly newly synthesized PtdIns from SR to the plasma membrane (35,36). As shown (Table 1), insulin normalized the SL PtdIns 4P 5-kinase activity while PtdIns 4-kinase was only partially corrected and remained significantly hypofunctional. It is thus possible that a defect in the catalytic domain of PtdIns 4-kinase may persist during insulin therapy. Since this enzyme is the rate limiting step in the PtdIns 4,5-P_2 biosynthetic pathway this could be, in part, a contributory factor for the failure of insulin to normalize SL PtdIns 4,5-P_2 content.

A number of diverse biochemical events are regulated by PtdIns 4,5-P_2 and are affected by the altered concentration of this lipid in the membrane (1,2). For example, the reduced PtdIns 4,5-P_2 could result in diminished activity of phosphoinositide-dependent phospholipase D1 and D2, which are important signaling enzymes that require PtdIns 4,5-P_2 as a cofactor (2,37). Of note, the decreased number of PtdIns 4,5-P_2 molecules could compromise the contractile performance of the heart by directly causing a depression of the inward rectifier K^+ channels (38), as well as of the SL Na^+ - Ca^{2+} exchanger and Ca^{2+} - pump activities (39,40). Therefore, a diminished amount of PtdIns 4,5-P_2 inside the SL membrane may be critical for cardiac dysfunction during diabetes.

Acknowledgement

This work was supported by a grant (VP) from the Heart and Stroke Foundation of Manitoba.

REFERENCES

1. S.B. Lee, and S.G. Rhee, Significance of PIP$_2$ hydrolysis and regulation of phospholipase C isozymes, *Curr. Opin. Cell Biol.* **7**, 183-189 (1995).
2. A. Toker, The synthesis and cellular roles of phosphatidylinositol 4,5-bisphosphate, *Curr. Opin. Cell Biol.* **10**, 254-261 (1998).
3. N. Mesaeli, J.M.J. Lamers, and V. Panagia, Phosphoinositide kinases in rat heart sarcolemma: biochemical properties and regulation by calcium, *Mol. Cell. Biochem.* **117**, 181-189 (1992).
4. B.C. Duckworth, and L.C. Cantley, PI 3-Kinase and receptor-linked signal transduction, in *Handbook of Lipid Research, Vol. 8: Lipid Second Messengers*, R. M. Bell, J. H. Exton, and S. M. Prescott, eds., Plenum Press, New York (1996), pp. 125-175.
5. T.P. Stanffer, Receptor-induced transient reduction in plasma membrane PtdIns (4,5) P$_2$ concentration monitored in living cells, *Curr. Biol.* **8**, 343-346 (1998).

6. S.G. Rhee, and Y.S. Bae, Regulation of phosphoinositide-specific phospholipase C isoenzymes, *J. Biol. Chem.* **272**, 15045-15048 (1997).

7. J.C. Gilbert, T. Shirayama, and A.J. Pappano, Inositol trisphosphate promotes Na-Ca exchange current by releasing calcium from sarcoplasmic reticulum in cardiac myocytes, *Circ. Res.* **69**, 1632-1639 (1991).

8. E.E. Quist, B.H. Foresman, R.Vasan, and C.W. Quist, Inositol tetrakisphosphate stimulates a novel ATP-dependent Ca^{2+} uptake mechanism in cardiac junctional sarcoplasmic reticulum, *Biochem. Biophys. Res. Commun.* **204**, 69-75 (1994).

9. H.W. De Jonge, H.A.A.Van Heugten, and J.M.J. Lamers, Signal transduction by the phosphatidylinositol cycle in myocardium, *J. Mol. Cell. Cardiol.* **27**, 93-106 (1995).

10. T. Saeki, J-B. Shen, and A.J. Pappano, Inositol-1,4,5-trisphosphate increases contractions but not L-type calcium current in guinea pig ventricular myocytes, *Cardiovasc. Res.* **41**, 620-628 (1999).

11. A.R. Marks, Intracellular calcium-release channels: regulators of cell life and death, *Am. J. Physiol.* **272**, H597-H605 (1997).

12. Y. Kijima, A. Saito, T.L. Jetton, M.A. Magnuson, and S. Fleischer, Different intracellular localization of inositol 1,4,5-trisphosphate and ryanodine receptors in cardiomyocytes, *J. Biol. Chem.* **268**, 3499-3506 (1993).

13. M. Puceat, and G. Vassort, Signalling by protein kinase C isoforms in the heart, *Mol. Cell. Biochem.* **157**, 65-72 (1996).

14. N.S. Dhalla, X. Liu, V. Panagia, and N. Takeda, Subcellular remodeling and heart dysfunction in chronic diabetes, *Cardiovasc. Res.* **40**, 239-247 (1998).

15. K.C. Tomlinson, S.M. Gardiner, R.A. Hebden, and T. Bennet, Functional consequences of streptozotocin-induced diabetes mellitus with particular reference to the cardiovascular system, *Pharmacol. Rev.* **44**, 103-150 (1992).

16. N. Rakienten, M.L. Rakienten, M.V. Nadkarni, Studies on the diabetogenic action of streptozotocin, *Cancer Chemother. Rep.* **29**, 91 (1963).

17. S.A. Williams, P.S. Tappia, C-H. Yu, M. Bibeau, and Panagia, Impairment of the sarcolemmal phospholipase D-phosphatidate phosphohydrolase pathway in diabetic cardiomyopathy, *J. Mol. Cell. Cardiol.* **30**, 109-118 (1998).

18. H.M. Piper, S.L. Jacobson, and P. Schwartz, Determinants of cardiomyocyte development in long-term primary culture, *J. Mol. Cell. Cardiol.* **20**, 825-835 (1998).

19. P.S. Tappia, S-Y. Liu, S. Shatadal, N. Takeda, N.S. Dhalla, and V. Panagia, Changes in sarcolemmal PLC isoenzymes in postinfarct congestive heart failure: partial correction by imidapril, *Am. J. Physiol.* **277**, H40-H49 (1999).

20. J.T.A. Meij, S. Suzuki , V. Panagia, and N.S. Dhalla, Oxidative stress modifies the activity of cardiac sarcolemmal phospholipase C, *Biochim. Biophys. Acta* **1199**, 6-12 (1994).

21. E.R. Chilvers, I.H. Batty, R.A. Challiss, P.J. Barnes, and S.R. Nahorski, Determination of mass changes in phosphatidylinositol 4,5-bisphosphate and evidence for agonist-stimulated metabolism of inositol 1,4,5-trisphosphate in airway smooth muscle, *Biochem. J.* **275**, 373-379 (1991).

22. S-Y. Liu, C-H. Yu, J-A. Hays, V. Panagia, and N.S. Dhalla, Modification of heart sarcolemmal phosphoinositide pathway by lysophosphatidylcholine, *Biochim. Biophys. Acta* **1349**, 264-274 (1997).

23. S.R. James, and C.P. Downes, Structural and mechanistic features of phospholipase C: effectors of inositol phospholipid-mediated signal transduction, *Cell. Signal.* **9**, 329-336 (1997).

24. W.D. Singer, H.A. Brown, and P.C. Sternweis, Regulation of eukaryotic phosphatidylinositol-specific phospholipase C and phospholipase D, *Annu. Rev. Biochem.* **66**, 475-509 (1997).

25. R.A. Henry, S.Y. Boyce, T. Kurz, and R.A. Wolf, Stimulation and binding of myocardial phospholipase C by phosphatidic acid, *Am. J. Physiol.* **263**, C1021-C1028 (1995).

26. N.S. Dhalla, Y-J. Xu, S-S. Sheu, P.S. Tappia, and V. Panagia, Phosphatidic acid: a potential signal transducer for cardiac hypertrophy, *J. Mol. Cell. Cardiol.* **29**, 2865-2871 (1997).

27. K. Okumura, N. Akiyama, H. Hashimoto, K. Ogawa, and T. Satake, Alteration of 1,2 diacylglycerol content in myocardium of diabetic rats, *Diabetes* **37**, 1168-1172 (1988).

28. T. Inoguchi, R. Battan, E. Handler, J.R. Sportsman, H. Heath, and G.L. King, Preferential elevation of protein kinase C isoform βII and diacylglycerol levels in the aorta and heart of diabetic rats: differential reversibility to glycemic control by islet cell transplantation, *Proc. Natl. Acad. Sci. USA* **89**, 11059-11063 (1992).

29. S. Das, and R.P. Rand, Diacylglycerol causes major structural transitions in phospholipid bilayer membranes, *Biochem. Biophys. Res. Commun.* **124**, 491-496 (1984).

30. S. Das, and R.P. Rand, Modification by diacylglycerol of the structure and interaction of various phospholipid bilayer membranes, *Biochemistry* **25**, 2882-2889 (1986).

31. S.R. James, S. Smith, A. Paterson, T.K. Harden, and C.P. Downes, Time-dependent inhibition of phospholipase Cβ-catalysed phosphoinositide hydrolysis: a comparison of different assays, *Biochem. J.* **314**, 917-921 (1996).

32. A.B. Tobin, G.B. Willars, and S.R. Nahorski, Regulation and desensitization of the phosphoinositidase C signaling pathway, in *Receptor Desensitization and Ca^{2+} Signaling*. M.K. Uchida, ed., Japan Sci Soc Press, (1996), pp181-206.
33. A.K. Srivastava, A possible role of oxidative stress-induced activation of phosphatidylinositol 3-kinase (PI3K) and mitogen-activated protein kinases (MAPK) in vascular dysfunction in diabetes. Proceedings of the International Conference on Diabetes and Cardiovascular Disease, Winnipeg, June3-6,1999, p48.
34. N. Makino, K.S. Dhalla, V. Elimban, and N.S. Dhalla, Sarcolemmal Ca^{2+} transport in streptozotocin-induced diabetic cardiomyopathy in rats, *Am. J. Physiol.* **253**, E202-E207 (1987).
35. R.A. Wolf, Synthesis, transfer and phosphorylation of phosphoinositides in cardiac membranes, *Am. J. Physiol.* **259**, C987-C994 (1990).
36. M.F. Roberts, Phospholipases: structural and functional motifs for working at an interface, *FASEB J.* **10**, 1159-1172 (1996).
37. M.A. Frohman, and A.J. Morris, Phospholipase D structure and regulation, *Chem. Phys. Lipids* **98**, 127-140 (1999).
38. C.L. Huang, S. Feng, and D.S. Hilgemann, Direct activation of inward rectifier potassium channels by PIP$_2$ and its stabilization by G$\beta\gamma$, *Nature* **391**, 803-806 (1997).
39. P. Caroni, M. Zurini, and A. Clark, The calcium-pumping ATPase of heart sarcolemma, *Ann. N. Y. Acad. Sci.* **402**, 402-421 (1982).
40. D.W. Hilgemann, and R. Ball, Regulation of cardiac Na, Ca exchange and K$_{ATP}$ potassium channels by the synthesis and hydrolysis of PIP$_2$ in giant membrane patches, *Science* **273**, 956-959 (1996).

TUMOR NECROSIS FACTOR-α, SPHINGOMYELINASE AND CERAMIDES ACTIVATE TYROSINE KINASE, p21RAS AND PHOSPHATIDYLINOSITOL 3-KINASE: IMPLICATIONS FOR GLUCOSE TRANSPORT AND INSULIN RESISTANCE

Atef N. Hanna, James Xu and David N. Brindley

Department of Biochemistry (Signal Transduction Laboratories),
Lipid and Lipoprotein Research Group,
University of Alberta,
Edmonton, Alberta, T6G 2S2
Canada

INTRODUCTION

Diabetes mellitus is one of the leading causes of morbidity in North America. Insulin resistance plays a key role in the pathogenesis of Type 2 diabetes[1]. Insulin resistance (defined as decreased ability of insulin to stimulate glucose uptake) is normally caused by a post-receptor defect in insulin signaling which leads to glucose transport into cells. The insulin signaling pathway responsible for glucose uptake involves sequential tyrosine phosphorylation of the insulin receptor (IR) and insulin receptor substrate-1 and -2 (IRS-1 and IRS-2) (Figure1). IRS-1 acts as a docking site by using specific phosphorylation motifs and SH2 domains and facilitates the activation of other proteins such as phosphatidylinositol 3-kinase (PI 3-kinase)[1].

PI 3-kinase exists as a heterodimer consisting of a p110 catalytic subunit and a p85 regulatory subunit[2]. PI 3-kinase phosphorylates the 3-position of the inositide ring thus producing a family of 3-phosphoinositides, e.g., phosphatidylinositol 3,4,5-trisphosphate (PIP3), which are potent lipid signaling molecules. In various cell types, PI 3-kinase is implicated in regulating cell growth and inhibiting apoptosis[3,4], intracellular vesicle trafficking and secretion[5-7] and cytoskeletal organization[8-10]. Downstream of PI 3-kinase stimulation is activation of ribosomal S6 kinase (pp70S6K), protein kinase B (PKB, or Akt) and PKC-ζ[11-14]. These activations are probably mediated through the stimulation of a PIP3-dependent kinase (PDK1) which phosphorylates the protein kinases in their activation loops[14,15] (Figure 1).

PI 3-kinase may also be regulated by Ras[16,17]. Alternatively, PI 3-kinase is stimulated by tyrosine kinase activation[18,19]. Also, activation of Ras leads to activation of the Raf/ MAP kinase pathway which is known to regulate gene expression[1] (Figure 1).

Activation of PI 3-kinase is essential for insulin to stimulate the movement of glucose transporters (mainly GLUT4) to the cell surface[20-22]. The increase in GLUT4 at the

Diabetes and Cardiovascular Disease: Etiology, Treatment and Outcomes
Edited by Aubie Angel *et al.*, Kluwer Academic/Plenum Publishers, 2001

191

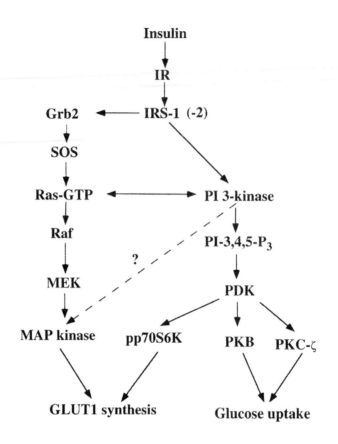

Figure 1. Some signaling pathways activated by insulin. The scheme emphasizes particularly some of the signaling pathways that might be activated as a result of the stimulation of PI 3-kinase.

plasma membrane is then responsible for insulin-dependent glucose uptake. Insulin resistance results from a decreased efficiency to stimulate this cascade. This can occur in sepsis, advanced cancer and trauma, partly as a result of TNFα action. TNFα is also secreted by adipose tissue and this secretion is implicated in insulin resistance associated with obesity[23,24].

TNFα has been reported to contribute to insulin resistance by increasing the serine phosphorylation of IRS-1 which inhibits the tyrosine kinase activity of IR[25] and impairs the association of IRS-1 with PI 3-kinase[26]. Decreases in the tyrosine phosphorylation of IRS-1 induced by TNFα were seen after incubation of rat hepatoma Fao cells for 1 h whereas 2 to 4 days was required for this to occur in 3T3-F442A adipocytes[25,26]. TNFα activates several signaling cascades including a stimulation of sphingomyelinases and consequent ceramide production[27]. Exogenous sphingomyelinase and cell-permeable (short-chain) ceramides have been shown to mimic some effects of TNFα in decreasing the insulin-dependent tyrosine phosphorylation of IRS-1[28,29] and activation of phosphoprotein phosphatase-1[30]. By contrast to these results, incubation of 3T3-L1 adipocytes with TNFα for 30-60 min had the opposite effect of increasing the tyrosine phosphorylation of IRS-1 and its binding of PI 3-kinase[31]. Other work with 3T3-L1 adipocytes ascribed the long-term effects of TNFα in producing insulin resistance to a decreased expression of IRS-1 and GLUT4 rather than decreased tyrosine phosphorylation of IRS-1[32]. Work from our Group demonstrated that cell-permeable ceramides increase rather than decrease PI 3-kinase activity associated with IRS-1 in 3T3-L1 adipocytes after a 12 h incubation[33]. We also measured insulin-dependent glucose uptake in parallel experiments in order to relate this to the signaling events. We showed that insulin-stimulated glucose uptake was decreased from 2 to 24 h. after treatment with C_2- and C_6-ceramides. We therefore concluded that the defect in insulin-stimulated glucose uptake that is caused by ceramides lies downstream of PI 3-kinase[33]. This conclusion was later confirmed by others[34]. The mechanism for prolonged activation of PI 3-kinase in 3T3-L1 adipocytes is not yet established.

The consequences of the ceramide-induced activation of PI 3-kinase in the adipocytes was the downstream activation of pp70 S6 kinase which was accompanied by an increase in MAP kinase activity[33]. These events were responsible for inducing the synthesis of the glucose transporter, GLUT1, which resulted in increased glucose uptake in the absence of insulin[33]. These effects of ceramides mimic those of TNFα which can increase the tyrosine phosphorylation of IRS-1, its binding of PI 3-kinase, synthesis of GLUT1 and basal glucose uptake by cells[33,35,36].

In the present work we investigated whether ceramides are able to stimulate PI 3-kinase in rat2 fibroblasts and, if so, to use this experimental system to determine the mechanism for the activation. We demonstrated that C_2-ceramide, but not dihydro-C_2-ceramide, activates PI 3-kinase transiently after 5 to 20 min through a pathway that involves tyrosine kinase activity and the activation of Ras. Treatment of the fibroblasts with TNFα or sphingomyelinase for 20 min also stimulated PI 3-kinase activity through activation of tyrosine kinase activity and Ras. This work therefore identifies a novel signaling pathway for TNFα and ceramide that could contribute to cellular responses such as increased glucose uptake in absence of insulin.

METHODS

Cell Culture

Rat2 fibroblasts were maintained in Dulbucco's Minimum Essential Medium (DMEM) supplemented with 10% fetal bovine serum, 100 units/ml penicillin and 100 µg of streptomycin/ml in a humidified atmosphere of 5% CO_2, 95% air at 37 °C until confluence. Rat2 fibroblasts stably expressing wildtype H-Ras and the dominant/negative mutant H-Ras (N17 Ras) were cultured in DMEM containing the appropriate drug selection using 0.6 mg of Geneticin (G418)/ml or 2.5 µg of puromycin/ml, respectively. N17 H-Ras is thought to form a stable inactive complex with Ras exchange factors and thereby prevents activation of endogenous Ras[37].

Immunoprecipitation and Immunoblotting

PI 3-kinase was immunoprecipitated from cell lysates (300 µg of protein) by adding 2 µg of anti-p85α and incubating for 6 h at 4 °C with constant gentle rocking followed by adding 40 µl of 50% protein A-Sepharose in phosphate buffered saline (PBS). The mixtures were incubated for overnight at 4°C. Immunoprecipitates were then washed three times and identical amounts of proteins were separated by SDS-PAGE as described by Laemmli[38] and were transferred to nitrocellulose membranes. The immunoreactive proteins were detected using anti-rabbit IgG linked to horseradish peroxidase and enhanced chemiluminescence and then analyzed densitometrically.

PI 3-kinase Assay

PI 3-kinase activity was determined by measuring the formation PI 3-[^{32}P]phosphate[39]. PI 3-kinase was immunoprecipitated by incubating the cell lysates with anti-p85α (2 µg), anti-phosphotyrosine (2 µg) or anti-pan Ras (5 µg) for 6 h at 4°C with constant gentle rocking followed by adding 40 μl of 50% protein A-Sepharose in PBS. The mixtures were incubated overnight at 4°C with constant gentle rocking. PI 3-kinase activity in the immunoprecipitate was assessed by measuring the incorporation of ^{32}P into PI 3-phosphate using PI as a substrate[33].

Activation of Ras

Ras-GTP was measured by using a non-isotopic method[40]. Briefly, fibroblasts overexpressing wildtype H-Ras were treated with different agents and then lysed. Cleared lysates were incubated for 30 min. at 4°C with 20-30 μg of glutathione-S-transferase-Ras binding domain (RBD) that was bound to glutathione Sepharose beads. After three washes with lysis buffer, bound proteins were resolved by SDS-PAGE on 11% gels and Ras was detected by immunoblotting with a pan Ras polyclonal antibody. Control experiments confirmed that Ras-GTP does not bind to glutathione-S-transferase alone.

RESULTS AND DISCUSSION

TNFα, sphingomyelinase and C$_2$-ceramide activate PI 3-kinase in Rat2 Fibroblasts

PI 3-kinase activity in cell lysates was assessed using an immune-complex kinase assay that employed an anti-p85 antibody to precipitate the enzyme and PI as a substrate. Treatment of rat2 fibroblasts with 40 μM C$_2$-ceramide, 10 ng/mL TNFα or 0.1 units of sphingomyelinase/mL stimulated PI 3-kinase activity by 4-6 fold after 20 min (Figure 2). It should be noted that these incubations contained 15 μM albumin which increases the amount of ceramide required to produce a biological effect.

We also assessed the PI 3-kinase activity associated with Ras after treatment with or without 40 μM C$_2$-ceramide for 20 min. Ceramide increased the PI 3-kinase activity that

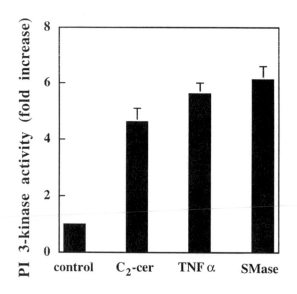

Figure 2. Activation of PI 3-kinase by C$_2$-ceramide, TNFa and sphingomyelinase. Confluent rat2 fibroblasts were incubated with 40 μM C$_2$-ceramide, TNFa (10 ng/mL) or sphingomyelinase (0.1 unit/mL) for 20 min. PI 3-kinase was immunoprecipitated with anti-p85 a and activity was measured by the phosphorylation of PI. Error bars illustrate SEM from 3 to 7 independent experiments.

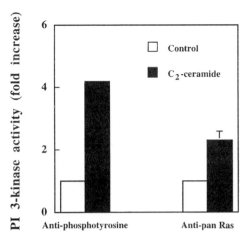

Figure 3. C_2-ceramide increases the precipitation of PI 3-kinase by anti-phosphotyrosine and anti-Ras antibodies. The figure shows PI 3-kinase activity in cell lysates as assessed by using an immune-complex kinase assay that employed an anti-phosphotyrosine or anti-pan Ras antibody to precipitate the enzyme and using PI as a substrate.

co-precipitated with Ras by about 3-fold after 20 min. PI 3-kinase was also assessed using anti-phosphotyrosine antibodies for precipitation. Under the latter conditions, PI 3-kinase activity in the immunoprecipitate increased by about 4.3-fold after 10 min following treatment with 40 μM C_2-ceramide (Figure 3). By comparison, the optimum increase in PI 3-kinase activity obtained after treating cells with 5 ng of PDGF/ml for 10 min was 6- to 8- fold.

TNFα, sphingomyelinase and C_2-ceramide activate PI 3-kinase in Rat2 Fibroblasts Through Stimulation of Tyrosine Kinase

Protein tyrosine phosphorylation could be involved at several levels in ceramide-induced activation of PI 3-kinase. For example, PI 3-kinase is activated through the binding of SH2 domains in the p85 subunit to tyrosine phosphorylated receptor or non-receptor proteins[41-43]. Therefore, we tested the effect of tyrosine kinase inhibitors on the activation of PI 3-kinase by TNFα, sphingomyelinase and C_2-ceramide. Rat2 fibroblasts were pretreated with 50 μM genistein or 1 μM PP1 for 1 h before adding 40 μM C_2-ceramide, 10 ng/mL TNFα or 0.1 units of sphingomyelinase/mL. These tyrosine kinase inhibitors blocked PI 3-kinase activation by TNFα, sphingomyelinase and C_2-ceramide (Figure 4 A). C_2-ceramide treatment also increased protein tyrosine phosphorylation including that of a protein of approximately 120 kDa. We, therefore, determined if this protein was FAK since this has been implicated in activation of PI 3-kinase[44]. C_2-ceramide and TNFα induced tyrosine phosphorylation of FAK (Figure 4B). In preliminary experiments we obtained evidence that tyrosine phosphorylated FAK becomes associated physically with PI -3-kinase following treatment of Rat2 fibroblasts with C_2-ceramide. This indicates that PI 3-kinase activation by TNFα, sphingomyelinase and ceramide, requires tyrosine kinase activity.

TNFα, Sphingomyelinase and C_2-ceramide Activate PI 3-kinase Through Increasing the Concentrations of Ras-GTP in Rat2 Fibroblasts

Ras-GTP can activate PI 3-kinase through binding to the p110 catalytic subunit[16-19]. We, therefore, investigated whether TNFα, sphingomyelinase and C_2-ceramide stimulates PI 3-kinase through Ras by using fibroblasts expressing N17 Ras which interferes with

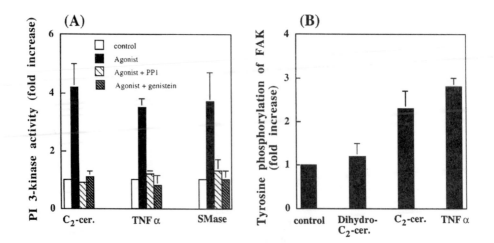

Figure 4. Activation of PI 3-kinase by C_2-ceramide, TNFa and sphingomyelinase involves activated tyrosine kinase activities. Panel A, Confluent rat2 fibroblasts were incubated with or without the tyrosine kinase inhibitors, 50 μM genistein and 1 μM PP1, for 1 h then treated with or without 40 μM C_2-ceramide, TNFa (10 ng/mL) or sphingomyelinase (0.1 unit/mL). Then PI 3-kinase activity was measured using PI as a substrate. Panel A shows that genistein and PP1 inhibit PI 3-kinase activation by C_2-ceramide, TNFa and sphingomyelinase.. Panel B shows the tyrosine phosphorylation of FAK obtained with anti-phosphotyrosine precipitation of 400 μg of lysate protein for each lane followed by immunoblotting with anti-FAK. Results are shown as means ± SEM from three independent experiments.

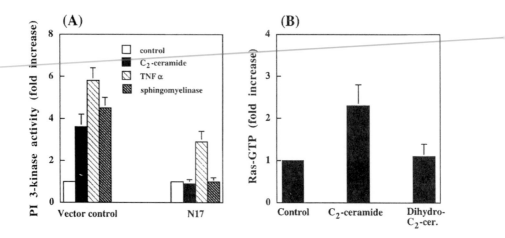

Figure 5. Activation of PI 3-kinase by C_2-ceramide, TNFa and sphingomyelinase requires activated Ras. Panel A, confluent rat2 fibroblasts expressing dominant negative Ras (N17) or vector control were incubated with 40 μM C_2-ceramide, TNFa (10 ng/mL) or sphingomyelinase (0.1 unit/mL) for 20 min. PI 3-kinase was immunoprecipitated with anti-p85 a and activity was measured by the phosphorylation of PI. Panel B shows that C_2-ceramide induces activation of Ras. Error bars illustrate SEM from 3 independent experiments.

activation of endogenous Ras by exchange factors[37]. C_2-ceramide (40 μM) and sphingomyelinase (0.1 unit/mL) did not increase PI 3-kinase activity significantly after a 10 min incubation in cells expressing N17 Ras compared to about a 4-fold increase of PI 3-kinase activity in the vector control cells (Figure 5A). However, the activations of PI 3-kinase by TNFα was inhibited by about 70% in fibroblasts expressing N17 Ras compared to control cells which implies that TNFα could partially stimulate PI 3-kinase by a Ras-independent pathway (Figure 5A). These results were confirmed by showing that C_2-ceramide, but not dihydro-C_2-ceramide, increased the concentration of Ras-GTP after 10 min (Figure 5B). This implies that full PI 3-kinase activation by TNFα, sphingomyelinase and ceramide requires activation of Ras.

CONCLUSION

Taken together, the present work establishes that TNFα, sphingomyelinase and C_2-ceramide all activate PI 3-kinase in rat2 fibroblasts. This process is dependent on tyrosine kinase activity and it involves an increase in the amount of Ras-GTP. Such a dual regulatory mechanism in other systems causes the synergistic stimulation of PI 3-kinase activity[18]. The novelty of the present study is that TNFα, sphingomyelinase and ceramides should initiate such a signaling pathway[45]. It is often expected that TNFα and ceramides will produce apoptosis, whereas, the activation of Ras and PI 3-kinase is more often associated with increasing cell survival or cell division. It should be remembered that in some cells, such as fibroblasts, TNFα and ceramides stimulate cell division as part of a wound-healing process and the development of fibrous tissue in inflammatory conditions. Activation of PI 3-kinase by TNFα may provide a mechanism for TNFα-induced proliferation of fibroblasts seen in various chronic inflammatory disorders. We have demonstrated that the fibroblasts treated with TNFα do, in fact, undergo cell division[45].

The activation of PI 3-kinase by ceramides and TNFα could also play an important role in regulating several cellular functions. For example, we demonstrated that cell-permeable ceramides and TNFα increase PI 3-kinase activity associated with IRS-1 in 3T3-L1 adipocytes which leads to increase glucose uptake in absence of insulin[33]. Cell-permeable ceramides and TNFα, therefore, have insulin-like effects especially in stimulating basal glucose uptake.

The observations that ceramides increase GLUT1 concentrations and basal glucose uptake (refs. 39-41 and our unpublished work) are compatible with the effect of TNFα in stimulating the peripheral uptake of glucose *in vivo* [46]. Furthermore, the expression of GLUT1 protein in plasma membranes prepared from skeletal muscle of obese diabetic SHR rats is increased by 40% compared to the lean genotype[47]. The idea that TNFα and ceramides exacerbate insulin resistance may seem paradoxical if these agents, on their own, stimulate glucose uptake and lipid synthesis. However, the problem with TNFα is that despite an increase in non-insulin stimulated (basal) glucose uptake, the insulin resistant tissue is unable to respond with sufficient glucose uptake to dispose of a post-prandial glucose load effectively. This may predispose to hyperglycemia and hyperinsulinemia after meals.

It is interesting to speculate that the increased glucose uptake in adipocytes that is produced by TNFα may be designed to enable the cells to store lipids effectively in conditions of semi-starvation when insulin concentrations are low. This may have provided an evolutionary advantage when food was in limited supply during many seasons of the year. However, this condition, with its attendant insulin resistance, becomes a health risk that contributes to obesity and Type 2 diabetes in affluent societies.

In conclusion, our work provides further mechanisms for explaining the effects of TNFα and ceramides in decreasing the importance of insulin as a regulator of metabolic balance in adipose tissue.

Acknowledgments

This work was supported by grants to DNB from the Heart and Stroke Foundation of Alberta and the Canadian Diabetes Association (in honour of Helen Margaret Clery).

DNB and AH are recipients of a Medical Scientist Award and a Research Fellowship from the Alberta Heritage Foundation for Medical Research, respectively. The results shown in Figure 5B are produced by Mr. Edmond Y.W. Chan and Dr. James C Stone. We are grateful to J. Biol. Chem. for permitting us to summarize results published in Ref. 45.

REFERENCES

1. C.R. Kahn, Insulin action, diabetogenes, and the cause of type II diabetes, *Diabetes* 43: 1066-1084 (1994).
2. R. Kapeller, and L.C. Cantley, Phosphatidylinositol 3-kinase, *BioEssays* 16: 565-   576 (1994).
3. S. Roche, M. Koegl, and S.A.Courtneidge, The phosphatidylinositol 3-kinase alpha is required for DNA synthesis induced by some, but not all, growth factors,   *Proc. Natl. Acad. Sci. USA* 91: 9185-9189 (1994).
4. K.L. Philpott, M.J. McCarthy, A. Klippel, and L.L. Rubin, Activated   phosphatidylinositol 3-kinase and Akt kinase promote survival of superior cervical   neurons, *J. Cell Biol.* 139: 809-815 (1997).
5. H.W. Davidson, Wortmannin causes mistargeting of procathepsin D. evidence for the involvement of a phosphatidylinositol 3-kinase in vesicular transport to lysosomes,   *J. Cell Biol.* 130: 797-805 (1995).
6. W.J. Brown, D.B. DeWald, S.D. Emr, H. Plutner, and W.E. Balch, Role for phosphatidylinositol 3-kinase in the sorting and transport of newly synthesized lysosomal enzymes in mammalian cells, *J. Cell Biol.* 130: 781-796 (1995).
7. S.M. Jones, and K.E. Howell, Phosphatidylinositol 3-kinase is required for the   formation of constitutive transport vesicles from the TGN, *J. Cell Biol.* 139: 339-   349 (1997).
8. C. Guinebault, B. Payrastre, C. Racaud-Sultan, H. Mazarguil, M. Breton, G.   Mauco, M. Plantavid, and H. Chap, Integrin-dependent translocation of   phosphoinositide 3-kinase to the cytoskeleton of thrombin-activated platelets involves specific interactions of p85 alpha with actin filaments and focal adhesion   kinase, *J. Cell Biol.* 129: 831-842 (1995).
9. M. Wymann, and A. Arcaro, Platelet-derived growth factor-induced   phosphatidylinositol 3-kinase activation mediates actin rearrangements in   fibroblasts, *Biochem. J.* 298: 517-520 (1994).
10. P. Rodriguez-Viciana, P.H. Warne, A. Khwaja, B.M. Marte, D. Pappin, P. Das,   M.D. Waterfield, A. Ridley, and J. Downward, Role of phosphoinositide 3-OH kinase in cell transformation and control of the actin cytoskeleton by Ras, *Cell* 89:   457-467 (1997).
11. M.M. Chou, and J. Blenis, The 70 kDa S6 kinase complexes with and is activated by the Rho family G proteins Cdc42 and Rac1, *Cell* 85: 573-583 (1996).
12. D. Stokoe, L.R. Stephens, T. Copeland, P.R.J. Gaffney, C.B. Reese, and G.F.   Painter, Dual role of phosphatidyl-3,4,5-trisphosphate in the activation of protein   kinase B, *Science* 277: 567-570 (1997).
13. H. Nakanishi, K.A. Brewer, and J.H. Exton, Activation of the isozyme of protein   kinase C by phosphatidylinositor 3,4,5-trisphosphate, *J Biol Chem* 268: 13-16   (1993).
14. J.A. Le Good, W.H. Ziegler, D.B. Parekh, D.R. Alessi, P. Cohen, and P.J. Parker,   Protein kinase C isotypes controlled by phosphoinositide 3-kinase through the   protein kinase PDK1, *Science* 281: 2042-2045 (1998).
15. D.R. Alessi, S.R. James, C.P. Downes, A.B. Holmes, P.R.J. Gaffney, C.B.   Reese, and P. Cohen, Characterization of a 3-phosphoinositide-dependent protein   kinase which phosphorylates and activates protein kinase B alpha, *Curr Biol* 7:   261-269 (1997).
16. R. Dhand, J. Downward, M.J. Fry, I. Gout, P. Rodriguez-Viciana, B.   Vanhaesebroeck, P.H. Warne, and M.D. Westefield, Phosphatidylinositol-3-kinase as a direct target of Ras, *Nature* 370: 527-532 (1994).
17. K. Yamauchi, K. Holt, and J.E. Pessin, Phosphatidylinositol 3-kinase functions upstream of Ras and Raf in mediating insulin stimulation of c-fos transcription, *J   Biol Chem* 268: 14597-14600 (1993).
18. P. Rodriguez-Viciana, P.H. Warne, B. Vanhaesebroeck, M.D. Waterfield, and J. Downward, Activation of phosphoinositide 3-kinase by interaction with Ras and by point mutation, *EMBO* 15: 2442-2451 (1996).
19. Q. Hu, A. Klippel, A.J. Muslin, W.J. Fantl, and L.T. Williams, Ras-dependent induction of cellular responses by constitutively active phosphatidylinositol-3 kinase, *Science* 268: 100-102 (1995).
20. D.A.E. Cross, D.R. Alessi, P. Cohen, M. Andjelkovich, and B.A. Hemmings, Inhibition of glycogen synthase kinase -3 by insulin mediated by protein kinase B, *Nature* 378: 785-789 (1995).

21. A.D. Kohn, S.C. Summers, M.J. Birnbaum, and R.A. Roth, Expression of a constitutively active Akt ser/thr kinase in 3T3-L1 adipocytes stimulates glucose uptake and glucose transporter 4 translocation, *J Biol Chem* 271: 31372-31378 (1996).

22. K. Ueki, R. Yamamoto-Honda, Y. Kaburagi, T. Yamauchi, K. Tobe, B.M. Burgering, P.J. Coffer, I. Komuro, Y. Akanuma, Y. Yazaki, and T. Kadowaki, Potential role of protein kinase B in insulin-induced glucose transport, glycogen synthesis, and protein synthesis, *J Biol Chem* 273: 5315-5322 (1998).

23. G.S. Hotamisligil, and B.M. Spiegelman, Tumor necrosis factor α: a key component of the obesity-diabetes link, *Diabetes* 43: 1271-1278 (1994).

24. G.S. Hotamisligil, A. Budavari, D. Murray, and B.M. Spiegelman, Reduced tyrosine kinase activity of the insulin receptor in obesity-diabetes, *J Clin. Invest.* 94: 1543-1549 (1994).

25. G.S. Hotamisligil, P. Peraldi, A. Budavari, R. Ellis, M.F. White, and B.M. Spiegelman, IRS-1-mediated inhibition of insulin receptor tyrosine kinase activity in TNFand obesity-induced insulin resistance, *Science* 271: 665-668 (1995).

26. H. Kanety, R. Feinstein, M.Z. Papa, R. Hemi, and A. Karasik, Tumor necrosis factor α-induced phosphorylation of insulin receptor substrate-1 (IRS-1), *J. Biol. Chem.* 270: 23780-23784 (1995).

27. Y.A. Hannun, The sphingomyelin cycle and the second messenger function of ceramide, *J. Biol. Chem.* 269: 3125-3128 (1994).

28. P. Peraldi, G.S. Hotamisligil, W.A. Burman, M.F. White, and B.M. Spiegelman, Tumor necrosis factor (TNF)- inhibits insulin signaling through stimulation of the p55 TNF receptor and activation of sphingomyelinase, *J. Biol. Chem.* 271: 13018-13022 (1996).

29. H. Kanety, R. Hemi, M.Z. Papa, and A. Karasik, Sphingomyelinase and ceramide suppress insulin-induced tyrosine phosphorylation of the insulin receptor substrate-1, *J Biol Chem* 271: 9895-9897 (1996).

30. N. Begum, and L. Ragolia, Effect of tumor necrosis factor-alpha on insulin action in cultured rat skeletal muscle cells, *Endocrinology* 137: 2441-2446 (1996).

31. D. Guo, and D.B. Donner, Tumor necrosis factor promotes phosphorylation and binding of insulin receptor substrate 1 to phosphatidylinositol 3-kinase in 3T3-L1 adipocytes, *J. Biol. Chem.* 271: 615-618 (1996).

32. J.M. Stephens, J. Lee, and P.F. Pilch, Tumor necrosis factor--induced insulin resistance in 3T3-L1 adipocytes is accompanied by a loss of insulin receptor substrate-1 and GLUT4 expression without a loss of insulin receptor-mediated signal transduction, *J. Biol. Chem.* 272: 971-976 (1997).

33. C.N. Wang, L. O'Brien, and D.N. Brindley, Effects of cell-permeable ceramides and tumor necrosis factor on insulin signaling and glucose uptake in 3T3-L1 adipocytes, *Diabetes* 47: 24-31 (1998).

34. S.A. Summers, L.A. Garza, H. Zhou, and M.J. Birnbaum, Regulation of insulin-stimulated glucose transporter GLUT4 translocation and Akt activity by ceramide, *Mol. Cell Biol.* 18: 5457-5464 (1998).

35. P. Cornelius, M. Marlowe, M.D. Lee, and P.H. Pekala, The growth factor-like effects of tumor necrosis factor α. Stimulation of glucose transport activity and induction of glucose transporter and immediate early gene expression in 3T3-L1 preadipocytes, *J Biol Chem* 265: 20506-20516 (1990).

36. D.A. Evans, D.O. Jacobs, and D.W. Wilmore, Tumor necrosis factor enhances glucose uptake by peripheral tissues, *Am J Physiol* 257: R1182-R1189 (1989).

37. L.A. Feig, and G.M. Cooper, Inhibition of NIH 3T3 cell proliferation by a mutant ras protein with preferential affinity for GDP, *Mol. Cell Biol.* 8: 3235-3243 (1988).

38. U.K. Laemmli, Cleavage of structural proteins during the assembly of the head of bacteriophage T4, *Nature* 227: 680-685 (1970).

39. F. Folli, M.J.A. Saad, J.M. Backer, and R.C. Kahn, Insulin stimulation of phosphatidylinositol 3-kinase activity and association with insulin receptor substrate 1 in liver and muscle of the intact rat, *J. Biol. Chem.* 267: 22171-22177 (1992).

40. S.J. Taylor, and D. Shalloway, (1996) Cell cycle-dependent activation of Ras, *Current Biol.* 6: 1621-1627 (1992).

41. C.L. Carpenter, and L.C. Cantley, Phosphoinositide kinases, *Curr. Opinion.Cell Biol.* 8: 153-158 (1996).

42. L.R. Stephens, T.R. Jackson, and P.T. Hawkins, Agonist-stimulated synthesis of phosphatidylinositol(3,4,5)-trisphosphate: a new intracellular signaling system?, *Biochim. Biophys. Acta* 1179: 27-75 (1993).

43. L. Varticovski, D. Harrison-Findik, M.L. Keeler, and M. Susa, Role of PI 3-kinase in mitogenesis, *Biochim. Biophys. Acta* 1226: 1-11 (1994).

44. H.C. Chen, P.A. Appeddu, H. Isoda, and J.L. Guan, Phosphorylation of tyrosine 397 in focal adhesion kinase is required for binding phosphatidylinositol 3-kinase, *J. Biol. Chem* 271: 26329-26334 (1996).

45. A.N. Hanna, E.Y.W. Chan, J. Xu, J.C. Stone, and D.N. Brindley, A novel pathway for tumor necrosis factor-a and ceramide signaling involving sequential activation of tyrosine kinase, p21ras and phosphatidylinositol 3-kinase, *J. Biol. Chem* 274: 12722-12729 (1999).

46. D.A. Evans, D.O. Jacobs, and D.W. Wilmore, Tumor necrosis factor enhances glucose uptake by peripheral tissues, *Am. J. Physiol.* 257: R1182-89 (1989).

47. A. Marette, C. Atgié, Z. Liu, U.J. Bukowiecki, and A. Klip, Differential regulation of GLUT1 and GLUT4 glucose transporters in skeletal muscle of a new model of type II diabetes, *Diabetes* 42: 1195-2001 (1993).

ANTIOXIDANTS, FREE RADICAL STRESS AND DIABETES

Shanti S. Rastogi and Ram B. Singh

Endocrine Point and Centre for Diabetes and Nutrition
Delhi, India and
Medical Hospital and Research Centre
Moradabad, India

INTRODUCTION

The DCCT, the UKPD and the DAGMI studies have demonstrated the role of hypoglycemic agents such as human insulin and metformin in the management of diabetes and its vascular complications and in decreasing mortality. However, many subjects died in the intervention groups of these studies indicating that beyond tight control of glucose, further intervention is necessary to reduce clinical events and progression of vascular disease. Increased consumption of refined sugar, total and saturated fat and linoleic acid rich oils and lower intake of n-3 fatty acids and antioxidant vitamins and coenzyme Q10 in the diet in association with smoking and sedentaryness have been suggested to be important risk factors of diabetes and cardiovascular disease (CVD).[1-3]

PREVALENCE OF DIABETES AND CARDIOVASCULAR DISEASE

The severity of vascular disease appear to be greater in diabetes than nondiabetes.[4] It has been suggested that increased free radical stress with changing diet and lifestyle resulting into greater metabolic susceptibility may be important in the pathogenesis of rapid emergence of diabetes and CVD among south Asians.[3,9,11] We reported that the prevalence of diabetes was 2.7% in rural and 6.0% in urban north Indians and 8% in urban south Indians.[9-11] In south Asian immigrants to industrialized countries, the prevalence of diabetes varies between 10-20% in different studies and the prevalence of coronary artery disease (CAD) is above 10%. Higher prevalence of diabetes and cardiovascular risk in Indian urban populations and in south Asian immigrants to developed countries has been suggested[9-11] to be due to insulin resistance syndrome as a result of free radical induced beta cell damage. In developed countries, the prevalence of diabetes is about 5% and almost half of the diabetes have some form of CVD. The risk of vascular disease in diabetics

Diabetes and Cardiovascular Disease: Etiology, Treatment and Outcomes
Edited by Aubie Angel et al., Kluwer Academic/Plenum Publishers, 2001

201

is two to three fold greater than in non-diabetics.

The prevalence of hypertension and CAD in Indian diabetics in a population study is not known. The unfavourable prognosis of diabetic patients has mainly been attributed to more pronounced left ventricular dysfunction, a high likelihood of reinfarction and sudden cardiac death. The unfavourable outcome may be due to more severe and diffuse CAD, diabetic cardiomyopathy, disturbed autonomic tone and abnormal fibrinolytic and platelet function as well as metabolic factors such as increased free radical stress, dyslipidemia and hyperinsulinemia. In our epidemiological study[10] among subjects aged 25-64 years, CAD was present in 11% rural and 25.4% urban diabetic men and 12.5% rural and 22% urban diabetic women. The prevalence of CAD among diabetics was 3-4 fold greater than in non-diabetics and among urban diabetics, CAD was three fold more common in men and two fold more in women than in rurals (Table 1). In another study[9] in which diabetes was diagnosed by reporting, hypertension (>140/90mmHg) was present in 35% of diabetics and 25% of non-diabetics in north Indian men and in 53% of diabetics and 34% of non-diabetics in south Indian men. Similar rates were noted among women (Table 2). Higher prevalence of diabetes and cardiovascular risk in people of south Asian origin are not explained by insulin resistance alone.

Table 1. Coronary artery disease in diabetes (n(%))

	Rural Diabetes	Without Diabetes	Urban Diabetes	Without Diabetes
Subjects(Men)	27	867	63	841
CAD	3 (11.1)	32 (3.7)	16 (25.4)	84 (9.9)
Subjects (Women)	24	851	45	857
CAD	3 (12.5)	20 (2.3)	10 (22.2)	53 (6.2)

Singh, Niaz, Rastogi, Int. J. Cardiol, 1998

Table 2. Hypertension in diabetes (n(%))

	North Indian Diabetes	Without Diabetes	South Indian Diabetes	Without Diabetes
Subjects (Men)	23	881	30	707
Hypertension	8 (34.7)	218 (24.7)	16 (53.3)	239 (33.8)
Subjects (Women)	17	885	25	735
Hypertension	6 (35.2)	196 (22.1)	12 (48.0)	222 (30.2)

Singh, Niaz, Rastogi, J. Diab. Assoc. India, 1996

Table 3. Vitamins status and lipid peroxides in diabetes

	Diabetes	Coronary Disease	No Risk Factors
Dietary Vitamins Intake		Mean (SD)	
Vitamin C (mg/100Kcal)	30.5 (3.2)**	28.8 (3.1)**	37.5 (3.8)
Vitamin E (mg/100Kcal)	4.2 (0.4)	3.1 (0.4)*	4.6 (0.6)
Vitamin A (Hg/1000Kcal)	225 (14)	216*	228 (19)
Beta-carotene (ug/1000Kcal)	624 (30)*	605 (21)**	693 (38)
Plasma Levels			
Vitamin C (mg/dl)	20.2 (2.8)**	21.6 (3.3)**	42.5 (4.5)
Vitamin E (mmol/L)	15.6 (2.7)*	15.2 (2.8)*	21.4 (3.2)
Vitamin E/cholesterol	2.88 (0.5)*	2.95 (0.47)*	4.2 (0.56)
Vitamin A (umol/L)	2.1 (0.23)	2.0 (0.24)	2.4 (0.25)
Beta-carotene (umol/L)	0.31 (0.05)**	0.33 (0.06)*	0.55 (0.08)
Lipid peroxides	2.86 (0.22)	2.82 (0.22)*	1.6 (0.20)

Singh, Niaz, Rastogi etal[12] Acta Cardial, 1994

ANTIOXIDANTS IN DIABETES AND CARDIOVASCULAR DISEASE

Free radicals stress is important in the pathogenesis of diabetes and cardiovascular disease.[3-7] In humans, the evidence concerning the role of antioxidants and free radicals in diabetes is limited. Antioxidant vitamin deficiency and increased lipid peroxidation have been observed in patients with diabetes compared to control subjects.[3-7] In one epidemiologic study in 152 adults, plasma levels of vitamin C and beta-carotene were inversely associated with diabetes and CAD.[12] (Table 3). Lipid peroxides which are indicator of free radical stress was higher in diabetes.

The Indian Lifestyle and Heart Study in Elderly[13] comprising 595 subjects, aged 50-84 years showed that 70 (11.7%) patients had diabetes and 72 (12.1%) CAD. One third of the diabetic patients also had CAD. Antioxidant vitamin consumption and plasma levels were significantly lower in patients with diabetes and those with CAD (Table 4). Glucose intolerance was associated with lower intake of vitamin C and E which is unlikely due to recent dietary modification. It is possible that poor intake of antioxidant vitamins may be a risk factor of glucose intolerance as well as diabetes and CAD. Indians cook their green leafy vegetables by frying and half of them use open frying pans which are likely to destroy the antioxidant content resulting into poor intake.[13] Lower intake and low plasma levels of vitamin E have also been observed in Finland.[14] In the Kuopio ischaemic heart disease risk factor study comprising 2682 men, the mean plasma vitamin E concentration was 19μmol/L which is similar to levels in Indians. In 566 (60%) men, the vitamin E intake was below the recommended 10mg/day. Follow-up after four years showed a strong independent association between low vitamin E status below median before follow up and an excess 3.9 fold risk of diabetes (n=45) in a cohort of men in eastern Finland. This finding supports the hypothesis that free radical stress has a role in non-insulin dependent diabetes mellitus. The strength of the association is remarkable and militates against a chance finding. Confounding with other risk factors was excluded. (Table 5)

Table 4. Vitamin status in glucose intolerance, diabetes and CAD in elderly subjects

Vitamins	Glucose Intolerance	Diabetes	CAD	No Risk Factors
Vitamin Intake (mg/1000 Kcal)				
Vitamin C	34.5 (4)*	32.6 (3.8)*	31.5 (4.1)*	41.6 (4.6)
Vitamin E	3.8 (0.4)*	3.8 (0.6)*	3.3 (0.5)*	4.7 (1.1)
Vitamin A				
(μg/1000Kcal)	236 (18)	228 (17)*	226 (19)**	240 (21)
Beta-carotene				
(μg/1000Kcal)	1115 (95)	1082 (95)**	1086 (86)**	1110 (98)
Plasma Levels (μmol/L)				
Vitamin C	32.6 (4.2)*	19.4 (3.1)**	20.3 (3.1)**	37.8 (5.6)
Vitamin E	18.1 (3.4)	14.2 (3.1)**	15.0 (2.6)**	20.2 (4.2)
Vitamin E/				
Cholesterol	3.8 (0.7)	2.72 (0.96)**	2.72 (0.56)**	3.9 (0.63)
Vitamin A	2.3 (0.2)	2.02 (0.21)**	2.02 (0.22)**	2.32 (0.21)
Beta-carotene	0.5 (0.08)	0.30 (0.05)**	0.31 (0.05)**	0.48 (0.09)
Lipid peroxides				
(mmol/ml)	1.61 (0.18)	2.61 (0.21)**	2.61 (0.23)**	1.5 (0.12)
2-hour plasma				
insulin (mμ/L)	30.6 (4.2)**	36.2 (4.6)**	35.0 (5)**	14.6 (3.8)

Singh, Niaz, Rastogi[13], Am J Cardiol, 1995

Table 5. Relative risk of diabetes associated with low plasma vitamin E concentration after adjustment of risk factors.

Risk Factor for Diabetes	Relative	95% Confidence Interval	P value
Lipid standardized vitamin E Below median (0.98)	3.90	1.76 to 8.61	0.0008
Age (years)	1.02	0.97 to 1.07	0.5401
Socioeconomic status	1.10	1.02 to 1.19	0.0122
Body mass index (Kg/m^2)	1.23	1.13 to 1.33	<0.0001
Cigarettes smoked daily	1.015	0.985 to 1.046	0.3274
Ratio of serum saturated fatty Acids to sum of monoeners polyenes	1.09	1.036 to 1.143	0.0007

Model X^2 = 71.82 (df=6), p<0.001. Salonen etal[14], BMJ, 1996

Table 6. Antioxidant vitamins in diabetes and acute coronary disease

μmol/L	Diabetes with Coronary Disease (n=21)	Coronary Disease without Risk Factors (n=50)	Diabetes (n=16)	Controls (n=110)
Vitamin C	3.0 (o.5)**	6.5 (1.4)*	24.6 (3.8)*	30.8 (4.1)
Vitamin E	13.0 (3.1)*	14.5 (3.5)*	16.4 (4)	18.3 (4.5)
Vitamin E/ Cholesterol	2.52 (0.4)*	2.62 (0.4)*	3.4 (0.6)	3.6 (0.6)
Vitamin A	1.73 (0.11)*	1.82 (0.14)*	2.01 (0.2)	2.31 (0.23)
Beta Carotene	0.12 (0.03)**	0.18 (0.04)*	0.46 (1)*	0.58 (1.2)
Lipid Peroxide	3.41 (0.8)*	2.8 (0.7)*	2.3 (0.3)*	2.30 (0.22)

Singh etal, Acta Cardiol[15]

Table 7. Antioxidant vitamin status in diabetes

Vitamin	Diabetes (n=54)	Controls (n=202)
Vitamin intakes (mg/day)		
Vitamin C	95 (8.5)*	125 (18)
Vitamin E	7.7 (1.2)*	9.2 (2.1)
Vitamin A	475 (66)*	578 (65)
Beta-carotene (μg/day)	1685 (212)*	2352 (305)
Plasma levels (μmol/L)		
Vitamin A	1.81 (0.2)*	2.23 (0.21)
Vitamin E	16.6 (2.1)*	19.2 (3.8)
Vitamin C	22.5 (3.5)*	27.4 (4.4)
Beta-carotene	0.46 (0.1)*	0.51 (0.1)
Lipid peroxides (nmol/ml)	2.7 (0.4)*	1.40 (0.2)

* = $p < 0.05$ Singh, Niaz, Rastogi etal[16]. J Nutr Environ Med, 1995.

There is greater evidence from case control studies regarding the role of antioxidants in diabetes. Singh etal[15] studied 109 patients with acute CAD and 182 controls. Plasma levels of antioxidant vitamins were inversely associated with diabetes and acute CAD compared to acute CAD without diabetes and control subjects (Table 6). In another case control study[16] among 54 patients of diabetes mellitus and 202 controls, dietary intake of vitamins and their plasma levels were significantly lower compared to control subjects. (Table 7)

OXIDATIVE STRESS

Oxidative stress seems to play an important role in the development of diabetes and CVD. In several of our clinical and epidemiological studies[12, 13] we have reported that lipid peroxides which is an indicator of free radical stress was significantly higher among diabetes and CVD patients compared to control subjects. Those subjects with any vascular complications, were associated with greater lipid peroxides compared to diabetics without complications (Table 6, 7)[15,16] Bambolkar and Sainani[17] also reported greater oxidative stress in diabetics with complications compared to uncomplicated diabetes (Table 8).

Antioxidant vitamin deficiency and free radical mechanisms have also been implicated in the pathogenesis of tissue damage in diabetes, atherosclerosis and thrombosis.[3-8] It has been speculated that as pancreatic beta-cells and arterial endothelial cells have low antioxidative enzyme activities they might be more sensitive to free radical injury.[4-7] Diabetes can be induced[18-20] in animals by free radical producing substances such as catalytic iron, alloxan and streptozocin and antioxidants may be prospective in preventing diabetes in animal experiments. Various sources of free radicals may modulate oxidative stress in diabetes (Table 9).

Superoxide, hydrogen peroxide and lipid peroxides are intermediate substances that are precursors of more reactive species such as hydroxyl radical.[3-6] Inhibitors of free radical generation are enzymes such as superoxide dismutase, catalase and peroxidases which limit accumulation of precursors. Other inhibitors that work by limiting concentration of free transition metal ions are transferin, ceruloplasmin, and albumin. They are catalysts of oxidation reactions. Free radical scavengers which limit hydroxyl radical damage by trapping reactive radicals in both hydrophilic and lipophilic

Table 8. Oxidative stress in different groups of diabetes

	Subjects	Diene Conjugates (OD units)	Lipid Peroxides (nmol/ml)	Glutathione (nmol/L)
Healthy	50	27 (3.6)	3.3 (0.7)	1.95 (0.13)
Diabetic without Complications	100	34 (5.6)*	5.4 (11)*	1.53 (0.16)*
Diabetes + Retinopathy	50	44 (6.7)*	6.2 (1.3)*	1.3 (0.08)*
Diabetes + CAD	50	43 (7.8)*	5.8 (1.1)*	1.43 (0.11)*
Diabetes + Nephropathy	50	46 (5.6)*	6.6 (1.1)*	1.26 (0.14)*

* = $p < 0.001$ Bambolker and Sainani, JAPI, 1995

Table 9. Sources of free radicals in diabetes

1. Non-enzymatic glycosylation of proteins.
2. Changes in the level of inflammatory mediators.
3. Monosaccharide auto-oxidation.
4. Polyol pathway activity, and alterations in sorbitol pathway activity.
5. Indirect production of free radicals through cell damage by other causes.
6. Reduced antioxidant reserve.
7. Metabolic stress due to change in energy metabolism.

cell membrane environments are vitamin C, glutathione and uric acid and vitamin E and ubiquinone respectively. Ubiquinone is a direct free radical scavenger as well as it also regenerates vitamin E after it converts into inactive tocopheroxyl form. Vitamin E is a highly potential antioxidant.

Streptozotocin and alloxan induced diabetes in experimental animals is caused by selective islet cell damage due to overproduction of free radicals.[18,19] Alloxan is taken up efficiently by the beta cells which produces free radicals by redox coupling with extracellular ascorbate and thiols (reductants) and low levels of antioxidants such as glutathione peroxidate and ubiquinol may facilitate the reaction. Alloxan induced beta cells damage can be prevented by hydroxyl radical scavengers, lipid soluble antioxidants and metal chelating agents.[18-20] Lipid soluble antioxidants are vitamin E and ubiquinol. Insulin secretion is regulated by prostaglandin metabolites including peroxides and their removal requires utilization of glutathione peroxidase, thereby making the islet cells inherently deficient in glutathione peroxidase and rendering them susceptible to free radical attack.

There is increased consumption of antioxidant vitamins, glutathione peroxidase, ubiquinol etc. by the body tissues in diabetes mellitus in the process of oxidant stress.[3-8] Plasma copper levels are higher and magnesium and zinc levels are lower in diabetes and CAD.[21-23] Free copper ions are known to catalyze ascorbate oxidation and compounds like aldos reductase inhibitor may block such reactions by blinding free copper ions.[24] Zinc deficiency is associated with insulin resistance and zinc therapy is capable of modulating insulin action.[25] Zinc may work as antioxidant through superoxide dismutase. Zinc deficiency may also decrease zinc/copper ratio and increase the adverse effects of copper ions on oxidant stress in diabetes. Diabetes mellitus is associated with increased availability of transition metals.

There is no evidence that once oxidative damage occurs, it may be reversed back to the native form. Modification of long-lived extracellular proteins and structural changes in tissues rich in proteins are associated with the development of complications in diabetes such as cataracts, microangiopathy, atherosclerosis and nephropathy.[7] The chemical and physical changes characteristic of collagen in diabetes are summarized (Table 11).

It is difficult to conclude that increased lipid peroxidation is a cause or effect of complications in diabetes. It may be more appropriate to consider lipid peroxidation as part of a continuous cycle of oxidative stress and damage. Recent studies indicated an increased oxidative stress and lower plasma level of carotenoids in patients with severe obesity.[26,27] Obesity is an independent risk factor of diabetes and this finding indicates that oxidative stress in obese subjects may be a risk factor of diabetes. In a recent study,[14] lower basal

Table 11. Chemical and physical changes in collagen in diabetes due to oxidative modifications.

Chemical	Physical
Increased gycation	Increased browning
Increased pentosidine	Increased fluorescence
Increased carboxymethylation	Increased mechanical strength
Increased cross-linking	Increased thermal stability
Maturation of reducible cross-linking	Decreased solubility
Resistance to enzymatic digestion	Resistance to denaturants

vitamin E levels were significantly associated with future development of diabetes. The above issue was addressed statistically by adjusting for measures of glucose metabolism at baseline. Besides fasting blood glucose concentration, the serum concentration of glycosylated protein as measured by fructosame value was available. If the baseline vitamin E level was influenced by a latent and unmanifested diabetes, the control for glucose status at baseline should have eliminated this effect certainly to the extent to which the validity and precision of these measurements allowed.

COENZYME Q (UBIQUINONE)

The discovery of coenzyme Q almost four decades ago has considerably promoted our understanding of membrane bound redox processes, proton distribution and energy conservation.[8] Coenzyme Q is found in plasma membranes, in all intracellular membranes and in low-density lipoproteins. Its content is very high in Golgi membranes and in lysosomal membranes. Since in diabetes, free radical inhibitory and scavenger system is compromised, coenzyme Q deficiency exacerbate the oxidative stress. Antioxidation of unsaturated lipids in plasma and membrane proteins results into deficiency of ubiquinol in the tissues which further enhances free radical damage in diabetes resulting into CVD. Ubiquinone is a lipid soluble scavenger similar to vitamin E and beta-carotene. It decreases hydroxyl radical damage by trapping reactive radicals in lipophilic cell membrane environment.[8,28-30] Coenzyme Q may be protective against cardiac damage, causing decrease in cardiac enzyme during bypass surgery.[32]

There are only a few studies showing the role of coenzyme Q10 in diabetes mellitus. In a study[33] of 120 patients with diabetes mellitus, 8.3% showed coenzyme Q deficiency compared with 1.9% of a group of healthy subjects. The incidence of coenzyme Q deficiency was 20% among patients receiving oral hypoglycemic agent indicating that these drugs might interfere with coenzyme Q metabolism. In another study[34], coenzyme Q7 was administered to 39 patients of diabetes in a dosage of 120mgm/day for a period ranging from 2-18 weeks. Fasting blood glucose decreased by 20% among 14 (36%) of 39 patients and by 30% among 12 (31%) of 39 patients. There was marked reduction (30%) in ketone bodies among 13 (59%) of 22 patients. Cessation of treatment was associated with increase in blood sugar in a few patients. The mechanism by which coenzyme Q modulates blood glucose is not clear. It is possible that coenzyme Q therapy induces synthesis of coenzyme Q dependent enzymes which in turn enhance carbohydrate metabolism. Coenzyme Q also regenerates vitamin E which indicates that coenzyme Q might improve insulin sensitivity and insulin action. This hypothesis is further suggested by the fact that the resistance of peripheral tissues to glucose uptake may be a consequence of permanently high lipid oxidation. The oxidation of lipids could be enhanced if the concentration of lipid soluble antioxidants such as ubiquinone and vitamin E are low. There are no published studies on the role of coenzyme Q in patients of diabetes associated with vascular disease. However in several studies, coenzyme Q has been demonstrated to provide beneficial effect in patients with angina, CAD, heart failure, hypertension and cardiomyopathy.[28-32]

Coenzyme Q is found in every plant and animal cell. However the amount of coenzyme Q through dietary supplementation appears to be too low to provide any clinical effects. The plasma level of coenzyme Q is more than two fold greater among vegetarians than in omnivores which indicates that a high intake of plant foods may preserve high coenzyme Q levels. Coenzyme Q deficiency may be a result of impaired synthesis, nutritional deficiency or increased tissue needs. In elderly subjects, there is increased requirements of coenzyme Q because of its declining levels with advancing age. A recent study[46] has demonstrated that treatment with coenzyme Q10 can modulate the chemical composition and quality of atheroma in experimental atherosclerosis in rabbits.

ANTIOXIDANT THERAPY

In humans, intervention trials on the role of antioxidants in diabetes are very limited.[33-39] However the role of antioxidant vitamin E, C and A and beta-carotene and coenzyme Q have been successfully examined in double blind randomized trials in the treatment and prevention of CAD and cancer. In a small, double blind randomized cross-over trial in 15 noninsulin, dependent diabetic and 10 healthy subjects, supplementation with 900mg vitamin E daily for four months reduced oxidative stress and improved insulin action in a euglycemic hyperinsulinimic glucose clamp.[35,36] Vitamin E reduced the area under the curve and increased the total body glucose disposal and non-oxidative glucose metabolism in both healthy and diabetes subjects. The Indian Experiment of Infarct survival[40] showed that a combination of vitamin E (40 mg/day), beta-carotene (25 mg/day), vitamin A (10000 units/day) and vitamin C (1000 mg/day) given for four weeks in patients with acute myocardial infarction (AMI) were beneficial. The Oxford study showed that vitamin E (400-800 mg/day) administered for 1 year was associated with significant decrease in the cardiac events in the intervention group compared to control group. It is possible that a greater case fatality rate in people of Indian origin with AMI may be due to increased oxidative stress among them.[41,42] In one randomized and controlled trial,[43] treatment with coenzyme Q10 in patients with AMI showed significant reduction in the cardiac events in the intervention group than control group. Serum levels of lipoprotein(a) as well blood pressures in known hypertensives showed significant decrease in the coenzyme Q group than control group.[44,45]

In view of above studies and the high risk of oxidative stress in diabetes, it is possible that the dosages of antioxidants in diabetes with CVD should be greater for prevention of oxidative stress and cardiovascular events. Vitamin E (400-500 mg/day), beta-carotene (20-50 mg/day), vitamin C (500-1000 mg/day) and coenzyme Q (100-300 mg/day), be administered without any significant side effects. However long term follow-up intervention trials would be necessary to demonstrate the benefit of antioxidants in the prevention of complications in diabetes and to assess whether above dose can be safely used. It may be prudent to advise 600 g/day of fruits, vegetable and legume and nuts such as almonds and walnuts (5-6 pieces) in conjunction with vegetable oils especially rich in n-3 fatty acids for primary prevention of diabetes and CVD because these foods are rich sources of antioxidants.[40]

REFERENCES

1. WHO Study Group. Diet, Nutrition and Prevention of Chronic Diseases. WHO, Geneva, 1990.
2. Indian Consensus Group. Indian Consensus for Prevention of Hypertension and Coronary Artery Disease. J Nutr Environ Med, 1996, 6:309-318.

3. Singh RB, Antioxidants, Free radical stress and coronary artery disease. J Intern Med India 1996, 7:23-24.
4. Malmberg K, for DEGAMI Study Group. Prospective randomized study of intensive insulin treatment on long term survival after acute myocardial infarction in patients with diabetes mellitus. BMJ 1997, 394:1512-15.
5. Packer L. The role of antioxidative treatment in diabetes mellitus. Diabetologia 1993, 36:1212-1213.
6. Wolff SP. Diabetes mellitus and free radicals. Free radicals, transition metals and oxidative stress in the etiology of diabetes mellitus and complications. Br Med Bull 1993, 49:642-652.
7. Baynes JW. Role of oxidative stress in development of complications in diabetes. Diabetes 1991, 40:405-412.
8. Cadnas E, Packer L. Handbook of Antioxidants. Marcel Dekker, Inc. New York, 1996, P. 157-203.
9. Singh RB, Beegon R, Rastogi V, Rastogi SS, Madhu SV, Clinical characteristics and hypertension among known patients of noninsulin dependent diabetes mellitus in north and south Indians. J Diab Asso India 1996, 36:45-50.
10. Singh RB, Rastogi V, Aslam M, Niaz MA, Rastogi SS. Diabetes mellitus and its determinants and risk ofcoronary artery disease in rural and urban populations of north India. Int J Cardio, 1998, 66:65-72.
11. Indian Consensus Group for Prevention of Diabetes. Diet and lifestyle guidelines and desirable levels of risk factors for prevention of diabetes and its vascular complications in Indians: A scientific statement of the International College of Nutrition. J Cardivas Risk 1997, 4:201-208.
12. Singh RB, Niaz MA, Gupta S, Rastogi SS etal. Diet, antioxidant vitamins, oxidative stress and risk of coronary disease. The Peerzada Prospective study. Acta Cardio 1994, 49:463-467.
13. Singh RB, Ghosh S, Niaz MA etal. Dietary intake, plasma levels of antioxidant vitamins and oxidative stress in relation to coronary artery disease in elderly subjects. Am J Cardio, 1995, 76:1233-1238.
14. Salonen JT, Nyyssonen K, Tuomainen TP, Maenpaa P, Korpela H, Kaplan GA, Lynch J, Helmrich SP, Salonen R. Increased risk of non-insulin dependent diabetes mellitus at low plasma vitamin E concentration: a four year follow up study in men. BMJ 1996, 311:1124-1127.
15. Singh RB, Niaz MA, Sharma JP, Kumar R, Bishnoi I, Beegom R. Plasma levels of antioxidant vitamins and oxidative stress in patients with acute myocardial infarction. Acta Cardio 1994, 49:441-452.
16. Singh RB, Niaz MA, Ghosh S etal. Dietary intake and plasma levels of antioxidant vitamins in health and disease: a hospital based case control study. J Nutr Environ Med, 1995, 5:235-242.
17. Bambolker S. Sainani GS. Evaluation of oxidative stress in diabetics with or without vascular complications. J Asso Phys India 1995, 43:10-12.
18. Malaisse WJ, Alloxan toxicity of the pancreatic beta cell: a new hypothesis. Biochem Pharmac 1982, 22:3527-2524.
19. Mendola J, Wright Jr JR, Lacy P: Oxygen Free radical scavengers and immune destruction of murine islets in allograft rejection and multiple low dose streptozotocin induced insulitis. Diabetes 1989, 38:379-385.
20. Flechner I, Maruta X, Burkart V, Kawai K, Kolb H, Kiesel U. Effects of radical scavengers on the development of experimental diabetes. Diabetes Res 1990, 13:67-73.
21. Mateo MCM, Bustamante JB, Cantalapiedra MAG. Serum, zinc, copper and insulin in diabetes mellitus, Biomed 1978, 29:56-58.
22. Noto R, Alicata R, Sfolgliano L. A study of cupremia in a group of elderly diabetics. Acta Diabetol Latina 1983, 20:81-85.
23. Singh RB, Niaz MA, Rastogi SS, Singh U, Agarwal P. Dietary and serum levels of antioxidant minerals in patients with acute myocardial infarction. Trace Elem Electrolytes 1995, 12:148-152.
24. Jiang ZY, Quong LZ, Eaton JW, Hunt JV, Koppenol WH, Wolf SP, Spirohydantoin inhibitors of aldose reductase inhibit iron and copper catalysed ascorbic oxidation in vitro. Biochem Pharmaco 1991, 42:1273-1278.
25. Kinlaw WB, Levine AS, Morley JE, Silvis SE, McClain CJ. Abmnormal zinc metabolism in type II diabetes mellitus. Am J Med 1983 75: 273-277.
26. Ohrvall M, Tengblad S, Vessby B. Lower tocopherol serum levels in subjects with abdominal obesity. J Intern Med 1993, 234:53-60.

27. Pipek R, Dankner G, Ben-Amotz A, Aviram M, Levy Y. Increased plasma oxidizability in subjects with severe obesity. J Nutr Environ Med 1996, 6:267-272.
28. Karlsson J, Diamant B, Edlund PO, Lund B, Folkers K, Theorell H. Plasma ubiquinone, alpha – tocopherol, and cholesterol in man. Int J Vit Nutr Res 1992, 62:160-164.
29. Karlsson J, Semb B. Muscle obiquinone and plasma antioxidants in effort angina. J Nutr environ Med 1996, 6:255-266.
30. Hofman-Bang C, Rehnqvist N, Swedberg K, Astrom H. Coenzyme Q10 as an adjunctive in treatment of congestive heart failure. J Am Coll Cardio 1992, 19 (Suppl):774-776.
31. Kamikawa T. Effects of coenzyme Q10 on exercise tolerance in chronic stable angina pectoris. Am J Cariol, 1985, 56:247-251.
32. Chelo M, Protection of coenzyme Q10 from myocardial reperfusion injury during coronary artery bypass grafting. Ann Thiorac Surg 1994, 58:1427-1482.
33. Kishi T. Bioenergetics in clinical medicine, XI, Studies on coenzyme Q and diabetes mellitus. J Med 1976, 7:307-312.
34. Shigeta Y, Izumik, Abe H. Effect of coenzyme Q7 treatment on blood sugar and ketone bodies of diabetics. J Vitaminol 1966, 12:293-297.
35. Paolisso G, D'Amore A, Giugliano D, Ceriell A, Varrichio M, D'Onofrio F. Pharmacologic doses of vitamin E improve insulin action in healthy subjects and non-insulin dependent diabetic patients. Am J Clin Nutr 1993, 57:650-656.
36. Caballero B. Vitamin E improves the action of insulin. Nutr Rev 1993, 51:339-340.
37. Packer L. The role of antioxidative treatment in diabetes mellitus workshop report. Diabetologia 1993, 36:1112-1114.
38. Sadikot SM, Raheja, BS. Vitamin E supplementation and oxidant stress in diabetes. J Diab Assoc India 1991, 31: 68-70.
39. Raheja BS, Sadikot SM. Vitamin C supplementation decreases oxidant stress and free radical damage in diabetes. J Diab Assoc India 1991, 31:79-81.
40. Singh RB, Niaz MA, Agarwal P, Beegom R, Rastogi SS. Effect of antioxidant rich foods on plasma ascorbic acid, cardiac enzyme and lipid peroxide levels in patients hospitalized with acute myocardial infarction. J Am Diet Assoc 1995, 95:775-580.
41. Wilkinson P, Sayer J, Lajik etal. Comparison of case fatality in south Asians and white patients after acute myocardial infarction: observational study. BMJ, 1996, 312:1330-1333.
42. Shaukat N, Lear J, Lowy A. etal. First myocardial infarction in patients at Indian subcontinent and European origin: comparison of risk factors, management and long term outcome. BMJ 1997, 314:639-642.
43. Singh RB, Wander GS, Rastogi A. etal. Randomized, double blind, placebo-controlled trial of coenzyme Q10 in patients with acute myocardial infarction. Cardiovas Drug Ther 1998, 12:347-353.
44. Singh RB, Niaz MA. Serum concentration of lipoprotein(a) decreases on treatment with hydrosoluble coenzyme Q10 in patients with coronary artery disease: discovery of a new role. Int. J Cardio 1999, 68:23-29.
45. Singh RB, Niaz MA, Rastogi SS, Shukla PK, Thakur AS. Effect of hydrosoluble coenzyme Q10 on blood pressures and insulin resistance in hypertensive patients with coronary artery disease. J Human Hyper 1999, 13:203-208.
46. Singh RB, Shinde SN, Chopra RK, Niaz MA, Thakur AS, Onouchi Z. Effect of coenzyme Q10 on experimental atherosclerosis and chemical composition and quality of atheroma in rabbits. Atherosclerosis, 2000, 148:275-282.

OXIDATIVE STRESS AND FUNCTIONAL DEFICIT IN DIABETIC CARDIOMYOPATHY

Pawan K. Singal, Adriane Belló-Klein,
Firoozeh Farahmand and Vic Sandhawalia

Institute of Cardiovascular Sciences
St. Boniface General Hospital Research Centre and
Department of Physiology, Faculty of Medicine,
University of Manitoba, Winnipeg, Manitoba, R2H 2A6, Canada

SUMMARY

When the equilibrium between free-radical production and cellular antioxidant defences is disturbed in favour of more free radicals, it causes oxidative stress which can promote cellular injury. Oxidative stress has been suggested to play a role in the pathogenesis of diabetic cardiomyopathy. In streptozotocin-induced diabetes, there is a decrease in antioxidant enzyme activities and an increase in myocardial lipid peroxidation. Probucol, an antioxidant, was found to improve cardiac function which may have been due to an increase in myocardial antioxidant enzyme activities and a decrease in lipid peroxidation in the diabetic animals. Some of the beneficial effects of probucol may also be due to an improvement in plasma insulin levels and a decrease in the plasma glucose. The diabetic state is also associated with endothelial dysfunction, retinopathy, neuropathy and renopathy. Some of these secondary complications may also be mediated by oxidative stress. It is suggested that diabetic cardiomyopathy is associated with an antioxidant deficit and that antioxidant therapy may be useful in improving cardiac function in diabetes.
Keywords: Antioxidant Enzymes; Lipid Peroxidation; Probucol; Heart Failure

INTRODUCTION

Heart dysfunction has been demonstrated in diabetic patients as well as experimental animals. The precise mechanism by which hyperglycemia induces this myocardial dysfunction is not fully understood. One proposal to explain this phenomenon is presented in this paper. It is focussed on the role of free radicals in the genesis of diabetic cardiomyopathy. This hypothesis is supported by the data obtained from diabetic-patients as well as animals studies. The involvement of free radicals in the secondary complications of diabetes is also explored in this concise review. Insulin therapy may normalize blood glucose levels but cannot completely avoid myocardial dysfunction. Thus it is necessary to investigate new therapies for treating and/or preventing this cellular injury. In the recent

Diabetes and Cardiovascular Disease: Etiology, Treatment and Outcomes
Edited by Aubie Angel et al., Kluwer Academic/Plenum Publishers, 2001

213

past, we have tested the efficacy of probucol as an antioxidant therapeutic agent in diabetic cardiomyopathy.

FREE RADICALS, ANTIOXIDANTS AND OXIDATIVE STRESS

In physiological conditions, > 95% of the oxygen consumed is tetravalently reduced, resulting in the formation of water and production of ATP to perform vital metabolic functions. This step is catalysed by cytochrome oxidase enzyme complex in the mitochondria. Less than 5% of the oxygen is reduced through the univalent reduction pathway where four electrons are added one at time. In this process, reactive oxygen species (ROS), including singlet oxygen, superoxide radical, hydrogen peroxide and hydroxyl radical are produced. These species have short half-lives, and can interact with different molecules, causing oxidative damage to tissues (1-3). ROS avidly react with unsaturated lipids in cellular membranes, starting lipid-radical chain reactions and producing lipoperoxides (4).

Living organisms have developed defence mechanisms to protect against oxidative damage to their tissues. One line of defence includes antioxidant enzymes such as superoxide dismutase (SOD), catalase (CAT) and glutathione peroxidase (GSHPx). SOD catalyses the dismutation of superoxide radical to hydrogen peroxide. There are several different types of SOD in mammalian tissues, but the two most abundant isoforms include manganese SOD present in mitochondria and copper-zinc SOD present in the cytosol (5). Hydrogen peroxide is removed by either CAT that is specific for hydrogen peroxide (H_2O_2) itself and by GSHPx that can also remove hydroperoxides. CAT has a peroxisomal localization and GSHPx has a form which is exclusively cytosolic (selenium-dependent) and another form that can be found in the mitochondrial matrix (selenium-independent) (6). CAT has been implicated in the detoxification of H_2O_2 at high concentrations (mM range) whereas GSHPx is effective at much lower concentrations (μM range) of H_2O_2 (3,7). Besides enzymatic antioxidants, cells have many other non-enzymatic defences such as tocopherols, carotenoids, uric acid, ascorbic acid, flavonoids, glutathione and other thiols. These substances act as a second line of defence, avoiding the propagation of the chain-reactions and because of this they are called chain-breaker antioxidants (8). When the damage has occurred, there are repair enzymes which can provide a third line of defence.

Changes in the protective cellular antioxidants in response to many physiological and pathological conditions, including age, exercise, and hypertrophy (2,9,10) have been reported. The enhanced generation of ROS and/or the reduction of antioxidant defences produce a situation called oxidative stress (11). Oxidative damage to tissues is a common end point of many different chronic diseases, such as atherosclerosis, diabetes, ischemia-reperfusion injury, and rheumatoid arthritis. Chemical modification of amino acids and lipids during lipid peroxidation results in the formation of many different products that can be detected experimentally and serve as indicators of oxidative stress, e.g. TBARS (thiobarbituric acid reactive substances), tert-butyl hydroperoxide initiated – chemiluminescence, oxygen uptake.

POTENTIAL SOURCES OF OXIDATIVE STRESS IN DIABETES

Oxidative stress may result from an overproduction of reactive oxygen species and/or decreased efficiency of inhibitory scavenger systems. The cause for the elevated oxidative stress in diabetes is not fully understood, however the autooxidation of glucose (12), the formation of advanced glycation end products (13) and the activation of NADPH-oxidase (14) have been suggested to play a role. Many of biochemical pathways that are strictly associated with hyperglycemia (glucose autooxidation, polyol pathway, prostanoid synthesis, protein glycation, SOD inactivation) can also increase the production of ROS (15). These may also include non-enzymatic glycosylation, monosaccharide autooxidation, other

metabolic changes, alterations in sorbitol pathway, and changes in the level of inflammatory mediators and the
status of antioxidant defence systems (12,13,16-18). Some drugs have been shown to block these pathways, preventing some diabetic complications and the list includes: aminoguanidine (inhibition of non-enzymatic glycation) (19), aldose reductase inhibitors (inhibition of polyol pathway) (18), vasodilators (prevention of hypoxia) and free radical scavengers such as alpha-lipoic acid (antioxidant effect). Different potential sources which may explain how hyperglycemia can cause increased formation of ROS and oxidative stress are schematically shown in figure 1.

AUTOOXIDATION OF FREE SUGARS

It has been shown that glucose, under physiological conditions, produces oxidants that possess reactivity similar to the hydroxyl radical (12). The process of glucose oxidation results in dicarbonyl compound formation which is accompanied by superoxide ($O_2^{\cdot-}$) production. As described above, superoxide radicals undergo dismutation to hydrogen peroxide and in the presence of transition metals it can also react with hydrogen peroxide leading to the production of extremely reactive hydroxyl radicals. That high glucose stimulates the generation of superoxide radicals from endothelial cells as a consequence of increased autooxidation of glucose and protein glycation has been demonstrated (12,20,21). Superoxide radical may quench nitric oxide, thus reducing the endothelial-dependent relaxation (15,22,23). On the other hand, endothelial dysfunction can produce excessive amount of nitric oxide which can be seen to react with the superoxide produced, resulting in the formation of peroxynitrite, a strong oxidant, and thus contributing to the oxidative stress. These data and the observation that the production of superoxide radical is not prevented by inhibitors of nitric oxide synthases, P-450-dependent oxygenase and lipo and cyclooxygenases suggest that the autooxidation of glucose may be one of the major sources of the reactive oxygen species in diabetes.

NON-ENZYMATIC REACTIONS

In autooxidative glycosylation, reducing sugar acts as a catalyst for oxidative chemical modification and cross linking of proteins (12,13,24). Furthermore, advanced glycation end product (AGE) which can be produced by aerobic, non-enzymatic glycation of protein in the presence of trace metals is accompanied by the production of ROS (25). The reactive oxygen species formed in the autooxidation of protein-bound products include superoxide and hydrogen peroxide (26). In addition, AGE products can stimulate the release of ROS from endothelium by a receptor-mediated process (27). Most of the proteins, under appropriate conditions, can undergo glycation if exposed to elevated glucose or glucose α-phosphate concentrations. In insulin requiring tissues of the diabetic subjects, intracellular proteins may be partially protected from glycation despite extracellular hyperglycemia because of poor glucose uptake (28). Nevertheless, at autopsy, tissue from diabetic subjects exhibit a generalized increase in glycation (25). It is important to note that the polyol pathway may also contribute to non-enzymatic glycation of proteins because fructose can bind non-enzymatically to proteins (so-called fructation), and fluorescence of collagen from diabetic animals is decreased by inhibitors of aldol reduction (18).

ALTERED ANTIOXIDANT PROFILE IN DIABETES

Many clinical and experimental studies suggesting the involvement of free radicals in diabetes are discussed below:

Human Studies

Sato et al. (29) have demonstrated that the level of lipid peroxides is increased in the plasma of diabetic patients. Plasma lipoproteins from diabetic patients are also more susceptible to oxidation (30,31). It has been shown that non-enzymatic glycosylation (glycation) of human CuZn superoxide dismutase leads to gradual inactivation of this enzyme *in vitro* as well as *in vivo* and the level of glycated CuZnSOD is increased in the erythrocyte of patients with diabetes mellitus (17). Levels of heat-shock protein 70 (HSP70), a stress-induced protein, are elevated in mononuclear cells of patients with diabetes (32). Furthermore, a powerful endogenous antioxidant, ubiquinol, is reduced in insulin dependent diabetes mellitus (IDDM) patients (33). In red blood cells of diabetic humans, changes such as an increase in glutathione reductase activity, a decreased susceptibility to oxidative glutathione depletion and an increased production of TBARS were observed. These changes correlated with the severity of diabetic complications (34).

Endothelial dysfunction is the major cause of vascular complications associated with diabetes (35). In diabetic patients, there is an increased incidence of atherosclerosis and hypertension, which can be explained by the vascular endothelium impaired synthesis of vasodilators and increased release of procoagulants and vasoconstrictors (22,23). It has been found that vascular cell adhesion molecule (VCAM)-1 expression is activated in non-insulin dependent diabetes mellitus (NIDDM) patients and the GSH/GSSG ratio is reduced. The therapy with N-acetyl-cysteine protected against the progression of vascular damage (36). Another event that is crucial to the pathophysiology of vascular disease is the transendothelial migration of monocytes as a result of phosphorylation of platelet endothelial cell adhesion molecule –1 (PECAM-1). This event can be induced by oxidative stress in human umbilical vein endothelial cells (37).

Free radicals also play a role in diabetic neuropathy (38). In these subjects, a novel conjugate of gamma-linolenic acid and alpha-lipoic acid has been used with encouraging results (39). Alpha lipoate is absorbed from diet and crosses the blood-brain barrier. This substance has potent antioxidant properties, regenerating other antioxidants like vitamins C and E and raising intracellular glutathione levels (40). Increased formation of isoprostanes (more specific parameter of oxidative stress than TBARS) was seen in diabetic patients and vitamin E supplementation modulated this change (14). All these findings on patients provide support for the concept that free radical production and decreased antioxidant reserve may play a role in diabetic complications.

Animal Studies

There are many experimental evidences that suggest the involvement of free radicals in the pathogenesis of diabetes. The oxidative stress may be amplified by an autocatalytic cycle of metabolic stress, tissue damage and cell death, leading to an increase in free radical production and compromised inhibitory and scavenger mechanism. It may mean that the secondary complications in diabetes may also be mediated by the oxidative stress. An increase in TBARS production was verified in many tissues, including heart, in STZ-diabetic rats (41-43). This increased oxidative stress was associated with many changes in the antioxidant enzyme activities. Wohaieb and Godin (44) found an increased activity in CAT and GSSG-reductase in the heart of STZ-diabetic rats. A similar result in the CAT activity was obtained in short-term STZ-induced diabetes in rats (41). These two observations may represent an early adaptive response to counter the oxidative stress. A reduction in SOD and CAT activities, an increase in glutathione-S-transferase, and a depletion of GSH content was observed in alloxan (ALX)-induced diabetes (45). Recently, an enhanced production of ROS in vivo in the diabetic state was detected by EPR (electron paramagnetic resonance) in STZ-diabetic rats (46).

ENDOTHELIAL DYSFUNCTION

Gene regulation in the cardiovascular tissues of diabetic subjects has also been reported to be altered. The activity of two redox-sensitive transcription factors, i.e. nuclear factor kappa B (NF-kappaB) and activating protein-1 (AP-1), were increased in STZ-diabetic rats. Probucol treatment prevented these changes, without changing plasma glucose concentration (47). Glucose also activates the transcription factor NF-kappaB and it is regarded as a key event in the modification of the vasculature in diabetes (14). There is now convincing data from animal studies showing that oxidative stress may play a role in the impairment of endothelial function, as well as in the development of perivascular fibrosis (38,48). The treatment with probucol resulted in partial restoration of endothelial function and noradrenaline-induced contraction in aorta of STZ-diabetic rats (49).

Endothelial dysfunction in diabetes may also be related to many other factors like activation of protein kinase C, hyperglycaemic pseudohypoxia, increased expression of transforming growth factor-beta and vascular endothelial growth factor, non-enzymatic glycation, activation of coagulation cascade, increased expression of tumor necrosis factor-alpha and high levels of insulin and insulin precursor molecules (35).

MYOCARDIAL DYSFUNCTION

Myocardial biochemical changes produced by STZ include the depletion of magnesium content as well as depression of K^+-stimulated sarcoplasmic reticular and myofibrillar ATPase activities (50). The ALX-induced diabetes is also associated with a significant decrease in magnesium levels and a slight elevation in myocardial calcium. ALX induces anatomical changes especially in mitochondria such as: swelling and fragmentation, with amorphous dense bodies, cristae appeared distorted and, in some cases, completely lysed (50). Myocardial functional changes observed in this model included: decreased left ventricular pressure, heart rate and rate of left ventricular pressure development (51). Heart dysfunction in chronic diabetes has been observed to be associated with depressed myofibrillar adenosine triphosphatase activities, abnormalities in the sarcoplasmic reticular, sarcolemmal calcium transport processes, and alterations in the expression of myosin isozymes and regulatory proteins as well as myosin phosphorylation (52).

There is some evidence suggesting the involvement of oxysterols, oxidation derivatives of cholesterol, in the development of diabetic cardiomyopathy (53). Enhanced glycation of protein and protein cross linking in heart sarcolemma may also participate in adaptive mechanisms that may be responsible for increased tolerance to calcium in diabetic cardiomyopathy (54). It was demonstrated that probucol can improve plasma lipids and cardiac performance in rats with experimental diabetes and may prevent diabetic cardiomyopathy (55-57).

In our studies on STZ-induced diabetes in rats, increased myocardial oxidative stress was indicated by increased lipid peroxidation and decreased antioxidant enzymes activities (catalase, superoxide dismutase and glutathione peroxidase). Hemodynamic studies revealed depressed left ventricular peak systolic pressure, and increased left ventricular end diastolic pressure (56,57). We found that probucol did not reverse the loss of weight induced by diabetes. Serum glucose levels of diabetic rats were about 450% of the control values which were reduced with probucol treatment, but were still significantly higher than the group that received only probucol. STZ administration induced a decrease of about 80% in insulin levels, whereas in the diabetic group that received probucol this reduction was about 62%. Probucol improved cardiac function in diabetic rats.

SOD activity was reduced about 50% in diabetic rats as compared to control. The group treated only with probucol had significantly more SOD than control. In the diabetic group, probucol caused small, but significant increase in SOD activity. Diabetic rats showed lower levels of GSHPx than control and probucol increased this enzyme activity. In addition, catalase was enhanced in diabetic rats as compared to control and this effect was amplified under probucol treatment. Lipid peroxidation was about 100% higher in diabetic group than in control. Probucol reduced these levels but they were still higher than control (56,57).

In conclusion, diabetic condition is associated with an overall decrease in "antioxidant reserve," an increase in lipid peroxidation and depressed cardiac function. In diabetic rats, probucol improved the endogenous "antioxidant reserve" and decreased myocardial lipid peroxidation. The beneficial effects of probucol in improving insulin, glucose levels and heart function may also be due, among other mechanisms, to its antioxidant properties.

Acknowledgments

Studies reported here were supported by the Canadian Diabetes Association and the Heart and Stroke Foundation of Manitoba. Dr. Singal is a Career Awardee of the Medical Research Council of Canada, Dr. Belló-Klein is supported by a scholarship from CAPES (an agency of the Brazilian Government) and Dr. Farahmand was supported by the Faculty of Graduate Studies, The University of Manitoba.

REFERENCES

1. Singal P.K., Petkau A., Gerrard J.M., Hrushovetz S., Foerster J., Free radicals in health and disease, *Mol Cell Biochem*. 84:121-2 (1988).
2. Kaul N., Siveski-Iliskovic N., Hill M., Slezak J., Singal P.K., Free radicals and the heart, *J Pharmacol Toxicol Methods* 30:55-67 (1993).
3. Yu, B.P., Cellular defenses against damage from reactive oxygen species, *Physiol Rev* 74(1):139-62 (1994).
4. Halliwell B. Oxidants and human disease: some new concepts. *FASEB J* 1:358-64 (1987).
5. McCord J.M., Fridovich I., Superoxide dismutase. An enzymatic function for erythrocuprein (hemecuprein), *J Biol Chem* 244:6049-55 (1969).
6. Chance B., Sies H., Boveris A., Hydroperoxide metabolism in mammalian tissues, *Physiol Rev* 59:527-605 (1979).
7. Travacio M.., Llesuy S., Antioxidant enzymes and their modification under oxidative stress conditions, *J Br Assoc Adv Sci* 48:9-13 (1996).
8. Burton G.W., Joyce A., Ingold K.U., Is vitamin E the only lipid soluble, chain breaking antioxidant in human plasma and erythrocyte membranes? *Arch Biochem Byophys* 221: 281-90 (1983).
9. Gupta M.., Singal P.K., Higher antioxidant capacity during a chronic stable heart hypertrophy, *Circ Res* 64:398-406 (1989).
10. Singal P.K., Hill M.F., Ganguly N.K., Role of oxidative stress in heart failure subsequent to myocardial infarction, *Linformation Cardiologique* 20:343-62 (1996).
11. Sies H. (ed). *Oxidative stress, oxidants and antioxidants*, London and New York. Academic Press, (1991).
12. Wolff S.P., Dean R.T., Glucose auto-oxidation and protein modification. The potential role of 'autoxidative glycosylation' in diabetes, *Biochem J* 1987245:243-50 (1987).
13. Bunn H.F., Nonenzymatic glycosylation of protein: relevance to diabetes, *Am J Med* 70: 1981;325-30 (1981).
14. Rosen P., Du X., Tschope D., Role of oxygen derived radicals for vascular dysfunction in the diabetic heart: prevention by alpha-tocopherol? *Mol Cell Biochem* 188 (1-2):103-11 (1998).
15. Giugliano D., Ceriello A., Paolisso G., Oxidative stress and diabetic vascular complications., *Diabetes Care* 19(3):257-67 (1996).
16. Thornalley P.J., Wolff S.P., Crabbe M.J., Stern A., The oxidation of oxyhaemoglobin by glyceraldehyde and other simple monosaccharides, *Biochem J* 217: 615-22 (1984).
17. Arai K., Maguchi S., Fujii S., Ishibashi H., Oikawa K., Taniguchi N. Glycation and inactivation of human Cu-Zn-superoxide dismutase. Identification of the in vitro glycated sites, *J Biol Chem* 262: 16969-72 (1987).

18. Suarez G., Rajaram R., Oronsky A.L., Gawinowicz M.A., Nonenzymatic glycation of bovine serum albumin by fructose (fructation). Comparison with the Maillard reaction initiated by glucose, *J Biol Chem* 264:3674-9 (1989).

19. Brownlee M., Ulassara H., Kooney A., Aminoguanidine prevents diabetes-induced arterial wall-protein cross linking, *Science* 232:1629-32 (1986).

20. Gillery P., Moinboisse J.C., Maquart F.X., Borel J.P., Glycation of proteins as a source of superoxide, *Diabetes Metab* 14(1):25-30 (1988).

21. Du X.L., Sui G.Z,, Stockklauser-Farber K., Weiss J., Zink S., Schwippert B., Wu Q.X., Tschope D., Rosen P., Introduction of apoptosis by high proinsulin and glucose in cultured human umbilical vein endothelial cells is mediated by reactive oxygen species, *Diabetologia* 41: 249-56 (1998).

22. Giugliano D., Ceriello A., Paolisso G., Diabetes mellitus, hypertension and cardiovascular disease: Which role for oxidative stress? *Metabolism* 44:363-8 (1995).

23. Tribe R.M., Poston L., Oxidative stress and lipids in diabetes: a role in endothelium vasodilator dysfunction? *Vas Med* 1(3):195-206 (1996).

24. Ahmed M.U., Thorpe S.R., Baynes J.W., Identification of N epsilon-carboxymethyllysine as a degradation product of fructoselysine in glycated protein. *J Biol Chem* 261: 4889-94 (1986).

25. Vogt B.W., Schleicher E.D., Wieland O.H., Epsilon-amino-lysine-bound glucose in human tissues obtained at autopsy. Increase in diabetes mellitus. *Diabetes* 31: 1123-7 (1982).

26. Sakurai T., Tsuchiya S., Superoxide production from nonenzymatically glycated protein. *FEBS Lett* 236: 406-10 (1988).

27. Yan S.D., Schmidt A.M., Anderson G.M., Zhang J., Brett J., Zou Y.S., Pinsky D., Stern D., Enhanced cellular oxidant stress by the interaction of advanced glycation end products with their receptors/binding proteins, *J Biol Chem* 269: 9889-97 (1994).

28. Higgins P.J., Garlick R.L., Bunn H.F., Glycosylated hemoglobin in human and animal red cells. Role of glucose permeability, *Diabetes* 31: 743-8 (1982).

29. Sato Y., Hotta N., Sakamoto N., Matsuoka S., Ohishi N., Yagi K., Lipid peroxide level in plasma of diabetic patients, *Biochem Med* 21:104 (1979).

30. Nishigaki I., Hagihara M., Tsunekawa H., Maseki M., Yagi K., Lipid peroxide levels of serum lipoprotein fractions of diabetic patients *Biochem Med* 25(3):373-8 (1981).

31. Babiy A.V., Gebicki J.M., Sullivan D.R., Willey K., Increased oxidizability of plasma lipoproteins in diabetic patients can be decreased by probucol therapy and is not due to glycation, *Biochem Pharmacol* 43:995 (1992).

32. Yabunaka N., Ohtsuka Y., Watanabe I., Noro H., Fujisaa H., Agishi Y., Elevated levels of heat-shock protein 70 (HSP70) in the mononuclear cells of patients with non-insulin-dependent diabetes mellitus, *Diabetes Res Clin Pract* 30(2):143-7 (1995).

33. McDonnell M.G., Archbold G.P., Plasma ubiquinol/cholesterol ratios in patients with hyperlipidaemia, those with diabetes mellitus and in patients requiring dialysis, *Clin Chim Acta* 253(1-2):117-26 (1996).

34. Godin D.V., Wohaieb S.A., Garnett M.E., Goumeniouk A.D., Antioxidant enzyme alterations in experimental and clinical diabetes, *Mol Cell Biochem* 84(2):223-31 (1988).

35. Stehouwer C.D., Lambert J., Donker A.J., Van Hinsbergh V.W., Endothelial dysfunction and pathogenesis of diabetic angiopathy, *Cardiovasc Res* 34(1): 55-68 (1997).

36. De Mattia G., Bravi M.C., Laurenti O., Cassone-Faldetta M., Proietti A., De Luca O., Armiento A., Ferri C., Reduction of oxidative tress by oral N-acetyl-L-cysteine treatment decreases plasma soluble vascular cell adhesion molecule-1 concentrations in non-obese, non-dyslipidaemic, normotensive patients with non-insulin-dependent diabetes, *Diabetologia* 41(11):1392-6 (1998).

37. Rattan V., Sultana C., Shen Y., Kalra V.K,. Oxidant stress-induced transendothelial migration of monocytes is linked to phosphorylation of PECAM-1, *Am J Physiol* 273(3)Pt1: E453-61 (1997).

38. Van Dam P.S., Van Asbeck B.S., Erkelens D.W., Marx J.J., Gispen W.H., Bravenboer B., The role of oxidative stress in neuropathy and other diabetic complications. *Diabetes Metab Rev*, 11(3):181-92 (1995).

39. Tomlinson D.R,. Future prevention and treatment of diabetic neuropathy. *Diabetes Metab*, 24(3):79-83 (1998).

40. Packer L., Tritschler H.J., Wessel K., Neuroprotection by metabolic antioxidant alpha-lipoic acid , *Free Radic Biol Med* 22(1-2):359-78 (1997).

41. Asayama K., Hayashibe H., Dobashi K., Niitsu T., Miyao A., Kato K., Antioxidant enzyme status and lipid peroxidation in various tissues of diabetic and starved rats, *Diabetes Res* 12:(2): 85-91 (1989).

42. Winkler R., Moser M., Alterations of antioxidant tissue defense enzymes and related metabolic parameters in streptozotocin-diabetic rats — effects of iodine treatment, *Wien Lin Wochenschr* 104(14):409-13 (1992).

43. Mukherjee B., Mukherjee J.R., Chatterjee M., Lipid peroxidation, glutathione levels and changes in glutathione-related enzyme activities in streptozotocin-induced diabetic rats, *Immunol Cell Biol* 72(2):109-14 (1994).

44. Wohaieb S.A., Godin D.V., Alterations in tissue antioxidant systems in the spontaneously diabetic (BB Wistar) rat, *Can J Physiol Pharmacol* 65(11):2191-5 (1987).
45. Kumar J.S., Menon V.P., Peroxidative changes in experimental diabetes mellitus, *Indian J Med Res* 96:176-81 (1992).
46. Sano T., Umeda F., Hashimoto T., Nawata H., Utsumi H., Oxidative stress measurement by in vivo electron spin resonance spectroscopy in rats with streptozotocin-induced diabetes, *Diabetologia* 41(11):1355-60 (1998).
47. Nishio Y., Kashiwagi A., Taki H., Shinozaki K., Maeno Y., Kojima H., Maegawa H., Haneda M., Hidaka H., Yasuda H., Horiike K., Kikkawa R., Altered activities of transcription factors and their related gene expression in cardiac tissues of diabetic rats, *Diabetes* 47(8):1318-25 (1998).
48. Rosen P., Ballhausen T., Bloch W., Addicks K., Endothelial relaxation is disturbed by oxidative stress in the diabetic rat heart: influence of tocopherol as antioxidant, *Diabetologia* 38(10):1157-68 (1995).
49. Karasu C., Acute probucol treatment partially restores vasomotor activity and abnormal lipid metabolism whereas morphological changes are not affected in aorta from long-term STZ-diabetic rats, *Exp Clin Endocrinol Diabetes* 106(3):189-96 (1998).
50. Bhimji S., Godin D.V., McNeill J.H., Insulin reversal of biochemical changes in hearts from diabetic rats, *Am J Physiol* 251(3):H670-5 (1986).
51. Bhimji S., Godin D.V., McNeill J.H., Biochemical and functional changes in hearts from rabbits with diabetes, *Diabetologia* 28(7):452-7 (1985).
52. Dhalla N.S., Liu X., Panagia V., Takeda N., Subcellular remodeling and heart dysfunction in chronic diabetes, *Cardiovasc Res* 40(2):239-47 (1998).
53. Matsui H., Okumura K., Mukawa H., Hibino M., Toki Y., Ito T., Increased oxysterol contents in diabetic rat hearts: their involvement in diabetic cardiomyopathy, *Can J Cardiol* 13(4):373-9 (1997).
54. Ziegelhoffer A., Ravingerova T., Styk J., Sebokova J., Waczulikova I., Breier A., Dzurba A., Volkovova K., Carsky J., Turecky L., Mechanisms that may be involved in calcium tolerance of the diabetic heart, *Mol Cell Biochem* 176(1-2):191-8 (1997).
55. Tada H., Oida K, Kutsumi Y., Shimada Y., Nakai T., Miyabo S., Effects of probucol on impaired cardiac performance and lipid metabolism in streptozotocin-induced diabetic rats, *J Cardiovasc Pharmacol* 20(2):179-86 (1992).
56. Kaul N., Siveski-Iliskovic N., Thomas T.P., Hill M., Khaper N., Singal P.K., Probucol improves antioxidant activity and modulates development of diabetic cardiomyopathy, *Nutrition* 11(5):551-4 (1995).
57. Kaul N., Siveski-Iliskovic N., Hill M., Khaper N., Seneviratne C., Singal P.K., Probucol treatment reverses antioxidant and functional deficit in diabetic cardiomyopathy, *Mol Cell Biochem* 160-161:283-8 (1996).

KETOSIS AND THE GENERATION OF OXYGEN RADICALS IN DIABETES MELLITUS

Sushil K. Jain[1] and Krishnaswamy Kannan[2]

Departments of [1]Pediatrics and [2]Medicine/Arthritis Center
Louisiana State University Health Sciences Center
Shreveport, LA 71130 USA

INTRODUCTION

The long-term complications of diabetes remain a major public health issue. Over the last decade, many of the biochemical pathways by which hyperglycemia may cause cellular damage have been studied. These include increased polyol pathway and associated changes in intracellular redox state, increased diacylglycerol synthesis with consequent activation of specific protein kinase C isoforms, increased nonenzymatic glycation of both intra- and extracellular proteins, and increased oxidative stress (1-11). Tissue injury then results from acute changes in protein function and chronic changes in protein expression. However, the molecular pathophysiology of altered membrane function and gene expression leading to tissue injury is still unclear. Type 1 diabetics frequently experience ketosis (hyperketonemia) because, in a state of insulin deficiency, body fuel is derived mainly from fat (12). The blood concentration of ketone bodies may reach 10 mM in diabetics with severe ketosis, compared with concentrations of less than 0.5 mM in normal individuals (12). It is known that ketosis can accelerate microangiopathy and underlying vascular disease and precipitate neuropathy in patients with long-duration diabetes (12). However, the underlying mechanisms by which ketosis promotes vascular disease in type 1 diabetic patients are unclear This chapter is focussed on the mechanisms that underlie the accelerated vascular disease and mortality in diabetic patients. To better differentiate among the complex interactions of various cell types, hormones and dynamic changes in the blood, we have used a cell culture model to accomplish the stated objectives. Specifically, this review discusses whether ketosis increases cellular oxidative stress/damage, and thereby promotes cell surface changes and adhesion between the monocytes and endothelial cells, a crucial step in the pathogenesis of vascular disease in diabetes.

KETOSIS AND OXIDATIVE STRESS

It is postulated that in diabetic patients, hyperglycemia burdens the cells with free radicals (10). This, coupled with the reduced activity of glucosylated-antioxidative enzymes, can cause increased oxidative stress and peroxidation of lipids (10). The levels of lipid

Diabetes and Cardiovascular Disease: Etiology, Treatment and Outcomes
Edited by Aubie Angel *et al.*, Kluwer Academic/Plenum Publishers, 2001

221

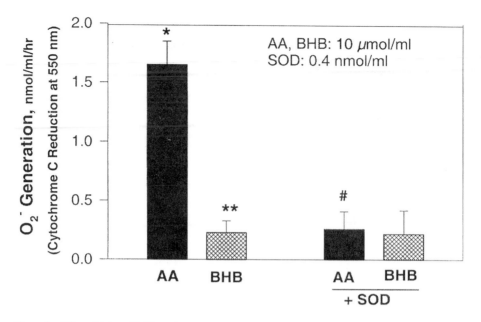

Figure 1. Effect of AA and BHB on the generation of superoxide radicals in a cell-free buffer solution. Figure taken from reference # 13.

peroxidation products in the blood are higher in diabetic patients in general (5,6,11) and much higher in diabetic patients with vascular disease (3).

Figure 1 shows the effects of acetoacetate (AA) and β-hydroxybutyrate (BHB) on cytochrome C reduction. There was a significant superoxide dismutase (SOD)-inhibitable reduction of cytochrome C (a measure of superoxide radicals generation) by AA but not by BHB, suggesting AA ability to generate oxygen radicals. The cytochrome C reduction was greater with increasing concentrations of acetoacetate (3.3-10 μmol/ml) and that acetoacetate levels as low as 3.3 μmol/ml, similar to those frequently encountered in diabetic patients, can generate superoxide anion radicals. In agreement with *in vitro* studies with cell-free solutions, cell culture studies showed that acetoacetate caused an increase in the cellular lipid peroxidation and growth inhibition of huam umbilical endothelial cells (13). Compared with controls, acetoacetate caused 12% growth inhibition at 5 μmol/ml, 40% inhibition at 10 μmol/ml, and 50% inhibition at 15 μmol/ml. The level of lipid peroxidation was 36.3$\pm$1.2, 56.4$\pm$1.7, 67.7$\pm$2.1 and 97.7$\pm$3.2 μmol/mg protein at 0 (control), 5, 10 and 20 μmol/ml acetoacetate concentrations, respectively. Changes at all the concentrations of acetoacetate were statistically significant compared with controls ($p<0.01$). Similarly, AA caused a dose-dependent growth inhibition and higher lipid peroxidation levels in cultured U937 cells, a premonocyte cell line (14).

The proposed mechanism by which AA can generate oxygen radicals and cause cellular lipid peroxidation may involve the formation of an ene-diol intermediate by the addition of $2H^+$ to two C=O groups in AA and its autoxidation that generate superoxide radicals. This can further undergo a Fenton reaction in the presence of Fe^{++} to form Fe^{+++} and hydroxyl radicals. Unlike β-hydroxybutyrate and acetone, the chemical structure of acetoacetate includes two keto groups. Whether this difference in chemical structure has anything to do with the potency of acetoacetate to generate oxygen radicals is not clear. Abnormalities in metabolism related to ketosis can increase extra-mitochondrial oxidation of fatty acids and generation of hydrogen peroxide, which in turn can also contribute to the increased oxidative stress in hyperketonemic diabetic patients. This hypothesis does not rule out the contribution of hyperglycemia but only proposes that hyperketonemia is another culprit contributing to the elevated oxidative stress in diabetes.

KETOSIS, OXIDATIVE STRESS AND APOPTOSIS

Reactive oxygen species (oxidative stress) are important regulators of apoptosis (14-17). Recent studies have demonstrated an antioxidant function of Bcl-2 (15,16). Bcl-2 can block programmed cell death and therby extend cell survival and promote cell growth. Bcl-2 does not appear to influence the generation of oxygen free radicals but does prevent oxidative damage to cellular constituents, including lipid membranes. Homo and heterodimerization of the Bcl-2 family members either promote or inhibit cell death. For example, the ratio of family members such as Bcl-2/Bax homo- or hetero-dimerization may determine the survival or death of cells following the apoptotic stimulus (17). Whether the expression or the ratio of Bcl2/Bax protein content is altered following exposure of cells to ketotic stress is not known. This area deserves exploration. It has recently become clear that mitochondrial changes, including disruption of the inner mitochondrial transmembrane potential constitute an early event of the apoptotic processes that preceed apoptosis as well as the apoptosis-associated exposure of phosphatidylserine (PS) residues on the plasma membrane surface (17). Using U937 cells as the *in vitro* model, we have shown the direct cytotoxic effects of AA on monocytes (14). Figure 2 illustrates an increase in apoptotic cell death (12.5% versus 2.3% in controls) in 20 μmol/ml AA-treated cells after 3 days. In addition, morphologically, AA-treated cells appeared swollen with increasing doses of AA. Thus, a plausible link between ketosis, oxidative stress and apoptosis is more likely a true event based on experimental evidence. Further research in this area may unravel the mechanistic aspects of this interaction.

OXIDATIVE STRESS, PS EXTERNALIZATION AND MONOCYTE
ADHESION TO ENDOTHELIAL CELLS

In normal cells including monocytes, endothelial cells and RBC, PS is present only in the inner membrane bilayer. Even a small fraction of the PS externalization would have profound effects on the interaction with endothelial cells that may promote adhesion as shown in studies with RBC (18). Membrane oxidative damage can result in the movement of PS from the inner to the outer membrane bilayer and adhesion of RBC to endothelial cells. (19,20). In addition, PS externalization at the outer surface of the membrane bilayer and characteristic changes in nuclear morphology and biochemistry are associated with apoptosis (21). The use of specific antibodies has suggested that an increase in the high-affinity receptor function of the CD11b/CD18 and CD14 proteins on monocytes also plays a role in monocyte adhesion to endothelial cells (22). In summary, ketosis mediated oxidtive stress can result in altered cell surface and altered cell-adhesion properties of monocytes, lymphocytes, platelets and endothelial cells.

MONOCYTE ADHESION TO ENDOTHELIAL CELLS AND
VASCULAR DISEASE OF DIABETES

Blood monocytes have the propensity to adhere to the vascular endothelium and release mediators, such as tumor necrosis factor-α, interleukin-1 and reactive oxygen species (22,23). The pathogenesis of atherosclerosis involves monocyte-endothelial cell interaction, inflammatory infiltration in the vessel wall, hyperlipidemia, cellular proliferation, fibrous plaque formation, and ultimately plaque rupture and occlusive thrombosis (9). The mechanisms by which diabetes enhance monocyte-endothelial cell interactions are not clear. Lipid peroxidation in endothelial cells may result in increased cell permeability, reduced cell viability, foam cell formation and adhesion to monocytes (24,25). The monocyte and

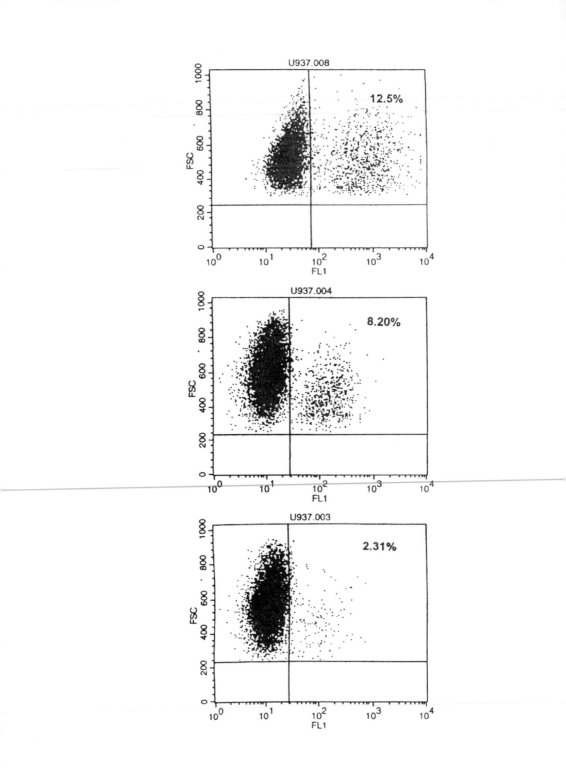

Figure 2. Histogram showing the effect of AA on apoptosis in U937 cells. U937 cells at a density of 5×10^5 /ml (24 hr culture) or 1×10^5 cells/ml were cultured in the presence of 0, 5, 10, 20 mM of AA for 72 hr. Data on media control, positive control (anti-Fas antibodies) and cells treated with 20 mM AA alone are presented in the histogram. The upper right hand corner of each histogram shows the percent apoptotic cell population scored in each treatment condition. Bottom Panel: Control; Middle Panel: Anti-Fas antibody control (positive); Top Panel: AA (20 mM). Figure taken from reference # 14.

endothelial cell dysfunction and increased adhesion between them is therefore a risk factor in the development of vascular disease (26). Studies showing a decrease in the occurrence of complications after supplementation with different antioxidants in diabetic animal models provide evidence that the cellular damage due to lipid peroxidation plays a role in the development of diabetic vascular disease (27).

In diabetic patients, monocytes are exposed to ketone bodies for a prolonged period of time, thus becoming targets of an oxidized environment similar to that of endothelial cells of the blood vessels. Since monocytes and endothelial cells interact at sites of vascular injury during inflammatory processes, such interactions result in the modulation of several biological functions of the two cell types, which include activation, adhesion, and release of pro-inflammatory cytokines. Peroxisome proliferator-activated receptor (PPAR) activators induce macrophage apoptosis by negatively interfering with the NFkappaB signaling pathway (28). It is therefore plausible to suggest that ketosis may initiate some of these pathological events.

Figure 3 summarizes a proposed scheme by which hyperketonemia can influence events leading to the atheroscerosis in diabetes. It appears that ketosis can cause increased generation of oxygen radicals and cellular lipid peroxidation, which in turn can induce phosphatidylserine externalization in the membrane bilayer and subsequently apoptosis. This is probably a cause for the enhanced monocyte adhesion to endothelium, a crucial step in the initiation of the atherosclerotic process.

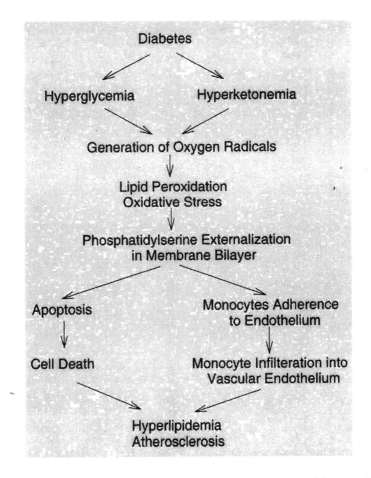

Figure 3. Proposed scheme for the effects of ketosis on lipid peroxidation and its potential role in the atherosclerosis of type-1 diabetic patients.

CONCLUSIONS

Ketosis is frequently encountered in type 1 diabetic patients. It is known that ketosis accelerates the vascular disease of diabetes. The mechanisms by which ketosis accelerates cellular dysfunctions are unclear. Specifically, this review discusses whether ketosis increases cellular oxidative stress/damage and thereby promotes cell surface changes and adhesion between the monocytes and endothelial cells, a crucial step in the pathogenesis of vascular disease in diabetes. A better understanding of the mechanisms that underlie the accelerated vascular disease will lead to new therapies.

Acknowledgments

This study was supported in part by a grant-in-aid from the American Heart Association (Southeast) and facilities and financial support of the Cancer Center and Arthritis Center of the Department of Medicine.

REFERENCES

1. DCCT Research Group. The absence of a glycemic threshold for the development of long-term complications: The perspective of the diabetes control and complications trial. *Diabetes* 45:1289 (1996).
2. S.M. Strowig and P. Raskin. Glycemic control and the complications of diabetes. Diab Rev 3:237 (1995).
3. A. Ceriello, R. Giacomello, G. Stel, E. Motz, C.Taboga, L. Tonutti, M. Pirisi, E. Falleti. and E. Bartoli. Hyperglycemia-induced thrombin formation in diabetes. The possible role of oxidative stress. Diabetes 44:924 (1995).
4. B. Tesfamariam and R.A. Cohen. Free radicals mediate endothelial cell dysfunction caused by elevated glucose. Amer J Physiol 262:H321 (1992).
5. J.W. Baynes. Role of oxidative stress in development of complications in diabetes. Diabetes 40: 405 (1991).
6. S.K. Jain, S.K. Krueger, R. McVie, J.J. Jaramillo, M. Palmer, and T. Smith. Relationship of blood thromboxane-B_2 with lipid peroxides and effect of vitamin E and placebo supplementation on TxB_2 and lipid peroxide levels in Type-1 diabetic patients. Diab Care 21:1511 (1998).
7. D. Koya, and G.L. King. Protein kinase C activation and the development of diabetic complications. Diabetes 47:859 (1998).
8. C.J. Mullarkey, D. Edelstein, and M. Brownlee. Free radical generation by early glycation products: A mechanism for accelerated atherogenesis in diabetes. Biochem Biophys Res Commun 173:932 (1990).
9. R. Klein. Hyperglycemia and microvascular and macrovascular disease in diabetes. Diab Care 18: 258 (1995).
10. S.K. Jain Hyperglycemia can cause membrane lipid peroxidation and osmotic fragility in human red blood cells. J Biol Chem 264:21340 (1989).
11. S.K. Jain, R. McVie, J. Duett, and J.J. Herbst: Erythrocyte membrane lipid peroxidation and glycosylated hemoglobin in diabetes. Diabetes 38:1539 (1989).
12. S.K. Jain and R. McVie. Hyperketonemia can increase lipid peroxidation and lower glutathione levels in human erythrocytes *in vitro* and in type-1 diabetic patients. Diabetes 48:1850 (1999).
13. S.K. Jain, K. Kannan, and G. Lim. Ketosis (acetoacetate) can generate oxygen radicals and cause increased lipid peroxidation and growth inhibition in human endothelial cells. Free Radical Biol Med 25:1083 (1998).
14. S.K. Jain, K. Kannan, and R. McVie. Effect of hyperketonemia on blood monocyttes in type-1 diabetic patients and apoptosis in cultured U937 monocytes. Antioxidants & Redox Signaling 1:211 (1999).
15. E. Yang and S.J. Korsmeyer. Molecular thanatopsis: a discourse on the Bcl-2 family and cell death. Blood 88 :386 (1996).
16. S.J. Korsmeyer, X. Yin, Z.N. Oltvai, D.J. Veis-Novack, and G.P. Linette. Reactive oxygen species and the regulation of cell death by the Bcl-2 gene family. Biochim Biophys Acta 1271:63 (1995).

17. K. Banki, E. Hutter, N.J. Gonchoroff, and A. Perl. Elevation of mitochondrial transmembrane potential and reactive oxygen intermediate levels are early events and occur independently form activation of caspases in fas signaling. J Immunol 162:1466 (1999).

18. R.K. Wali, S. Jafe, D. Kumar, N. Sorgenete, and V.K. Kalra. Increased adherence of oxidant-treated human and bovine erythrocytes to cultured endothelial cells. J Cell Physiol 133:25 (1987).

19. S.K. Jain. The accumulation of malonyldialdehyde, a product of fatty acid peroxidation, can disturb aminophospholipid organization in the membrane bilayer of human erythrocytes. J Biol Chem 259:3391 (1984).

20. S.K. Jain. In vivo externalization of phosphatidylserine and phosphatidylethanolamine in the membrane bilayer and hypercoagulability by the lipid peroxidation of erythrocytes in rats. J Clin Invest 76:281 (1985).

21. A.M. Gardner, F.H. Xu, C. Fady, F.J. Jacoby, D.C. Duffey, Y. Tu, and A. Lichtenstein. Apoptotic vs nonapoptotic cytotoxicity induced by hydrogen peroxide. Free Rad Biol Med 22:73 (1997).

22. V. Rattan, C. Sultana, Y. Shen, and V.K. Kalra. Oxidant stress-induced transendothelial migration of monocytes is linked to phosphorylation of PECAM-1. Amer J Physiol 273:E453 (1997).

23. J.W. Larrick, and S.C. Wright. Cytotoxic mechanism of tumor necrrosis factor-alpha. FASEB J 4: 3215 (1990).

24. S.K. Jain, N. Mohandas, M.R. Clark, and S.B. Shohet. The effect of malonyldialdehyde, a product of lipid peroxidation, on the deformability, dehydration, and ^{51}Cr-survival of erythrocytes. Brit J Haematol 53:247 (1983).

25. S.K. Jain, K.M. Morshed, K. Kannan, K.E. McMartin, and J.A. Bocchini. Effect of elevated glucose concentrations on cellular lipid peroxidation and growth of cultured human kidney proximal tubule cells. Mol Cell Biochem 162:11 (1996).

26. V. Rattan, Y. Shen, C. Sultana, D. Kumar, and V.K. Kalra. Diabetic RBC-induced oxidant stress leads to transendothelial migration of monocyte-like HL60 cells. Amer J Physiol 273:E369 (1997).

27. S.K. Jain. Should high-dose vitamin E supplementation be recommended to diabetic patients. Diab Care 22:1242 (1999).

28. G. Chinetti, S. Griglio, M. Antonucci, I.P.Torra, P. Delerive, A. Majd, J.C. Fruchart, J. Chapman, J. Najib, and B. Staels. Activation of prolifertor-activated receptors alpha and gamma induces apoptosis of human monocyte-derived macrophages. J Biol Chem 273:25573 (1998).

EFFECT OF DIABETES MELLITUS ON HEMODYNAMIC AND CARDIOMETABOLIC CORRELATES IN EXPERIMENTAL MYOCARDIAL INFARCTION

Suresh K. Gupta,[1] Dharamveer S.Arya,[1] Uma Singh[1] and Kewal K.Talwar[2]

[1]Cardiovascular Laboratory, Department of Pharmacology
[2]Department of Cardiology,
All India Institute of Medical Sciences,
New Delhi-110029, India.

INTRODUCTION

It is well documented that diabetic patients are more prone than the general population to cardiovascular disease.[1-5] Diabetes has been repeatedly found to be associated with an increased mortality from vascular disease.[6-10] However, there is mounting evidence to suggest that an abnormality of the myocardium may play a more important role than accelerated coronary atherosclerosis.[1,11-14] Among the increased prevalence of cardiovascular complications encountered in diabetes is an increased incidence of congestive heart failure and myocardial infarction.[2-5,13,15-18]

Although there have been numerous experimental studies relating to metabolic abnormalities in the hearts of diabetic animals, limited work has been done on the functional status of the diabetic heart.

In the human studies on heart function it is difficult to discriminate between abnormalities due to structural changes in coronary vessels or malfunction of myocardial cells secondary to the diabetic state. Hence, the animal model might prove useful. Studies on isolated hearts from rats with streptozotocin (STZ) -or alloxan-induced diabetes have shown a number of myocardial alterations in mechanics, metabolism, structure and response to ischemia[19,20]. Because catecholamines have been suggested to contribute to the propagation of the ischemic necrosis[17,21], the effect of isoproterenol (ISO), a strong ß-receptor agonist on the cardiometabolic status and function of the diabetic rat heart was studied.

High doses of ISO have been shown to lead to myocardial necrosis in experimental animals. This effect is thought to be mediated through an excessive calcium influx to the myocardial cell leading to toxic cell death[22,23].

The present study was designed to study the cardiovascular complications of diabetes mellitus by addressing the abnormalities of the diabetic myocardium in rats (made diabetic by intravenous injection of STZ) by examining: (1) the effect of diabetes on the hemodynamic variables and cardiometabolic correlates and (2) the altered responsiveness

Diabetes and Cardiovascular Disease: Etiology, Treatment and Outcomes
Edited by Aubie Angel et al., Kluwer Academic/Plenum Publishers, 2001

229

of the myocardium to the cardiotoxic effects of isoproterenol.

MATERIALS AND METHODS

Diabetic Rat Model

Albino male Wistar rats 170-250 g in body weight were made diabetic with a single intravenous injection of streptozotocin (STZ) 65 mg/kg (Sigma Chemical Co. St. Louis, Mo, USA)[24,25]. Streptozotocin was dissolved in 0.1 M citrate buffer (pH adjusted to 4.5), and less than 1 ml per rat was injected via the tail vein within 20 minutes of its preparation. Control animals from the same initial group were injected with citrate buffer alone. The experimental animals were maintained on standard laboratory feed and water *ad libitum* throughout the study period.

Blood Sugar, Body Weight and Heart Weight

Seventy-two hours after STZ administration and, thereafter, at weekly intervals, blood was drawn from the tail vein of ether-anesthetized control and diabetic animals for measurement of non-fasting blood glucose concentration (by the standard O-toluidine reagent method). Animals with a non-fasting blood glucose level of more than 350 mg/dl were included in the study. Body weights and heart weights of the experimental animals were also recorded at weekly intervals.

Cardiac Lesions

Method of inducing myocardial ischemic necrosis. Typical infarct-like cardiac lesions were produced by administration of isoproterenol (ISO) 85 mg/kg subcutaneously for two consecutive days, at 24 hour interval, according to the method of Rona et al.[22] Hearts were removed and embedded in paraffin, Hematoxylin and eosin stained paraffin-sections (5 μ thick) were graded in a blind fashion. ISO induced cardiac lesions were visible on light microscope. Severity of heart lesions was judged essentially according to the method of Rona et al,[22] with slight modification (Photographs of sections not shown here).

Grade 0	:	No lesions
Grade 1	:	Mottling of apex and distal parts of the left ventricle by intermingled pale and dark streaks
Grade 2	:	Well demarcated necrotic tissue areas limited to apex
Grade 3	:	Large infarct-like necrosis involving at least one-third of left ventricle and extending to adjacent right ventricle
Grade 4	:	Large infarct-like necrosis involving more than half of left ventricle, interventricular septum and extending to the distal portions of the right ventricle.

Study Protocol

The experimental animals were divided randomly into the following groups :

Group I	:	Control non-diabetic animals
Group II	:	STZ-treated diabetic animals.
Group III	:	ISO-treated non-diabetic animals with myocardial lesions
Group IV	:	STZ-diabetic rats treated with ISO:(i) four weeks (STZ+ISO-4) and (ii) six weeks (STZ+ISO-6) after induction of diabetes.

Study with diabetic rats was extended to an eight week period after STZ injection but without ISO administration; to assess the serum glucose levels, body weight and heart weight of the animals with diabetic state of 8 weeks duration. A period of 4 to 6 weeks stabilization to the diabetic state was allowed prior to subsequent isoproterenol treatment followed by biochemical studies (at 4 weeks) and hemodynamic measurements (at 6 weeks) of STZ-induced diabetes.

At the end of the experimental period (in each protocol) the animals were sacrificed by decapitation and the blood glucose was again determined.

The experimental protocol was worked out with strict adherence to the Institute Animal Care Guidelines.

Hemodynamic Measurements

The hemodynamic study was performed six weeks after STZ injection in rats which were anesthetized with urethane (1.5g/kg) intraperitoneally. A midline incision was made in the neck and a tracheostomy performed. The rats were mechanically ventilated with room air using small rodent ventilator (INCO, Ambala, India). The respiratory rate and tidal volume were adjusted in order to maintain arterial blood gases within the normal range.

The right jugular vein was cannulated for infusion of saline/ fluids. The right carotid artery was cannulated and connected to a pressure transducer for the measurement of arterial blood pressure. A left thoracotomy was performed and the heart was exposed. A short 22 gauge metal cannula positioned through the posterior part of apex of the heart was introduced into the left ventricular cavity to measure left ventricular pressure from which left ventricular end-diastolic pressure (LVEDP) and the maximal rate of change of left ventricular pressure [LV peak positive (+) dP/dt and negative (-) dP/dt] were derived by electronic differentiation. Both arterial and left ventricular pressures were measured by Statham P23ID pressure transducers and were monitored and recorded on a Grass 7D Polygraph (Grass Instruments, Quincy, Mass, USA). Heart rate was recorded from Standard limb II electrocardiogram monitored and recorded on the Grass Polygraph.

Biochemical Studies

Metabolite and enzymatic assays. Experimental animals were sacrificed 4 weeks after STZ injection and the heart was rapidly frozen in liquid nitrogen. The deproteinized perchloric acid extract of heart tissue was used for estimation of the following: myocardial adenosine triphosphate (ATP) and creatine phosphate (CP) estimated by the method of Lamprecht et al,[26] myocardial lactate levels estimated by the method of Gaweher and Bergmeyer[27]. Myocardial glycogen was estimated by the phenol-sulphuric acid method of Siu LO et al.[28]

Serum LDH activity. Blood was collected by cardiac puncture and serum lactate dehydrogenase (LDH) was estimated.[29] Protein content of cardiac tissue samples was estimated by the method of Lowry et al[30].

Data Analysis

A one way analysis of variance and Student's *t* test were performed for statistical analysis. All data are expressed as mean ± standard error (SEM) with the number of experiments involved. For all data in this study a p value of less than 0.05 was considered as a statistically significant difference.

Table 1. Serum glucose, body weight and heart weight in rats with STZ-induced diabetes

GROUPS	Serum glucose (mg/dl)	Body Weight (BW:g)	Heart Weight (HW:g)	BW/HW (g/mg)
4 weeks study				
Control (n=12)	131.61 ± 9.2	260.00 ± 8.41	0.61± 0.01	2.20 ± 0.11
Diabetic (n=10)	545.50 ± 56.60***	189.20 ± 8.0*	0.53± 0.01	2.64± 0.01
8 weeks study				
Control (n=6)	162.0± 18.0	453.5± 9.0	0.84± 0.03	2.00± 0.09
Diabetic (n=6)	623.50± 53.9***	258.0 ± 15.4**	0.75± 0.04*	2.85± 0.17

Body weight was measured throughout the experimental period i.e. 4 weeks study and 6 weeks study, but only the final values taken before sacrifice of animals are indicated. Values are expressed as mean ± SEM; n = number of animals; * = $p<0.05$; ** = $p<0.01$; *** = $p<0.001$ as compared to control values.

RESULTS

Blood Glucose, Body Weight and Heart Weight

Streptozotocin (STZ)-induced diabetes of 4 and 8 weeks resulted in loss of body weight in the diabetic animals. Effects of 4 and 8 weeks diabetes on blood glucose levels, body weight and heart weight are shown in Table 1. Body weight measurements prior to STZ treatment and at the time of sacrifice revealed significant ($p<0.05$, 4 weeks study and $p<0.01$, 8 weeks study) decreases in the rate of growth of STZ-treated animals relative to the age-matched controls. The heart weight to body weight ratios were slightly higher in the diabetic rats than in controls. Diabetic rats failed to gain weight and the difference in body weight between diabetic animals and controls increased progressively until they were killed in accordance to the experimental protocol. Blood glucose determination revealed a significant ($p<0.001$) hyperglycemic state in the 4-week and 8 week STZ-treated animals as compared to the controls.

Morphological Changes in Diabetic and Non-Diabetic Rat Hearts

Hearts of rats from the control group and STZ-treated group showed no gross lesions. ISO treatment caused a well demarcated necrotic area limited to the apex in two rats. Three rats showed large infarct-like necrosis involving at least one-third of left ventricle. Three of the total eight hearts examined in ISO-treated group revealed large infarct-like necrosis involving more than half of left ventricle, interventricular septum and extending to distal part of right ventricle. Diabetic groups treated with ISO 4 and 6 weeks after STZ injection respectively showed no gross lesions (Table 2).

Table 2. Gross heart lesions in rats of different groups of the study

GROUPS	Total Number of rats	Number of rats showing different grade (Gr.) of lesions					Average degree of lesions (mean ± SEM)
		Gr.4	Gr.3	Gr.2	Gr.1	Gr.0	
CON[a]	8	0	0	0	0	8	0
STZ [b] (65mg/kg,i.v.)	7	0	0	0	0	7	0 NS[f] (CON vs STZ)
ISO[c] (85mg/kg,s.c.)	8	3	3	2	0	0	3.87±0.25 *p<0.001* (CON vs ISO)
STZ + ISO-4[d]	6	0	0	0	0	6	0 *p<0.01* (ISO vs STZ+ISO-4)
STZ + ISO-6[e]	6	0	0	0	0	6	0 *p<0.01* (ISO vs STZ+ISO-6)

[a]Control group
[b]Streptozotocin-treated group
[c]Isoproterenol-treated group
[d]STZ+ISO-4 = 4 weeks diabetes + ISO
[e]STZ+ISO-6 = 6 weeks diabetes + ISO
[f]NS = Non-significant;
s.c. = Subcutaneous; i.v. = Intravenous.

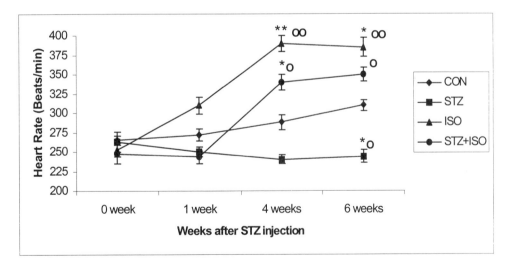

Figure 1. Time course of changes in heart rate in (a) control (non-diabetic) group (CON); (b) streptozotocin-induced diabetic group (STZ); (c) isoproterenol-treated myocardial infarction group (ISO); and (d) STZ + ISO combination group. Values are expressed as mean ± SEM. Verticle bars indicate SE. Number of animals (n) used for hemodynamic measurements were 15, 15, 12 and 10 in CON group; 15,11,10 and 8 in STZ group; 15,13,10 and 10 in ISO group and 15,12,10,8 in STZ + ISO group during hemodynamic studies at 0 week (baseline value), 1 week, 4 weeks and 6 weeks (after STZ/vehicle injection) respectively; * = $p<0.05$; ** = $p<0.01$ as compared to control value of corresponding time period; O = $p<0.05$; OO = $p<0.01$ as compared to initial (baseline) value before STZ and/or ISO injection respectively.

Table 3. The effect of 6 weeks of streptozotocin-induced diabetes and ß-adrenergic inotropic stimulation on various cardiovascular variables in rats undergoing thoracotomy

PARAMETERS	CON[a] (n=10)	STZ[b] (n=8)	ISO[c] (n=10)	STZ + ISO[d] (n=8)
1. Heart rate (beats/min)	310 ± 10	244 ± 8*	385 ± 12*	350 ± 9
2. Blood pressure (mm Hg)				
(i) Systolic	128 ± 7	151 ± 11*	99 ± 8*	102 ± 9
(ii) Diastolic	83 ± 9	72 ± 6	81 ± 10	70 ± 7
3. Left ventricular end diastolic pressure (mm Hg)	1.8 ± 0.08	3.9 ± 0.18**	4.8 ± 0.16**	4.0 ± 0.17**
4. Maximal rate of change of left ventricular pressure (mm Hg/s)				
(i) Positive (+) LV dP/dt $_{max}$	4860 ± 350	2400 ± 200*	4000 ± 280	3600 ± 230**
(ii) Negative (-) LV dP/dt $_{max}$	3800 ± 300	1850 ± 210*	3125 ± 250	2380 ± 220**

[a]Control group
[b]Streptozotocin-treated group
[c]Isoproterenol-treated group
[d] Streptozotocin + isoproterenol treated group
Values are expressed as mean ± SEM
* = $p<0.05$; ** = $p<0.01$; as compared to control value
n = number of animals.

Hemodynamics

The effect of STZ-induced diabetes on hemodynamic variables are shown in Figures 1, 2 and Table 3. Hemodynamic studies revealed that heart rate (Figure 1) and the maximal rate of change of left ventricular pressure, positive and negative (Table 3) was significantly ($p<0.01$) reduced in diabetic animals, as compared with non-diabetic controls. Blood pressure (Figure 2) showed a decreasing trend in all the experimental groups except the STZ- treated group in which this parameter was significantly ($p<0.05$) elevated as compared to the controls. The ISO-treated group showed significant ($p<0.05$) tachycardia and a significant ($p<0.01$) elevation of left ventricular end diastolic pressure (LVEDP). LVEDP, was also found to be significantly ($p<0.01$) elevated in the diabetic groups. The STZ + ISO group did not show profound contractile abnormality; as assessed by the LV (+) dP/dt$_{max}$ and LV (-) dP/dt$_{max}$; however, this group showed nearly the same degree of tachycardia as the ISO alone group though these values were not significant.

Biochemical Studies

High energy phosphates, (HEPs): Adenosine triphosphate (ATP) and Creatine

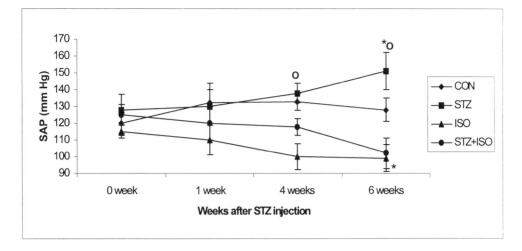

Figure 2. Time course of changes in systolic arterial blood pressure (SAP) in the experimental groups ennumerated in legend of Figure 1. Values are expressed as mean ± SEM. Vertical bars indicate SE; * = p<0.05 as compared to control value of corresponding time period; O = p<0.05 as compared to initial (baseline) value before STZ and/or ISO injection respectively.

phosphate (CP). The administration of STZ significantly reduced the myocardial, ATP (p<0.001) and CP (p<0.05) content as compared to the control values. Administration of ISO significantly lowered myocardial ATP (p<0.001) and CP (p<0.01) in the non-diabetic rats. Administration of ISO to rats with 4 weeks diabetes resulted in significantly lower values of ATP as compared with the controls. However, the values of CP in the combination group were comparable with the control values.

Myocardial lactate. Following administration of ISO, the deleterious substrate lactate was found to accumulate to a significant (p<0.001) level in the non-diabetic rat hearts. However no such elevated levels on account of increased accumulation were observed in the STZ and STZ + ISO groups, as compared to the control values (Table 4).

Myocardial glycogen. It was observed that the glycogen content of the diabetic hearts was significantly (p<0.001) higher than that of non-diabetic rat hearts (Table 4). There was a significant (p<0.001) depletion of this parameter following ISO-administration in the non-diabetic rats. Similar trend was not seen in the diabetic group with ISO treatment (STZ + ISO). (Table 4)

Serum Lactate dehydrogenase (LDH) activity. There was no significant difference in the serum LDH activity in the diabetic or control rats (Figure 3) when estimated 4 weeks after STZ injection. Administration of ISO to non-diabetic animals resulted in a significant (p<0.001) increase in serum LDH activity levels as compared to the control group values. However, serum LDH activity of diabetic animals was not markedly altered after ISO administration 4 weeks after STZ treatment.

DISCUSSION

Clinical, pathological and epidemiological data have shown the existence of a diabetic cardiomyopathy independent of atherosclerotic coronary artery disease[2]. It has been reported that a sizable fraction of diabetic subjects has preclinical cardiac dysfunction[3,9,10].

235

Table 4. Myocardial metabolites/substrate levels in different groups of the study (4 week study)

PARAMETERS	CON[a] (n=12)	STZ[b] (n=10)	ISO[c] (n=10)	STZ + ISO (n=10)
ATP[d] (μ mol/g dry wt of tissue)	7.51 ± 0.22	2.20 ± 0.20***	2.65 ± 0.33***	2.23 ± 0.15***
CP[e] (μ mol/g dry wt of tissue)	5.65 ± 0.32	2.47 ± 0.29*	2.08 ± ± 0.24**	3.93 ± 0.43
Lactate (mol/g) dry wt of tissue)	2.22 ± 0.19	2.32 ± 0.15	12.23 ± 0.12	2.69 ± 0.48***
Glycogen (mg/g dry wt. of tissue)	3.60 ± 0.20	6.70 ± 0.53***	1.89 ± 0.20***	3.43 ± 0.32

[a]Control group
[b]Streptozotocin-treated group
[c]Isoproterenol-treated group
[d]Adenosine triphosphate
[e]Creatine phosphate
Values are expressed as mean ± SEM
* = p<0.05; ** = p<0.01; *** = p<0.001 compared to control value

In human studies on heart function, it is difficult to discriminate between abnormalities due to structural changes in coronary vessels (small or large) or due to impaired functioning of the myocardial cells. Here the animal model proves useful. Because it is clear that chemical, biochemical and functional abnormalities are closely interrelated, the present study relates to the multiplicity of levels of structural and functional organization at which alterations may be investigated, in order to gain a better understanding of events leading to experimental diabetic cardiomyopathy.

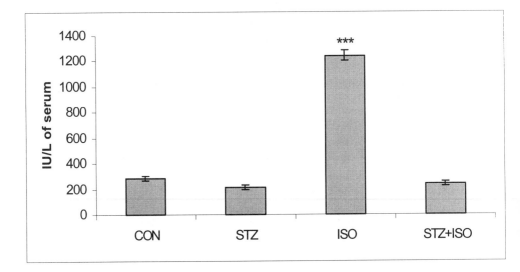

Figure 3. Serum lactate dehydrogenase activity 4 weeks after STZ injection in the experimental groups enumerated in Figure 1. Values are expressed as mean ± SEM; Columns represent mean values; Vertical bars indicate SE; *** = p<0.001 as compared to control value.

Rakieten et al[31] first reported that streptozotocin, like alloxan, causes diabetes in rats and dogs by selectively destroying the pancreatic β-cells. A later study[25] confirmed this in many species. The diabetogenic effect of STZ is more reproducible and the metabolic changes are much closer to those existing in human diabetes[32]. Hence, STZ is considered the drug of choice for the induction of experimental diabetes[24,25].

Diabetes is known to result in a number of alterations, the most prominent ones being those of abnormal carbohydrate and fat metabolism. Elevated levels of glucose in the blood of diabetics may alter enzyme activities by inducing glycosylation of the enzymes, eventually leading to or contributing towards functional alterations of the heart.

In the present study, treatment with STZ resulted in a diabetic state characterized by hyperglycemia and loss of body weight as early as 3 days after treatment. The diabetic rats also showed signs of hyperphagia, polydipsia, and polyuria. Elevated blood glucose levels were maintained for the entire duration of the study in agreement with previous studies [13,19]. The diabetic state produced in the present study was associated with decreased rate of growth. Similar to earlier studies[15,33] STZ-induced depressions in myocardial function and several abnormalities of biochemical parameters were not found to be present in the non-diabetic rats. It has been reported earlier that there is no direct cardiotoxic effect of STZ[34-36] and abnormalities encountered in this condition are primarily due to lack of insulin and its metabolic consequences.

Hemodynamic variables were assessed 6 weeks after diabetes induction in rats, because alterations in cardiac performance occur 6 weeks after the onset of diabetes[37]. In the present study the results regarding the effects of STZ diabetes on blood pressure and heart rate are consistent with previous reports[38-41]. In our study systolic arterial blood pressure increased progressively after STZ-treatment. Heart rate in the present study was reduced within 1 week after STZ injection. Similar results have been reported in earlier studies[39,41]. Though some workers are of the opinion that the underlying mechanisms of bradycardia are obscure[38], others have speculated that the decrease in heart rate may be due to hypothyroidism[39], reduced myocardial lipid metabolism[11,40] or due to alterations in SA nodal electrical activity as a result of hyperglycemia[41]. However, the exact mechanism(s) by which bradycardia is produced has not yet been fully elucidated.

Myocardial contractile dysfunction is a major manifestation of diabetes mellitus. In the present study analysis of the hemodynamic results revealed that the major mechanical defects relate to left ventricular pressure development, and the rate of relaxation as measured by LV negative (-) dP/dt_{max}. An earlier report on studies in dogs[11] with milder diabetes also demonstrated depressed ventricular functional responses to increasing preload and also suggested decreased diastolic compliance. Investigations in humans mainly employing non invasive techniques also suggest that relaxation is impaired in hearts of diabetic subjects[5,42]. Although numerous studies have evidenced myocardial dysfunction in diabetes specific investigations of dynamics in which preload and afterload are known have rarely been reported. In an investigation on isolated working rat heart[15] which assessed hemodynamics similar to the present study, these critical parameters have been assessed alongwith the ventricular dynamics. The results of both studies are comparable.

Diabetes results in a number of diverse alterations in cardiac metabolism. To define how critical biochemical parameters relate to alterations in cardiac function in experimental diabetes, the cardiometabolic status of the diabetic and non-diabetic rat heart were assessed. In the present study diabetic rats were found to have serum LDH activity levels comparable to the control group. This enzyme activity levels are not altered in chronic disease states. Glycogen content of the diabetic hearts showed a twofold increase as compared to the hearts of control rats. High levels of citrate are known to accumulate in the diabetic hearts. This causes a pronounced inhibition of phosphofructokinase (PFK), a key regulatory enzyme of glycoysis. Despite a marked restriction of glucose uptake in diabetic rats high tissue levels of fructose-6-phosphate and glucose-6-phosphate accumulate. This process shifts the pathway of glycogen turnover towards storage of this polysaccharide. In the present study lactate production by the heart of diabetic rats was similar to the hearts of controls. A significant depletion in the concentration of the high energy phosphates ATP and CP as compared to controls was seen in the present study. This could be due to calcium overloading of the diabetic cells as a consequence of altered membrane permeability and defective Ca^{2+} handling by the sarcoplasmic reticulum. Increased cellular Ca^{2+} may lead to an activation of ATP-dependent processes attenuation leading to depletion of ATP and CP concentrations.

Previous studies have shown that myocardial lesions can be produced in rats and dogs when ISO a potent synthetic catecholamine is injected[22]. ISO-induced lesions were called infarct-like by Rona et al[22] as it grossly resembled human myocardial infarction. Catecholamines have been reported to have cardiotoxic effects at the membrane level and produce damage of endothelial wall, resulting calcium overload leads to hypercontraction of cardiac muscle and mitochondrial calcification. All these mechanisms lead to coagulative myocytolysis. Ingebretsen and associaties[43] have reported altered mechanical response of the isolated diabetic rat heart to isoproterenol in addition to an attenuation of the isoproterenol-induced increase in myocardial cyclic AMP levels. The present study evidences an abnormal response to strong β-receptor stimulation in experimental diabetes, this finding is in accordance to earlier reports[23,44]. STZ induced diabetic rats are protected against the cardiotoxic effect of ISO, however they show the same degree of tachycardia. In the present study ISO administration to control rats resulted in severe myocardial necrosis and profound deleterious metabolic alterations. As mentioned above, ISO administration to STZ diabetic rats failed to produce myocardial necrosis. Neither did lactate accumulate in the ISO administered diabetic heart nor were the serum LDH levels significantly altered. Lactate levels were comparable in diabetic and non-diabetic hearts.

Diabetic rats are characterized by a depressed cardiac performance[45]. In the present study altered cardiac function in rats with 6 weeks STZ-induced diabetes and biochemical correlates of these functional abnormalities have been demonstrated. In conjunction with these findings the present study illustrated the earlier reported protection of the myocardium against the cardiotoxic effect of ISO in diabetic rats. Clearly there is need to further explore the details of the relationship between diabetes and cardiovascular disease.

REFERENCES

1. T. Ledet, B. Neubauer, N.J. Christensen, and K. Lundback. Diabetic cardiomyopathy *Diabetologia*. **16** : 207-209 (1979).
2. W.B. Kannel, M. Hjortland, and W.P. Castelli. Role of diabetes in congestive heart failure. The Framingham study. *Am J Cardiol*. **34** : 29-35 (1974).
3. S.S. Ahmed, G.A. Jaferi, R.M. Narang, and T.J. Regan. Preclinical abnormality of left ventricular function in diabetes mellitus. *Am Heart J*. **89** : 153-158 (1975).
4. L.M. Shapiro, A.P. Howat, and M.M. Calter. Left ventricular function in diabetes mellitus I: methodology and prevalence and spectrum of abnormalities. *Br Heart J*. **45** :122-128 (1981).
5. T.J. Regan, M.M. Lyons, S.S. Ahmed, G.E. Levinson, H.A. Oldewurtel, M.R. Ahmed, and B. Haider. Evidence of cardiomyopathy in familial diabetes mellitus. *J Clin Invest*. **60** : 885-889 (1977).
6. W.B. Kannel. Role of diabetes in cardiac disease: conclusions from population studies, in: *Diabetes and the Heart*. S. Zoneraich, ed., Charles C. Thomas, Springfield; 97-112 (1978).
7. M.J. Garcia, P.M. McNamara, T. Gordon, and W.B. Kannel. Morbidity and mortality in diabetics in the Framingham population: Sixteen year follow-up study. *Diabetes* **23** :105-111 (1974).
8. R. Bradley, and J.W. Brytogie. Survival of diabetic patients after myocardial infarction. *Am J Med*. **20** : 207-215 (1956).
9. J.C. Wili and M. Casper. The contribution of diabetes to early deaths from ischemic heart disease. US gender and racial comparisons. *Am J Public Health*. **86** : 576-579 (1996).

10. A.H. Zargar, A.I. Wani, S.R. Masoodi, B.A. Laway, and M.I. Bashir. Mortality in diabetes mellitus – data from a developing region of the World. *Diabetes Res Clin Practice.* **43** : 67-74 (1999).

11. T.J. Regan, P.O. Ettinger, M.I. Khan, M.U. Jesrani, M.M. Lyons, H.A. Oldewurtel, and M. Weber. Altered myocardial function and metabolism in chronic diabetes mellitus without ischemia in dogs. *Circ Res.* **35** : 222-237 (1974).

12. D. Feuvray, J.A. Idell-Wenger, J.R. Neely. Effects of ischemia on rat myocardial function and metabolism in diabetes. *Circ Res.* **44** : 322-329 (1979).

13. F.S. Fein, L.B. Kornstein, J.E. Strobeck, J.M. Capasso, and E.H. Sonnenblick. Altered myocardial mechanics in diabetic rats. *Circ Res.* **47** : 922-933 (1980).

14. A.G. Tahiliani and J.H. McNeill. Diabetes- induced abnormalities in the myocardium. *Life Sci.* **38** : 959-974 (1986).

15. S. Penpargkul, T. Schaible, T. Yipintsoi and J. Scheuer. The effects of diabetes on performance and metabolism of rat hearts. *Circ Res.* **47** : 911-921 (1980).

16. R.Vadlamudi, and J.H. McNeill. Cardiac function in normal and diabetic rats. *Proc West Pharmacol Soc.* **23** : 29-31 (1980).

17. S. Ramanadham, and T.E. Tenner Jr. Alterations in cardiac performance in experimentally-induced diabetes. *Pharmacology.* **27** : 130-139 (1983).

18. S. Ramandham, and T.E. Tenner Jr. Basal developed force and inotropic characteristics of myocardial tissue isolated from streptozotocin diabetic animals. *Proc West Pharmacol Soc.* **27** : 197-200 (1984).

19. R. Vadlamudi, R.L. Rodgers, J.H. McNeill. The effect of chronic alloxan- and streptozotocin-induced diabetes on isolated rat heart performance. *Can J Physiol Pharmacol.* **50** : 902-911 (1982).

20. R. Vadlamudi, and J.H. McNeill. Effect of chronic streptozotocin-induced diabetes on cardiac performance in rats. *Proc West Pharmacol Soc.* **24** : 73-77 (1981).

21. A.P. Waldenstrom, A.C. Hjalmarson, Thornell L. A possible role of noradrenalin in the development of myocardial infarction : an experimental study in the isolated rat heart. *Am Heart J.* **95** : 43-47 (1978).

22. G. Rona, C.I. Chappel, , T. Blazas and R. Gaudry. An infarct-like myocardial lesion and other toxic manifestations produced by isoproterenol in the rat. *Arch Pathol.* **67** : 443-455 (1959).

23. O. Gotzsche. Decreased myocardial calcium uptake after isoproterenol in streptozotocin-induced diabetic rats. *Lab Invest.* **48** : 156-161 (1983).

24. A. Junod, A.E. Lambert, L. Orci, R. Pictet, A.E. Gonet, and A.E. Reynold. Studies of the diabetogenic action of streptozotocin. *Proc Soc Exp Biol Med.* **126** : 201-205 (1967).

25. C.C. Rerup. Drugs producing diabetes through damage of the insulin secreting cells. *Pharmacol Rev.* **22** : 485-518 (1970).

26. W. Lamprecht, F. Stein, F. Heinz, H. Weisser, and F. Heinz. Determination of creatine phosphate and adenosine triphosphate with creatine kinase, phosphoglycerate kinase and glyceraldehyde phosphate dehydrogenase, in: *Methods of Enzymatic Analysis,* H.U. Bergmeyer, ed., Academic Press, New York 1776-1778 (1974).

27. K. Gawehr, H.U. Bergmeyer. Lactate determination, in: *Methods of Enzymatic Analysis,* H.U. Bergmeyer, ed., Academic Press, New York 1492-1495 (1974).

28. L.O. Siu, J.C. Russel, and A.W. Taylor. Determination of glycogen in small tissue samples. *J Appl Physiol.* **28** : 234-236 (1970).

29. F. Wroblewski, and J.S. LaDue. Lactic dehydrogenase activity in blood. *Proc Soc Exp Med.* **90** : 210-213 (1955).

30. O.H. Lowry, N.J. Rosenbrough, A.L. Farr, and R.J. Randall. Protein measurement with folin phenol reagent. *J Biol Chem.* 265-275 (1951).

31. N. Rakieten, M.L. Rakieten, M.V. Nadkarni. Studies on the diabetogenic action of streptozotocin. *Cancer Chemother Rep.* **29** : 91-98 (1963).

32. K.R.L. Mansford, and L.H. Opie. A comparison of metabolic abnormalities in diabetes mellitus induced by streptozotocin or by alloxan. *Lancet.* **i** : 670-671 (1968).

33. S. Ramanadham, A. Doroudian, and J.H. McNeill. Myocardial and metabolic abnormalities in streptozotocin-diabetic Wistar and Wistar-Kyoto rats. *Can J Cardiol.* **6** : 75-82 (1990).

34. J Tisne-Versailles, M. Constantin, J.C. Lamar, and B. Pourrias. Cardiotoxicity of high doses of isoproterenol on cardiac hemodynamics and metabolism in SHR and WHY rats. *Arch Int Pharmacodyn.* **273** : 142-154 (1985).

35. Ramanadham S, Decker P, and Tenner TE Jr. Effect of insulin replacement on

streptozotocin-induced effects in the rat heart. *Life Sci.* **33** : 289-296 (1983).

36. T. Takamura, H. Ando, Y. Nagai, H. Yamashita, E. Nohara, and K. Kobayashi. Pioglitazone prevents mice from multiple low-dose streptozotocin-induced insulitis and diabetes. *Diabetes Res Clin Practice.* **44** : 107-114 (1999).

37. A.G. Tahilitani, and J.H. McNeill. Prevention of diabetes-induced myocardial dysfunction in rats by methyl palmoxirate and triiodothyronine treatment. *Can J Physiol Pharmacol.* **63** : 925-931(1985).

38. B. Rodrigues, R.K. Goyal, and J.H. McNeill. Effects of hydralazine on streptozotocin-induced diabetic rats : prevention of hyperlipidemia and improvement in cardiac function. *J Pharmacol Exptl Ther.* **237** : 292-299 (1986).

39. D.W. Garber, A.W. Everett, and J.R. Neely. Cardiac function and myosin ATPase in diabetic rats treated with insulin T_3 and T_4. *Am J Physiol.* **244** : H592-H598 (1983).

40. D.J. Hearse, D.E. Steward, E.D. Chain. Diabetes and the survival and recovery of the anoxic myocardium. *J Mol Cell Cardiol.* **7** : 397-406 (1975).

41. J. Senges, J. Brachman, D. Pelzer, C. Hasslacher, E. Weihe, and W. Kubler. Altered cardiac automaticity and conduction in experimental diabetes mellitus. *J Mol Cell Cardiol.* **12** : 1341-1351 (1980).

42. S. Rubler, J. Dlugash, Y.Z. Yuceoglu, T. Kumral, A.W. Branwood, and A.Grishman. New type of cardiomyopathy associated with diabetic glomerulosclerosis. *Am J Cardiol.* **30** : 595-602 (1972).

43. W.R. Ingebretsen Jr, C. Peralta, M. Monsher, L.K. Wagner, and C.G. Ingebretsen. Diabetes alters the myocardial cAMP protein kinase cascade system. *Am J Physiol.* **240** : H375-H382 (1981).

44. C.E. Heyliger, G.N. Pierce, P.K. Singal, R.E. Beamish, and N.S. Dhalla. Cardiac alpha and beta adrenergic receptor alterations in diabetic cardiomyopathy. *Basic Res Cardiol.* **77** : 610-618 (1982).

45. N.S. Dhalla, G.N. Pierce, I.R. Innes, and R.E. Beamish. Pathogenesis of cardiac dysfunction in diabetes mellitus. *Can J Cardiol.* **1** : 263-281 (1985).

CARDIAC FUNCTION IN PERFUSED HEARTS FROM DIABETIC MICE

Darrell D. Belke,[1] Terje S. Larsen,[2] and David L. Severson[1]

[1]Faculty of Medicine
University of Calgary
Calgary, AB, Canada T2N 4N1

[2]Institute of Medical Biology
University of Tromsø
N-9037 Tromsø, Norway

INTRODUCTION

Non-insulin dependent (type 2) diabetes mellitus accounts for more than 90% of all cases of diabetes. An increased incidence of cardiovascular diseases is the most common complication of NIDDM.[1,2] The cardiac complications associated with NIDDM are due to both increased coronary heart disease secondary to atherosclerosis[3] and a specific diabetic cardiomyopathy resulting in ventricular dysfunction.[4]

Experimental studies with animal models of diabetes allow an assessment of the direct deleterious effects of a diabetic cardiomyopathy in the absence of atherosclerotic coronary artery disease. However, most reports of diabetes-induced cardiac dysfunction have used insulin-deficient (type 1) diabetic animals;[5,6] relatively few studies on cardiac performance have been conducted with NIDDM animal models exhibiting insulin resistance.[7]

The genetically diabetic C57BL/KsJ (db/db) mouse provides an animal model of NIDDM, characterized by obesity, hyperglycemia and insulin resistance with hyperinsulinemia.[8] The purpose of this study was to evaluate parameters of cardiac contractile function in isolated perfused working hearts from diabetic (db/db) mice relative to lean heterozygote control (db/+) mice. The effect of an inotropic stimulus, isoprenaline acting on cardiac β-adrenergic receptors, was also examined.

METHODS

Working mouse hearts were perfused as described in detail by Larsen et al.[9] Briefly, this required cannulation of the aorta for an initial retrograde Langendorff perfusion while the left atrium was cannulated through the pulmonary vein. The perfusion was then switched to working mode at a preload (left atrial filling pressure) of 15 mm Hg and an

Diabetes and Cardiovascular Disease: Etiology, Treatment and Outcomes
Edited by Aubie Angel et al., Kluwer Academic/Plenum Publishers, 2001

241

afterload of 50 mm Hg. The perfusion solution consisted of a Krebs-Henseleit bicarbonate buffer (118.5 mM NaCl, 25 mM NaHCO$_3$, 4.7 mM KCl, 1.2 mM MgSO$_4$, 1.2 mM KH$_2$PO$_4$, 2.5 mM CaCl$_2$ and 0.5 mM EDTA, gassed with 95% O$_2$ and 5% CO$_2$) containing 11 mM glucose and 0.4 mM palmitate (complexed to 3% albumin).

Left ventricular function was monitored by measuring intraventricular pressures recorded from a cannula inserted through the apex of the perfused heart into the left ventricle;[9] left ventricular developed pressures (LVDevP) were calculated from the difference between peak left ventricular systolic pressures and left ventricular end-diastolic pressures (LVEDP). Cardiac output (CO) was obtained from the sum of aortic (afterload line) and coronary (effluent dripping from the heart) flows. Cardiac power (LVDevP x CO) was also calculated over the 60 min perfusion period.

Heart rate was controlled by electrical pacing of the right atrium. For hearts perfused under basal conditions (absence of isoprenaline), pacing was at 360 bpm; the pacing rate was increased to 450 bpm when 1 µM isoprenaline (+ Iso) was added to the perfusion solution to control heart rate precisely in the presence of a chronotropic stimulus. Since perfused working mouse hearts exhibit a decline in cardiac function at heart rates greater than 400 bpm,[9] the positive inotropic effect of isoprenaline may have been underestimated slightly.

RESULTS

Larsen et al.[9] reported that cardiac performance of working Swiss-Webster mouse hearts was stable over 60 min of perfusion with two oxidizable substrates, glucose and a fatty acid (palmitate), added to the perfusate. Similar results are shown in Table 1 for control (db/+) hearts at 10 and 60 min of perfusion in the working mode.

Perfused working hearts from diabetic (db/db) hearts demonstrated marked cardiac dysfunction. Cardiac power in db/db hearts was reduced to 45% and 30% of control at perfusion times of 10 and 60 min, respectively (Table 1). Several parameters of left ventricular contractility were altered in perfused hearts from diabetic (db/db) hearts (Table 2). LVDevP was decreased by 24%, from 72 mm Hg in control (db/+) hearts to 55 mm Hg in diabetic (db/db) hearts; + dP/dt was decreased by 31% in db/db hearts (from 3.6 mm Hg/s x 10^{-3} to 2.5 mm Hg/s x 10^{-3}). LVEDP was much higher (22 mm Hg) in diabetic perfused hearts compared to control hearts (12 mm Hg).

Hearts were also perfused in the presence of 1 µM isoprenaline (+ Iso) to determine if both control and diabetic hearts exhibited an inotropic response to this β-adrenergic agonist (Table 2). In control (db/+) perfused hearts, isoprenaline increased LVDevP by

Table 1. Cardiac power measurements for perfused working hearts from control (db/+) and diabetic (db/db) mice.

PARAMETER	PERFUSION TIME (min)	CONTROL (db/+)	DIABETIC (db/db)
Cardiac Power (mJ/min)	10	56.0 ± 8.8	25.0 ± 8.8*
	60	59.3 ± 9.1	17.9 ± 5.5**

Results are mean ± SE (n=6 for both groups of hearts). *p<0.05   **p<.01

242

Table 2. Cardiac function in working hearts from control (db/+) and diabetic (db/db) mice, perfused in the absence (-Iso) and presence of 1 µM isoprenaline (+Iso).

PARAMETER	CONTROL (db/+)		DIABETIC (db/db)	
	-Iso (7)	+Iso (7)	-Iso (7)	+Iso (3)
LVDevP (mm Hg)	72 ± 7	88 ± 6*	55 ± 7‡	75 ± 6*
+dP/dt (mm Hg/s x 10^{-3})	3.6 ± 0.4	5.2 ± 0.6*	2.5 ± 0.4‡	4.1 ± 0.8*
LVEDP (mm Hg)	12 ± 2	4 ± 1*	22 ± 3‡	15 ± 3*‡

Results are mean ± SE for the number of perfused hearts indicated in parentheses.
*p<0.05 for perfusions with isoprenaline (+Iso) *versus* basal perfusion (-Iso)
‡p<0.05 for diabetic (db/db) hearts *versus* corresponding control (db/+) heart perfusions

22% and + dP/dt by 44%, and significantly decreased LVEDP from 12 mm Hg to 4 mm Hg. Similar changes in contractility were observed when diabetic (db/db) hearts were perfused with isoprenaline. The β-adrenergic agonist increased LVDevP and + dP/dt by 36% and 64%, respectively, to values that were no longer significantly different from contractile measurements in control hearts perfused with isoprenaline. Thus, the inotropic response to isoprenaline in perfused db/db hearts counter-acted some of the deleterious effects of diabetes on basal cardiac contractile performance. In the case of LVEDP measurements, however, although isoprenaline caused a significant reduction from 22 mm Hg to 15 mm Hg., this value was still significantly elevated compared to LVEDP measured in control hearts perfused with isoprenaline (4 mm Hg).

DISCUSSION

The availability of genetic models of disease in mice due to naturally-occurring mutations and the increasing ability to create genetically-engineered mice has stimulated efforts in developing techniques to assess murine cardiac performance.[10] The isolated perfused working mouse heart allows phenotypic analysis of cardiac function in an *ex vivo* model where preload, afterload, heart rate and substrate supply can be controlled without neuorhumoural influences.[9] Various indices of cardiac contractile performance (cardiac power, LVDevP, + dP/dt and LVEDP) are stable over 60 min perfusion times (ref. 9 and Table 1). An inotropic response to isoprenaline with increased LVDevP and + dP/dt and reduced LVEDP was observed (Table 2), indicating that mouse hearts perfused under normoxic conditions have sufficient cardiac reserve to response to a β-adrenergic agonist.

The pathophysiology of NIDDM includes both insulin resistance and impaired β-cell function,[11,12] resulting in concomitant hyperglycemia and hyperinsulinemia. Previous investigations into cardiac function have, however, largely been restricted to animal models of obesity and insulin resistance without overt signs of diabetes such as hyperglycemia. Rosen et al.[13] observed no reduction in cardiac mechanical performance in perfused hearts from obese Zucker rats; in fact, left ventricular pressure and + dP/dt values were increased significantly. Cardiac function has not been assessed as yet in Zucker diabetic fatty (ZDF) rats,[14] a model of obesity complicated by diabetes. The JRC:LA-cp corpulent rat is obese with marked insulin resistance and glucose intolerance resulting in modest non-fasting hyperglycemia.[15] Under specific perfusion conditions of reduced calcium concentrations (to 1.8 mM) and the presence of high concentrations of insulin (2 mU/mL), perfused JCR:LA-cp rat hearts exhibited either no reduction in heart function[15] or slightly decreased parameters of active cardiac contractile function with an increase in resting tension.[16] Finally, a chemically-induced model of NIDDM has been developed by Schaffer[17] in which a defect in insulin secretion precedes peripheral insulin resistance; mechanical dysfunction was a relatively late manifestation in this NIDDM model.

Perfused working hearts from diabetic (db/db) mice exhibited clear signs of cardiac dysfunction, with reductions in cardiac power (Table 1) and evidence of impaired left ventricular contractility from reductions in LVDevP and + dP/dt, together with elevated LVEDP (Table 2). Therefore, manifestation of cardiac dysfunction in NIDDM (diabetic cardiomyopathy) may require both insulin resistance and impaired β-cell function to produce marked hyperglycemia, in contrast to the models of obesity with insulin resistance only which exhibited no reductions in cardiac contractility.[13,15] The reduction in cardiac contractility observed in this db/db mouse model of NIDDM is similar to the diabetic cardiomyopathy observed consistently in type 1 (insulin-deficient) models of diabetes.[5,18]

The stimulatory effect of β-adrenergic agonists on cardiac contractility is diminished in insulin-deficient diabetic hearts.[5,19,20] In contrast, perfused working db/db hearts had a significant inotropic response to isoprenaline that normalized the depressed values for LVDevP and dP/dt observed under basal conditions (Table 2). In the case of LVEDP, however, although isoprenaline produced a significant reduction that in absolute terms was similar to the fall in LVEDP observed in control hearts perfused with isoprenaline, LVEDP in diabetic hearts was still significantly elevated in comparison to isoprenaline-treated control hearts.

In summary, perfused hearts from db/db mice, a genetic model of NIDDM, demonstrated considerable cardiac dysfunction with reduced left ventricular contractility. Part of this reduction in cardiac contractile performance could be reversed by perfusing with isoprenaline. A challenge for future investigations will be to identify the mechanistic basis for the reduction in basal contractility in perfused db/db hearts, and to establish interventions that can prevent or reverse cardiac dysfunction observed in situations of NIDDM.

REFERENCES

1. D.M. Nathan, J. Meigs, and D.E. Singer, The epidemiology of cardiovascular disease in type 2 diabetes mellitus: how sweet it is…or is it? *Lancet* 350(Suppl 1):4-9 (1997).
2. M. Laakso, and S. Lehto, Epidemiology of macrovascular disease in diabetes, *Diabetes Rev* 5:294-315 (1997).
3. M. Syvänne, and M-R. Taskinen, Lipids and lipoproteins as coronary risk factors in non-insulin-dependent diabetes mellitus, *Lancet* 350(Suppl 1):20-23 (1997).
4. F.S. Fein, Diabetic cardiomyopathy, *Diabetes Care* 13(Suppl 4):1169-1179 (1990).
5. K.C. Tomlinson, S.M. Gardiner, R.A. Hebden, and T. Bennett, Functional consequences of streptozotocin-induced diabetes mellitus, with particular reference to the cardiovascular system, *Pharmacol Rev* 44:103-179 (1992).
6. B. Rodrigues, M.C. Cam, and J.H. McNeill, Myocardiac substrate metabolism: implications for diabetic cardiomyopathy, *J Mol Cell Cardiol* 27:169-179 (1995).
7. G.N. Pierce, T.G. Maddaford, and J.C. Russell, Cardiovascular dysfunction in insulin-dependent and non-insulin-dependent animal models of diabetes mellitus, *Can J Physiol Pharmacol* 75:343-350 (1997).
8. D.L. Coleman, Diabetes-obesity syndromes in mice, *Diabetes* 31(Suppl 1):1-6 (1982).
9. T.S. Larsen, D.D. Belke, R. Sas, W.R. Giles, D.L. Severson, G.D. Lopaschuk, and J.V. Tyberg, The isolated working mouse heart: methodological considerations, *Pflüg Arch* 437:979-985 (1999).
10. G. Christensen, Y. Wang, and K.R. Chien, Physiological assessment of complex cardiac phenotypes in genetically engineered mice, *Am J Physiol* 272:H2513-H2524 (1997).
11. H. Beck-Nielsen, and L.C. Groop, Metabolic and genetic characterization of prediabetic states. Sequence of events leading to non-insulin-dependent diabetes mellitus, *J Clin Invest* 94:1714-1721 (1994).

12. Patti M-E, Kahn CR. Transgenic animal models: insights into the pathophysiology of NIDDM, *Diabetes Rev* 5:149-164 (1997).
13. P. Rösen, L. Herberg, and H. Reinauer, Different types of postinsulin receptor defects contribute to insulin resistance in hearts of obese Zucker rats, *Endocrinology* 119:1285-1291 (1986).
14. R.H. Unger, How obesity causes diabetes in Zucker diabetic fatty rats, *Trends Endocrinol Metab* 7:276-282 (1998).
15. G.D. Lopaschuk, and J.C. Russell, Myocardial function and energy substrate metabolism in the insulin-resistant JCR:LA corpulent rat, *J Appl Physiol* 71:1302-1308 (1991).
16. T.G. Maddaford, J.C. Russell, and G.N. Pierce, Postischemic cardiac performance in the insulin-resistant JCR:LA-*cp* rat, *Am J Physiol* 273:H1187-H1192 (1997).
17. S.W. Schaffer, Cardiomyopathy associated with noninsulin-dependent diabetes, *Mol Cell Biochem* 107:1-20 (1991).
18. C.E. Flarsheim, I.L. Grupp, and M.A. Matlib, Mitochondrial dysfunction accompanies diastolic dysfunction in diabetic rat heart, *Am J Physiol* 271:H192-H202 (1996).
19. R.V.S.V. Vadlamudi, and J.H. McNeill, Effect of experimental diabetes on isolated rat heart responsiveness to isoproterenol, *Can J Physiol Pharmacol* 62:124-131 (1993).
20. S. Gando, Y. Hattori, Y. Akaishi, J. Nishihira, and M. Kanno, Impaired contractile response to *beta* adrenoceptor stimulation in diabetic rat hearts: alterations in *beta* adrenoceptors-G protein-adenylate cyclase system and phospholamban phosphorylation, *J Pharmacol Exper Ther* 282:475-484 (1997).

MG^{2+}-DEPENDENT ATPASE ACTIVITY IN CARDIAC MYOFIBRILS FROM THE INSULIN-RESISTANT JCR:LA-CP RAT

Tarun Misra[1], James C. Russell[2], Tod A. Clark[1] and Grant N. Pierce[1]

[1]Division of Stroke & Vascular Disease, St. Boniface General Hospital Research Centre, and the Department of Physiology, University of Manitoba, R2H 2A6
[2]Department of Surgery, University of Alberta, Edmonton, Alberta, T6G 2R7

SUMMARY

There is a great deal of information presently available documenting a cardiomyopathic condition in insulin-deficient models of diabetes. Less information is available documenting a similar status in non insulin-dependent models of diabetes. We have studied the functional integrity of the myofibrils isolated from hearts of JCR:LA rats. The JCR:LA rat is hyperinsulinemic, hyperlipidemic, glucose intolerant and obese. As such, it carries many of the characteristics found in humans with non insulin-dependent diabetes mellitus. These animals also have many indications of heart disease. However, it is not clear if the hearts suffer from vascular complications or are cardiomyopathic in nature. We examined Mg^{2+} - dependent myofibrillar ATPase in hearts of JCR:LA-cp/cp rats and their corresponding control animals (+/?) and found no significant differences (P> 0.05). This is in striking contrast to the depression in this activity exhibited by cardiac myofibrils isolated from insulin-deficient models of diabetes. Our data demonstrate that myofibrillar functional integrity is normal in JCR:LA-cp rats and suggest that these hearts are not in a cardiomyopathic state. Insulin status may be critical in generating a cardiomyopathic condition in diabetes.

INTRODUCTION

The diabetic condition has now been conclusively associated with a cardiomyopathic condition. Defects in cardiac contractile performance in the absence of vascular complications have been reported by a number of laboratories (5,10,22,27,28,31). These lesions have been associated with defects in the function of a variety of subcellular membrane systems including mitochondria, sarcoplasmic reticulum and sarcolemma (2,6-8,12,16,18,19,23,27,29,33,37,40). These membranes are responsible for among other things, the regulation of ionic homeostasis within the cardiomyocyte (5,21,25). The changes in protein function within these membranes in

Diabetes and Cardiovascular Disease: Etiology, Treatment and Outcomes
Edited by Aubie Angel et al., Kluwer Academic/Plenum Publishers, 2001

diabetic hearts have been suggested to contribute to the contractile dysfunction (21,22,25).

One of the most important groups of proteins involved in the contractile process are the myofibrils. The integrated coupling of actin and myosin in concert with the movements of several other regulatory myofibrillar proteins directly results in force generation in the heart (38). An alteration in the function of any of the myofibrillar proteins will result in a change in the coordinated interaction of these proteins that will ultimately disrupt the contractile process. Myofibrillar ATPase activity is critical to this process. Defects in this activity have been closely correlated to cardiac contractile dysfunction under a variety of pathological conditions (6,11,19,24). Conversely, conditions of enhanced cardiac contractile performance have been associated with increased myofibrillar ATPase activity (1,38). Because of this close association, myofibrillar ATPase activity has often been used as a marker to identify a cardiomyopathic condition (22,23,38).

The identification of a cardiomyopathic condition in diabetes has been limited by two important factors. First, the model of diabetes used to characterize this pathological state has been insulin-dependent (type I). Very few studies have investigated cardiac function and subcellular organelle integrity in a non insulin-dependent diabetic model. This is unfortunate because it is the predominant form of diabetes in humans today. Secondly, although the cardiomyopathy has now been identified in diabetics, we have been unable to identify the causative stimulus. The accompanying hyperlipidemia (14,32), hyperglycemia (3), or insulin status (22,26) of the diabetic animals have all been suggested to play important causative roles in the diabetic cardiomyopathy. However, it has not been possible as yet to conclusively establish which one of these factors is causative on its own.

The purpose of the present study was to assay the functional integrity of myofibrillar Mg^{2+}ATPase activity in hearts from JCR:LA-cp rats. These animals are hyperinsulinemic, hyperlipidemic, glucose intolerant, obese and insulin resistant (34-36). They are thought to be an ideal model to mimic the non-insulin dependent diabetic condition in humans who have all of these same conditions (9,15,17,34-36). In addition, the JCR:LA-cp rats experience small spontaneous myocardial infarctions (34-36). Because of the strikingly different metabolic profile for the JCR:LA-cp rat and the streptozotocin-induced diabetic rat (that is conventionally used in the diabetes field as a model of insulin dependent diabetes), we believed it may provide valuable mechanistic insight to evaluate the status of myofibrillar functional integrity in hearts from JCR:LA-cp rats.

METHODS

Animals: Male JCR:LA-cp rats were bred in the established breeding colony at the University of Alberta, until they reached 3 or 6 months of age. The animals had food (Laboratory Rodent Diet, PMI feeds, St. Louis, MO.) and water availability ad libitum and were maintained on a 12:12 light dark schedule in a 50% humidity environment on woodchip bedding in polycarbonate cages. Care and treatment of the animals conformed to the Guidelines of the Canadian Council on Animal Care and was approved by the animal welfare committees at the appropriate institutions. The JCR:LA-cp/cp homozygous animals exhibited obesity, hyperinsulinemia, and glucose intolerance (34-36). The control group consisted of JCR:LA heterozygotes (cp/+) or homozygous +/+ rats which are not affected, showing none of the above traits.

Myofibril isolation: Cardiac myofibril isolation was achieved by differential centrifugation (23,24). 1mM dithiothreitol, 1mM phenylmethylsulfonyl fluoride, and 1μM leupeptin were present in all isolation solutions. Suspension of the final fraction occurred in 0.1M KCl, 20mM imidazole (pH 7.0), 1mM dithiothreitol, and was stored up to a maximum of 48hrs post isolation. Assays to determine the purity of the final fraction consisted of succinic dehydrogenase, mannose-6-phosphatase, and Na^+-K^+ ATPase as described previously (4,13).

Myofibril ATPase assay & protein assay: Measurement of the Mg^{2+} dependent ATPase activity was carried out at 37°C for 5mins in a medium of 20mM imidazole (pH 7.0), 2mM $MgCl_2$, 2mM Na_2ATP, 10mM NaN_3, 1mM EGTA, and 50mM KCl. Myofibrillar protein concentration was measured as previously described (4,23,24). The reaction was initiated with the addition of 50μg of myofibrillar protein and ceased upon addition of 1ml ice-cold 12% trichloroacetic acid. Measurement of inorganic phosphate liberation was as described previously (23). Enzyme activity was measured as a function of reaction time.

Statistics: A two-tailed students t-test was used to determine statistical significance (P<0.05).

RESULTS

Myofibrils were isolated from hearts of JCR:LA-cp rats and the lean control animals. We could detect no appreciable Na^+, K^+ - ATPase activity, succinic dehydrogenase activity or oxalate-supported Ca^{2+} uptake in these myofibrillar fractions. This would suggest that membraneous contamination of the isolated myofibrils was minimal. Furthermore, myofibrillar yield was similar between the two groups (66±7mg/g wet tissue weight in the +/? controls rats versus 63±2mg/g wet tissue weight in the cp/cp rats). This finding would again support the contention that the myofibrillar fractions were not differentially contaminated.

Mg^{2+}-dependent ATPase activity in cardiac myofibrils was examined as a function of varying reaction times in the 3 month old JCR:LA rats. There was a linear increase in activity from 1-20 minutes (Figure 1). There were no significant differences in Mg^{2+} - ATPase activity between the two groups at any of the time points examined.

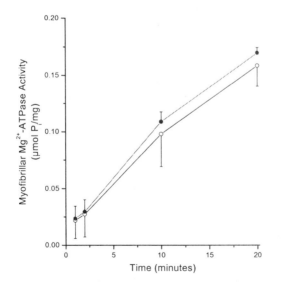

Figure 1. Myofibrillar Mg^{2+}-ATPase activity as a function of reaction time in 3 month old lean (o) and corpulent (•) JCR:LA-cp rats. Values represent the mean ±SEM for 4-6 animals

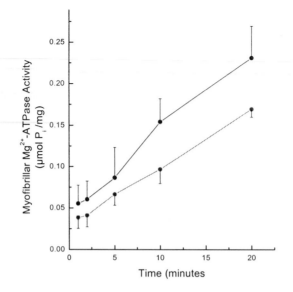

Figure 2. Myofibrillar Mg2+-ATPase activity as a function of reaction time in 6 month old lean (o) and corpulent (•) JCR:LA-cp rats. Values represent the mean ±SEM for 4-6 animals.

Myofibrillar Mg^{2+} ATPase activity was also measured in 6 month old JCR:LA rats as a function of reaction time (Figure 2). Although there was a trend for a depressed activity in cp/cp rats in comparison to their control counterparts, this did not achieve statistical significance at any of the time points examined.

DISCUSSION

Our results demonstrate that myofibrillar Mg^{2+} dependent ATPase activity was unaltered in the JCR:LA-cp rats despite a disturbed metabolic profile. It was possible that contractile protein function may become altered as the duration of diabetes lengthened. This was demonstrated by JCR:LA-cp rats previously with regard to their response to an ischemic challenge (17). However, this was not a factor in the present study. Increasing the age of the animals did not reveal any significant affects in myofibrillar Mg^{2+} ATPase activity. This finding was also not influenced by a significant or differential contamination of the myofibrillar fraction with other subcellular organelles.

Our findings confirm and extend a previous study examining myofibrillar Ca^{2+} ATPase activity and sarcoplasmic reticular function in JCR:LA-cp rats (20). In that study (20), there were no significant differences observed between the lean and corpulent rats in these activities. Our results are in striking contrast to those observations obtained in insulin-dependent models of diabetes. Myofibrillar Mg^{2+}-dependent ATPase activity was significantly depressed in hearts from streptozotocin-induced, insulin-deficient diabetic animals (2,6-8,16,18,19,23,24,27,29,33,39).

The differences in the response of the Mg^{2+} ATPase activity in myofibrils from the two models of diabetes suggest that there may be an association of the integrity of the protein with the metabolic profile of the animal. The primary metabolic difference between JCR:LA-cp rats and chemically-induced models of diabetes is the insulin concentration and function. JCR:LA-cp rats have abnormally high basal concentrations of insulin and exhibit profound insulin resistance (9,15,17,34-36). Chemically-induced diabetic rats exhibit extremely low circulatory insulin levels (11). It is possible that the low insulin concentration may induce a depression in myofibrillar function and, conversely, high levels may preserve function despite the presence of other metabolic abnormalities. It is known that insulin-like growth factors may alter cardiac contractile performance when over-expressed (30). Conversely, it is still possible that the modest hyperglycemia exhibited by the JCR:LA-cp rats is insufficient to induce myofibrillar defects. This will require further study. It is clear from our results that the further use of alternative models of diabetes may provide unique and valuable information regarding heart disease and provide further insight into the key factors that may be responsible for this disease in the diabetic population.

Acknowledgements

Grants from the Heart & Stroke Foundation of Manitoba and Alberta, and a grant from the Canadian Diabetes Association in honour of Agnes Dorothy Knudsen supported this work. T. Misra was supported by a studentship from the Manitoba Medical Services Foundation. T. Clark was a Bronfman Scholar. G. N. Pierce was a Senior Scientist of the Medical Research Council of Canada.

REFERENCES

1. Barany, M., ATPase activity of myosin correlated with speed of muscle shortening, J.Gen.Physiol., 50, 197, 1967.
2. Belcastro A.N., J.S. Gilchrist, and J.A. Scrubb, G. Arthur. Calcium-supported calpain degradation rates for cardiac myofibrils in diabetes. Mol Cell Biochem 135:51-60, 1994.
3. Cross, H.R., L.H. Opie, G.K. Radda, and K. Clarke. Is high glycogen content beneficial or detrimental to the ischemic heart? Circ.Res. 78:482-491,1996.
4. Czubryt, M.P., B. Ramjiawan, J.S.C. Gilchrist and G.N. Pierce. The presence and partitioning of calcium binding proteins in hepatic and cardiac nuclei. J Mol Cell Cardiol 28: 455-465, 1996.
5. Dhalla N.S., G.N. Pierce, I.R. Innes and R.E. Beamish. Pathogenesis of cardiac dysfunction in diabetes mellitus. Can J Cardiol 1:263-281, 1985.
6. Dillmann, W.H. Diabetes mellitus induces changes in cardiac myosin of the rat. Diabetes 29:579-582, 1980.
7. Dillmann, W.H. Fructose feeding increases Ca++-activated myosin ATPase activity and changes myosin isoenzyme distribution in the diabetic rat heart. Endocrinology 114: 1678-1685, 1984.
8. Dillmann, W.H. Influence of thyroid hormone administration on myosin ATPase activity and myosin isoenzyme distribution in the heart of diabetic rats. Metabolism 31: 199-204, 1982.
9. Dolphin P.J., R.M. Amy, and J.C. Russell: Effect of age on serum lipids and lipoproteins of male and female JCR:LA-corpulent rats. Biochim Biophys Acta 1042:99-106, 1990.
10. Fein F.S. and E.H. Sonnenblick. Diabetic cardiomyopathy. Prog. Cardiovasc. Dis. 27: 255-270, 1985.
11. Fein,F.S., J.E. Strobeck, A.Malhotra, J. Scheuer, and E.H. Sonnenblick. Reversibility of diabetic cardiomyopathy with insulin in rats. Circ.Res. 49:1251-1261,1981.
12. Ganguly, P.K., G.N. Pierce, K.S. Dhalla and N.S. Dhalla. Defective sarcoplasmic reticular calcium transport in diabetic cardiomyopathy. Am. J. Physiol. 244:E528-E535, 1983.
13. Gilchrist, J.S.C. and G.N. Pierce. Identification and purification of a calcium-binding protein in hepatic nuclear membranes. J Biol Chem 268: 4291-4299, 1993.
14. Kannel W.B., McGee D.L. Diabetes and cardiovascular risk factors. The Framingham Study. Circulation 1979;59:8-13.
15. Lopaschuk G.D. and J.C. Russell. Myocardial function and energy substrate metabolism in the insulin-resistant JCR:LA corpulent rat. J Appl Physiol 71:1302   -1308, 1991.
16. MacLean I.M., R.V. Rajotte, and A.N. Belcastro. Insulin and islet cell transplants: effects on diabetic rat cardiac myofibril ATPase. Am J Physiol 252:E244-E247, 1987.
17. Maddaford T.G., J.C. Russell, and G.N. Pierce. Postischemic cardiac performance in the insulin-resistant JCR:LA-cp rat. Am J Physiol 273:H1187-H1192, 1997.
18. Malhotra A, J.P. Mordes, L. McDermott, and T.F. Schaible. Abnormal cardiac biochemistry in spontaneously diabetic Bio-Breeding/Worcester rat. Am J Physiol 249:H1051-H1059, 1985.
19. Malhotra A, S. Penpargkul, F.S. Fein, E.H. Sonnenblick, and J. Scheuer. The effect of streptozotocin-induced diabetes in rats on cardiac contractile proteins. Circ Res 49:1243-1250, 1981.

20. Misra, T., J.S.C. Gilchrist, J. C. Russell, and G. N. Pierce. Cardiac myofibrillar andsarcoplasmic reticulum function are not depressed in insulin-resistant JCR:LA-cp rat. Am J Physiol. 276 (Heart Circ.Physiol. 45):H1811-H1817, 1999.

21. Penpargkul, S, F. Fein, E.H. Sonnenblick and J. Scheuer. Depressed cardiac sarcoplasmic reticular function from diabetic rats. J Mol Cell Cardiol 13:303-309, 1981.

22. Pierce G.N., R.E. Beamish and N.S. Dhalla. Heart Dysfunction in Diabetes, Boca Raton, FL, CRC Press, 1988, p.1-245

23. Pierce G.N. and N.S. Dhalla. Mechanisms of the defect in myofibrillar function during diabetes. Am J Physiol 248:E170-E175, 1985.

24. Pierce G.N. and N.S. Dhalla. Cardiac myofibrillar ATPase activity in diabetic rats. J Mol Cell Cardiol 13: 1063-1069, 1981.

25. Pierce G.N., Dhalla N.S. Mitochondrial abnormalities in diabetic cardiomyopathy. Can J Cardiol;1:48-54, 1985.

26. Pierce, G.N., P.K. Ganguly, A. Dzurba and N.S. Dhalla. Modification of the function of cardiac subcellular organelles by insulin. In: Advances in Myocardiology, edited by N.S. Dhalla and D.J. Hearse, 1985, p. 113-125.

27. Pierce G.N., M.K. Lockwood, and C.D. Eckhert. Cardiac contractile protein ATPase activity in a diet induced model of noninsulin dependent diabetes mellitus. Can. J. Cardiol. 5: 117-120, 1989.

28. Pierce, G.N., T.G. Maddaford and J.C. Russell. Cardiovascular dysfunction in insulin-dependent and non-insulin-dependent animal models of diabetes mellitus. Can. J. Physiol. Pharmacol. 75: 343-350, 1997.

29. Pollack, P.S., A. Malhotra, F.S. Fein, and J. Scheuer. Effects of diabetes on cardiac contractile proteins in rabbits and reversal with insulin. Am J Physiol 251: H448- H454, 1986.

30. Redaelli, G., A. Malhotra, B. Li, P. Li, E. H. Sonnenblick, P. A. Hofmann and P. Anversa. Effects of constitutive overexpression of insulin-like growth factor-1 on the mechanical characteristics and molecular properties of ventricular myocytes. Circ Res. 82:594-603, 1998.

31. Regan T.J. Congestive heart failure in the diabetic. Annu Rev Med 34:161-168, 1983.

32. Rodrigues, B., M.C. Cam and J.H. McNeill. Myocardial substrate metabolism: implications for diabetic cardiomyopathy. J. Mol. Cell Cardiol. 27:169-179, 1995.

33. Rupp H., V. Elimban, and N.S. Dhalla. Modification of myosin isozymes and SR Ca $(^{2+})$-pump ATPase of the diabetic rat heart by lipid-lowering interventions. Mol Cell Biochem 132:69-80, 1994.

34. Russell J.C., S.K. Ahuja, V. Manickavel, R.V. Rajotte, and R.M. Amy. Insulin resistance and impaired glucose tolerance in the atherosclerosis-prone LA/N corpulent rat. Arteriosclerosis 7:620-626, 1987.

35. Russell J.C. and R.M. Amy. Early atherosclerotic lesions in a susceptible rat model: the LA/N-corpulent rat. Atherosclerosis 60:119-129, 1986.

36. Russell J.C., D.G. Koeslag, P.J. Dolphin and R.M. Amy. Prevention of myocardial lesions in JCR:LA-corpulent rats by nifedipine. Arteriosclerosis 10:658-664, 1990.

37. Schaffer, S.W., M.S. Mozaffari, M. Artman and G.L. Wilson. Basis for myocardialmechanical defects associated with non-insulin-dependent diabetes. Am J Physiol 256:E25-E30, 1989.

38. Scheuer, J. and A.K. Bhan. Cardiac contractile proteins: Adenosine triphosphatase activity and physiological function. Circ Res 45: 1-12, 1979.

39. Takeda, N., I.M.C. Dixon, T. Hata, V. Elimban, K.R. Shah and N. S. Dhalla. Sequence of alterations in subcellular organelles during the development of heart dysfunction in diabetes. Diabetes Res. Clin. Pract. 30:S113-S122, 1996.

40. Yu, Z., G. F. Tibbits and J. H. McNeill. Cellular functions of diabetic cardiomyocytes: contractility, rapid-cooling contracture, and ryanodine binding. Am. J. Physiol. 266: H2082-H2089, 1994.

CYCLIC NUCLEOTIDE PHOSPHODIESTERASE FAMILIES IN INTRACELLULAR SIGNALING AND DIABETES

Claire Lugnier

Pharmacologie et Physico-Chimie des Interactions Moléculaires et Cellulaires, CNRS UMR 7034, Université Louis Pasteur de Strasbourg, Faculté de Pharmacie, 67401 Illkirch, France.

INTRODUCTION

Cyclic nucleotide phosphodiesterases (PDE), by hydrolyzing cyclic AMP (cAMP) and cyclic GMP (cGMP), play a major role in intracellular signal transduction and participate in the regulation of pathophysiological states. This enzymatic system, is made up of at least 10 gene families (PDE1 to PDE10), differently distributed in tissues (Lugnier et al., 1983) and subcellular compartments and characterized by different substrate affinities and sensitivities to endogenous effectors (cGMP and calcium-calmodulin). The most studied families are PDE1 to PDE5. They are selectively inhibited by specific and very potent inhibitors (Beavo et al., 1994; Stoclet et al., 1995). These enzymes, when present in specific tissues implicated in pathophysiological states, are up- or down-regulated by various phosphorylating processes or by protein induction (Dousa, 1999). Therefore the altered PDE family could be a therapeutic target for the studied disease. PDE3 and PDE4 may represent new classes of drug targets for diabetes since it was reported that insulin-induced phosphorylation activates PDE3 (Degerman et al., 1990) and that PDE4 inhibitors may prevent installation of diabetes (Liang et al., 1998). Since these two PDE families play a major role in cardiovascular functions (Stoclet et al., 1995), PDE3 and PDE4 inhibitors may be especially useful in cardiovascular diseases associated to diabetes.

CYCLIC NUCLEOTIDE PHOSPHODIESTERASES

Family Classification

Multiple PDEs are expressed in mammalian cells. They play an important role downstream receptors in the regulation of intracellular concentrations of cAMP and cGMP which in turn modulate phosphorylations and consequently major physiological responses. These PDEs are now classified in 10 families on the basis of their gene, their structural and kinetic characteristics (Table 1), (Beavo et al., 1994; Dousa, 1999; Fujishige et al., 1999; Soderling et al., 1999). Their differential tissue distribution and their selective inhibitors provide a basis for the search for therapeutically useful compounds. Since characterizations of PDE7 to PDE10 are very recent, studies on PDE involvement in signal transduction concern mainly PDE1 to PDE5 which are the major PDE isoforms in mammalian tissues.

Diabetes and Cardiovascular Disease: Etiology, Treatment and Outcomes
Edited by Aubie Angel et al., Kluwer Academic/Plenum Publishers, 2001

253

Table 1. PDE gene families

Short name	PDE isozyme gene family	Number of gene products	Number of splice products
PDE1	CaM-dependent PDEs	3	9+
PDE2	cGMP-stimulated PDEs	1	2
PDE3	cGMP-inhibited PDEs	2	2+
PDE4	cAMP-specific PDEs	4	15+
PDE5	cGMP-specific PDEs	2	2
PDE6	photoreceptor PDEs	3	2
PDE7	cAMP-specific PDEs	2	2
PDE8	cAMP-specific PDE	1	1
PDE9	cGMP-specific PDE	1	1
PDE10	cAMP/cGMP PDEs	2?	2 or 3

These different PDEs share common structural determinants: a catalytic domain encompassing a region of 270 aminoacids, a N-terminal regulatory domain and a carboxy terminal domain. They are characterized by their substrate specificity, their regulation by endogenous modulators and their sensitivities to selective inhibitors (Stoclet et al., 1995):
- **PDE1** hydrolyses both cAMP and cGMP and is activated by Ca-calmodulin complex; there is no good specific inhibitor at present time;
- **PDE2** hydrolyses both cAMP and cGMP and is allosterically activated by cGMP in the μM range, it is selectively inhibited by EHNA (an inhibitor of adenosine deaminase);
- **PDE3** hydrolyses cAMP and at a lower velocity cGMP, therefore cAMP hydrolysis is competitively inhibited by cGMP ($K_i = 0.2 \ \mu M$), it is specifically inhibited by cilostamide;
- **PDE4** hydrolyses specifically cAMP and is specifically inhibited by rolipram;
- **PDE5** hydrolyses cGMP and is specifically inhibited by zaprinast (Lugnier et al., 1986).

PDE Families in Cardiovascular Functions

Heart. In heart, cAMP has a positive inotropic effect related to cAMP dependent protein kinase activation. Four major families have been identified in cardiac tissue: PDE1, PDE2, PDE3 and PDE4. Among them PDE1 and PDE2 hydrolyse both cAMP and cGMP and are positively allosterically regulated, whereas PDE3 and PDE4 preferentially hydrolyse cAMP. PDE3 inhibitors such as milrinone, SK&F 94120 induce an increase of contractile force in guinea pig heart (Muller et al., 1990a), whereas PDE4 inhibitors induce only a positive inotropy in the presence of PDE3 inhibitors or low amount of forskolin (a direct activator of adenylyl cyclase). This suggests that PDE4 participates in the regulation of cAMP only when cAMP levels are elevated (Muller et al., 1990b). Since cGMP is able to stimulate PDE2 as well as to inhibit PDE3, cGMP could either potentiates or inhibits cardiac inotropy depending on the relative proportions of PDE2 and PDE3 in the species considered (Muller et al., 1990a). Nevertheless PDE3 inhibitors are effective in heart failure. In blood platelets, PDE3 is the only PDE form hydrolysing mainly cAMP and their specific inhibitors are potent antiaggregant agents.

Blood Vessels. Opposite to the heart, both cAMP and cGMP induce relaxation of blood vessels. In smooth muscle cAMP is hydrolysed by PDE3 and PDE4, whereas cGMP is hydrolysed by PDE1 and PDE5. PDE distribution in blood vessels differs from the heart since smooth muscle contains PDE5 but does not contain PDE2. Therefore an increase in cGMP in this tissue is not able to increase hydrolysis of cAMP, but rather increases cAMP content by inhibiting PDE3. By studying the effect of specific PDE3 and PDE4 inhibitors on precontracted aorta, we showed that PDE3 are potent endothelium-independent vasorelaxant agents whereas, PDE4 inhibitors are endothelium-dependent vasorelaxant agents (Komas et al.,

1991; Lugnier and Komas 1993). Furthermore, in absence of endothelium, PDE4 inhibitors are able to relax smooth muscle and increase cAMP level, only in the presence of agents increasing cGMP level or of specific inhibitors of PDE3 (Komas et al., 1991; Lugnier and Komas, 1993; Eckly and Lugnier, 1994) (Figure 1).

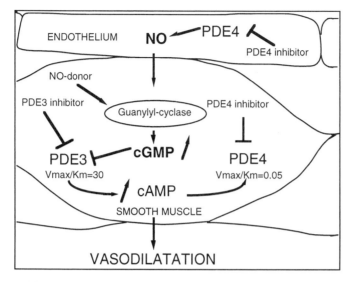

Figure 1. NO participates to the cross-talk between PDE3 and PDE4. Enzyme inhibition is indicated by a stopped line, whereas activation is indicated by an arrow.

Since PDE3 has a lower K_m value and a higher V_{max} value for cAMP than PDE4, PDE3 is firstly implicated in the cAMP hydrolysis. It is concluded that cGMP by inhibiting PDE3 increases intracellular cAMP level allowing PDE4 to participate in cAMP degradation and to be inhibited by PDE4 inhibitors (Figure 1).

It is well known that endothelium which lines smooth muscle cells participates mainly in the regulation of vasodilatation by producing nitric oxide (NO) which in turn stimulates guanylyl cyclase and consequently increases cGMP level. Therefore, cGMP increase related to the presence of endothelium may explain the endothelium-dependent vasorelaxing effect of PDE4 inhibitors (Komas et al., 1991; Lugnier and Komas, 1993; Eckly and Lugnier, 1994). A similar effect is observed in the presence of NO donors such as molsidomine and sodium nitroprussiate (Figure 1).

In endothelium PDE2 and PDE4 are the sole PDE isoforms present (Lugnier and Schini 1990). By studying cyclic nucleotide levels in condition modulating NO production, surprisingly we observed in cultured endothelial cells incubated with L-arginine (substrate of nitric oxide synthase, NOS) that rolipram (selective PDE4 inhibitor) is able to increase cGMP level. Since this could not be observed in the control condition or in the presence of L-NAME, an inhibitor of NOS, and since rolipram does not inhibit cGMP hydrolysis, it was concluded that PDE4 inhibitors may upregulate endothelial NOS (Kessler and Lugnier, 1995). We were the first to demonstrate this mechanism and we suggest that it could also participate to the endothelium-dependent relaxing effect of PDE4 inhibitors.

Long term treatment with PDE3 and PDE4 inhibitors in cardiovascular tissues have potential beneficial effects in atherosclerosis since they inhibit basal smooth muscle cell proliferation (Johnson-Mills et al., 1998) as well as insulin-induced cell proliferation (Takahashi et al., 1992; Souness et al., 1992) and cell migration (Palmer et al., 1998). For instance milrinone, which is a PDE3 and PDE4 inhibitor, suppresses intimal thickening (Kondo et al., 1999). PDE3 and PDE4 inhibitors also prevent endothelial cell proliferation (Leitman et al., 1986) which is a key event in angiogenesis (Folkmann, 1995). Therefore they could also be helpfull in diabetic retinopathy.

PDE Families in Diabetes

Variations of PDE Activities Related to Diabetes.   In the seventies, the first studies showing variation of PDE activity in experimental model of diabetes were performed mainly in non cardiovascular tissues such as fat, liver and pancreas in which insulin plays a major role. It was reported that insulin stimulates particulate cAMP-PDE in adipocytes (Manganiello and Vaughan, 1973) and that diabetes decreases cAMP-PDE activity in this tissue (Solomon, 1975). Glyburide, an hypoglycemic agent, was shown to restore the normal PDE activity in liver and fat (Solomon et al., 1986). These data markedly suggested that PDEs could be involved in diabetes.

Liver, Fat Tissues and Pancreas.   The regulation of PDE3 in adipocytes by insulin was very well studied step by step in collaborative studies performed by E. Degerman and V. Manganiello teams. They showed that in intact rat fat cells, insulin and isoprenaline activate by phosphorylation the cGMP-inhibited low-K_m cAMP phosphodiesterase (presently named PDE3) (Degerman et al., 1990). This phosphorylation is mediated by phosphatidylinositol 3-kinase which plays an essential role (Rahn et al., 1994). Furthermore, phosphorylation of PDE3 plays a key role in the antilipolytic action of insulin (Eriksson et al., 1995). Only one residue of PDE3B, serine[302], was phosphorylated after insulin or isoproterenol treatment (Rahn et al., 1996). This process of phosphorylation participates in the phosphorylation cascade inducing anti-lipolytic effect of insulin which includes protein kinase B (PKB) downstream of phosphatidylinositol 3-kinase (Wijkander et al., 1998). In the same way, it was shown that in pancreatic β-cells, leptin causes the activation of PDE3B which leads to inhibition of insulin secretion (Zhao et al., 1998).

PDE1 represents another isoform which has been reported to be altered in diabetes. PDE1 activity and its endogenous activator, calmodulin, are decreased in liver and fat tissues from spontaneous as from streptozotocin-induced diabetic rats (Solomon et al., 1986). At the opposite, insulin stimulates PDE1 in the liver via calmodulin (Smoake et al., 1995). Studies concerning the implication of PDE1 are rare, since good specific PDE1 inhibitors are not available.

Cardiovascular Tissues.   No study was performed in cardiovascular tissues showing alteration of PDE activities in diabetic heart. However, it was shown that heart isolated from non-insulin-dependent diabetic rat exhibited reduced responsiveness to the β-adrenergic agonist isoproterenol which is independent of adenylyl cyclase but was related to defective response of cAMP-dependent protein kinase (PKA) (Schaffer et al., 1991). This suggests that cAMP-PDE activity could be activated in cardiomyopathy and consequently the decrease of cAMP hydrolysis could decrease inotropic force. Furthermore it was shown that in human platelets insulin stimulates PDE3 via serine phosphorylation (Lopez-Aparicio et al., 1993). In aorta of the JCR:La-cp rat it was recently shown that PDE3 activity and PDE3A mRNA are increased 2 and 3 fold in comparison with the lean rat and it was hypothetized that this increase might contribute to accelerated atherosclerosis in diabetes (Nagaoka et al., 1998).

Kidney.   Since the eighties, Dousa and colleagues have studied nephrogenic diabetes insipidus and particularly implications of cyclic AMP catabolism. They suggest that abnormally high activity of cAMP phosphodiesterase may cause unresponsiveness to the diuretic vasopressin (Homma et al., 1991). This was related to the higher activity of PDE4 in collecting ducts (Takeda et al., 1991). Studies performed on renal epithelial cell line showed that overexpression of PDE4 induced vasopressin resistance (Yamaki et al., 1993).

Cellular Signaling in Diabetes.   Hyperglycemia, a major pathological factor in diabetes, induces oxidative stress and consequently cardiovascular diseases (Baynes and Thorpe, 1999). This is mainly due to the generation of oxygen derived radicals which results from auto-oxidation of glucose, advanced glycation end products (AGE), activation of receptor for AGE (RAGE) and also from NADPH-oxidase and NOS (Rösen et al., 1998). These radicals, by activating NFKB, modify gene expression and particularly increase production of tumor necrosis factor-α (TNFα) and interleukin-1 (IL-1). This mechanism is ascertained since high level of circulating TNFα is associated to human type 2 diabetes (insulin resistant) (Zinman et al., 1999) and since it was shown that cytokine antibodies prevent the development of diabetes in transgenic mice (André-Schmutz et al., 1999).

In pancreatic islets which produce insulin, local expression of TNFα promotes diabetes by enhancing presentation of islet antigens which leads to tissue destruction (Green et al., 1998). It is well kown that TNFα upregulates inducible NOS (iNOS) which produces NO and that excessive production of NO generates superoxide anions. The dual physiological and pathophysiological role of NO in pancreatic β-cells was recently reviewed (Spinas, 1999). This author suggests that the constitutively expressed endothelial NOS (eNOS), in α-cells or endothelial cells, stimulates insulin in a paracrine manner, whereas iNOS (which synthetizes NO 1000 fold more than eNOS) causes β-cell injury resulting in insulin-dependent diabetes.

In the same way, it was reported that cAMP as well as specific PDE3 inhibitors stimulate insulin release (Parker et al., 1995; Shafiee-Nick et al., 1995). This mechanism could be implicated in the insulin secretagogue effect of NO (Figure 2). As reported above for PDE3 in smooth muscle, NO by increasing cGMP level could inhibit PDE3 present in human islets of Langerhans (Parker et al., 1995) and therefore could increase cAMP level. This may represent the physiological effect of NO. However, when NO is overproduced by iNOS, consequently to TNFα increase, the resulting superoxide anions induce β-cell necrosis and suppress insulin secretion.

In vascular smooth muscle cells, it was shown that hyperglycemia, which increased superoxide generation, induced NFKB activation and consequently activated VCAM-1 promoter (Yerneni et al., 1999; Figure 2). VCAM-1 plays a key early step in atherosclerosis by mediating the recruitment and retention of monocytes in the subendothelial space. Furthermore superoxide anions related to hyperglycemia stimulate NO production in endothelial cells (Graier et al., 1999). These reciprocal effects of oxidative stress could induce an inflammatory process which is not easily reversed when already well installed.

PDE4 and Inflammation. PDE4 family merges as a new target for anti-inflammatory drugs (Torphy and Undem, 1991), since specific PDE4 inhibitors are able to inhibit cytokine production, especially TNFα in many inflammatory cells and to inhibit superoxide anions and hydroperoxide productions (Barnette et al., 1995). Furthermore, PDE4 is upregulated in inflammation processes such as asthma, atopic dermatitis and particularly in diabetes insipidus (Takeda et al., 1991). Currently pharmaceutical companies are developing new very potent and specific PDE4 inhibitors as anti-inflammatory compounds. For instance, Ariflo® which is under clinical investigation and developed by SmithKline Beecham, acts in the nanomolar range on PDE4 (Barnette et al., 1998). In our laboratory we have also synthetized new PDE4 inhibitors structurally unrelated to rolipram (Bourguignon et al., 1997) which are very potent *in vivo* and *in vitro* to inhibit TNFα release and inflammatory cell recruitment (Boichot et al., 2000). These PDE4 inhibitors should be therefore beneficial for breaking oxidative stress induced in diabetes (Figure 2).

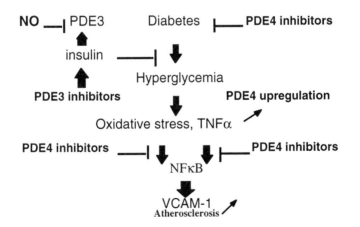

Figure 2. Possible involvement of PDE3 and PDE4 in diabetes. Stopped line indicates inhibition, whereas arrow indicates activation.

PDE INHIBITORS ARE POTENTIAL DRUGS FOR DIABETES

According to their various effects in signal transduction, PDE3 and PDE4 inhibitors should be beneficial not only in preventing diabetes but also in treating associated cardiovascular diseases as well as cardiovascular alterations, such as atherosclerosis, hypertension and cardiomyopathy. Figure 2 illustrates the various possible targets of PDE3 and PDE4 inhibitors. As reported above, PDE3 inhibitors by stimulating insulin secretion should be helpfull for type 2 diabetes. Reciprocally it was shown that a novel insulin secretagogue is a PDE3/PDE4 inhibitor (Leibowitz et al., 1995). PDE3 inhibitors are effective in man since they are able to increase lipolysis in adipose tissue but not in skeletal muscle (Moberg et al., 1998; Enoksson et al., 1998). PDE3 inhibitors are also antiproliferative, therefore they could prevent atherosclerosis associated to diabetes. Furthermore, PDE3 inhibitors which are endothelium-independent relaxing agents (Komas et al., 1991) and positive inotropic agents (Muller et al., 1990a) are used in heart failure. Additionally a PDE3 inhibitor, the antiplatelet drug cilostazol (Pletaal®; Kawamura et al., 1985) is successfully used for arthritis and claudication in Japan (Dawson et al., 1998). This compound is also able to prevent high D-glucose induced endothelial cell death (Morishita et al., 1997).

PDE4 inhibitors, a new class of anti-inflammatory drugs, similarly to the antibody against TNFα (André-Schmutz et al., 1999), are able to prevent the development of diabetes NOD mice. In agreement with its potency on isolated PDE4, rolipram is 100 fold more potent than pentoxifylline to prevent autoimmune diabetes, this effect was still apparent over 10 weeks after withdrawal of the drug treatment (Liang et al., 1998). In patients known to be at risk of developing diabetes, the administration of PDE4 inhibitors could be considered to arrest the progression of insulitis and prevent disease since it was reported that in autoimmune diabetes the transition from benign to pernicious insulitis requires an islet cell response to TNFα (Pakala et al., 1999). In diabetic patients pentoxifylline administration reduces proteinuria and TNFα (Navarro et al., 1999). Furthermore since PDE4 inhibitors are effective in cardiovascular function in presence of NO donors or in presence of PDE3 inhibitors (Lugnier and Komas 1993; Stoclet et al., 1995), they should be beneficial in atherosclerosis, hypertension and cardiomyopathy. Also, since TNFα operates during the development of proliferative diabetic retinopathy (Limb et al., 1999), PDE4 inhibitors should be in this case effective. PDE4 inhibitors are also able to inhibit superoxide production (Barnette et al., 1995) which mainly results from oxidative stress secondarily to hyperglycemia.

All together, it seems that PDE3 and PDE4 inhibitors should represent new classes of compounds with potential therapeutical effects on diabetes development and on their associated cardiovascular diseases. Therefore re-investigations with new generations of very potent and specific PDE 3 and PDE4 inhibitors (for review Stoclet et al., 1995) as well as molecular biology studies should be run to ascertain the respective roles of PDE3 and PDE4 in diabetes. Since PDE3 seems to be involved in the insulin mechanism and PDE4 in the TNFα and superoxide productions, it is plausible that a mixed PDE3/PDE4 inhibitor would be the answer.

Acknowledgements:

Dr Thérèse Keravis is acknowledged for critical reading of the manuscript. Dr Claire Lugnier is supported by CNRS.

REFERENCES

André-Schmutz, I., Hindelang, C., Benoist, C., and Mathis, D., 1999, Cellular and molecular changes accompanying the progression from insulitis to diabetes, *Eur. J. Immunol.* 29:245.

Barnette, M.S., Manning, C.D., Cieslinski, L.B., Burman, M., Christensen, S.B., and Torphy, T.J., 1995, The ability of phosphodiesterase IV inhibitors to suppress superoxide production in guinea pig eosinophils is correlated with inhibition of phosphodiesterase IV catalytic activity, *J. Pharmacol. Exp. Ther.* 273:674.

Barnette, M.S., Christensen, S.B., Essayan, D.M., Grous, M., Prabhakar, U., Rush, J.A., Kagey-Sobotka, A., and Torphy, T.J., 1998, SB 207499 (Ariflo), a potent and selective second generation phosphodiesterase 4 inhibitor: in vitro anti-inflammatory actions, *J. Pharmacol. Exp. Ther.* 284:420.

Baynes, J.W., and Thorpe, S.R., 1999, Role of oxidative stress in diabetes complications: a new perspective on old paradigm, *Diabetes* 48:1.

Beavo, J.A., Conti, M., and Heaslip, R.J., 1994, Multiple cyclic nucleotide phosphodiesterases, *Mol. Pharmacol.* 46:399.

Boichot, E., Wallace, J.L., Germain, N., Lugnier, C., Lagente, V., and Bourguignon, J.J., 2000, Anti-inflammatory activities of a new series of selective phosphodiesterase 4 inhibitors derived from 9-benzyladenines, *J. Pharmacol. Exp. Ther.* 292:647.

Bourguignon, J.J., Désaubry, L., Raboisson, P., Wermuth, C.G., and Lugnier, C., 1997, 9-benzyladenines: potent and selective cAMP phosphodiesterase inhibitors, *J. Med. Chem.* 40:1768.

Dawson, D.L., Cutler, B.S., Meissner, M.H., and Strandness, D.E. Jr., 1998, Cilostazol has beneficial effects in treatment of intermittent claudication: results from a multicenter, randomized, prospective, double-blind trial, *Circulation* 98:678.

Degerman, E., Smith, C.J., Tornquist, H., Vasta, V., Belfrage, P., and Manganiello, V.C., 1990, Evidence that insulin and isoprenaline activate the cGMP-inhibited low-Km cAMP phosphodiesterase in rat fat cells by phosphorylation, *Proc. Natl. Acad. Sci. U.S.A.* 87:533.

Dousa, T.P., 1999, Cyclic-3',5'-nucleotide phosphodiesterase isozymes in cell biology and pathophysiology of the kidney, *Kidney Int.* 55:29.

Eckly, A.E., and Lugnier, C., 1994, Role of phosphodiesterases III and IV in the modulation of vascular cyclic AMP content by the NO/cyclic GMP pathway, *Br. J. Pharmacol.* 113:445.

Enoksson, S., Degerman, E., Hagstrom-Toft, E., Large, V., and Arner, P., 1998, Various phosphodiesterase subtypes mediate the in vivo antilipolytic effect of insulin on adipose tissue and skeletal muscle in man, *Diabetologia* 41:560.

Eriksson, H., Ridderstrale, M., Degerman, E., Ekholm, D., Smith, C.J., Manganiello, V., Belfrage, P., and Tornsqvist, H., 1995, Evidence for the key role of the adipocyte cGMP-inhibited cAMP phosphodiesterase in the antilipolytic action of insulin, *Biochim. Biophys. Acta* 1266:101.

Folkmann, J., 1995, Angiogenesis in cancer, vascular, rheumatoid and other diseases, *Nature Med.* 1:27.

Fujishige, K., Kotera, J., Michibata, H., Yaasa, K., Takebayashi, S.I., Kumura, K., and Omori, K., 1999, Cloning and characterization of a novel human phosphodiesterase that hydrolyzes both cAMP and cGMP (PDE10A), *J. Biol. Chem.* 274:18438.

Graier, W.F., Simecek, S., Kukovetz, W.R., and Kostner, G.M., 1996, High D-glucose-induced changes in endothelial Ca^{2+}/EDRF signaling are due to generation of superoxide anions, *Diabetes* 45:1386.

Green, E.A., Eynon, E.E., and Flavell, R.A., 1998, Local expression of TNFα in neonatal NOD mice promotes diabetes by enhancing presentation of islet antigens, *Immunity* 9:733.

Homma, S., Gapstur, S.M., Coffey, A., Valtin, H., and Dousa, T.P., 1991, Role of cAMP-phosphodiesterase isozymes in pathogenesis of murine nephrogenic diabetes insipidus, *Am. J. Physiol.* 261:F345.

Johnson-Mills, K., Arauz, E., Coffey, R.G., Krzanowski, J.J. Jr., and Polson, J.B., 1998, Effect of CI-930 [3-(2H)-pyridazinone-4,5-dihydro-6-[4-(1H-imidazolyl) phenyl]-5-methyl monohydro chloride] and rolipram on human coronary artery smooth muscle cell proliferation, *Biochem. Pharmacol.* 56:1065.

Kawamura, K., Watanabe, K., and Kimura, Y., 1985, Effect of cilostazol, a new antithrombotic drug, on cerebral circulation, *Arzneim-Forsch./Drug Res.* 35:1149.

Kessler, T., and Lugnier, C., 1995, Rolipram increases cyclic GMP content in L-arginine-treated cultured bovine aortic endothelial cells, *Eur. J. Pharmacol.* 290:163.

Komas, N., Lugnier, C., and Stoclet, J.C., 1991, Endothelium-dependent and independent relaxation of the rat aorta by cyclic nucleotide phosphodiesterase inhibitors, *Br. J. Pharmacol.* 104:495.

Kondo, K., Umemura, K., Miyaji, M., and Nakashima, M., 1999, Milrinone a phosphodiesterase inhibitor, suppresses intimal thickening after photochemically induced endothelial injury in the mouse femoral artery, *Atherosclerosis* 142:133.

Leibowitz, M.D., Biswas, C., Brady, E.J., Conti, M., Cullinan, C.A., Hayes, N.S., Manganiello, V.C., Saperstein, R., Wang, L.H., Zafian, P.T., and Berger, J.,1995, A novel insulin secretagogue is a phosphodiesterase inhibitor, *Diabetes* 44:67.

Leitman, D.C., Fiscus, R.R., and Murad, F., 1986, Forskolin, phosphodiesterase inhibitors, and cyclic AMP analogs inhibit proliferation of cultured bovine aortic endothelial cells, *J. Cell. Physiol.* 127:237.

Liang, L., Beshay, E., and Prud'homme, G.J., 1998, The phosphodiesterase inhibitors pentoxifylline and rolipram prevent diabetes in NOD mice, *Diabetes* 47:570.

Limb, G.A., Soomro, H., Janikoun, S., Hollifield, R.D., and Shilling, J., 1999, Evidence for control of tumour necrosis factor-alpha (TNFα) activity by TNF receptors in patients with proliferative diabetic retinopathy, *Clin. Exp. Immunol.* 115:409.

Lopez-Aparicio, P., Belfrage, P., Manganiello, V.C., Kono, T., and Degerman, E., 1993, Stimulation by insulin of a serine kinase in human platelets that phosphorylates and activates the cGMP-inhibited cAMP phosphodiesterase, *Biochem. Biophys. Res. Commun.* 193:1137.

Lugnier, C., Stierlé, A., Beretz, A., Schoeffter, P., Le Bec, A., Wermuth, C.G., Cazenave, J.P., and Stoclet, J.C., 1983, Tissue and substrate specificity of inhibition by alkoxy-aryl-lactams of platelet and arterial smooth muscle cyclic nucleotide phosphodiesterase, *Biochem. Biophys. Res. Commun.* 113: 954.

Lugnier, C., Schoeffter, P., Le Bec, A., Strouthou, E., and Stoclet, J.C., 1986, Selective inhibition of cyclic nucleotide phosphodiesterases of human, bovine and rat aorta, *Biochem. Pharmacol.* 35:1743.

Lugnier, C., and Schini, V.B., 1990, Characterization of cyclic nucleotide phosphodiesterases from cultured bovine aortic endothelial cells, *Biochem. Pharmacol.* 39:75.

Lugnier, C., and Komas, N., 1993, Modulation of vascular cyclic nucleotide phosphodiesterases by cyclic GMP: role in vasodilatation, *Eur. Heart. J.* 14:141.

Manganiello, V.C., and Vaughan, M., 1973, An effect of insulin on cyclic 3':5'- monophosphate phosphodiesterase activity in fat cells, *J. Biol. Chem.* 248:7164.

Moberg, E., Enoksson, S., and Hagstrom-Toft, E., 1998, Importance of phosphodiesterase 3 for the lipolytic response in adipose tissue during insulin-induced hypoglycemia in normal man, *Horm. Metab. Res.* 30:684.

Morishita, R., Higaki, J., Hayasi, S.I., Aoki, M., Nakamura, S., Moriguchi, A., Matsushita, H., Matsumoto, K., Nakamura, T., and Ogihara, T., 1997, Role of hepatocyte growth factor in endothelial regulation: prevention of high D-glucose-induced endothelial cell death by prostaglandins and phosphodiesterase type 3 inhibitor, *Diabetologia* 40:1053.

Muller, B., Lugnier, C., and Stoclet, J.C., 1990a, Implication of cyclic AMP in the positive inotropic effects of cyclic GMP-inhibited cyclic AMP phosphodiesterase in the regulation of cardiac contraction, *J. Cardiovasc. Pharmacol.* 15:444.

Muller, B., Lugnier, C., and Stoclet, J.C., 1990b, Involvement of rolipram-sensitive cyclic AMP phosphodiesterase in the regulation of cardiac contraction, *J. Cardiovasc. Pharmacol.* 16:796.

Nagaoka, T., Shirakawa, T., Balon, T.W., Russell, J.C., and Fujita-Yamaguchi, Y., 1998, Cyclic nucleotide phosphodiesterase 3 expression in vivo: evidence for tissue-specific expression of phosphodiesterase 3A or 3B mRNA and activity in the aorta and adipose tissue of atherosclerosis-prone insulin-resistant rats, *Diabetes* 47:1135.

Navarro, J.F., Mora, C., Rivero, A., Gallego, E., Chahin, J., Macia, M., Mendez, M.L., and Garcia, J., 1999, Urinary protein excretion and serum tumor necrosis factor in diabetic patients with advanced renal failure: effect of pentoxifylline administration, *Am. J. Kidney Dis.* 33:458.

Pakala, S.V., Chivetta, M., Kelly, C.B., and Katz, J.D., 1999, In autoimmune diabetes the transition from benign to pernicious insulitis requires an islet cell response to TNFα, *J. Exp. Med.* 189:1053.

Palmer, D., Tsoi, K., and Maurice, D.H., 1998, Synergistic inhibition of vascular smooth muscle cell migration by phosphodiesterase 3 and phosphodiesterase 4 inhibitors, *Circ. Res.* 82:852.

Parker, J.C., VanVolkenburg, M.A., Ketchum, R.J., Brayman, K.L., and Andrews, K.M., 1995, Cyclic AMP phosphodiesterases of human and rat islet of Langerhans: contributions of type III and IV to the modulation of insulin secretion, *Biochem. Biophys. Res. Commun.* 217:916.

Rahn, T., Ridderstrale, M., Tornqvist, H., Manganiello, V., Fredrikson, G., Belfrage, P., and Degerman, E., 1994, Essential role of phosphatidylinositol 3-kinase in insulin-induced activation and phosphorylation of the cGMP-inhibited cAMP phosphodiesterase in rat adipocytes, *FEBS Lett.* 350:314.

Rahn, T., Rönnstrand, L., Leroy, M.J., Wernsted, C., Tornqvist, H., Manganiello, V.C., Belfrage, P., and Degerman, E., 1996, Identification of the site in the cGMP-inhibited phosphodiesterase phosphorylated in adipocytes in response to insulin and isoproterenol, *J. Biol. Chem.* 271:11575.

Rösen, P., Du, X., and Tschöpe, D.,1998, Role of oxygen derived radicals for vascular dysfunction in the diabetic heart: prevention by α-tocopherol? *Mol. Cell. Biochem.* 188:103.

Schaffer, S.W., Allo, S., Punna, S., and White, T., 1991, Defective response to cAMP-dependent protein kinase in non-insulin-dependent diabetic heart, *Am. J. Physiol.* 261:E369.

Shafiee-Nick, R., Pyne, N.J., and Furman, B.L., 1995, Effects of type-selective phosphodiesterase inhibitors on glucose-induced secretion and islet phosphodiesterase activity, *Br. J. Pharmacol.* 115:1486.

Smoake, J.A., Moy, G.M.M., Fang, B., and Solomon, S.S., 1995, Calmodulin-dependent cyclic AMP phosphodiesterase in liver plasma membranes: stimulated by insulin, *Arch. Biochem. Biophys.* 323:223.

Soderling, S.H., Bayuga, S.J., and Beavo, J.A., 1999, Isolation and characterization of a dual-substrate phosphodiesterase gene family: PDE10A, *Proc. Natl. Acad. Sci. U.S.A.* 96:1071.

Solomon, S.S., 1975, Effect of insulin and lipolytic hormones on cyclic AMP phosphodiesterase activity in normal and diabetic rat adipose tissue, *Endocrinology* 96:1366.

Solomon, S.S., Deaton, J., Shankar, T.P., and Palazzolo, M., 1986, Cyclic AMP phosphodiesterase in diabetes, effect of glyburide, *Diabetes* 35:1233.

Souness, J.E., Hassall, G.A., and Parrott, D.P., 1992, Inhibition of pig aortic smooth muscle cell DNA synthesis by selective type III and type IV cyclic AMP phosphodiesterase inhibitors, *Biochem. Pharmacol.* 44:857.

Spinas, G.A., 1999, The dual role of nitric oxide in islet β-cells, *News Physiol. Sci.* 14: 49.

Stoclet, J.C., Keravis, T., Komas, N., and Lugnier, C., 1995, Cyclic nucleotide phosphodiesterases as therapeutic targets in cardiovascular diseases, *Exp. Opin. Invest. Drugs* 4:1081.

Takahashi, S., Oida, K., Fujiwara, R., Maeda, H., Hayashi, S., Takai, H., Tamai, T., Nakai, T., and Miyabo, S., 1992, Effect of cilostazol, a cyclic AMP phosphodiesterase inhibitor, on the proliferation of rat aortic smooth muscle cells in culture, *J. Cardiovasc. Pharmacol.* 20:900.

Takeda, S., Lin, C.T., Morgano, P.G., McIntyre, S.J., and Dousa, T.P., 1991, High activity of low-Michaelis-Menten constant 3',5'-cyclic adenosine monophosphate-phosphodiesterase isozymes in renal inner medulla of mice with hereditary nephrogenic diabetes insipidus, *Endocrinology* 129:287.

Torphy, T.J., and Undem, B.J., 1991, Phosphodiesterase inhibitors: new opportunities for treatment of asthma, *Thorax* 46:512.

Wijkander, J., Landstrom, T., Manganiello, V., Belfrage, P., and Degerman, E., 1998, Insulin-induced phosphorylation and activation of phosphodiesterase 3B in rat adipocytes: possible role for protein kinase B but not mitogen-activated protein kinase or p70 S6 kinase, *Endocrinology* 139:219.

Yamaki, M., McIntyre, S., Murphy, J.M., Swinnen, J.V., Conti, M., and Dousa, T.P., 1993, ADH resistance of LLC-PK$_1$ cells caused by overexpression of cAMP-phosphodiesterase type-IV, *Kidney Int.* 43:1286.

Yerneni, K.K.V., Bai, W., Khan, B.V., Medford, R.M., and Natarajan, R., 1999, Hyperglycemia-induced activation of nuclear transcription factor KB in vascular smooth muscle cells, *Diabetes* 48:855.

Zhao, A.Z., Bornfeldt, K.E., and Beavo, J.A., 1998, Leptin inhibits insulin secretion by activation of phosphodiesterase 3B, *J. Clin. Invest.* 102:869.

Zinman, B., Hanley, A.J.G., Harris, S.B., Kwan. J., and Fantus, I.G., 1999, Circulating tumor necrosis factor-α concentrations in a native canadian population with high rates of type 2 diabetes mellitus, *J. Clin. Endocrinol. Metab.* 84:272.

ALTERATIONS IN G-PROTEIN-LINKED SIGNAL TRANSDUCTION

IN VASCULAR SMOOTH MUSCLE IN DIABETES*

Madhu B. Anand-Srivastava, Rui Wang and Yi Yong Liu

Department of Physiology
Faculty of Medicine
University of Montreal
Montreal, Quebec, Canada

ABSTRACT

The present studies were undertaken to determine the levels of stimulatory and inhibitory guanine nucleotide regulatory proteins (Gs and Gi respectively) and their relationship with adenylyl cyclase activity in aorta from 5-day streptozotocin-induced diabetic (STZ) rats. The levels of $Gi\alpha$-2 as determined by immunoblotting techniques using AS/7 antibody were significantly decreased by about 60% in STZ as compared to control rats, whereas the levels of $Gs\alpha$ were not altered. In addition, the stimulatory effect of cholera toxin (CT) on GTP-sensitive adenylyl cyclase was not different in STZ as compared to control rats. On the other hand, the stimulatory effects of $GTP\gamma S$, isoproterenol, glucagon, forskolin (FSK) and sodium fluoride on adenylyl cyclase were enhanced in STZ-rats. Furthermore, $GTP\gamma S$ inhibited FSK-stimulated adenylyl cyclase activity in a concentration-dependent manner (receptor independent functions of Gi) in control rats which was almost completely abolished in STZ rats. In addition, receptor-mediated inhibition of adenylyl cyclase by angiotensin II (AII), oxotremorine and atrial natriuretic peptide (ANP) was attenuated in STZ rats. These results suggest that the decreased expression of $Gi\alpha$, but not of $Gs\alpha$, may be responsible for the observed altered responsiveness of adenylyl cyclase to hormonal stimulation and inhibition in STZ-rats. It may thus be suggested that the decreased Gi activity may be one of the possible mechanisms responsible for the impaired vascular functions in diabetes.

INTRODUCTION

Cardiovascular complications of diabetes mellitus are responsible for most of morbidity and mortality associated with the disease. The adenylyl cyclase/cyclic AMP (cAMP) system is believed to be one of the biochemical mechanisms participating in the

Diabetes and Cardiovascular Disease: Etiology, Treatment and Outcomes
Edited by Aubie Angel *et al.*, Kluwer Academic/Plenum Publishers, 2001

263

regulation of cardiovascular function. The adenylyl cyclase system is composed of three components: receptor, catalytic subunit and stimulatory (Gs) and inhibitory (Gi) guanine nucleotide regulatory proteins[1, 2]. The stimulation and inhibition of adenylyl cyclase by hormones are mediated by two distinct G-proteins, Gs and Gi respectively that couple the receptor to the catalytic subunit. The G-proteins are heterotrimeric and are composed of α, β and γ subunits. The specificity of G-proteins is attributed to α subunits. Molecular cloning has revealed four different forms of Gsα resulting from the differential splicing of one gene [3-5] and three distinct forms of Giα; Giα-1, Giα-2 and Giα-3 encoded by three distinct genes [6-8]. All three forms of Giα (Giα-3) have been reported to be implicated in adenylyl cyclase inhibition [8] and activation of atrial K^+ channels [9]. In addition, five different β subunits of 35-36 kDa and seven γ subunits of 8-10 kDa have been identified by molecular cloning [10, 11]. Several functions of the complex $\beta\gamma$ subunit have been reported such as anchoring the G-protein to the membrane [10], stimulation of type II and IV enzyme [12], inhibition of Ca^{2+}/calmodulin or Gs-activated type I enzyme and activation of muscarinic-gated atrial K^+ channels [13]. Molecular cloning has also revealed eight different types of adenylyl cyclases but only types V and VI have been identified in heart and aorta [14-16].

The adenylyl cyclase/cAMP system has been implicated in both the control of heart contractility [17, 18] and vascular smooth msucle tone [19, 20]. Several abnormalities in the expression of G-proteins and adenylyl cyclase regulation have been demonstrated in various pathophysiological conditions, such as heart failure, hypertension and hypothyroidism [21-25]. The defective G-protein and adenylyl cyclase activity in STZ-induced acute diabetic liver has also been reported [26-29]. However, there are no reports that document alterations in the levels of G-proteins and their relationship with adenylyl cyclase in aorta from short time streptozotocin-induced diabetic (STZ) rats.

The present studies were therefore undertaken to determine the levels of G proteins (Gi and Gs) and their relation with adenylyl cyclase stimulation and inhibition in aorta from short-term STZ rats.

MATERIALS AND METHODS

Animal Preparation

Male Sprague-Dawley (SD) rats (200 g) (6-8 weeks-old) were maintained on standard rat chow and tap water and libitum with 12h light/dark cycles in a quiet environment. Diabetes was induced by intraperitoneal injection of streptozotocin (STZ, 60 mg/kg body weight), dissolved in sodium citrate buffer (pH 4.5). Age-matched control rats were injected with an equal volume of buffer solution. Blood glucose levels were monitored 5 days after the injection using a dextrometer (Ames). Streptozotocin-injected rats with blood glucose levels in excess of 26 mM were considered to be diabetic rats (STZ) and used in this study. The blood glucose level of control rats was 5.5 mM.

Preparation of Aorta Washed Particles

Aorta washed particles were prepared as described previously [23]. The dissected aortae were quickly frozen in liquid N_2 and pulverized to a fine powder, in a percussion mortar cooled in liquid N_2. They were stored at -70°C until assayed. After homogenization in a motor-driven Teflon/glass homogenizer in a buffer containing 10 mM-Tris/HCl and 1 mM-EDTA (pH 7.5), the homogenate was centrifuged at 16000 g for 10 min. The supernatant fraction was discarded, and the pellet was finally suspended in 10 mM-Tris/HCl/1 mM-EDTA and used for determination of adenylyl cyclase activity.

Cholera Toxin (CT) Treatment

Aorta washed particles were treated with CT as described previously [23].

Immunoblotting

Immunoblotting of G-proteins was performed as described earlier [23]. After SDS/PAGE, the separated proteins were electrophoretically transferred to nitrocellulose paper (Schleicher and Schuell) with a mini transfer apparatus (Bio-Rad) at 100 V for 1 hour or a semi-dry transblot apparatus (Bio-Rad) at 15 V for 45 min. After transfer, the membranes were washed twice in phosphate-buffered saline (PBS) and were incubated in PBS containing 3% BSA at room temperature for 2 hours. The blots were then incubated with antisera against G-proteins in PBS containing 1% BSA and 0.1% Tween-20 at room temperature for 2 h. The antigen-antibody complexes were detected by incubating the blots with goat anti-rabbit IgG (Bio-Rad) conjugated with horseradish peroxidase for 2 hours at room temperature. The blots were washed three times with PBS before reaction with enhanced-chemiluminescence (ECL) Western-blotting detection reagents from Amersham. Quantitative analysis of the G-proteins was performed by densitometric scanning of the autoradiographs employing the enhanced laser densitometer (LKB Ultrscan XL) and quantified using the gel Scan XL evaluation software (version 2.1) from Pharmacia (Quebec, Canada).

Adenylyl Cyclase Activity Determination

Adenylyl cyclase activity was determined by measuring $[^{32}P]$-cAMP formation from $[\alpha^{32}]ATP$, as described previously [23]. The assay medium containing 50 mM-glycylglycine, pH 7.5, 0.5 mM-MgATP, $[\alpha^{-32}P]ATP(1-1.5 \times 10^6$ c.p.m.), 5 mM $MgCl_2$ (in excess of the ATP concentration), 100 mM NaCl, 0.5 mM-cAMP, 1 mM 3-isobutyl-1-methylxanthine, 0.1 mM EGTA, 10 μM-guanosine 5'-[γ-thio]triphosphate (GTPγS) (or otherwise indicated), and an ATP regenerating system consisting of 2 mM-phosphocreatine, 0.1 mg of creatine kinase/ml and 0.1 mg of myokinase/ml in a final volume of 200 μl. Incubations were initiated by addition of the membrane preparation (30-70 μg) to the reaction mixture, which had been thermally equilibrated for 2 min at 37°C. The reactions, conducted in triplicate for 10 min at 37°C, were terminated by addition of 0.6 ml of 120 mM-zinc acetate. cAMP was purified by co-precipitation of other nucleotides with $ZnCO_3$, by addition of 0.5 ml of 144 mM Na_2CO_3 and subsequent chromatography by the double-column system, as described by Salomon et al.[30]. Under the assay conditions used, adenylyl cyclase activity was linear with respect to protein concentration and time of incubation. Protein was determined essentially as described by Lowry et al. (with crystalline BSA as standard) [31].

RESULTS

Effect of GTPγS on Adenylyl Cyclase Activity

Guanine nucleotides stimulate or inhibit adenylyl cyclase activity by interacting with G proteins. In order to investigate if G-proteins are impaired in aorta from STZ-rats, the effect of GTPγS on adenylyl cyclase activity was examined and the results are shown in Figure 1. GTPγS stimulated adenylyl cyclase activity in aorta from both STZ and control rats in a concentration-dependent manner; however, the extent of stimulation was significantly greater in STZ than control. GTPγS at 10 μM stimulated adenylyl cyclase activity by about 12-fold in STZ, whereas about 7-fold stimulation was observed in CTRL.

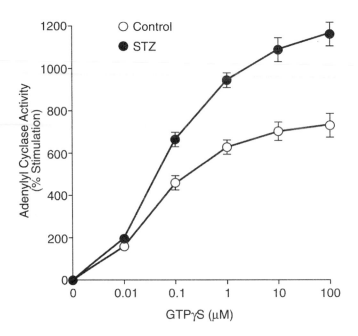

Figure 1. Effect of GTPγS on adenylyl cyclase activity in aorta from STZ-induced 5-day diabetic rats. Adenylyl cyclase activity was determined in aorta from control (CTRL) and STZ-induced diabetic rats (STZ)in the absence or presence of various concentrations of GTPγS as described in the «Materials and Methods». Values are means ± S.E.M. of three separate experiments. Basal enzyme activities in CTRL and STZ were 101.5 ± 8 and 61 ± 5 pmol of cAMP/10 min per mg of protein respectively. Six animal were utilized for each experiment.

These results indicate that G-protein may be impaired in STZ.

G-protein levels

In order to investigate if the increased responsiveness of adenylyl cyclase to GTPγS in aorta from STZ as compared to control rats was due to the increased levels of Gsα or decreased levels of Giα, the levels of G-proteins were determined by immunoblotting using specific antibodies; AS/7 antibodies against Giα-1 and Giα-2 and RM/1 antibodies against Gsα. As shown in Figure 2, AS/7 antibodies recognized a single protein of 40 KDa referred to Giα-2 (Giα-1 is absent in aorta [32]) from both control and STZ rats, however, the relative amount of immunodetectable Giα-2 was significantly decreased in STZ as compared to control rats by about 60% as determined by densitometric scanning. On the other hand, the levels of Gsα protein were not altered in STZ rats (in arbitrary units CTRL 1.4 ± 0.1, STZ, 1.5 ± 0.15 (n = 3).

To corroborate our results with the functions of G-proteins, the effect of cholera toxin (CT) on adenylyl cyclase activity was investigated. CT stimulated adenylyl cyclase in aorta from both control and STZ rats, however, the percent stimulation was not significantly different in two groups (data not shown). These results suggest that the functions of Gsα in aorta were also not altered in STZ rats.

Hormonal Regulation of Adenylyl Cyclase

Since the levels and functions of Gsα were not altered in STZ rats, it was of interest

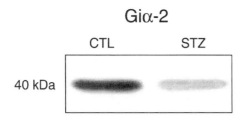

Figure 2. Quantification of Gsα-2 proteins by immunoblotting in aorta from control (CTL) and STZ-induced rats (STZ). The membrane proteins (50 μg) from CTL and STZ were separated on SDS-PAGE and transferred to nitrocellulose which was then immunoblotted using AS/7 antibody specific for Giα-2 as described in the «Materials and Methods». The autoradiograph is representative of 3 separate experiments.

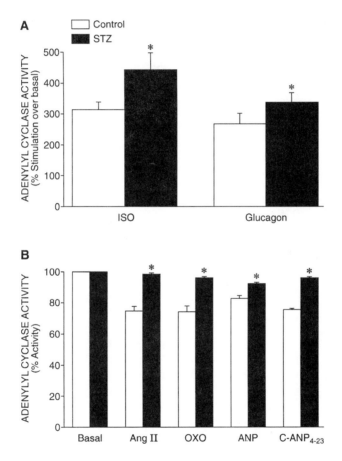

Figure 3. Effects of various agonists on adenylyl cyclase activity in aorta from control (CTRL) and STZ-induced diabetic rats (STZ). Adenylyl cyclase activity was determined in the presence of 10 μM GTP alone or in combination with 50 μM isoproterenol (ISO) or 1 μM glucagon (GLU) (A) or 10 μM GTPγS alone (basal) or in combination with 10 μM angiotensin II (Ang II), 50 μM oxotremorine (OXO) 0.1 μM atrial natriuretic peptide (ANP) or 0.1 μM ring deleted ANP (C-ANP$_{4-23}$) (B) as described in «Materials and Methods». Values are the means ± S.E.M. of three separate experiments. Six animals from each group were utilized for each experiment. Adenylyl cyclase activities in the presence of GTP in CTRL and STZ rats were 198 ±32.7 and 192 ± 26.6 pmol cAMP (mg protein. 10 min)$^{-1}$ respectively and in the presence of 10 μM GTPγS were 831 ± 27 and 540 ± 21 pmol cAMP (mg protein.10 min)$^{-1}$ respectively. *P < 0.05.

to investigate if Gs mediated hormonal stimulations were also unaltered in STZ rats. Results shown in Figure 3A demonstrate that isoproterenol and glucagon, stimulated adenylyl cyclase activity in aorta from both the groups, however, the extent of stimulation was significantly augmented in STZ-diabetic rats as compared to control rats. For example, isoproterenol and glucagon stimulated adenylyl cyclase activity by about 300% and 250% respectively in control and about 450% and 350% respectively in STZ rats. In addition, FSK- and NaF-stimulated enzyme activities were also augmented in STZ-rats (data not shown).

Adenylyl cyclase activity is regulated by dual pathways; stimulatory and inhibitory, mediated by Gsα and Giα respectively. Since the levels of Giα proteins were decreased in STZ rats, it was of interest to examine if the functions of Giα were also attenuated in these rats. For this reason, the receptor-dependent and receptor independent functions of Gi were studied and the results are shown in Figure 3B. and Figure 4 respectively. Angiotensin II (Ang II), oxotremorine (OXO), atrial natriuretic peptide (ANP$_{99-126}$) and ring deleted peptide of ANP (C-ANP$_{4-23}$) that inhibit adenylyl cyclase through Gi [33-35] inhibited the enzyme activity by about 20%, 24%, 21% and 24% in control rats; which was almost completely attenuated in STZ rats (Figure 3B). Similarly, GTPγS inhibited FSK-stimulated activity in a concentration-dependent manner in control rats which was almost completely attenuated in STZ rats, suggesting a correlation between the decreased levels and decreased functions of Gi in STZ rats.

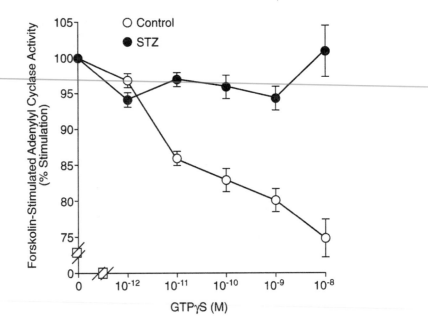

Figure 4. Effect of GTPγS on forskolin-stimulated adenylyl cyclase activity in aorta from control and STZ-induced diabetic rats (STZ). Adenylyl cyclase activity was determined in the absence or presence of 100 μM FSK alone or in combination with various concentrations of GTPγS in aorta from control (O) and STZ rats (●) as described in the «Materials and Methods». Values are means ± SEM of 3 separate experiments. Six animals were utilized for each experiment. Adenylyl cyclase activity in the presence of 100 μM FSK in aorta from control and STZ rats were 603 ± 25 and 381 ± 27 pmol cAMP (mg protein.10 min)$^{-1}$ respectively.

DISCUSSION

In the present studies, we demonstrate for the first time that adenylyl cyclase activity, its responsiveness to various hormones as well as the levels of Giα but not of Gsα are altered in aorta from STZ rats as compared with control rats.

A significant increase in the responsiveness of adenylyl cyclase to GTPγS stimulation in aorta from STZ rats as compared to control rats may be attributed to the increased sensitivity of Gsα or increased levels of Gsα or decreased levels of Giα in aorta from STZ rats. However, our results did not demonstrate any changes in the levels or functions of Gsα in STZ rats and suggest that the Gsα may not be responsible for the increased sensitivity of adenylyl cyclase to GTPγS stimulation.

Since the levels of Giα-2 were decreased in aorta from STZ rat, it may be possible that the decreased level of Giα-2 may be responsible for the enhanced stimulation of adenylyl cyclase by GTPγS in STZ rat. The decreased levels of Giα-2 were also reflected in the decreased functions, as has been demonstrated by an attenuation of the inhibitory responses of Ang II, OXO, ANP and C-ANP on adenylyl cyclase activity. However, it appears that a partial decrease (~ 60%) in the levels of Giα-2 observed in aorta from STZ as compared to control rats may be enough to uncouple the hormone receptors from adenylyl cyclase system or alternatively, some other mechanisms at the receptor level, such as receptor down regulation, may also be responsible for a complete attenuation of inhibitory responses on adenylyl cyclase. In this context, the down regulation of ANP receptors in various models of hypertension and congestive heart failure has been demonstrated in various tissues including platelets [36, 37].

Taken together, it is suggested that the decreased levels of Giα-2 in aorta from STZ rat may partly be responsible for the attenuated receptor-mediated inhibition of adenylyl cyclase by ANG II, OXO, ANP, C-ANP and receptor-independent inhibition, i.e. the inhibition of forskolin stimulated adenylyl cyclase activity by low concentration of GTPγS.

The hyperresponsiveness of adenylyl cyclase of aorta from STZ rat to ISO and glucagon stimulation as compared to control rats may be attributed to the upregulation of hormone receptors or increased levels of Gsα. However, several studies have shown a down-regulation or no change in the number of stimulatory hormone receptors in various cardiovascular diseases [38]. Furthermore, since no alterations in the levels and functions of Gsα were observed in STZ, the enhanced stimulation of adenylyl cyclase by ISO and glucagon cannot be explained by Gsα. Based on our results in STZ rats, it is possible that the augmented responsiveness of adenylyl cyclase to ISO and glucagon in STZ rats may be attributed to decreased levels of Giα-2 proteins. In this regard, pertussis toxin and amiloride which inactivate the Gi protein have been shown to augment the stimulatory responses of hormones on adenylyl cyclase[33, 39]. Similarly, the enhanced stimulation of adenylyl cyclase by FSK and NaF in aorta from STZ rat as compared to CTRL rats may be due to the hypersensitivity of the catalytic subunit of the adenylyl cyclase system per se or to the decreased expression of Giα-2 or both. The Gi-mediated regulation of FSK-stimulated enzyme activity has been shown previously[33, 39]. On the other hand, the requirement of Gs and guanine nucleotides for the FSK activation of adenylyl cyclase has also been reported [40]. Since the present studies do not demonstrate any alteration in Gsα, the increased sensitivity of adenylyl cyclase to FSK stimulation in diabetes cannot be attributed to the Gs activity. Taken together, the data indicate that the decreased levels of Giα-2 in aorta from STZ rats may partly be responsible for the observed augmentation of the FSK-sensitive adenylyl cyclase activity.

In conclusion, the expression of Giα is decreased in aorta from STZ, whereas the levels of Gsα were not altered. The decreased expression of Giα-2 appears to explain, in part, the attenuated responsiveness of adenylyl cyclase to inhibitory hormones and augmented responsiveness to stimulatory hormones and agents that activate adenylyl cyclase by receptor-independent mechanisms. It is suggested that the decreased expression of Giα in aorta from STZ may be one of the mechanisms responsible for the impaired cardiovascular function in diabetes.

Abbreviations

ANP, atrial natriuretic peptide (99-126), C-ANP$_{4-23}$, a ring deleted analog of atrial natriuretic peptide; C-ANP$_{4-23}$,[des(Gln18,Ser^{19},Gln^{20},Leu^{21},Gly^{22})ANP$_{4-23}$-NH$_2$]. Gi inhibitory gaunine nucleotide regulatory protein, GTPγS, guanosine 5'-0-(3-thiotriphoshate), FSK, forskolin, AII, angitoensin II.

Acknowledgements

We would like to thank Christiane Laurier for her valuable secretarial help.

Footnotes

*   This work was supported by grant from Medical Research Council of Canada

REFERENCES

1. Neer EJ. Heterotrimeric G proteins. Organizers of transmembrane signals. *Cell* 1995; 80:249-257.
2. Fleming JW, Wisler PL, Watanabe AM. Signal transduction by G-proteins in cardiac tissues. *Circulation* 1992;85:420-433.
3. Murakami T, Yasuda H. Rat heart cell membranes contain three substrate for cholera toxin-catalyzed ADP-ribosylation and a single substrate for Pertussis toxin-catalyzed ADP-ribosylation. *Biochem. Biophys. Res. Commun.* 1986;138:1355-1361.
4. Robishaw JD, Smigel MD, Gilman AG. Molecular basis for two forms of the G-protein that stimulate adenylate cyclase. *J. Biol. Chem.* 1986;261:9587-9590.
5. Bray P, Caster A, Simons C, Guo V, Puckett C, Hamholz J, Spiegel A, Nirenberg H. Human cDNA clones for four species of Gsα signal transduction protein. *Proc. Natl. Acad. Sci. U.S.A.* 1986;83:8893-8897.
6. Itoh H, Kozaka T, Magata S, Nakamura S, Katada T, Ui M, Iwai S, Ohtsuka E, Kawasaki H, Suzuki K, Kaziro Y. Molecular cloning and sequence determination of cDNAs for α subunits of the guanine nucleotide-binding proteins Gs, Gi and Go from brain. *Proc. Natl. Acad. Sci. U.S.A.* 1986;83:3776-3780.
7. Itoh H, Toyama R, Kozasa T, Tsukamoto T, Matsuoka M, Kaziro Y. Presence of three distinct molecular species of Gi protein: a subunit structure of rat cDNA and human genomic DNAs. *J. Biol. Chem.* 1988;263:6656-6664.
8. Wong YH, Conklin BB, Bourne HR. G2-mediated hormonal inhibition of cyclic AMP accunulation. *Science* 1992;255:339-342.
9. Yatani A, Mattera R, Codina J. The G-protein gated atrial K$^+$ channels is stimulated by three distinct Giα subunits. *Nature* 1988;336:680-682.
10. Simon MI, Strathmann MP, Gautam N. *Science* 1991;252:802-808.
11. Cali JJ, Balcueva EA, Rybalkin I, Robishaw JD. Selective tissue distribution of G protein γ subunits, including a new form of the γ subunits identified by cDNA cloning. *J. Biol. Chem.* 1992;267:24023-24027.
12. Tang W-J, Gilman AG. Type-specific regulation of adenylyl cyclase by G protein βγ subunits. *Science* 1991; 254:1500-1503.
13. Wickman KD, Iniguez-Liuhi JA, Davenport PA, Taussig R, Krapivinski GB, Linder ME, Gilman AG, Clapham DE. Recombinant G-protein βγ subunit activate the muscarinic-gated atrial potassium channel. *Nature* 1994;368:255-257.
14. Tang W-J, Gilman AG. Adenylyl cyclase. *Cell* 1992;70:869-872.
15. Premont RT, Chen J, Ma H-W, Ponnapalli M, Iyengar R. Two members of a widely expressed subfamily of hormone-stimulated adenylyl cyclases. *Proc. Natl. Acad. Sci U.S.A* 1992;89:9809-9813.
16. Katsushika S, Chen L, Kawabe J-I, Nilakantan R, Halnon NJ, Homcy CJ, Ishikawa Y. Cloning and

characterization of a sixth adenylyl cyclase isoform: type V and VI constitute a subgroup within the mammalian adenylyl cyclase family. *Proc. Natl. Acad. Sci. U.S.A* 1992;89:8774-8778.

17. Katz AM, Tada M, Kirchberger MA. Control of calcium transport in the myocardium by the cyclic AMP-protein kinase system. *Adv. Cyclic Nucleotide Res.* 1975;5:453-472.

18. Keely SL Jr, Lincoln TM, Corbin JD. Interaction of acetylcholine and epinephrine on heart cyclic AMP-dependent protein kinase. *Am. J. Physiol.* 1978;234:H432-H438.

19. Triner L, Vulliemoz Y, Verosky M, Habif DV, Nahas VV. Adenylyl cyclase phosphodiesterase system in arterial smooth muscle. *Life Sci* 1972; 11:817-824.

20. Bär H-P. Cyclic nucleotides and smooth muscle. *Adv. Cyclic nucleotide Res.* 1974;4:195-237.

21. Feldman AM, Cates AE, Veazey WB, Hershberger RE, Bristow MR, Baughman KL, Baumgartner WA, Dop CV. Increase of the 40,000 mol wt pertussis toxin substrate (G-protein) in the failing human heart. *J Clin Invest* 1988;82:189-197.

22. Malbon CC, Rapiejko PJ, Watkins DC. Permissive hormone regulation of hormone-sensitive effector systmes. *Trends Pharmacol Sci* 1988;9:33-36.

23. Anand-Srivastava MB. Enhanced expression of inhibitory guanine nucleotide regulatory protein in spontaneously hypertensive rats: relationship to adenylate cyclase inhibition. *Biochem J* 1992;288:79-85.

24. Thibault C, Anand-Srivastava MB. Altered expression of G-protein mRNA in spontaneously hypertensive rats. *FEBS Lett* 1992;313:160-164.

25. Anand-Srivastava MB, de Champlain , Thibault C. DOCA-salt hypertensive rat hearts exhibit altered expression of G-protiens. *Am J Hypertens* 1993;6:72-75.

26. Lynch CJ, Blackmore PF, Johnson EH,Wange RL, Krone, PK, Exton JH. Guanine nucleotide binding regulatory proteins and adenylate cyclase in livers of streptozotocin- and BB/Wor-diabtic rats. Immunodetection of Gs and Gi with antisera prepared against synthetic peptides. *J Clin Invest* 83:2050-2062.

27. Bushfield M, Griffiths SL, Strassheim D, Tang E, Shakur Y, Lavan B, Houslay MD. Guanine-nucleotide-binding proteins in diabetes and insulin-resistant states. *Biochem Soc Symp* 1990; 56:137-154.

28. Gawler D, Milligan G, Spiegel AM, Unson CG, Houslay MD. Aboltion of the expression f inhibitory guanine nucleotide regulatory protein Gi activity in diabetes. *Nature* 1987;327:229-232.

29. Bushfield M, Griffiths SL, Murphy GJ, Pyne, NJ, Knowler JT, Milligan G, Parker PJ, Mollner S, Houslay MD. Diabetes-induced alterations in the expressio, functioning and phosphorylation state of the inhibitory guanine nucleotide regulatory protein Gi-2 in hepatocytes. *Biochem J* 1990;271:365-372.

30. Salomon Y, Londos C, Rodbell M. A highly sensitive adenylate cyclase assay. *Anal Biochem* 1974;58:541-548.

31. Lowry OM, Rosebrough NJ, Farr AL, Randall RJ. Protein measurement with the folin phenol reagent. *J Biol Chem* 1951;193:265-275.

32. Jones DT, Reed RR. Molecular cloning of five GTP-binding protein cDNA species from rat olfactory neuroepithelium. *J Biol Chem* 1987; 262:14241-14249.

33. Anand-Srivatava MB, Srivastava AK, Cantin M. Pertussis toxin attenuates atrial natriuretic factor-mediated inhibtion of adenylate cyclase. Involvement of inhibitory guanine nucleotide regulatory protein. *J Biol Chem* 1987;262:4931-4934.

34. Anand-Srivastava MB, Sairam MR, Cantin M. Ring-deleted analogs of atrial natriuretic factor inhibits adenylyl cyclase/cAMP system: possible coupling of clearance atrial natriuretic factor receptors to adenylate cyclase/cAMP signal transduction system. *J Biol Chem* 1990;265:8566-8572

35. Anand-Srivastava MB. Angiotensin II receptors negatively coupled to adenylate cyclase in rat myocardial sarcolemma: involvement of inhibitory guanine nucleotide protein. *Bniochem Pharmacol* 1989;38:489-496.

36. Swithers SE, Stewart RE, McCarty R. Binding sites for atrial natriuretic factor (ANF) in kidneys and adrenal glands of spontaneously hypertensive (SHR) rats. *Life Sci* 1987;1673-1681.

37. Schiffrin EL. Decreased density of binding sites for atrial natriuretic peptide on platelets of patients with severe congestive heart failure. *Clin Sci* 1988;74:213-218.

38. Limas C, Limas CJ. Reduced number of β-adrenergic recpetors in the myocardium of spontaneously hypertensive rats. *Biochem Biophys Res Commun* 1978;83:710-714.

39. Anand-Srivastava MB. Amiloride interacts with guanine nucletoide regulatory proteins and attenuates the hormonal inhibition of adenylate cyclase. *J Biol Chem* 1989;264:9491-9496.

40. Hildebrandt JD, Hanoune J, Birnbaumer J. Guanine nucleotide inhibition of cyc-S49 mouse lymphoma cell membrane adenylyl cyclase. *J Biol chem* 1982;257:14723-14725.

MECHANISM OF HDL LOWERING IN INSULIN RESISTANT STATES

Gary F. Lewis[1], Shirya Rashid[1], Kristine D. Uffelman and Benoît Lamarche[2]

[1]Department of Medicine, Division of Endocrinology, University of Toronto, Toronto, Canada
[2]Department of Food Sciences and Nutrition and Lipid Research Center, Laval University Hospital Research Center
Ste-Foy, Quebec, Canada

INTRODUCTION

Hypertriglyceridemia and low plasma HDL-cholesterol (HDL-c) are the lipid abnormalities that typically occur as a consequence of insulin resistant conditions, including abdominal obesity, impaired fasting glucose and Type 2 diabetes. HDL-c and apolipoprotein A-1 (apo A-1, the major protein moiety of HDL particles) are inversely associated with plasma triglycerides (TG). In fact, the majority of individuals who have HDL-c levels below the 10th percentile for age and gender have some degree of fasting and/or postprandial hypertriglyceridemia, insulin resistance and abdominal obesity. Hypertriglyceridemia is due predominantly to elevated very low density lipoprotein (VLDL) production by the liver in the fasting state and delayed clearance of intestinally-derived chylomicrons and hepatically-derived VLDL in the postprandial state. In hypertriglyceridemic states there is active lipid exchange between TG-rich lipoproteins (VLDL and chylomicrons) and HDL. We hypothesise that TG enrichment of HDL particles, followed by lipolytic modification by HL, enhances the clearance of HDL particles from the circulation, ultimately lowering plasma HDL-c concentrations. Since we have recently reviewed in detail the various lines of evidence in support of this hypothesis,[1] the present brief review will summarize only our own recent work in this area.

POSTPRANDIAL HDL CHANGES IN INSULIN RESISTANT AND DIABETIC HUMANS

In a series of studies we characterized the postprandial changes in TG-rich lipoproteins and HDL.[2,3,4,5,6] The studies were performed in; 1. healthy lean,[5] 2. obese, insulin resistant, non-diabetic,[5] 3. type 2 diabetic,[6] 4. type 1 diabetic individuals [3,4] and 5. in individuals with isolated low HDL-c[7] . We made the following general observations regarding postprandial changes in HDL.

Diabetes and Cardiovascular Disease: Etiology, Treatment and Outcomes
Edited by Aubie Angel *et al.*, Kluwer Academic/Plenum Publishers, 2001

273

The TG content of fasting HDL particles in normolipidemic individuals is usually extremely low, constituting no more than 3 to 5% by mass. Due to cholesteryl ester transfer protein (CETP)-mediated exchange of HDL core lipids with the core lipids of TG-rich lipoproteins, the TG content of HDL may approximately double at the peak of postprandial lipemia (usually 3 to 5 hours after ingestion of fat.) HDL phospholipids increase proportionately and cholesteryl ester declines in the postprandial state. Hypertriglyceridemic diabetic and non-diabetic individuals have TG enrichment of their HDL in the fasting state (typically the TG content of HDL may be in the order of 10 to 20% by weight, depending on the magnitude of hypertriglyceridemia) and the HDL particles are predominantly small and of the HDL_3 subclass. In hypertriglyceridemia individuals HDL becomes further enriched with TGs (up to 20 to 25% by weight) in the postprandial state. The magnitude of TG-enrichment of HDL is determined predominantly by the magnitude of the hypertriglyceridemia (ie, the pool size of the TG rich lipoproteins) and CETP mass is usually not rate-limiting in most physiological conditions.

Since the postprandial TG enrichment of HDL particles occurs predominantly by CETP-mediated heteroexchange of TG for cholesteryl ester (CE), there is a reciprocal decrease in HDL CE at the peak of postprandial lipemia. HDL-c levels therefore decline postprandially in a mirror image to the elevation of plasma TGs (reaching a nadir usually at 3 to 5 hours following ingestion of a high fat mixed meal). HDL-c levels return slowly to baseline over the ensuing hours. Interestingly there is no significant decline in plasma apo A1 postprandially, suggesting that there is no major decline in HDL particle numbers acutely in the postprandial state. We and others have found positive correlations between fasting and postprandial TGs and the magnitude of HDL TG enrichment and inverse correlations between HDL TG enrichment and fasting plasma HDL-c concentration. This latter observation raised the question of a potential causal relationship between HDL-TG enrichment and the lowering of plasma HDL-c concentration, an observation which lead to the mechanistic studies described below.

THE EFFECT OF LIPOLYSIS ON HDL IN HUMANS

O'Meara et al[8] administered an intravenous bolus of heparin to humans at the peak of postprandial lipemia, to stimulate intravascular lipolysis. They found that in normolipidemic individuals there was very little change in HDL size, composition and subclass distribution after rapid lipolysis induced by IV heparin. In contrast, hypertriglyceridemic individuals had marked changes in HDL size and composition after IV heparin, with the formation of small HDL particles (HD3c.) The quantity of small particles formed after lipolysis was directly related to the preheparin HDL TG content. An unresolved question arising from that study was whether the transformation of HDL particles with heparin was an intrinsic property of the individual's HDL, or whether this process could be modified with lipid-lowering therapy, presumably by altering the composition of the HDL particles. We proceeded to examine whether the generation of lipolysis-induced small HDL particles in hypertriglyceridemic individuals can be reduced after 3 months of TG-lowering treatment with gemfibrozil.[9] TG-lowering therapy resulted in a reduction of plasma TG's and HDL TG content, an increase in fasting HDL-c, and proportionately fewer HDL3c particles formed post-heparin, administered at the peak of postprandial lipemia. These results showed that the postprandial increase in TG levels in hypertriglyceridemic subjects is associated with increased production of small HDL particles when lipolysis is stimulated, and that lipid-lowering therapy can contribute to favourably reduce this postprandial production of small HDL particles. The logical question to arise from these observations was whether these small, lipolytically modified HDL particles, formed from lipolysis of TG-rich HDL, are cleared more rapidly from the circulation, thus contributing to an overall lowering of HDL-c in hypertriglyceridemic states.

HDL KINETIC STUDIES IN A RABBIT MODEL

To address this question, we turned to the rabbit model. Because rabbits are naturally deficient in hepatic lipase (HL), the fate of human lipoproteins injected into the rabbit circulation can be traced, with minimal further *in vivo* modification by this key catalytic enzyme. We modified the size and composition of HDL *in vivo* in hypertriglyceridemic humans by administering an IV bolus of heparin 5 hours after an oral fat load, to stimulate the release of endothelial lipases.[10] Large TG-rich preheparin HDL and small, lipolytically modified, postheparin HDL particles were isolated from the human subjects, radiolabeled, and their clearance rates determined in New Zealand white rabbits. The fractional catabolic rate (FCR) of the small, postheparin HDL particles was 45% greater than that of the larger, TG-rich postprandial particles when the tracers were injected sequentially into the rabbit. In a second study in NZW rabbits[11] we examined the impact of particle size and lipid composition in determining the metabolic clearance of human HDL, in the absence of substantial in vivo modification of the particles by HL. Small and large HDL particles were isolated either from normo- or hypertriglyceridemic humans by gel filtration chromatography and were labeled with either ^{125}I or [131]I. The clearance of the HDL tracers was determined over approximately 72 hours following injection into NZW rabbits. Surprisingly, it was the large HDL particles which were cleared more rapidly than the small particles which, in contrast to the study described above, were not lipolytically modified. In addition, there was no difference in the FCR of HDL isolated from normo- and hypertriglyceridemic humans. There was also no correlation between the TG content of HDL and its FCR. These results, combined with our previous observations, support the hypothesis that triglyceride enrichment of HDL, in the absence of substantial lipolytic modification, is not sufficient to enhance the clearance of HDL from the circulation. Stated another way, TG enrichment of HDL is necessary, but not sufficient, to enhance the metabolic clearance of apo A1-associated with HDL.

HDL KINETIC STUDIES IN HUMANS

The studies described above took advantage of the fact that rabbits have a natural deficiency of HL, which allowed us to examine the clearance of human HDL apo A1 in the absence of substantial further *in vivo* lipolytic modification. The disadvantage and limitation of such interspecies studies, however, is that the relevance of these findings for human physiology is questionable. Humans have abundant HL activity and there are a number of additional important differences in lipoprotein physiology between humans and rabbits. To overcome these limitations, we studied the effect of TG-enrichment of human HDL on the clearance of HDL-associated apo A1 in humans.[12]

HDL was isolated from the plasma of normolipidemic men in the fasting state and following a five hour intravenous infusion of a synthetic triglyceride emulsion, Intralipid. The Intralipid infusion resulted in a physiological ~2-fold increase in the TG content of HDL. Each tracer was then whole labeled with ^{125}I or ^{131}I and injected into the subject. Apo A1 in TG-rich HDL was cleared 26% more rapidly than apo A1 in fasting HDL. A strong correlation between the Intralipid-induced increase in the TG content of HDL and the increase in HDL apo A1 FCR reinforced the importance of TG enrichment of HDL in enhancing its metabolic clearance. Most of this difference was attributed to the clearance of lipoproteins containing only apo A1, without A2 (LpA1). The HDL compositional changes that occurred with Intralipid infusion in our study were very similar to those generally seen after an oral fat load. The 5 hr Intralipid infusion resulted in a slight, but non-significant, decrease in the cholesterol content of HDL, unaltered apo A-I or A-II concentrations, but a significant decrease in apo C-III and E levels. Therefore, it is possible that part of the increased FCR of apo A-I from triglyceride enriched HDL may be attributed to changes in components other than the triglyceride content of the particle. Our study did not allow us to identify a precursor-product relationship between large and small HDL particles and there was no size difference between normal and triglyceride enriched HDL. Therefore, we were not able to determine if the triglyceride enrichment of HDL enhanced the formation of small HDL particles arising from the hydrolysis of large HDL. Results from our study, however, support the concept that triglyceride enrichment of HDL, directly or indirectly, enhances the metabolic clearance of the particles in humans, a species with significant hepatic lipase activity. This was the first direct demonstration in humans that TG enrichment of HDL enhances the clearance of HDL apo A1 from the circulation. This phenomenon could provide an important mechanism explaining how HDL apo A1 and HDL-c are lowered in hypertriglyceridemic states.

SUMMARY AND FUTURE DIRECTIONS

The results of our studies and those of others (reviewed in [1]) provide strong evidence for an important role of TG-enrichment of HDL in enhancing its metabolic clearance, presumably contributing to an overall lowering of HDL-c plasma concentrations. This mechanism is likely to play an important role in hypertriglyceridemic states, which are commonly associated with insulin resistance. It is unlikely that a single pathophysiological mechanism, such as this, can be invoked to explain all cases of low HDL-c, and other mechanisms have also been shown to be important.

The effect of HDL-TG enrichment on the important pathway of selective cholesteryl ester uptake by liver and steroidogenic tissues has not yet been examined in detail, and our present studies (not discussed) are designed to examine that issue. The precise mechanism by which HDL TG-enrichment enhances particle clearance is also not known, and will likely become the subject of intense examination in ensuing years. Our present working hypothesis is that HDL TG-enrichment enhances the particle's susceptibility to lipolysis by hepatic lipase, but the biochemical mechanism by which this occurs and the mechanism by which lipolytic modification of TG-rich HDL enhances HDL clearance are presently not known. It is still possible that TG-enrichment of HDL may be a marker of more fundamental biochemical conformational changes in lipids and apolipoproteins affecting the particle stability, thereby enhancing particle clearance and lowering plasma HDL-c in insulin resistant and hypertriglyceridemic states.

REFERENCES

1. B.Lamarche, S.Rashid, and G.F.Lewis, HDL metabolism in hypertriglyceridemic states. An overview., *Clin. Chim. Acta* 286:145 (1999).
2. G.F.Lewis, Postprandial lipoprotein metabolism in diabetes mellitus and obesity. *J. Atheroscler. Thromb.* 2 Suppl 1:S34 (1995).
3. G.F.Lewis and V.G.Cabana, Postprandial changes in high-density lipoprotein composition and subfraction distribution are not altered in patients with insulin- dependent diabetes mellitus, *Metabolism* 45:1034 (1996).
4. G.F.Lewis, N.M.O'Meara, V.G.Cabana, J.D.Blackman, W.L.Pugh, A.F.Druetzler, J.R.Lukens, G.S.Getz, and K.S.Polonsky, Postprandial triglyceride response in type 1 (insulin-dependent) diabetes mellitus is not altered by short-term deterioration in glycaemic control or level of postprandial insulin replacement, *Diabetologia* 34:253 (1991).
5. G.F.Lewis, N.M.O'Meara, P.A.Soltys, J.D.Blackman, P.H.Iverius, A.F.Druetzler, G.S.Getz, and K.S.Polonsky, Postprandial lipoprotein metabolism in normal and obese subjects: comparison after the vitamin A fat-loading test, *Journal of Clinical Endocrinology & Metabolism* 71:1041 (1990).
6. G.F.Lewis, N.M.O'Meara, P.A.Soltys, J.D.Blackman, P.H.Iverius, W.L.Pugh, G.S.Getz, and K.S.Polonsky, Fasting hypertriglyceridemia in noninsulin-dependent diabetes mellitus is an important predictor of postprandial lipid and lipoprotein abnormalities, *J. Clin. Endocrinol. Metab.* 72:934 (1991).
7. N.M.O'Meara, G.F.Lewis, V.G.Cabana, P.H.Iverius, G.S.Getz, and K.S.Polonsky, Role of basal triglyceride and high density lipoprotein in determination of postprandial lipid and lipoprotein responses, *J. Clin. Endocrinol. Metab.* 75:465 (1992).

8. N.M.O'Meara, V.G.Cabana, J.R.Lukens, B.Loharikar, T.M.Forte, K.S.Polonsky, and G.S.Getz, Heparin-induced lipolysis in hypertriglyceridemic subjects results in the formation of atypical HDL particles, *J. Lipid Res.* 35:2178 (1994).
9. G.F.Lewis, K.D.Uffelman, B.Lamarche, V.G.Cabana, and G.S.Getz, Production of small HDL particles after stimulation of *in vivo* lipolysis in hypertriglyceridemic individuals. Studies before and after triglyceride-lowering therapy., *Metabolism* 47:234 (1998).
10. G.F.Lewis, B.Lamarche, K.D.Uffelman, A.C.Heatherington, L.W.Szeto, M.A.Honig, and H.R.Barrett, Clearance of postprandial and lipolytically modified human HDL in rabbits and rats., *J. Lipid Res.* 38:1771 (1997).
11. B.Lamarche, K.D.Uffelman, G.Steiner, P.H.R.Barrett, and G.F.Lewis, Analysis of particle size and lipid composition as determinants of the metabolic clearance of human high density lipoproteins in a rabbit model., *J. Lipid Res.* 39:1162 (1998).
12. B.Lamarche, K.D.Uffelman, A.Carpentier, J.S.Cohn, G.Steiner, P.H.R.Barrett, and G.F.Lewis, Triglyceride-enrichment of HDL enhances the in vivo metabolic clearance of HDL-apo A-1 in healthy men., *J.Clin.Investig.* 103:1191 (1999).

INSULIN TREATMENT POST MYOCARDIAL INFARCTION:
THE DIGAMI STUDY

Klas Malmberg, Anna Norhammar, Lars Rydén
Department of Cardiology
Karolinska Hospital
Stockholm, Sweden

INTRODUCTION

During a review of the unselected diabetic patients with acute MI at our institution in the mid 80's, we found that 22% of our patients had diabetes, and an even more striking finding was that more than 50% have died within one year[1]. One can argue that this was before the introduction of modern treatment strategies but even recent data confirm an almost doubled 35-day mortality rate in diabetic patients who have suffered an acute MI compared to non-diabetics[2]. After that we planned for the DIGAMI study which was completed in 1994. The results of this study have been published elsewhere.[3, 4,5]

Reviewing the literature regarding most the common cause of death in patients with diabetes and acute myocardial infarction the most common cited is myocardial pump failure[6, 7]. Potential mechanistic explanations of this is a more vulnerable non-infarct area resulting in an impaired compensatory hemodynamic response to injury. This may be due to metabolic perturbations associated with the diabetic state but also to an impaired vascular reserve. The second most cited cause of death is myocardial re-infarction which could be due to more extensive coronary atherosclerosis and/or that patients with diabetes are more prone to thrombus formation.[1, 6,8,9]

Over the past years there has been a renewed interest regarding GIK therapy in acute MI. A recent meta-analysis of several studies including almost 2000 predominantly non-diabetic patients has recently been published. It suggests an in-hospital relative mortality reduction of 28 %, corresponding to 49 saved lives per 1000 treated, by using GIK treatment[10] . Furthermore the authors stated that GIK treatment might be even more important in the area of reperfusion, since experimental studies have indicated that GIK treatment has the potential to protect ischemic myocardium before reperfusion for 10 hours or more. This is supported by the recently published ECLA pilot trial showing a trend towards a non-significant reduction in major and minor in-hospital events in patients allocated to GIK. However, among the 252 patients who underwent reperfusion therapy there was a significant 66% reduction in mortality and a consistent trend towards fewer in-hospital events in the GIK group compared the controls[11].

Diabetes and Cardiovascular Disease: Etiology, Treatment and Outcomes
Edited by Aubie Angel et al., Kluwer Academic/Plenum Publishers, 2001

POSSIBLE MECHANISMS FOR THE BENEFICIAL GIK EFFECT

The prevailing opinion regarding the mechanism of the effect of metabolic treatment centers around the favorable effect of insulin and glucose on ischemic and reperfusion metabolism. Insulin promotes glucose oxidation, which is known to be beneficial in the ischemic situation. An increase in the amount of available glycolytic substrate increases the anaerobic ATP synthesis and attenuates the ischemia induced ATP decrease. Furthermore, it has been suggested that agents that support glucose oxidation could reduce post-ischemic contractile dysfunction.

Increased levels of circulating free fatty acids (FFA) due to high sympathetic activity also characterize acute myocardial ischemia. FFA oxidation is potentially detrimental in the setting of myocardial ischemia due to an increased oxygen demand and to a direct inhibition of glucose oxidation, which is more favorable in the ischemic situatuion. Furthermore, increased utiliztion of FFA during ischemia also causes accumulation of toxic FFA-metabolites wich further may induce membrane damage, provoke arrhythmias and exacerbate mechanical dysfunction. Metabolic support by GIK could decrease both circulating FFA levels and myocardial FFA uptake[12].

Patients with diabetes have impaired glucose oxidation and increased FFA utilization due to a relative or absolute insulin deficiency and hence the above discussed metabolic pertubarations may be even more important in diabetics during an acute ischemic event. The post-ischemic myocardial contractile dysfunction and the increased frequency of overt heart failure reported in diabetics may be a result of these metabolic derangements.

There is also clear indications that insulin treatment in patients with diabetes could favorably affect the coagulation system. Diabetes is associated with enhanced platelet activation and aggregability, increased plasminogen activator inhibitor-1 (PAI-1) activity, and increased fibrinogen concentrations, among other aberrations of the coagulation system. Insulin therapy has been shown to reduce the increased production of thromboxane A$_2$ and decrease PAI-1 activity in patients with type 2 diabetes and may therefore positively influence the high re-infarction rate linked to this patient group.[13, 14] Clinical outcomes data with regard to these effects are not available.

THE DIGAMI STUDY

Based on these principles, we postulated that exogenous insulin administration during and after acute myocardial infarction in patients with diabetes would favorably influence the development of pump failure, the susceptibility to re-infarction, and therefore, mortality. The DIGAMI study was designed to evaluate the effect of insulin therapy on survival in patients with diabetes suffering acute myocardial infarction. Eligible patients were those with suspected acute myocardial infarction and admission blood glucose over 11 mmol/l , with or without known diabetes. Before randomization, all patients were stratified according to cardiovascular risk and according to prior insulin treatment. Patients were randomized to either intravenous insulin-glucose infusion for at least 24 hours, followed by multi-dose subcutaneous insulin treatment for at least three months or to a control group, which received "conventional treatment". The protocol utilized "conventional treatment" for the control arm, which was left to the discretion of the treating physician. That means that most patients in the control arm continued with their ongoing pre-randomized treatment. However, the responsible study physician could reinforce the antidiabetic treatment; that is, institute oral therapy or insulin treatment if clinically indicated. Pre-randomized insulin treatment was never withdrawn in the control group. Standard therapy for acute MI was applied to all subjects, and the protocol emphasized the use of thrombolytic therapy when indicated (50% of enrolled patients), aspirin (80%), and beta-blockers (70%) as tolerated. The primary end-point in the this study was 3-month mortality, and the secondary end-point was one-year mortality.

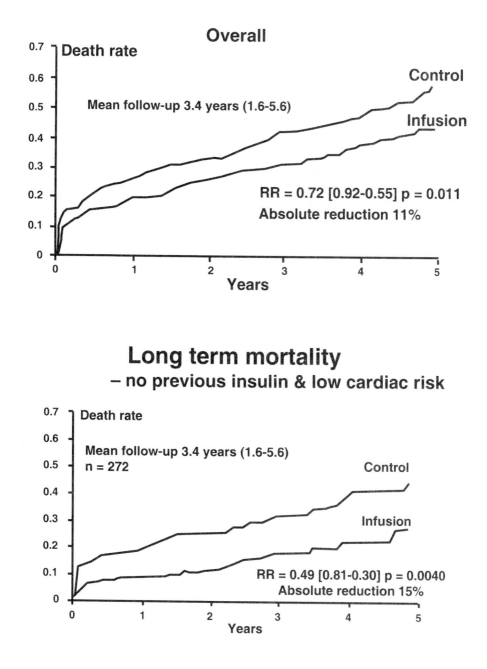

Figure 1. Panel A and B

Long-term mortality for all patients (A) and stratum 1 (B) from the paper:
Malmberg K. Prospective randomized study of intensive insulin treatment on long-term survival after acute myocardial infarction in patients with diabetes mellitus. British Medical Journal 1997; 314: 1512-1515.

There were 1240 eligible patients screened during the enrollment period, half of which were excluded due to pre-defined exclusion criteria. The excluded patients were somewhat older and more often female. These excluded patients were entered into a registry, and their age-adjusted one-year mortality was similar to the "conventional therapy" arm. 620 patients were randomized to the study. The groups were well balanced with regard to baseline characteristics. The mean age was 68 years and around 60% were men. Notably, this was a rather sick population, with 40% having prior myocardial infarction, 50% with a history of angina, 50% with hypertension, 20% with previously diagnosed heart failure, and 23% were smokers. The mean duration of diabetes was 10 years and the majority of patients had type 2 diabetes. Around 45% of the patients were being treated with oral diabetic therapy at enrollment and about 1/3 were receiving insulin. This breakdown of diabetic treatment at study entry is representative of the current practice in Sweden. Glycated hemoglobin averaged 8%, which is notably lower than that found among diabetics in the United States. Admission blood glucose averaged 15.5 mmol/liter, and was the same between treatment arms. There was no difference in serum potassium between the groups at presentation, but there was a slight but expected decrease in the infusion group secondary to the effects of insulin on potassium flux.

The blood glucose curve in the infusion patients had a rather fast decline, with an average blood glucose of 7 mmol/l by six hours. The curve then leveled off and finally rose a bit. 15% of the infusion group (42 patients) had at least one episode of hypoglycemia, which was pre-defined as a blood glucose below 3mmol/l with or without symptoms. Most patients did not report any symptoms during the hypoglycemia, and no direct harmful effects of hypoglycemia were noted acutely or during the 12 months of follow up. The infusion group stayed almost three days longer in the hospital, which was presumably due to injection training.

At hospital discharge, 80% were receiving aspirin, with most of the remaining 20% receiving warfarin. 70% of all patients were discharged on beta blockers and 30% on ACE inhibitors. The beneficial effect of ACE inhibitors became evident during the study, so the patients receiving ace inhibitors in the study represented a group with the more congestive heart failure. There was no difference between the groups at discharge or during one year of follow-up in these medications.

The compliance to insulin treatment was good, and among all patients, almost 90% randomized to the infusion group were receiving insulin at hospital discharge, compared to 44% in the control group. At one year, more than 70% of the infusion group were still on insulin, compared to about 50% of the control group on insulin. The increasing prevalence of insulin use over the 12 months of follow-up in the control group presumably reflects the natural course of type 2 diabetes. The difference as regards insulin treatment between the two study groups was even more pronounced among stratum 1 patients. In that predefined subgroup containing 272 patients without prior insulin treatment and at low cardiovascular risk, 81% randomized to the infusion group were on insulin at hospital discharge, compared to 15% in the control group. At one year, 66% of the infusion group were still on insulin, compared to about 24% of the control group. This difference was also reflected by a significantly more pronounced absolute reduction in HbA1c after one year of -1.3% compared to -0.5% the control group. Among all DIGAMI patients the reduction in HbA1c was -0.9% in the treatment group compared to -0.4% in the control group (p<0.001).

Figure 1 gives the long-term mortality curves. There was an early separation between the mortality curves favoring the insulin treatment arm. The mortality at one year was significantly reduced from 26% in the control group to 19% in the infusion group. This is a significant difference , but with broad confidence intervals. The long-term data (3.4 years of follow-up), shows a persistent relative mortality reduction of 25% (p=0.011) in the insulin treated group. This corresponds to an absolute mortality reduction of 11%.

Returning to the pre-defined strata regarding cardiovascular risk and prior insulin usage, the largest stratum included those patients without prior insulin treatment and at a low overall risk prior to randomization (stratum 1). This comprised 272 of the patients. It was a younger group which had been treated with oral anti-diabetic (64%), diet (15%), or was newly diagnosed (21%), and with approximately the same blood glucose control as the other strata. As expected, there was a much lower mortality in both groups within this stratum compared with the other strata. However, it was this group which demonstrated the largest effect from the insulin therapy. At hospital discharge, there was a 58% mortality reduction (p<0.05) in this stratum. This benefit was sustained throughout the follow-up, with a 50% reduction at 12 months. From the long-term mortality curves (Figure 1b), there appears to be a further separation between the curves within this stratum during the 3.4 years of follow-up, with a highly significant 45% mortality reduction (33% vs 18%; p=0.004).

There are limitations this study. There was a much lower overall mortality than was predicted in the power calculation during the design of this study. This is probably due to the prevalent use of thrombolytics, aspirin, and beta-blockers within the study. This low mortality decreased the power of the study to detect a difference at 3 months, which was the primary endpoint. Another limitation involves the issue of mechanism of benefit. The data does demonstrate trends favoring the insulin group with regard to cardiac enzyme peaks, LV function, and arrhythmia. Furthermore, we cannot separate the effect of the acute therapy compared with the ongoing therapy over the course of the study. In addition, it is possible that oral agents are detrimental as suggested by UGDP-study, and a potential interpretation could be that oral hypoglycemics were actually causing harm instead of insulin causing benefit. To address this issue would require a placebo arm, which is impossible because most of the patients require some kind of blood glucose lowering therapy. Some of these limitations should be addressed in our follow-up study, the DIGAMI II, for which we are currently enrolling.

In summary, several recent epidemiological reports suggest that hyperglycemia per se is a determinant for the development of macrovascular disease in patients with diabetes. Biochemical perturbations related to diabetes and hyperglycemia may also be of major importance during the acute infarction period with subsequent impaired myocardial hemodynamic response to the injury. Furthermore, they may increase the risk for early reocclusion. Theoretically, strict metabolic control by means of insulin treatment could improve these metabolic alterations and data from the DIGAMI study strongly supports this theory.

REFERENCES

1. Malmberg K, Ryden L. Myocardial infarction in patients with diabetes mellitus. Eur Heart J 1988; 9: 256-64
2. Woodfield SL, Lundergan CF, Reiner JS, et al. Angiographic findings and outcome in diabetic patients treated with thrombolytic therapy for acute myocardial infarction: the GUSTO-I experience. J Am Coll Cardiol 1996;28:1661-1669
3. Malmberg K, Ryden L, Efendic S, Herlitz J, Nicol P, Waldenstrom A, Wedel H, Welin L. A randomized trial of insulin-glucose infusion followed by subcutaneous insulin treatment in diabetic patients with acute myocardial infarction: Effects on one year mortality. J Am Coll Cardiol 1995; 26:57-65
4. Malmberg K, Ryden L, Hamsten A, Herlitz J, Waldenstrom A, Wedel H. Effects of insulin treatment on cause-specific one-year mortality and morbidity in diabetic patients with acute myocardial infarction. Eur Heart J 1996; In press

5. Malmberg K. Prospective randomized study of intensive insulin treatment on long-term survival after acute myocardial infarction in patients with diabetes mellitus. British Medical Journal 1997; 314: 1512-1515

6. Stone P, Muller J, Hartwell T, Yourk B, Rutherford J, Parker C, Turi Z, Strauss W, Willerson J, Robertson T. The effect of diabetes mellitus on prognosis and serial left ventricular function after acute myocardial infarction: Contribution of both coronary disease and diastolic left ventricular dysfunction to the adverse prognosis. J Am Coll Cardiol 1989; 14: 49-57

7. Jaffe A, Spadaro J, Schechtman K, Roberts R, Geltman E, Sobel B. Increased congestive heart failure after myocardial infarction of modest extent in patients with diabetes mellitus. Am Heart J 1984; 108: 31-37

8. Karlson BW, Herlitz J, Hjalmarson A. Prognosis of acute myocardial infarction in diabetic and non-diabetic patients. Diabet Med 1993; 10: 449-54

9. Barbash GI, White HD, Modan M, Van der werf WF. Significance of diabetes mellitus in patients with acute myocardial infarction receiving thrombolytic therapy. J Am Coll Cardiol 1993; 22: 707-713

10. Fath-Ordoubadi F, Beatt K. Glucose-Insulin-Potassium therapy for treatment of acute myocardial infarction. An overview of randomized placebo controlled trials. Circulation 1997; 96: 1152-1156.

11. Diaz R, Paolasso EA, Piegas LS et al. Metabolic modulation of acute myocardial infarction. The ECLA glucose-insulin-potassium pilot trial. Circulation 1998; 98: 2227-2234.

12. Glucose-insulin-potassium in acute myocardial infarction. The time has come for a large, prospective trial. Apstein CS, Taegtmeyer H. Circulation 1997; 96: 1074-1077.

13. Jain SK, Nagi DK, Slavin BM, Lumb PJ, Yudkin JS. Insulin therapy in type 2 diabetic subjects suppresses plasminogen activator inhibitor (PAI-1) activity and proinsulin-like molecules independently of glycemic control. Diabet Med 1993; 10: 27-32

14. Davi G, Catalan I, Averna M, Notarbartolo A, Sartrano A, Ciaboattoni G, Patrono C. Thromboxane biosynthesis and platelet function in type 2 diabetes mellitus. New Engl J Med 1990; 322:1769-1774

RESPONSE TO ISCHEMIA AND ENDOGENOUS MYOCARDIAL PROTECTION IN THE DIABETIC HEART

Tanya Ravingerova, Radovan Stetka, Miroslav Barancik, Katarina Volkovova*, Dezider Pancza, Attila Ziegelhöffer, Jan Styk.

Institute for Heart Research, Slovak Academy of Sciences; *Research Institute of Nutrition, Bratislava, Slovak Republic

INTRODUCTION

Diabetic patients are more prone to develop congestive heart failure and/or ischemic heart disease. Myocardial dysfunction is often attributed to diabetic cardiomyopathy that has been described in various clinical and experimental settings[1,2]. Deteriorations of heart contractile function as well as rhythm disorders are caused by the alterations in the cell membranes ion transport systems responsible for the maintenance of the homeostasis of Na^+, K^+ and Ca^{2+} and abnormal Ca^{2+}-handling[3,4,5,6].

Intracellular calcium overload has been suggested as one of the main factors that determine the severity of ischemic injury and exacerbate the damage of the heart caused by reperfusion in the normal heart[7]. From that point of view, it appears that diabetic hearts should be more vulnerable to ischemia/reperfusion. However, experimental data suggest that susceptibility of the diabetic hearts to ischemia may be increased, decreased or unchanged[8].

Prolonged ischemia induces profound alterations in the heart metabolism, function and ultrastructure. On the contrary, brief episodes of ischemia have been found to protect the hearts of different species (dogs, rabbits, rats, guinea pigs) against subsequent prolonged ischemia, an adaptive phenomenon termed as ischemic preconditioing[9]. Protection can be manifested by a reduced size of infarction[10], improved postischemic contractile recovery[11], as well as by suppression of malignant ischemia- and reperfusion-induced arrhythmias[12].

The studies of preconditioning are usually performed on normal healthy animals, whereas relatively little is known whether mechanisms of adaptation of the heart to ischemia are modified in the diseased myocardium. Some authors suggest that preconditioning is "a healthy heart phenomenon"[13], while others observed preconditioning-induced protection in the the diabetic hearts as well[15].

The present study was designed to investigate whether response to ischemia and ischemic preconditioning are modified with the time course of diabetes mellitus. We have chosen a rat model of streptozotocin-induced diabetes of different duration, and ischemia-induced malignant arrhythmias in the isolated heart as a main end-point of protection. Our results suggest that increased diabetic rats are less sensitive to ischemia-induced

Diabetes and Cardiovascular Disease: Etiology, Treatment and Outcomes
Edited by Aubie Angel et al., Kluwer Academic/Plenum Publishers, 2001

285

arrhythmias in the early period of the disease. Development of diabetic cardiomyopathy partially attenuates this protective effect but does not suppress a potential for ischemic preconditioning.

MATERIALS AND METHODS

Animals

All studies were performed in accordance with the Guide for the care and use of laboratory animals published by the US National Institutes of Health (NIH publication No 85-23, revised 1996). Male Wistar rats (250-300g body weight), fed a standard diet and tap water *ad libutum*, were used for all studies.

Diabetes was induced by a single i.v. injection of streptozotocin (45 mg/kg), whereas control animals received an equal amount of vehicle. Following 1 week (acute phase of diabetes) and 9 weeks (chronic phase), the diabetic animals, as well as the control ones were sacrificed and all experiments were performed in isolated perfused hearts.

Perfusion technique

Rats were anaesthetised (sodium pentobarbitone, 40 mg/kg, i.p.) and given heparin (500 IU, i.p.). Hearts were rapidly excised, placed in ice-cold perfusion buffer, cannulated via the aorta and perfused in the Langendorff mode at a constant perfusion pressure of 70 mm Hg and at 37°C. Perfusion solution was a modified Krebs-Henseleit buffer gassed with 95% O_2 and 5% CO_2 (pH 7.4) containing (in mM): NaCl 118.0; KCl 3.2; $MgSO_4$ 1.2; $NaHCO_3$ 25.0; NaH_2PO_4 1.18; $CaCl_2$ 2.5; glucose 11.1. Solution was filtered through a 5 μm porosity filter (Millipore) to remove contaminants.

An epicardial electrogram (EG) was registered by means of two stainless steel electrodes attached to the apex of the heart and the aortic cannula and continuously recorded (Mingograph ELEMA-Siemens, Solna, Sweden). Heart rate was calculated from the EG. Coronary flow was measured by a timed collection of coronary effluent. Left ventricular pressure was measured by means of a latex water-filled balloon inserted into the left ventricle via the left atrium (adjusted to obtain end-diastolic pressure of 5-10 mm Hg) and connected to a pressure transducer (P23 Db Pressure Transducer, Gould Statham Instruments, Inc.). Left ventricular developed pressure (LVDP, systolic minus diastolic pressure), rates of positive and negative pressure development (+dP/dt and –dP/dt) as the indexes of contraction and relaxation, as well as heart rate, coronary flow and pressure-rate product (PRP; LVDP x HR) were used to assess cardiac function.

Arrhythmias were analysed in accordance with Lambeth Conventions[15]. In this study we focused on the measurement of the incidences of ventricular tachycardia (VT) and fibrillation (VF) as well as of their duration. VF lasting more than 2 min was considered as sustained. Severity of arrhythmias was evaluated by means of arrhythmia score ranging from a score of 1 (given to the hearts with ventricular premature beats only) to 5 (for the hearts with sustained VF).

Experimental protocols

After 30 min equilibration, all hearts were assigned to one of the following protocols:
1. Test ischemia/reperfusion
After additional 15 min perfusion, both, diabetic and control hearts (n = 12 per group) were subjected to a test ischemic challenge. Regional ischemia was induced by a ligature placed around the left anterior descending coronary artery close to its origin and a traction-type plastic occluder. After 30 min, the ligature was released to permit 10 min lasting

reperfusion. Efficacy of occlusion and reperfusion was confirmed by a fall in coronary flow at the onset of ischemia of about 40% and its recovery upon reperfusion Further verification was performed by dye exclusion technique and measurement of an ischemic zone size[16].

2. Ischemic preconditioning

After equilibration, diabetic and control hearts (n = 12 per group) were subjected to one cycle of ischemic preconditioning consisting of 5 min ischemia and 10 min reperfusion, prior to test ischemia/reperfusion.

Data were expressed as means ± SEM. A one-way analysis of variance (ANOVA) was applied to test for significant differences between the groups followed by the unpaired Student's t-test, with p<0.05 considered as significant. Non-Gaussian distributed variables were compared using χ^2 test.

RESULTS

Development of diabetes

After 1 and 9 weeks blood glucose levels increased to 17.4±0.7 mM and 23.8±0.9 mM, as compared to 5.74±0.1 and 5.43±0.26 mM in respective age-matched controls.

In the diabetic rats, body weight loss was observed already after 1 week of the disease and even more markedly after 9 weeks (Table 1). Heart weight was moderately decreased only in the chronic phase. However, relative heart weight (heart weight/body weight ratio) was progressively increased at 1 and 9 weeks as compared to the respective age-matched controls.

Cardiac function in the diabetic hearts

Evaluation of cardiac function in the Langendorff preparation before the onset of ischemia revealed a gradual and significant reduction of heart rate and coronary flow with the time course of the disease (Table 2).

Although there were no differences in LVDP between the groups, both +dP/dt and –dP/dt, as well as PRP were consistently lower in both diabetic groups, especially in the chronic one, indicating impaired myocardial performance, as well as the rates of contraction and relaxation, due to a gradual development of heart failure.

Table 1. Body and heart weight in the rats after 1 and 9 weeks of streptozotocin-induced diabetes mellitus.

Parameters	1 week		9 weeks	
	control	Diabetic	control	diabetic
body wt. (g)	329±6	286±14*	362±10	259±22*
heart wt. (mg)	800±50	875±30	920±10	838±16*
heart wt./ body wt. (mg/g)	2.43±0.1	3.06±0.3*	2.54±0.1	3.2±0.2*

Data are means±SEM (n = 24 in each group). *-p<0.05; diabetic animals vs respective age-matched non-diabetic controls.

Table 2. Myocardial function in Langendorff-perfused rat hearts after 1 and 9 weeks of streptozotocin-induced diabetes mellitus.

Parameters	1 week		9 weeks	
	control	diabetic	control	diabetic
HR	300±11	266±9*	320±8	203±8*#
CF	13.6±1.5	11.9±0.8	12.2±0.6	8.6±0.4*#
LVDP	94±4	75±20	90±2	79±14
+dP/dt	3320±180	2407±280*	2881±187	1918±130*#
-dP/dt	1959±160	1577±150*	1826±50	1291±77*#
PRP	27570±1300	20534±2070*	25800±1250	15720±1600*#

Data are means±SEM (n = 24 in each group). HR - heart rate (beats/min); CF - coronary flow (ml/min); LVDP - left ventricular developed pressure (mmHg); +dP/dt and –dP/dt - rates of positive and negative pressure development (mm Hg/s); PRP - pressure and rate product (mmHg x beats/min).*-p<0.05; diabetic hearts vs respective age-matched non-diabetic controls. #-p<0.05; 9 weeks diabetic vs 1 week diabetic hearts.

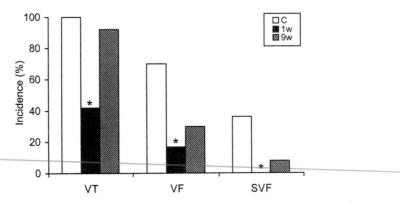

Figure 1. Effect of streptozotocin-induced diabetes on susceptibility to ischemic arrhythmias in isolated rat hearts. C - non-diabetic control hearts (n=12); 1w - acute diabetic hearts (n=12), 9w - chronic diabetic hearts (n=13). VT - ventricular tachycardia, VF - ventricular fibrillation, SVF - sustained ventricular fibrillation (lasting >2 min). Data are % of incidence evaluated by means of χ^2 test. *-p<0.05; diabetic hearts vs age-matched non-diabetic controls.

Susceptibility to ischemia-induced arrhythmias

In this model of LAD occlusion, severe ventricular arrhythmias peak between the 10 and 20 minutes of ischemia (Figure 1). In the non-diabetic controls, VT was observed in all the hearts, and 70% of the hearts exhibited VF (total incidence including transient VF, as well as sustained VF in 36% of the hearts). In the 1 week diabetic hearts, the incidence of VT was lower (42% vs 100% in the controls), and only transient VF occured in 17% of the hearts, whereas sustained VF was completely abolished (p<0.05). However, in the chronic phase of the disease, alterations in cardiac function were accompanied by an exacerbation of arrhythmias: incidence of VT increased and appeared to be similar to that in the non-diabetic controls, the total incidence of VF (non-sustained and sustained) was also moderately increased to 30% including sustained VF in 8% of the hearts, so that the differences between the diabetic and non-diabetic control hearts observed at 1 week waned at 9 weeks.

Effect of ischemic preconditioning on susceptibility to arrhythmias

In the non-diabetic hearts, ischemic preconditioning markedly suppressed the incidence and severity of arrhythmias (Figure 2). Incidence of VT was decreased to 33% and VF was totally abolished (p<0.05). In the diabetic hearts at 1 week, this intervention, however, failed to induce any additional antiarrhythmic protection. Incidence of VT (Fig. 2, top) did not differ significantly from that in the non-preconditioned diabetic hearts (58% vs 42%; p>0.05). Total incidence of VF (Figure 2, bottom) was 50% (vs 17% in the non-preconditioned diabetic hearts) and sustained VF occured in 25% of the hearts (not shown).

In the 9 weeks diabetic hearts, the effect of preconditioning on arrhythmias was more pronounced and comparable with that in the control hearts. Incidence of VT was reduced to 50% (Figure 2, top).

Different from the ineffective suppression of VF in the acute diabetic hearts, only a short episode of transient VF occured in one of ten hearts (Fig. 2, bottom).

Figure 3 demonstrates the effect of preconditioning on the severity of arrhythmias in the 1 and 9 weeks diabetic hearts, evaluated by means of arrhythmia score, that corresponded to the above findings. Severity of arrhythmias was significantly lower in the 1 week diabetic group than in the controls (2.25 ± 0.35 vs 4.1 ± 0.3; p<0.05) reflecting an enhanced resistance of the hearts to ischemia in the acute phase of the disease (Figure 3, middle). Development of diabetic cardiomyopathy was associated with an increase of severity (Figure 3, right), although it was still lower than in the non-diabetic controls (3.25 ± 0.2 vs 4.1 ± 0.3; p<0.05).

Preconditioning reduced the severity of arrhythmias in the controls (from the score 4.1 ± 0.3 to 1.7 ± 0.3; p<0.05).

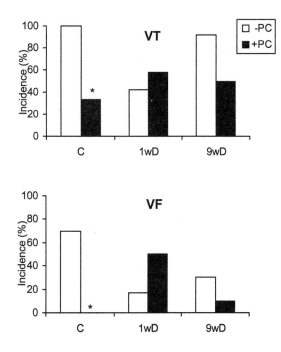

Figure 2. Effect of preconditioning on susceptibility to ischemic arrhythmias in isolated rat hearts after and 9 weeks of diabetes mellitus. Abbreviations as in Fig. 1. In the control group, the data were pooled from the non-diabetic hearts age-matched with 1 and 9 weeks diabetics. Filled bars - preconditioned hearts; open bars - non-preconditioned hearts. Data are % of incidence evaluated by means of χ^2 test. *-p<0.05; preconditioned vs non-preconditioned hearts.

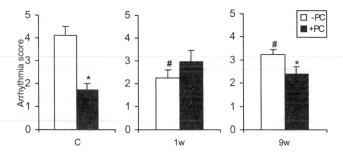

Figure 3. Effect of preconditioning on the severity of arrhythmias evaluated by arrhythmia score in isolated rat hearts with acute and chronic diabetes mellitus. C - controls, 1w - acute diabetes, 9w - chronic diabetes. Data are means of 12 to 13 experiments in each group $\pm$S.E.M. Filled bars - preconditioned hearts, open bars - non-preconditioned hearts. *-p<0.05; preconditioned vs non-preconditioned hearts; #-p<0.05; diabetic hearts vs non-diabetic controls.

At 1 week, severity of arrhythmias in the preconditioned diabetic hearts did not differ from that in the non-preconditioned ones (2.95$\pm$0.5 vs 2.25$\pm$0.35; p>0.05). On the contrary, at 9 weeks of diabetes, the hearts benefited more from preconditioning and severity of arrhythmias was reduced (from the score 3.25$\pm$0.2 to 2.4$\pm$0.3; p<0.05).

DISCUSSION

Although a large body of evidence accumulated in clinical studies of diabetic cardiomyopathy suggests an increased risk of myocardial infarction and a rate of mortality, experimental results point out to either increased or decreased susceptibility to ischemic injury in different experimental settings. Furthermore, it is not very clear whether mechanisms of adaptation to ischemia are operating in the pathologically altered myocardium. Results of this study demonstrate that diabetic hearts in the early phase of the disease are more resistant to ischemia-induced severe ventricular arrhythmias than non-diabetic controls. One week of diabetes (with significantly elevated blood glucose level) already caused myocardial dysfunction manifested by a significant reduction of heart rate and rates of contraction and relaxation, as well as of pressure-rate product, although LVDP and coronary flow were still unchanged (Table 2). However, in these hearts, the incidence and duration of VT and total VF was lower, and sustained VF was totally abolished during 30 min regional ischemia, the intervention which induces a high incidence of ventricular arrhythmias in the normal heart (Figure 1). One of the major determinants of arrhythmogenesis is the size of an involved (ischemic) area[17]. However, we can disregard this factor since there were no differences in the size of the occluded zone (area at risk) between the groups. Tosaki et al.[13] have demonstrated a lower incidence of reperfusion-induced arrhythmias in the rat heart in the early phase of diabetes, as well as improved functional recovery upon reperfusion. Tani and Neely[18] have pointed out to the attenuation of myocardial postischemic dysfunction in the diabetic rat hearts as early as 48 hours after the administration of streptozotocin. It is suggested that processes related to the alterations in glucose metabolism and to the regulation of the intracellular pH might be responsible for the reduced sensitivity to ischemia in the diabetic hearts[19]. A decreased accumulation of glycolitic products on one hand and a reduced activity of Na^+/H^+- and Na^+/Ca^{2+}-exchangers[4,5] on the other hand, may account for the reduced rate of Ca^{2+} influx and cellular uptake upon reperfusion associated with lower arrhythmogenesis and improved contractility[13,18]. In addition, numerous mechanisms, such as activation of protein kinase C[20] can trigger endogenous protection that may be considered as „metabolic preconditioning".

Development of the disease leads to a gradual attenuation of antiarrhythmic protection due to persisting metabolic alterations. Massive intracellular accumulation of toxic intermediates of fatty acids metabolism (e.g. acylcarnitine and long chain acyl-CoA) within sarcolemma has been suggested to alter biophysical properties of the cell membrane and cause electrophysiological derangements (like cell-to-cell uncoupling) as well as deterioration of the membrane-bound ion transporting enzymes[21]. Inhibition of Na^+/K^+- and Ca^{2+}- ATPases in the cardiac sarcolemma of the diabetic hearts might be expected to enhance susceptibility to ischemia- and reperfusion-induced arrhytthmias[22]. Some authors found a suppression of initial protection with the time course of the disease associated with an increased calcium accumulation in the myocardium[13], while others point out to the increased resistance to ischemia even after longer duration of the disease[23]. These conflicting data may be partially explained by the differences between the species, severity of different protocols utilizing regional, global, low-flow ischemia, or hypoxia and the choice of the end-points studied[8].

In this study, ishaemic preconditioning by one cycle of ischemia/reperfusion effectively suppressed ischemia-induced arrhythmias in the normal hearts, while it did not confer any additional protection in the acute phase of diabetes. It seems that enhanced resistance to ischemia in the early period of diabetes might „mask" the effect of classical ischemic preconditioning since they may share some common mechanisms, such as activation and translocation of protein kinase C[24] as well as opening of KATP channels[25].

In the chronic phase of the disease, when arrhythmogenesis was increased, these hearts benefited more from preconditioning since the incidence and severity of arrhythmias were reduced in a way comparable with the preconditioned non-diabetic controls (Figures 2, 3) indicating that potential for ischemic preconditioning was still preserved. This is different from the study by Tosaki et al.[13] demonstrating a lack of preconditioning protection in the chronic phase of diabetes. The latter, however, can be attributed to the differences between the mechanisms of ischemia- and reperfusion-induced events[22,26], and to a different model utilized (working hearts, global ischemia versus Langendorff-perfused hearts and regional ischemia).

In chronic diabetes, glucose transport and utilization are severely impaired[21]. On the other hand, it is known that brief ischemic episodes cause the depletion of glycogen stores and reduced rate of production of ATP as well as of glycolytic metabolites and lower acidosis[9], whereas glycogen recovery is associated with a loss of protection[27]. Recently, it has been demonstrated that in the diabetic hearts, despite a higher glycogen content, preconditioning induces a more efficient depletion of myocardial glycogen stores and a lower lactate production contributing thus to a greater extent of myocardial protection than in the normal hearts[28]. So far, it is difficult to differentiate whether it is a real effect of ischemic preconditioning itself, or still preserved diabetes-induced „metabolic preconditioning", or a combination of both, that may account for the protective effect.

In conclusion, the results of this study show that early period of diabetes is associated with an increased resistance of the rat heart against ischemia-unduced arrhythmias. This protective effect is partially attenuated in the chronic phase of the disease associated with the development of diabetic cardiomyopathy. Preconditioning does nor confer any additional protection in the early phase, whereas the hearts can benefit more in the chronic phase of diabetes, due to persisting potential for preconditioning.

Acknowledgements

This study was suppoted, in part, by VEGA grant No. 2/6094/99.

REFERENCES

1. Kannel WB, McGee DL. Diabetes and cardiovascular risk factors. The Framingham Study. Circulation 1979;59:8-13.
2. Fein FS, Kornstein LB, Strobeck LJ, Capasso JM, Sonnenblick EH. Altered myocardial mechanics in diabetic rats. Circ Res 1980;47:922-933.
3. Ganguly PK, Pierce GN, Dhalla KS, Dhalla NS. Defective sarcoplasmic reticular calcium transport in diabetic cardiomyopathy. Am J Physiol 1983;244:E528-E535.
4. Khandoudi A, Bernard M, Cozzone P, Feuvray D.Intracellular pH and role of Na^+/H^+ exchange during ischemia and reperfusion of normal and diabetic rat hearts. Cardiovasc Res 1990;24:873-878.
5. Pierce GN, Ramjiawan B, Dhalla NS, Ferrari R. Na^+/H^+ exchange in cardiac sarcolemmal vesicles isolated from diabetic rats. Am J Physiol 1990;258:H255-E261.
6. Dhalla NS, Pierce GN, Panagia V, Singal PK, Beamish RE. Calcium movements in relation to heart function. Basic Res Cardiol 1982;77:117-139.
7. Opie LH. Myocardial ischemia, reperfusion and cytoprotection. Rev Port Cardiol 1996;15(10):703-708.
8. Paulson D. The diabetic heart is more sensitive to ischemic injury. Cardiovasc Res 1997;34:104-112.
9. Murry CE, Jennings RB, Reimer KA. Preconditioning with ischemia: a delay of lethal cell injury in ischemic myocardium. Circulation 1986;74:1124-1136.
10. Liu GS, Downey JM. Preconditioning against infarction in rat heart does not involve pertussis toxin sensitive G protein. Cardiovasc Res 1993;27:608-611.
11. Cave AC. Preconditioning induced protection against postischemic contractile dysfunction: characteristics and mechanisms. J Mol Cell Cardiol 1995;27:969-979.
12. Vegh A, Komori S, Szekeres L, Parratt JR. Antiarrhythmic effects of preconditioning in anaesthetised dogs and rats. Cardiovasc Res 1992;26:487-495.
13. Tosaki A, Engelman DT, Engelman RM, Das DK. The evolution of diabetic response to ischemia/reperfusion and preconditioning in isolated working rat hearts. Cardiovasc Res 1996;31:526-536.
14. Bouchard JF, Lamontagne D. Protection afforded by preconditioning in the diabetic heart against ischemic injury. Cardiovasc Res 1998;37:82-90.
15. Walker MJA, Curtis MJ, Hearse DJ, Campbell RWF, Janse MJ, Yellon DM, Cobbe SM, Coker SJ, Harness JB, Harron DWG, Higgins AJ, Julian DJ, Lab MJ, Manning AS, Northover BJ, Parratt JR, Riemersma RA, Riva E, Russel DC, Sheridan DJ, Winslow E, Woodward B. The Lambeth conventions: guidelines for the study of arrhythmias in ischemia, infarction, and reperfusion. Cardiovasc Res 1988;22:447-455.
16. Ravingerova T, Tribulova N, Slezak J, Curtis MJ. Brief, intermediate and prolonged ischemia in the crystalloid perfused rat heart: Relationship between susceptibility to arrhythmias and degree of ultrastructural injury. J Mol Cell Cardiol 1995;27:1937-1951.
17. Curtis MJ. Characterisation, utilisation and clinical relevance of isolated perfused heart models of ischemia-induced ventricular fibrillation. Cardiovasc Res 1998;39:194-215.
18. Tani M, Neely JR. Hearts from diabetic rats are more resistant to in vitro ischemia: possible role of altered Ca^{2+} metabolism. Circ Res 1988;62: 931-940.
19. Feuvray D, Lopaschuk GD. Controversies on the sensitivity of the diabetic heart to ischemic injury: the sensitivity of the diabetic heart to ischemic injury is decreased. Cardiovasc Res 1997;34:113-120.
20. Malhotra A, Reich D, Reich D, Nakouzi A, Sanghi V, Geenen DL, Buttrick PM. Experimental diabetes is associated with functional activation of protein kinase C   and phosphorylation of troponin I in the heart, which are prevented by angiotensin II receptor blockade. Circ Res 1997;81:1027-1033.
21. Rodrigues B, Cam MC, McNeill JH. Myocardial substrate metabolism: implications for diabetic cardiomyopathy. J Mol Cell Cardiol 1995;27:169-179.
22. Curtis MJ, Hearse DJ. Ischemia-induced and reperfusion-induced arrhythmias differ in their sensitivity to potassium: Implications for the mechanisms of initiation and maintenance of ventricular fibrillation. J Mol Cell Cardiol 1989;21:21-40.
23. Gamble J, Lopaschuk GD. Glycolysis and glucose oxidation during reperfusion of ischemic hearts from diabetic rats. Biochim Biophys Acta Mol Basis Dis 1994;1225:191-199.
24. Mitchell MB, Meng X, Ao L, Brown JM, Harken AH, Banerjee A. Preconditioning of isolated rat heart is mediated by protein kinase C. Circ Res 1995;76:73-81.
25. Gross GJ, Auchampach JA. Blockade of ATP-sensitive potassium channel prevents myocardial preconditioning in dogs. Circ Res 1992;70:223-233.
26. Hearse DJ. Myocardial protection in ischemia and reperfusion. Medicographia 1996;18:22-29.

27.   Wolfe CL, Sievers RE, Visseren FLJ, Donnelly TJ. Loss of myocardial protection after
       preconditioning correlates with the time course of glycogen recovery within the
       preconditioned segment. Circulation1993;87:881-892.
28.   Tatsumi T, Matoba S, Kobara M, Keira N, Kawahara A, Tsuruyama K, Tanaka T, Katamura M,
       Nakagawa C, Ohta B, Yamahara Y, Asayama J, Nakagawa M. Energy metabolisms after
       ischemic preconditioning in streptozotocin-induced diabetic rat hearts. J Am Coll Cardiol
       1998;31: 707-715.

TYPE 2 DIABETES: PHARMACOLOGICAL INTERVENTION IN AN ANIMAL MODEL

James C. Russell

Department of Surgery
275 Heritage Medical Research Centre
University of Alberta
Edmonton, Alberta

INTRODUCTION

The state of insulin resistance and the accompanying hyperinsulinemia are strong correlates of cardiovascular disease, even in the absence of overt diabetes. Insulin resistance is the central component of the metabolic syndrome, accompanied by abdominal obesity, hypertension, and hypertriglyceridemia. It is a serious and growing problem in prosperous societies throughout the world and is a major contributor to atherosclerotic disease and the ischemic sequelae.[1-4] The metabolic syndrome is the established stage of a silent—and generally unrecognized—malignant process that leads to vasculopathy and atherosclerosis over a period of several years. This stage proceeds without any overt hyperglycemia or diabetes, yet contributes greatly to the ultimate complication, cardiovascular disease.

The recognized components of the metabolic syndrome reflect the complex multifactorial and polygenetic nature of the origins of end-stage cardiovascular disease. The silent nature of most dyslipidemias and of insulin resistance allows the disease process to progress asymptomatically until an individual has lost the compensating ability to maintain hyperinsulinemia and presents with a frank Type 2 diabetes. At this stage, the vascular damage is well established, with atherosclerosis and functional vasculopathy giving a thrombogenic and vasospastic status. Effective treatment regimens will require recognition of the different stages of the progression of vascular disease. Ideally, treatment should begin at the earliest stages of insulin resistance, well before full development of the hyperinsulin-emic state so that the vascular system is not damaged by high insulin levels. Because this is very difficult to achieve in practice, treatment that can reverse the insulin resistance is critical. For the patient who is diagnosed late in the process, and who presents with hyperinsulinemia and perhaps overt diabetes and vascular damage, any potential treatment must also minimize the vascular dysfunction and ischemic sequelae.

The strategies for treating insulin resistance-mediated cardiovascular disease can be analyzed in terms of the metabolic and functional aspects towards which they are directed. In the first instance, insulin-sensitizing agents may offer a preventative approach. The current absence of any established treatment for insulin resistance is a major clinical shortcoming that has prompted intensive efforts to develop new insulin-sensitizing agents. Established insulin resistance-related vascular disease, on the other hand, requires treatment directed at preventing the vasospasm and thrombus formation and minimizing ischemic damage. Animal studies conducted in our laboratory over recent years provide grounds for optimism in regard to each of these approaches.

ANIMAL MODELS OF ATHEROSCLEROSIS

Diabetes and Cardiovascular Disease: Etiology, Treatment and Outcomes
Edited by Aubie Angel et al., Kluwer Academic/Plenum Publishers, 2001

Considerable progress has been made in understanding the role of hypercholesterolemic states on atherogenesis, largely through the use of animal models.[5] Most such animal models involve the use of very high cholesterol diets to rapidly induce lesions in species that are normally resistant to atherogenesis.[6–9] These high-cholesterol diets induce an extremely abnormal and problematic status in species, such as rabbits, that do not normally consume significant amounts of cholesterol. None of the hypercholesterolemic models provides a good analogue for the large segment of the human population with normal lipoprotein receptors, only modestly elevated levels of plasma cholesterol, and yet at high risk for cardiovascular disease.[10] This group is essentially composed of individuals with the obesity/insulin resistance/hypertriglyceridemia syndrome.

THE RAT

Due to its size and relatively low costs, the rat has become one of the most widely used mammalian animal models. Although a small animal, it is still large enough to permit physiological and metabolic studies that are not practical in smaller species such as the mouse. Furthermore, while the rat is not phylogenetically close to humans, it shares many characteristics with us, including an omnivorous diet. The glucose-insulin metabolism of the rat is also very similar to that of humans. However, there are significant differences in lipid/lipoprotein status, with serum total cholesterol being much lower in the rat (<50 mg/100 ml). The majority of the cholesterol is carried in the HDL fraction, and VLDL and LDL contents are correspondingly low. This pattern, in normal rats, is unfavourable to atherogenesis and has strengthened the view that this species is not a good animal model for the study of atherosclerosis. However, the recent development and characterization of genetic rat models that are atherosclerosis prone proves that this is not the case. In particular, rats incorporating the two mutant genes leading to obesity, the *fa*, or fatty Zucker, and the *cp*, or corpulent rats, have provided the bases for several animal models of insulin resistance and hyperlipidemia.

THE JCR:LA-cp RAT

Background

The JCR:LA-cp strain of rats is one of a number of strains incorporating the autosomal recessive *cp* gene first isolated by Koletsky.[11,12] The gene was bred into two inbred strains at the National Institutes of Health by Hansen, and then two congenic strains, the LA/N-cp and SHR/N-cp, were created through repeated backcrossing.[13] At an early stage (the fifth backcross), nucleus breeding stock of the LA/N-derived line was donated to the author and became the basis for a closed outbred colony. This colony retains some 3% genetic contribution from the original Koletsky strain. It is maintained through a formal breeding protocol[14] so as to retain the gene pool and not inadvertently select out certain (unknown) genes. This protocol is essential, as the spontaneous development of cardiovascular disease is unique to rats of this colony and the trait is clearly polygenetic.

Genetic Defect

In common with the other strains incorporating the *cp* gene,[15] the JCR:LA-cp rats, if homozygous for the *cp* gene (cp/cp), are obese, insulin resistant, and hypertrigly-ceridemic.[16–19] Rats that are heterozygous (+/cp) or homozygous normal (+/+) are lean and are not distinguishable from the parent LA/N strain in any respect. The *cp* gene has been shown to be a stop codon in the extracellular domain of the leptin receptor (ObR).[20] This leads to a complete absence of the ObR in the plasma membrane of the cp/cp animals. In contrast, the other obese rat gene, the *fa*, has been shown to result in an amino acid substitution, also in the extracellular domain of the ObR, that leads to a 10-fold reduction in binding affinity for leptin. Thus, the fa/fa rat is leptin resistant as opposed to having no functional receptor. There are also major metabolic and pathophysiological differences between cp/cp and fa/fa animals.[21–23] Most critically, the JCR:LA-cp strain is unique in the spontaneous development of atherosclerosis and myocardial ischemia. Neither the fa/fa Zucker[22] nor the cp/cp rats of the other *cp* strains develops cardiovascular disease,[15] confirming the complex polygenetic character of this disease.

The *ob* gene, coding for leptin itself, of the cp/cp rat is structurally normal and leptin levels are dramatically elevated ($\approx$ 30-fold). The adipocyte signal to the central nervous system is not recognized, as expected in the absence of the ObR, and the levels of neuropeptide Y (the strongest known mediator of eating) are significantly elevated in the arcuate nucleus of the hypothalamus.[24,25] Leptin also downregulates insulin secretion from the pancreas in normal animals.[26] The cp/cp rat exhibits an extreme hypersecretion of insulin that is much greater than that of the fa/fa rat,[21] consistent with the leptin-resistant status of the fa/fa rat and absent-receptor status of the cp/cp rat.

Metabolism

Animals of the JCR:LA-cp strain that are cp/cp are detectably obese at 3 weeks of age. A modest hyperinsulinemia is present at 4 weeks and develops rapidly after 5 weeks of age.[27] The insulin resistance develops such that, in the male cp/cp rats at 8 weeks of age, there is no insulin-mediated glucose uptake or turnover.[17] Increased muscle triglyceride concentrations are present in the cp/cp rats at 4 weeks, even before the development of the insulin resistance.[17] As triglycerides are known to reduce insulin sensitivity, this may be the origin of the insulin resistance. The cp/cp females, on the other hand, are only mildly affected and show both a much more modest hyperinsulinemia and only reduced insulin-mediated glucose turnover and peripheral uptake.[17,28] The profound peripheral insulin resistance in the cp/cp males leads to the diversion of glucose, derived from a carbohydrate diet, to triglyceride synthesis and VLDL secretion into the plasma.[18,29] Thus the marked VLDL hyperlipidemia is due to an elevated secretion of VLDL and not to reduced clearance.[18,19] The modestly increased cholesterol levels are due to the obligatory cholesterol content of the VLDL particles and flowthrough to the HDL fraction.[19]

Vasculopathy

Male cp/cp rats exhibit a hypercontractile response of the arterial vessels to norepi-nephrine and an impaired relaxant ability.[30,31] The greater vasoconstriction appears to be due, in part, to inadequate nitric oxide release from the endothelium.[32] Nitric oxide-mediated relaxation of arteries from cp/cp rats is also deficient at the smooth muscle cell level, indicating that the obese, insulin-resistant state contributes to impaired vascular function of both endothelial and smooth muscle cell origins. A defective response to nitric oxide may be an important contributor to vasospasm. The impairment of vascular function develops as the hyperinsulinemic state becomes established. The vascular dysfunction of the cp/cp rat is associated with increased phosphodiesterase (PDE3A) activity in the aorta.[33] The role of PDEs in vascular function and nitric oxide metabolism is just beginning to be unravelled, but appears to be important in the cp/cp rat. In addition, the aorta of the cp/cp rat exhibits elevated activity of the matrix metalloproteinase MMP-2 when the animals are given a dietary cholesterol challenge, which exacerbates the vascular damage. MMPs hydrolyze tissue elements, allowing cells such as macrophages and smooth muscle cells to migrate. These vessel wall changes are consistent with the hyperproliferative and hyperactive charac-ter of the aortic smooth muscle cells of the cp/cp rat.[34]

Fibrinolytic System

The fibrinolytic system is an important element of the pathophysiological processes leading to atherosclerosis, vascular occlusion, and myocardial damage. Plasminogen, which lyses fibrin or intracellular clots, is activated by the activators t-PA and u-PA, that are in turn inhibited by plasminogen activator inhibitor-1 (PAI-1). Elevated levels of PAI-1 are associated with thrombotic phenomena,[35] and we have shown increased plasma concentra-tions of PAI-1 and greater mRNA expression in the hearts of male cp/cp rats.[36] Moreover, cultured aortic rings from male cp/cp rats secrete significantly more PAI-1 into the medium than do those from either male +/+ or female cp/cp animals. These findings are consistent with observations of thrombus accumulation in the arterial system of the cp/cp rat.[37,38]

Atherosclerosis

Male cp/cp rats develop frank atherosclerotic lesions from an early age, with raised intimal lesions being present in the aortic arch of 100% of the rats by 9 months of age.[37-39] Marked endothelial damage, including areas of desquamation, are also evident on scanning electron microscopy. Adherent macrophages are common, especially on raised lesions where active penetration of the endothelium occurs. Occlusive thrombi are also seen in both the coronary and major abdominal arteries. Accompanying the vascular lesions is a cumulative progression of ischemic lesions in the myocardium.[37,39] Transmission electron microscopy reveals that the raised intimal lesions strongly resemble developing atherosclerotic lesions on large vessels in humans, and neither resembles the massive foam cell lipid-laden lesions of the cholesterol-fed rabbit.[40] The presence of ischemic lesions in the hearts of cp/cp rats was demonstrated early in our study of the animals.[38] The lesions are present in young (12-week-old) male cp/cp rats at a low frequency and their numbers increase with age. They vary from early-stage necrosis through to old, scarred lesions that represent a cumulative record of tissue damage.[39]

PHARMACOLOGICAL INTERVENTIONS

Insulin-Sensitizing Agents

The growing recognition of the importance of the metabolic syndrome in human disease has led to efforts to develop pharmaceutical agents that would facilitate weight reduction and/or increase insulin sensitivity. There has been some success in this. For instance, drugs such as benfluorex have both lipid-lowering and insulin-sensitizing effects,[29,41,42] and we have shown that it not only improves insulin sensitivity, but reduces vascular dysfunction and lesions and largely prevents the development of myocardial lesions in the cp/cp rat.[42] Similarly, D-fenfluramine has insulin-sensitizing effects in the cp/cp rat, essentially normalizes the hyperplasticity of the islets of Langerhans, reduces the severity of aortic lesions, and protects the heart from ischemic damage.[43]

The compound β,β'-tetramethylhexadecanedioic acid (MEDICA 16) is a fatty acid analogue that has potent hypotriglyceridemic properties. Treatment of the cp/cp rats from the time of weaning (3 weeks of age) with MEDICA 16 normalizes food intake and body weight gain, prevents the early accumulation of triglyceride in muscle tissue, and markedly delays and blunts development of the hyperinsulinemia.[27] This finding is consistent with the suggested role of triglycerides in the development of insulin resistance. MEDICA 16 also causes mitochondrial uncoupling with an increase in respiration.[44] When cp/cp rats are treated from 6 weeks of age, by which time the insulin resistance has been established, triglyceride levels are reduced by 80%, insulin levels are halved, the hyperplastic islets of Langerhans are essentially normalized, and atherosclerotic lesions are largely prevented.[45]

The binding of various agents to the peroxisome proliferator activator receptor (PPAR) sites has effects on many intracellular functions, including insulin metabolism. MEDICA 16 is a PPAR-α agonist and this may contribute to the insulin-sensitizing effects and improvements in vascular function in the cp/cp rat. Similarly, fenofibrate, a PPAR-γ agonist developed as an antihypertriglyceridemic compound, improves insulin sensitivity, but without reducing the VLDL hyperlipidemia. Troglitazone, another PPAR agonist, also reduces insulin levels, but has no effect on plasma lipid concentrations or vascular hypercontractility. These preliminary results indicate that the PPAR system plays a role in the metabolic dysfunction of the insulin-resistant cp/cp rat, but do not as yet allow for any conclusions regarding the mechanisms.

Recently, a novel oral agent, S15261, has been reported to increase insulin sensitivity in the aging Sprague Dawley rat.[46] This compound contains an ester linkage that is cleaved by plasma esterases, yielding the fragments Y415 and S15511. Previous results have suggested that Y415 has glucose-clearing effects, whereas S15511 may have insulin-sensitizing properties. Treatment of cp/cp rats with S15261 or S15511 resulted in highly significant reductions in food intake and body weights, whereas Y415 did not significantly change either. In comparison, troglitazone caused a small increase in food intake with no effect on body weight. Treatment with S15261 or S15511 decreased fed plasma insulin levels, while Y415 had no significant effect. Meal tolerance tests have revealed that treatment with S15261 or S15511 essentially prevents the marked postprandial peak in insulin levels seen in JCR:LA-cp rats,[47] whereas Y415 had no significant effect. Troglita-zone only halved the insulin response to the test meal. S15261 decreased the expression of two hepatic gluconeogenic enzymes (PEPCK and glucose-6-phosphase) and stimulated the expression of genes involved in glucose utilization through glucokinase and lipogenesis (acyl-CoA carboxylase and fatty acid synthase). In comparison, the known insulin-sensitizing agent S15261 also reduced the expression of genes regulating hepatic long-chain fatty acid oxidation (carnitine palmitoyltransferase I) and ketogenesis (hydroxymethyl-glutaryl-CoA synthase). S15261, but not troglitazone, reduced the exaggerated contractile response of mesenteric resistance vessels to norepinephrine and increased maximal nitric oxide-mediated relaxation. Thus S15261, through its product, S15511, increases insulin sensitivity, decreases insulin levels, reduces the vasculopathy of the JCR:LA-cp rat, and may be expected to be protective against cardiovascular disease.

Calcium Channel Antagonists

Calcium channel antagonists are widely used for the inhibition of vascular contraction and treatment of hypertension. However, calcium is intimately involved in physiological functions other than muscle contraction, particularly as an essential co-factor for many enzymes. We have demonstrated that the dihydropyridine, nifedipine, reduces plasma triglycerides by 50% and prevents the formation of myocardial lesions.[48] Similar hypolipidemic, antiatherosclerotic, and cardioprotective effects were seen with another dihydropyridine, nisoldipine. In this study, and in another involving the metabolic effects of only benzothiazepine calcium channel antagonists, we included female cp/cp rats.[49,50] In male cp/cp rats, the two classes of agents had very similar effects on lipid metabolism. In female cp/cp animals, in contrast, neither class of calcium channel antagonists caused any decrease in plasma triglycerides, but did result in a 50% increase in VLDL cholesterol esters.[50] These findings illustrate the complex interactions between the insulin-resistant state, metabolic dysfunction, sex, and cardiovascular disease. They clearly emphasize the need for careful preclinical studies of pharmacological agents in the appropriate animal models.

Angiotensin-Converting Enzyme Inhibitors

Angiotensin-converting enzyme inhibitors, especially captopril, are extensively and successfully used for the control of hypertension. They have also been reported to have cardioprotective effects in the presence of myocardial infarcts.[51] We have studied the effects of captopril on metabolism, particularly on the vascular and myocardial lesions in the cp/cp rat. Long-term treatment did not change plasma levels of insulin or triglycerides, but did result in a 40% reduction in cholesterol, both esterified and unesterified, and in phospho-lipids.[52] Vascular lesion frequency was unreduced, but the highly hyperplastic and fibrosed islets of Langerhans were largely normalized, and myocardial lesion frequency was greatly reduced. It appears that captopril has quite general protective properties against ischemic tissue injury. This effect is probably mediated through the inhibition of bradykinin degradation by captopril.

Probucol

Probucol is an agent with both hypolipidemic and antioxidant properties that has been considered to be cardioprotective.[53] Treatment of cp/cp rats caused only a transient reduction in insulin levels at 12 weeks of age and a marked reduction in the islet hyperplasia. There was no other metabolic improvement, especially in lipid levels. This is not surprising in view of the hypertriglyceridemic, rather than hypercholesterolemic, character of the dyslipidemia of the cp/cp rat. There was similarly no reduction in the severity of lesions of the aortic arch. The raised intimal lesions seen in probucol-treated cp/cp rats were clearly more severe than those of the control rats and were the worst seen in any experimental group. However, there was a marked reduction in the frequency of myocardial lesions. Thus, probucol is able to inhibit ischemic injury, even without any improvement in metabolic status or reduction in atherosclerosis. This may reflect improvements in endothelial cell or smooth muscle cell function or antioxidant-mediated protection against ischemia.

SUMMARY

The results of our pharmaceutical interventions are summarized in Table 1. A striking aspect of the responses obtained in the JCR:LA-cp rat is that end-stage vascular and myocardial disease responds to a range of different interventions. Reduction of the insulin resistance and hyperinsulinemia by MEDICA 16, D-fenfluramine, or even by intensive physical activity[54] clearly addresses the core dysfunction of the cp/cp rat and inhibits the whole pathophysiological process. However, the prevention of vasospasm or reduction of ischemic injury by captopril or probucol is effective in preventing advanced damage to both the pancreas and the heart. These findings are encouraging, suggesting that a variety of approaches may well be effective in preventing the consequences of insulin resistance in humans. We may find

Table 1. Pharmacological interventions in the JCR:LA-cp rat

Agent	Action	Metabolic effects		Vascular effects	Myocardial effects
		Insulin	Lipids		
Benfluorex	Insulin sensitizer	Insulin, IR ↓	TG ↓	Athero ↓, VF ↑	Lesions ↓↓
D-fenfluramine	Insulin sensitizer	Insulin, IR ↓	TG ↓	Athero ↓, VF ↑	Lesions ↓↓
MEDICA 16	Triglyceride inhibitor	Insulin, IR ↓↓	TG ↓↓	Athero ↓, VF ↑	Lesions ↓↓
Fenofibrate	Antihypertri-glyceridemic	Insulin, IR ↓	NE	NK	NK
Troglitazone	Insulin sensitizer	Insulin, IR ↓	NE	NK	NK
S15261	Insulin sensitizer	Insulin, IR ↓↓	NE	VF ↑	NK
Nifedipine	Ca^{++} channel antagonist	NE	TG ↓	Athero ↔	Lesions ↓
Nisoldipine	Ca^{++} channel antagonist	NE	TG ↓	Athero ↔	Lesions ↓
Diltiazem	Ca^{++} channel antagonist	NE	TG ↓	NK	NK
Captopril	ACE inhibitor	Islets ↓	Cholesterol ↓	Athero ↔	Lesions ↓
Probucol	Antioxidant	Islets ↓	NE	Athero ↔	Lesions ↓
Ethanol	Oxydizable substrate	Insulin ↓, Islets ↓	CE ↓	NK	Lesions ↓↓

Athero, atherosclerosis; CE, cholesterol esters; IR, insulin resistance; NE, no effect; NK, not known; TG, triglyceride; VF, vascular function.

that a combination of treatments may provide enhanced protection for susceptible individuals.

CONCLUSIONS

Our results covering the various aspects of the pathophysiology of the insulin resistance syndrome and a wide range of pharmaceutical interventions confirm the value of the cp/cp rat as a model for the study of insulin resistance and cardiovascular disease. The animals exhibit the range of metabolic dysfunctions seen in humans with the obesity/insulin resistance syndrome. Most importantly, they also show spontaneous development of atherosclerotic lesions of the aorta and other arteries, along with a vasculopathy that leads to vasospasm and thrombosis. This is reflected in the ischemic lesions of the heart, the critical end-stage of cardiovascular disease. The vascular disease appears to be particularly dependent upon the hyperinsulinemia, and any intervention resulting in a major reduction in plasma insulin levels is antiatherosclerotic and cardioprotective. On the other hand, the VLDL hyperlipidemia is an essential component of the syndrome and appears to contribute strongly to the vasculopathy and vessel damage. From an overall perspective, the cardiovascular disease in these animals appears to be multifactorial and probably polygenetic—a situation that almost undoubtedly exists in the human population as well.

The findings from our pharmaceutical interventions help reveal the critical role of high insulin levels in cardiovascular disease in this model. They also reveal a strikingly similar pattern of responses between the cp/cp rat and humans to all agents studied. In many cases, there are few data on human responses at a level comparable to that which can be obtained with a short-lived animal model such as the cp/cp rat. Nonetheless, the similarity is very clear and gives us confidence that responses found to new agents in the cp/cp rat will be good predictors of human responses. This will be a crucial point as the importance of the insulin resistance syndrome in human disease and mortality becomes more widely appreciated. Effective new therapeutic approaches will require better understanding of the underlying pathophysiological mechanisms, as well as animal models that will permit screening and preclinical experimentation. The cp/cp rat offers such a model and in a small, short-lived species, permitting relatively rapid and efficient study of a chronic disease process.

REFERENCES

1. P.Z. Zimmet, D.J. McCarty, and M.P. de Courten. The global epidemiology of non-insulin-dependent diabetes mellitus and the metabolic syndrome (Review). *J. Diab. Complic.* 11:60 (1997).
2. G.M. Reaven. Role of insulin resistance in human disease. *Diabetes* 37:1595 (1988).
3. G. Steiner. Hypertriglyceridemia and carbohydrate intolerance: Interrelations and therapeutic implications. *Am. J. Cardiol.* 57(suppl.):27G (1986).
4. R.W. Stout. Overview of the association between insulin and atherosclerosis. *Metabolism* 34:7 (1985).
5. D. Vesselinovitch. Animal models of atherosclerosis, their contributions and pratfalls. *Artery* 5:193 (1979).
6. R.B. Wilson, R.H. Miller, C.C. Middleton, and D. Kinden. Atherosclerosis in rabbits fed a low cholesterol diet for five years. *Arteriosclerosis* 2:228 (1982).
7. C.E. Hunt and L.A. Duncan. Hypercholesterolemia and atherosclerosis in rabbits fed low-level cholesterol and lecithin. *Br. J. Exp. Pathol.* 66:35 (1985).
8. C.W.M. Adams, N.E. Miller, R.S. Morgan, and S.N. Rao. Lipoprotein levels and tissue lipids in fatty-fibrous atherosclerosis induced in rabbits by two years of cholesterol feeding at a low level. *Atherosclerosis* 44:1 (1982).
9. R.W. St. Clair. Metabolic changes in the arterial wall associated with atherosclerosis in the pigeon. *Fed. Proc.* 42:2480 (1983).
10. G. Steiner. Hyperinsulinemia and hypertriglyceridemia. *J. Int. Med.* 736(suppl.):23 (1994).
11. S. Koletsky. Obese spontaneously hypertensive rats: A model for the study of atherosclerosis. *Exp. Mol. Pathol.* 19:52 (1973).
12. S. Koletsky. Pathological findings and laboratory data in a new strain of obese hypertensive rats. *Am. J. Pathol.* 80:129 (1975).
13. D.D. Greenhouse, O.E. Michaelis IV, and R.G. Peterson. The development of fatty and corpulent rat strains, in: *New Models of Genetically Obese Rats for Studies in Diabetes, Heart Disease and Complications of Obesity.* C.T. Hansen, O.E. Michaelis IV, eds., National Institutes of Health, Bethesda (1988).
14. S.M. Poiley. A systematic method of breeder rotation for non-inbred laboratory animal colonies. *Animal Care Panel* 10:159 (1960).
15. J.C. Russell, R.M. Amy, O.E. Michaelis, S.M. McCune, and A.A. Abraham. Myocardial disease in the corpulent strains of rats, in: *Frontiers in Diabetes Research: Lessons from Animal Diabetes III.* E. Shafrir, ed., Smith-Gordon, London, UK (1990).
16. P.J. Dolphin, B. Stewart, R.M. Amy, and J.C. Russell. Serum lipids and lipoproteins in the atherosclerosis prone LA/N-corpulent rat. *Biochim. Biophys. Acta* 919:140 (1987).
17. J.C. Russell, S.E. Graham, and M. Hameed. Abnormal insulin and glucose metabolism in the JCR:LA-corpulent rat. *Metabolism* 43:538 (1994).
18. J.C. Russell, D.G. Koeslag, R.M. Amy, and P.J. Dolphin. Plasma lipid secretion and clearance in hyperlipidemic JCR:LA-corpulent rats. *Arteriosclerosis* 9:869 (1989).
19. J.E. Vance and J.C. Russell. Hypersecretion of VLDL, but not HDL, by hepatocytes from the JCR:LA-corpulent rat. *J. Lipid Res.* 31:1491 (1990).
20. X.S. Wu-Peng, S.C. Chua, Jr., N. Okada, S.-M. Liu, M. Nicolson, and R.L. Leibel. Phenotype of the obese Koletsky (*f*) rat due to Tyr763Stop mutation in the extracellular domain of the leptin receptor (Lepr). *Diabetes* 46:513 (1997).
21. R.A. Pederson, R.V. Campos, A.M.J. Buchan, C.B. Chisholm, J.C. Russell, and J.C. Brown. Comparison of the enteroinsular axis in two strains of obese rats: The fatty Zucker and JCR:LA-corpulent. *Int. J. Obes.* 15:461 (1991).
22. R.M. Amy, P.J. Dolphin, R.A. Pederson, and J.C. Russell. Atherogenesis in two strains of obese rats. The fatty Zucker and LA/N-corpulent. *Atherosclerosis* 69:199 (1988).
23. C.B. Chan, R.M. McPhail, M.T. Kibenge, and J.C. Russell. Increased glucose phosphorylation activity correlates with insulin secretory capacity of male JCR:LA-corpulent rat islets. *Can. J. Physiol. Pharmacol.* 73:501 (1995).
24. G. Williams, H. Cardoso, J. Domin, M.A. Ghatei, J.C. Russell, and S.R. Bloom. Disturbances of regulatory peptides in the hypothalamus of the JCR:LA-corpulent rat. *Diabetes Res.* 15:1 (1990).
25. G. Williams, L. Shellard, D.A. Lewis, P.E. McKibbin, H.D. McCarthy, D.G. Koeslag, and J.C. Russell. Hypothalamic neuropeptide Y disturbance in the obese cp/cp JCR:LA-corpulent rat. *Peptides* 13:537 (1992).
26. V. Emilsson, Y.L. Lim, M.A. Cawthorne, N.M. Morton, and M. Davenport. Expression of the functional leptin receptor in RNA in pancreatic islets and directly inhibitory action of leptin on insulin secretion. *Diabetes* 46:313 (1997).
27. J.C. Russell, J. Bar-Tana, G. Shillabeer, D.C.W. Lau, M. Richardson, L.M. Wenzel, S.E. Graham, and P.J. Dolphin. Development of insulin resistance in the JCR:LA-cp rat: Role of triacylglycerols and effects of MEDICA 16. *Diabetes* 47:770 (1998).
28. J.C. Russell, S.K. Ahuja, V. Manickavel, R.V. Rajotte, and R.M. Amy. Insulin resistance and impaired glucose tolerance in the atherosclerosis-prone LA/N-corpulent rat. *Arteriosclerosis* 7:620 (1987).
29. J.C. Russell, S.E. Graham, P.J. Dolphin, and D.N. Brindley. The effects of benfluorex on serum triacyl-glycerols and insulin sensitivity in the corpulent rat. *Can. J. Physiol. Pharmacol.* 74:879 (1996).

30. S.F. O'Brien, J.D. McKendrick, M.W. Radomski, S.T. Davidge, and J.C. Russell. Vascular wall reactivity in conductance and resistance arteries: Differential effects of insulin resistance. *Can. J. Physiol. Pharmacol.* 76:72 (1998).

31. J.D. McKendrick, E. Salas, G.P. Dubé, J. Murat, J.C. Russell, and M.W. Radomski. Inhibition of nitric oxide generation unmasks vascular dysfunction in JCR:LA-cp rats. *Br. J. Pharmacol.* 124:361 (1998).

32. S.F. O'Brien, J.C. Russell, and S.T. Davidge. Vascular wall dysfunction in JCR:LA-cp rats: Interaction of age and insulin resistance. *Am. J. Physiol.* 46:C987 (1999).

33. T. Nagaoka, T. Shirakawa, T.W. Balon, J.C. Russell, and Y. Fujita-Yamaguchi. Cyclic nucleotide phosphodiesterase III (PDE3) expression *in vivo*. Evidence for tissue-specific regulation of PDE3A or 3B mRNA expression in adipose tissue and aorta of atherosclerosis-prone insulin resistant rats. *Diabetes* 47:1135 (1998).

34. P.M. Absher, D.J. Schneider, J.C. Russell, and B.E. Sobel. Increased proliferation of explanted vascular smooth muscle cells: A marker presaging atherogenesis. *Atherosclerosis* 131:187 (1997).

35. J.B. McGill, D.J. Schneider, C.L. Arfken, C.L. Lucore, and B.E. Sobel. Factors responsible for impaired fibrinolysis in obese subjects and NIDDM patients. *Diabetes* 43:104 (1994).

36. D.J. Schneider, P.M. Absher, D. Neimane, J.C. Russell, and B.E. Sobel. Fibrinolysis and atherogenesis in the JCR:LA-cp rat in relation to insulin and triglyceride concentrations in blood. *Diabetologia* 41:141 (1998).

37. J.C. Russell and R.M. Amy. Myocardial and vascular lesions in the LA/N-corpulent rat. *Can. J. Physiol. Pharmacol.* 64:1272 (1986).

38. M. Richardson, A.M. Schmidt, S.E. Graham, B. Achen, M. DeReske, and J.C. Russell. Vasculopathy and insulin resistance in the JCR:LA-cp rat. *Atherosclerosis* 138:135 (1998).

39. J.C. Russell. The atherosclerosis-prone JCR:LA-corpulent rat, in: *Atherosclerosis X: Proceedings of the 10th International Symposium on Atherosclerosis*. F.P. Woodford, J. Davignon, A. Sniderman, eds., Elsevier Science, Amsterdam (1995).

40. M. Richardson, E.M. Kurowska, and K.K. Carroll. Early lesion development in the aortas of rabbits fed low-fat, cholesterol-free, semipurified casein diet. *Atherosclerosis* 107:165 (1994).

41. J.C. Russell, D.G. Koeslag, P.J. Dolphin, and R.M. Amy. Beneficial effects of acarbose in the atherosclerosis prone JCR:LA-corpulent rat. *Metabolism* 42:218 (1993).

42. J.C. Russell, S.E. Graham, P.J. Dolphin, R.M. Amy, G.O. Wood, and D.N. Brindley. Antiatherogenic effects of long-term benfluorex treatment in male insulin resistant JCR:LA-cp rats. *Atherosclerosis* 132:187 (1997).

43. J.C. Russell, P.J. Dolphin, S.E. Graham, R.M. Amy, and D.N. Brindley. Improvement of insulin sensitivity and cardiovascular outcomes in the JCR:LA-cp rat by D–fenfluramine. *Diabetologia* 41:380 (1998).

44. O. Hermesh, B. Kalderon, and J. Bar-Tana. Mitochondria uncoupling by a long chain fatty acid analogue. *J. Biol. Chem.* 273:3937 (1998).

45. J.C. Russell, R.M. Amy, S.E. Graham, P.J. Dolphin, G.O. Wood, and J. Bar-Tana. Inhibition of atherosclerosis and myocardial lesions in the JCR:LA-cp rat by β, β'-tetramethylhexadecanedioic acid (MEDICA 16). *Arterioscler. Thromb. Vasc. Biol.* 15:918 (1995).

46. J. Duhault, S. Berger, M. Boulanger, O.D. Zuana, F. Lacour, and M. Wierzbicki. General pharmacology of S15261, a new concept for treatment of diabetes. *Arzneim. Forsch.* 48:734 (1998).

47. J.C. Russell, D. Ravel, J.-P. Pégorier, P. Delrat, R. Jochemsen, S.F. O'Brien, S.E. Graham, S.T. Davidge, and D.N. Brindley. Beneficial insulin-sensitizing and vascular effects of S15261 in the insulin-resistant JCR:LA-cp rat. *Diabetes,* submitted.

48. J.C. Russell, D.G. Koeslag, P.J. Dolphin, and R.M. Amy. Prevention of myocardial lesions in JCR:LA-corpulent rats by nifedipine. *Arteriosclerosis* 10:658 (1990).

49. J.C. Russell, P.J. Dolphin, S.E. Graham, and R.M. Amy. Cardioprotective and hypolipidemic effects of nisoldipine in the JCR:LA-cp rat. *J. Cardiovasc. Pharmacol.* 29:586 (1997).

50. J.C. Russell, S. Graham, B. Stewart, and P.J. Dolphin. Sexual dimorphism in the metabolic response to the calcium channel antagonists, diltiazem and clentiazem, by hyperlipidemic JCR:LA-cp rats. *Biochim. Biophys. Acta* 1258:199 (1995).

51. W. Linz, P.A. Martorana, and B.A. Scholkens. Local inhibition of bradykinin degradation in ischemic rat hearts. *J. Cardiovasc. Pharmacol.* 15:S99 (1990).

52. J.C. Russell, S.E. Graham, R.M. Amy, and P.J. Dolphin. Inhibition of myocardial lesions in the JCR:LA-corpulent rat by captopril. *J. Cardiovasc. Pharmacol.* 31:971 (1998).

53. J.C. Russell, S.E. Graham, R.M. Amy, and P.J. Dolphin. Cardioprotective effect of probucol in the atherosclerosis-prone JCR:LA-cp rat. *Eur. J. Pharmacol.* 350:203 (1998).

54. J.C. Russell, R.M. Amy, V. Manickavel, P.J. Dolphin, W.F. Epling, D. Pierce, and D. Boer. Prevention of myocardial disease in the JCR:LA-corpulent rat by running. *J. Appl. Physiol.* 66:1649 (1989).

55. P.M. Absher, D.J. Schneider, L.C. Baldor, J.C. Russell, and B.E. Sobel. The retardation of vasculopathy induced by attenuation of insulin resistance in the corpulent JCR:LA-cp rat is reflected by decreased vascular smooth muscle cell proliferation in vivo. *Atherosclerosis* 143:245 (1998).

302

THE DIABETIC HEART AND CARDIAC GLYCOSIDES

Makoto Nagano

Jikei University School of Medicine

INTRODUCTION

The diabetic heart develops easily heart failure than non-diabetic heart. The genesis of this problems has been examined and discussed worldwide from the view-point of micro and macro angiopathies, cardiac mechanics, energy and electrolyte metabolism and molecular biology.[1] Also the influence of drugs on diabetic and non-diabetic failing hearts is different. In this paper, I would like to show about Diabetic heart and digitalis, which has clinically not been discussed.

DIABETIC FAILING HEART AND DIGITALIS EFFECT

The low effect of digitalis preparations on diabetic heart was the first interest of my clinical work for 45 years. 45 years ago my first patient in the hospital ward was a female diabetes mellitus with congestive heart failure which was treated with digitalis purpurea. This patient was the connection to my life work on diabetes mellitus. I published an article on this patient in a Japanese Medical Journal in 1960.[2] Her ECG showed an old myocardial infarction. But even in earlier phases, she never complained of anginal pain as sign of acute myocardial infarction. It was a so-called silent myocardial infarction. The silent myocardial infarction has been discussed widely since the 1970's, but its concept was already reported in the Journal "Diabetes" by Marble of Joslin Clinic in 1954.[3] The genesis of the diabetic painless myocardial infarction was understood to be by diabetic neuropathy. But, in my article in 1960, I wrote that the ECG change, the old myocardial infarction without anginal pain was a result of the accumulation of myocardial microscars, which were induced due to capillaropathy. It was commonly held that atherosclerosis of the large extramural coronary arteries, non-specific macroangiopathy are intimately involved in the pathogenesis of heart dysfunction in the diabetic patient.

Since the 1970's several pathological studies by Rubler[4] Regan et al[5] have indicated that diabetic cardiomyopathy may be the consequence of microangiopathy. But, I already reported the role of microangiopathy for

Diabetes and Cardiovascular Disease: Etiology, Treatment and Outcomes
Edited by Aubie Angel et al., Kluwer Academic/Plenum Publishers, 2001

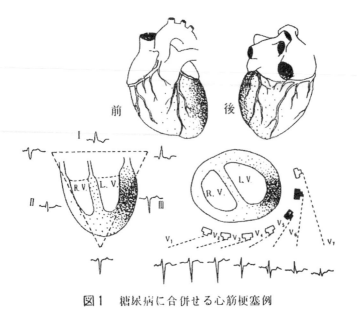

図1　糖尿病に合併せる心筋梗塞例

Figure 1. The illustration of pathological scar formation and ECG changes of the autopsy-patient.

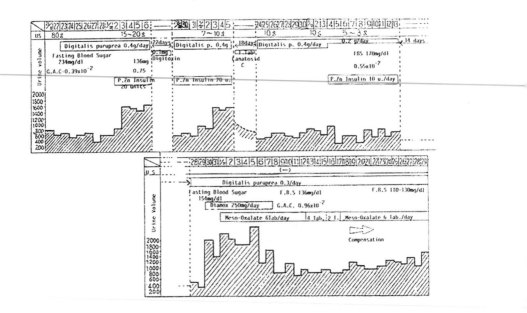

Figure 2. The time course and treatment of the patient. The effective maintenance dose of digitalis purpurea for this patient was 0.3 – 0.4 gram/day.

diabetic heart failure in 1960. The title of my article was "Diabetic heart disease and its treatment". Unfortunately, it appeared only in the Japanese Medical Journal in 1960. Therefore it remained virtually unknown outside Japan. Figure 1 shows the illustration of pathological scar formation and ECG changes of the autopsy-patient. Extramural coronary arteries were almost undamaged. The small black points showed microscar formation due to

304

capillaropathy.   Congestive heart failure of this patient was treated with digitalis purpurea.

Figure 2 shows time course and treatment of the patient. Back then, the only therapeutically effective drug for heart failure was cardiac glycoside. The presently used diuretics were not on the market yet. Only diamox, carbonic anhydrase inhibitore was used.   Generally, before 1955, patients with congestive heart failure in Japan were treated with digitalis purpurea. Primary dose was 0.3 g/day and after digitalis saturation the maintenance dose was 0.1 g/day. But for this patient, we needed to give 0.3 or 0.4 gram of digitalis purpurea per day as effective maintenance dose. These amounts were 3 or 4 times higher than the usual maintenance dose of digitalis purpurea. Additionally, the active effect of digitalis purpurea on the diabetic failing heart was quite small. As we know, if cardiac glycoside is overdosed, toxic signs
will appear. But this patient showed no symptoms of digitalis intoxication. Why was this large amount of digitalis necessary for this diabetic patient?

I examined the correlation of the maintenance dose of digitalis purpurea with the Glucose assimilation Index of diabetic patients. Figure 3 shows the maintenance does of digitalis purpurea per day for diabetic failing heart. In generally, the maintenance dose of digitalis purpurea is 0.1 or 0.05 g/day. To diabetic heart patients, it was necessary to give a higher dose for treatment. The front row show the maintenance dose of each cases. Nevertheless, these amounts of digitalis purpurea have shown non effect on diabetic failing hearts treated without insulin. A positive digitalis effect on diabetic hearts appeared

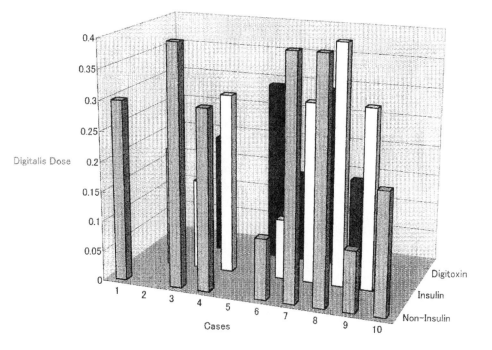

Figure 3. The maintenance dose of digitalis purpurea / day for diabetic failing heart. It was necessary to give a higher dose for treatment. The front row shows digitalis dose of diabetic patient without insulin treatment. The middle row: with insulin treatment. The back row: digitoxin treatment.

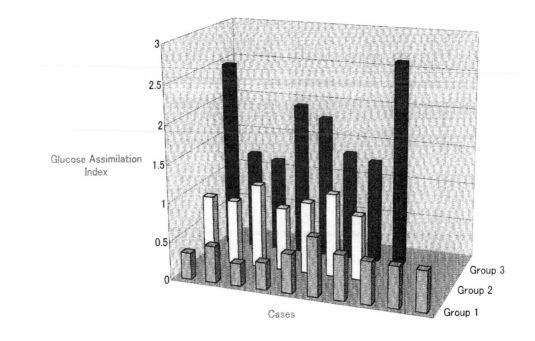

Figure 4. The correlation of glucose assimilation index with the effect of digitalis purpurea. Group 1: diabetic failing heart. Group 2: non-diabetic hypertensive failing heart. Group 3: failing heart with valvular disease.

only after additional insulin treatment. The columns of middle row show this group. As you can see, for the digitalis action to appear after insulin treatment, the dose of digitalis purpurea had to be higher than the normal maintenance dose. The back row columns show the maintenance dose of digitoxin. Digitoxin showed on active effect on the diabetic failing heart without insulin treatment, but the maintenance dose was also higher than that for the non-diabetic heart. A possible reason could be that Sodium-Potassium ATPase activity in the sarcolemma of the diabetic heart decreased compared to the non-diabetic heart.[6] Figure 4 shows the correlation of glucose assimilation index with the effect of digitalis purpurea in each group, diabetic falling heart (group 1 in Figure 4), non-diabetic hypertensive heart failure (group 2) and heart failure with valvular disease (group 3). The vertical axis shows the glucose assimilation index which is a sign for the glucose tolerance grade of the patients. Diabetic cases (group 1) had a low index value and valvular disease cases (group 3) a high index value of glucose assimilation. In the non-diabetic hypertensive heart failure, this index value was between the other 2 groups. All cases in Figure 4 were treated with digitalis purpurea or Lanatoside C.

Both cardiac glycosides have glucose in the terminal position of the glycoside-structure. Comparing the effect of cardiac glycosides on each group, these cardiac glycosides show not enough effect on diabetic failing heart. Therefore, at the patients with a high index value of glucose assimilation in the non-diabetic group, especially with valve diseases, the effect of cardiac glycosides on the failing heart appeared rapidly with a low dose of digitalis. These findings shows that the digitalis effect on diabetic failing hearts increased with insulin treatment.

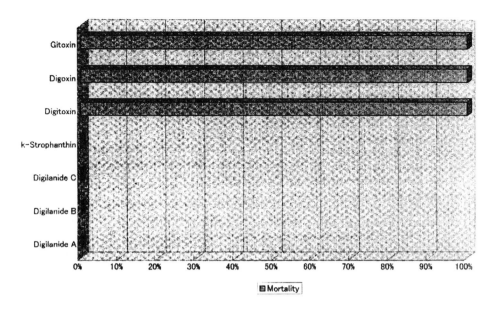

Figure 5. Stucture-activity relationship of cardiac glycosides on 72 hour chick embryo heart (Keyl & Dragstedt).

CARDIAC GLYCOSIDES AND INSULIN EFFECT

Keyl and Dragstedt[7] have observed the structure-activity relationship. of 2 groups of cardiac glycosides on 72 hour chick embryo hearts. The first group is a digilanide A, B, C and k-strophanthin group, and the second is a digitoxin, digoxin and gitoxin group.In the second group cardiac glycosides have no glucose in the terminal position of the glycoside structure. Figure 5 shows that in the first group cardiac glycoside had no influence on the mortality of the chick embryo. Keyl observed that a number of cardiac glycosides with d-glucose in the terminal position of sugar were inactive on the mortality of 72 hour chick embryo hearts as compared with the second group of cardiac glycoside, des-glucose derivatives.

Figure 6 shows the effect of insulin on the activity of the first group of cardiac glycosides, digilanide A, B, C and k-strophanthin on the 72 hour chick embryos. Insulin has augmented the activity of these cardiac glycosides on the mortality. In 1952, Levine and Goldstein[8] observed that insulin is a factor which influences the penetration of the sugar with specific stereochemical configuration into the cell. Insulin augments the rate of disappearance of simple sugars, having the configuration of d-glucose in the first three carbon atoms.

Figure 7 shows the mortality of k-strophanthin on chick embryos of varying age.[9] K-strophanthin become active when the embryos reach an age of 9 days. On the 9th day ages, endogenous pancreatic function appears in the chick embryo. So it seems highly probably that the endogenous insulin is involved and influences the mortality effect of the first group of cardiac glycosides. For the active appearance of cardiac glycoside compounds containing glucose, the existence of insulin is very important.

Figure 8 shows an experiment consisting of observations regarding the effect of insulin on non-diabetic and diabetic mice mortalitites by Lanatoside C. The insulin was intraperitoneal injected, 1 micro unit per

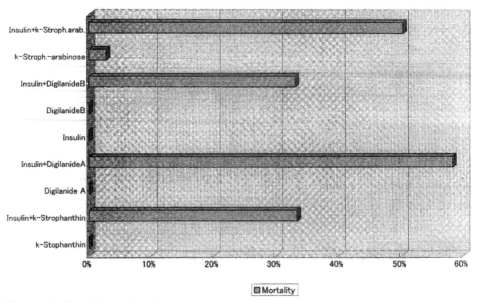

Figure 6. The effect of insulin on the activity of certain cardiac glycosides on the 72 hour chick embryos.

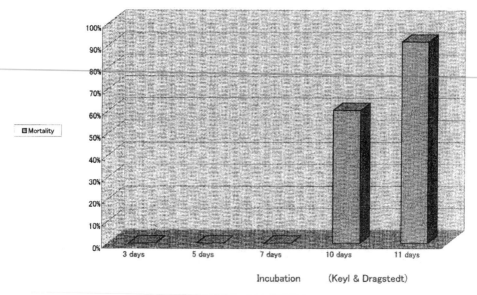

Figure 7. Cardiac glycoside (DigilanideC)-24 hour mortality data for chick embryo (Keyl & Draggiest).

gram of body weight of normal and diabetic mice. These insulin doses alone showed no influence on the mortality of both mice groups. The effect of gamma/gram of body weight of Lanatoside C on diabetic mice showed the same mortality grade as 8 gamma Lanatoside C on normal non-diabetic mice.

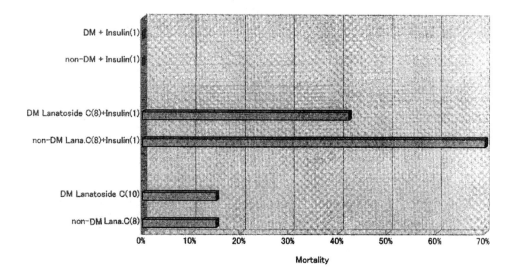

Figure 8. The effect of insulin on the activity of Landslide C on non-diabetic and diabetic mice.

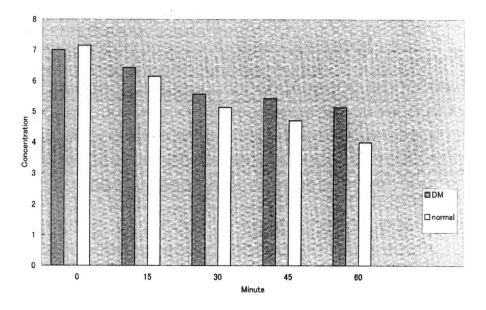

Figure 9. Lanatoside C levels in serum of diabetic and non-diabetic rats after intravenous administration of Lanatoside C.

These findings show that the effect of Lanatoside C on the diabetic heart is weaker than on the non-diabetic heart. In the center of this slide, the administration of the same dose of Lanatoside C and insulin shows a smaller effect on the diabetic heart in comparison to the non-diabetic heart. These findings support that the presence of insulin is very important for the appearance of the cardiac activity of cardiac glycoside having d-Glucose in the terminal position.

Looking at the different effect and appearance of cardiac glycosides with and without d-glucose on the terminal position, it may be possible that these d-glucose plays an important role in the inhibition of the digitalis receptor.

From these clinical and experimental findings, we tried to make a quantitative measurement of serum levels of cardiac glycosides. Figure 9 shows the intravenous tolerance curve of Lanatoside C in normal and streptozotosin diabetic rats. The assimilation grade of Lanatoside C in diabetic rats was smaller than that in normal non-diabetic rats. These findings support our old clinical findings of the relation between diabetes mellitus and the effect of cardiac glycosides.

REFERENCES

1. Nagano M and Dhalla NS. The Diabetic Heart edt. Nagano & Dhalla. Raven Press NY 1991.
2. Nagano M, Kawamura M, Nakamura T et al. Diabetic hypertension and heart, and its therapy. Nippon Rinshou (Japanese Clinical Journal) 18:1169-1184, 1965.
3. Marble A. Coronary artery disease in the diabetic. Diabetes 4:290-297, 1954.
4. Rubler DS, Ingash J, Yuceoglu YZ et al. New type of cardiomyopathy associated with diabetic glomerulosclerosis. Am J Cardiol 30:595:-602, 1972.
5. Regan TJ, Lyons MM, Ahmed SS et al. Evidence for cardiomyopathy in familial diabetes mellitus. J Clin Invest 60: 885-899, 1977.
6. Imanaga I, Kanegaw Y, Kanei R et al. Cardiac sarcolemma Na+ K+ ATPase activity in diabetic dog. In The Diabetic Heart. Edt. By Nagano M & Dhalla NS. Raven Press Ltd. NY. 1991.
7. Keyl AC and Dragstedt CA. The relationship of the sugar moiety of the cardiac glycosides to their toxicity on the intact embryonic chick heart. J Pharm Exp Therap 100: 411-414, 1954.
8. Levine R and Goldstein MS. Action of insulin on transfer of sugar across cell membrane: the common chemical configuration of sugars affected by the hormone. Fed Pro 11: 56, 1952.
9. Keyl AC and Dragstedt CA. Influence of insulin on action of cardiac glycosides on the intact embryonic chick heart. J Pharm Exp Therap 112: 129-132, 1956.

HYPERGLYCEMIA-INDUCED PROTEIN KINASE SIGNALING PATHWAYS IN VASCULAR SMOOTH MUSCLE CELLS: IMPLICATIONS IN THE PATHOGENESIS OF VASCULAR DYSFUNCTION IN DIABETES

Ashok K. Srivastava[1]

Research Centre,
Centre hospitalier de l'Université de Montréal (CHUM) - Hôtel-Dieu
Department of Medicine, University of Montreal
Montréal (Québec) H2W 1T8, Canada

INTRODUCTION

Vascular dysfunction is among the most common complications associated with diabetes,[1-3] and chronic hyperglycemia appears to be an important contributor in this process.[3] However, the precise mechanism(s) responsible for hyperglycemia-induced vascular dysfunction remain(s) poorly characterized. Non-enzymatic glycation, enhanced production of diacylglycerol (DAG), an activator of some isozymic forms of protein kinase C (PKC) and increased oxidative stress have been implicated as possible mediators of this response.[2-4] A role of oxidative stress in vascular disease associated with diabetes has been advanced by the recent demonstration that hyperglycemia enhances the proliferation of vascular smooth muscle cells (VSMC),[5, 6] which is blocked by antioxidants.[6] Furthermore, it has been shown that therapy of experimental diabetes models and diabetic human subjects with ascorbic acid, vitamin E and other antioxidants is able to reverse some cardiac abnormalities of diabetes.[7-9]

At the molecular level, several signaling pathways, activated by oxidative stress, and linked to cell growth and proliferation, have been identified.[10-12] Interestingly, some of these pathways are also stimulated in response to hyperglycemia in VSMC. The objective of this article is to provide an overview of key studies on hyperglycemia-induced signal transduction pathways in VSMC in relation to its implication in the development of vascular dysfunction in diabetes.

[1] Research Centre, Centre hospitalier de l'Université de Montréal
Hôtel-Dieu - CHUM
3840 St.Urbain Street
Montréal (Québec) H2W 1T8
Tel.: (514) 843-2917; FAX: (514) 843-2911
E-mail: Srivasta@ere.umontreal.ca

Diabetes and Cardiovascular Disease: Etiology, Treatment and Outcomes
Edited by Aubie Angel *et al.*, Kluwer Academic/Plenum Publishers, 2001

Hyperglycemia and PKC

PKC is a serine/threonine protein kinase comprised of at least 11 isozymic forms.[13-14] These isozymic forms have been classified as classical novel and atypical. Classical PKCs (α, βI, βII, and γ) are activated by Ca^{2+}, DAG, phosphatidylserine (PS) and the tumor promoter phorbol 12-myristate 13-acetate (PMA). Novel PKCs (δ, ϵ, η, μ, and θ) are activated by DAG, PS and unsaturated fatty acids, while atypical PKCs (ζ, λ, and ι) are insensitive to DAG but are activated by PS and phosphatidylinositides (reviewed in [14-16]). PKCs have been implicated in a wide variety of cellular responses, including growth, differentiation, gene expression, angiogenesis, contractility, and vesicle trafficking.[13]

Increases in PKC activity and DAG levels have been demonstrated in several tissues from diabetic animals (reviewed in [4, 17-20]). In aortic and vascular cells, the PKC-βII and PKC-δ isoforms have been shown to be activated in diabetic rats as well as in response to hyperglycemia.[4, 17-20] Most of these studies investigated the chronic effect of high glucose concentrations (15-25 mM) on DAG levels and PKC activities. For example, in VSMC from the rat aorta, incubation with 22 mM glucose for 3 days increased DAG levels by 50%, compared to VSMC incubated with 5.5 mM glucose.[19] In these studies, the protein content of membrane-associated PKC-βII rose by about 110% whereas no change in PKC-α level was detected.[19] Interestingly, intraperitoneal injection of the antioxidant α-tocopherol to diabetic animals or incubation of VSMC with α-tocopherol prevented the DAG and PKC elevation due to diabetes and hyperglycemia.[19] These and other investigations suggest a role of oxidative stress in diabetes/hyperglycemia-induced responses.[3, 4]

In a recent study, hyperglycemia was shown to activate total PKC activity in particulate fractions of VSMC, which was almost completely blocked by pretreatment of cells with the antioxidants probucol and D-α-tocopherol.[6] These authors also reported that hyperglycemia increased platelet-derived growth factor (PDGF)-BB-mediated migration, growth and DNA synthesis in VSMC, which could be significantly attenuated by antioxidants as well as by the protein kinase C inhibitor calphostin C.[6] In this regard, it is noteworthy that incubation of rabbit aortic medial smooth muscle cells with 27.5 mM glucose for 5 days augmented PDGF-BB binding activity as well as particulate total PKC activity, which could be completely suppressed by staurosporine, a general inhibitor of PKC.[21]

The attenuating effect of probucol and D-α-tocopherol on hyperglycemia-induced DAG-PKC activity in VSMC may be mediated by the activation of DAG-kinase.[20] DAG-kinase can phosphorylate DAG and, thus, decrease the level of active DAG available to stimulate PKC.[20] An increase of total cellular PKC in cultured human VSMC has also been demonstrated in response to high glucose.[22] Results showing that an orally active inhibitor of PKC-β, LY33353, reversed some of the vascular abnormalities in diabetic rats have strengthened the proposed role of PKC as a mediator of diabetic vascular complications.[23]

It should be emphasized that the acute effects of hyperglycemia on PKC appear to be quite different since the treatment of A10 cells, a rat aortic VSMC line, with 25 mM glucose for 6 hours decreased the expression of protein and mRNA levels of PKC-βII without altering PKC-βI levels.[24] Thus, the gene expression of various isoforms of PKCs under hyperglycemia is complex and warrants detailed investigation under acute and chronic conditions.

Hyperglycemia and Mitogen-activated Protein Kinases

Mitogen-activated protein kinases (MAPK) are serine/threonine protein kinases, which are activated in response to a variety of external stimuli, including growth factors, hormones and stress. MAPK have been classified into several subfamilies: MAPK ERK 1/2 (extracellular signal-regulated kinases 1 and 2), P38^{mapk}, JNK/SAPK (c-Jun NH$_2$-terminal kinase/stress-activated protein kinase), ERK 3/4, ERK 5 (reviewed in [25, 26]). MAPK are activated by dual phosphorylation on both tyrosine and threonine residues by dual specificity protein kinases known as MAPKK or MEK (mitogen extracellular signal-regulated kinase kinase).[25] The sequential upstream signaling molecules to MEK are Raf, serine/threonine kinase, and ras, a small GTP-binding protein.[26] MAPKs phosphorylate downstream cytosolic and nuclear substrate/transcription factors, such as p90^{rsk}, and many transcription factors, such as c-Jun, ATF-2, Elk-1, CHOP, CREB, and MEF-2.[26-35] P90^{rsk} phosphorylates ribosomal proteins and participates in protein synthesis,[36] whereas the phosphorylation of transcription factors by MAPK leads to activation of several genes involved in growth and differentiation.[26] Thus, activation of the MAPK pathway can potentially result in increased growth, gene expression and proliferation of VSMC in response to hyperglycemia. However, it was only recently that studies on the effect of hyperglycemia on MAPK pathways were initiated. In porcine VSMC, hyperglycemia (25 mM glucose) markedly stimulated the activation state of ERK 1/2, JNK/SAPK as well as p38^{mapk}, compared with cells exposed to normal glucose (5.5 mM).[37] The impact of hyperglycemia on ERK and JNK/SAPK activation was detectable within 1 hour of cell treatment whereas at least 3-hour exposure was required to elicit any stimulatory effect on p38^{mapk} activity.[37] High glucose was also found to enhance the DNA-binding activity of activating protein 1 (AP-1) after long-term (5-10 days) culture of VSMC. Another study examined the effect of hyperglycemia on ERK 1/2 and p38^{mapk} activity in rat aortic VSMC.[38] It was demonstrated that treatment of VSMC with high glucose (16.5 mM) for 72 hours increased the activation status of p38^{mapk} by about 3-4-fold, compared to cells treated with normal glucose (5.5 mM).[38] However, no effect on ERK 1/2 activation was seen under these conditions. It was also shown that hyperglycemia-induced activation of p38^{mapk} was blocked by a general inhibitor of PKC and not by 20 nM LY33353, which specifically suppresses PKC-β at this concentration,[23] suggesting the involvement of a PKC isoform other than PKC-β in the response.[38]

Hyperglycemia and Transcriptional Nuclear Factor Kappa βeta

In addition to transcription factors such as c-Jun, ATF-2, Elk-1, CHOP, CREB and MEF-2, which are nuclear proteins phosphorylated and activated by MAPK to mediate gene expression, growth and transformation, transcriptional nuclear factor kappa beta (NF-kβ) has been implicated in the regulation of several genes linked to growth, adhesion and inflammation (reviewed in [39, 40]). However, in contrast to nuclear transcription factors, NF-kβ is a cytoplasmic protein existing as a heterodimeric complex composed of 50-kD (p50) and 65-kD (p65) subunits.[39, 40] In the cytoplasm, NF-kβ remains associated with the inhibitory proteins IKβα and β, which mask the nuclear translocation signal of NF-kβ. Phosphorylation of IKβs in specific serine residues catalyzed by IKβ kinases leads to its ubiquitination and subsequent degradation, resulting in dissociation of the NF-kβ-IKβ complex, which can then be translocated to the nucleus to regulate gene transcription.[41] The effect of hyperglycemia on NF-kβ activity in porcine VSMC was examined recently and it was shown that treatment with high glucose (25 mM)) for two passages enhanced the DNA-binding activity of NF-kβ by about 50%, compared to cells treated with normal glucose (5.5 mM).[42] Hyperglycemia also increased nuclear expression of the p65 subunit of NF-kβ, which could be further potentiated by several cytokines and growth factors such as tumor necrosis factor α (TNFα) and epidermal growth factor (EGF).[42] In line with a potential role of PKC in hyperglycemia-induced responses, these investigators also demonstrated that calphostin C, a PKC inhibitor, could completely attenuate NF-kβ activation by high glucose, whereas a non-selective protein tyrosine kinase inhibitor, genistein, had no effect.[42] Since NF-kβ has been implicated as a potential initiator of atherosclerotic lesions[43, 44] and antisense-oligonucleotides to the p65 subunit of NF-kβ have been shown to block VSMC proliferation as well as cell adhesion in response to balloon catheter injury,[45] it is possible that NF-kβ contributes to abnormal vascular function in diabetes and under hyperglycemic conditions.

Hyperglycemia and Angiotensin II (AII)-induced Signaling

AII is a vasoactive peptide which, exerts myriad effects on VSMC, including cell growth, migration and hypertrophy, and has been implicated in vascular dysfunction.[46] In this context, it **Figure 1.** A simplified schematic model depicting some of the protein kinase signaling pathways activated by hyperglycemia in vascular smooth muscle cells. The transcription factors are shown inside the nucleus (N) and appear in italics. Further details are given in the text. Abbreviations: PTPase: protein tyrosine phosphatase; DAG-PKC: diacylglycerol-protein kinase C; R/NR-PTK: receptor/non-receptor protein tyrosine kinase; MAPK pathways: (mitogen-activated protein kinase pathways include small GTP-binding proteins, mitogen-activated protein kinase kinase (MAPKK such as c-raf) and MAPKK (MEK); ERK: extracellular signal-regulated kinase; JNK: c-Jun N-terminal kinase; SAPK: stress-activated protein kinase; NF-kB: nuclear factor kappa beta; CBP: creb-binding protein; PI3-K: phosphatidylinositol 3-kinase; PI3,4,5,P₃: phosphatidylinositol 3,4,5,triphosphate; PDK 1/2: phosphatidylinositol phosphate-dependent kinase 1/2; PKC-zeta: protein kinase C-zeta; PKB: protein kinase B; mTOR: mammalian target of rapamycin; p70ˢ⁶ᵏ: 70-kD ribosomal S-6-kinase; p90ʳˢᵏ: 90-kD ribosomal S-6-kinase.

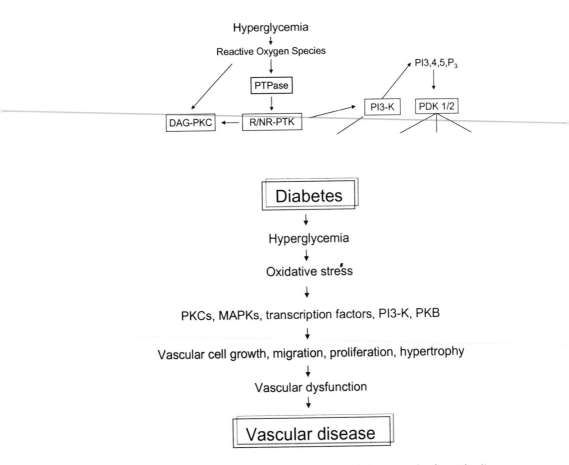

Figure 2. Summary of the key steps which might lead to diabetes-associated vascular disease.

is interesting that recent work has demonstrated an interaction between hyperglycemia and AII-induced signaling. In porcine VSMC, short-term (0.5 hr) hyperglycemia, compared to normoglycemia, increased AII-stimulated ERK 1/2 and p38[maapk] activation by about 2-fold.[37] In these studies, longer incubation (24 hours) with high glucose exerted an additive effect on AII-induced responses to p38[maapk] and AP-1 binding activity.[37] Similarly, when the effect of hyperglycemia on AII-induced activation of Janus-activated kinase (JAK) was investigated with signal transducers and activators of the transcription (STAT) pathway in rat aortic VSMC, high glucose was shown to cause more than a 2-fold increase in AII-stimulated JAK and STAT phosphorylation relative to low glucose-treated cells.[47] In these studies, hyperglycemia per se slightly augmented basal JAK and STAT phosphorylation.[47] The mechanism by which it enhances and potentiates the effect of AII was not addressed by these investigators.[37, 46] In fact, based on results showing that 20 mM glucose down-regulated AII binding in VSMC,[48] one would expect that hyperglycemia would attenuate AII-induced signaling responses. However, since hyperglycemia is associated with heightened expression of the PDGF-β-receptor,[21] and PDGF receptor activation induces JAK and STAT phosphorylation,[49] it is possible that enhancement of AII signaling by high glucose is mediated through this mechanism. Thus, hyperglycemia is likely to modulate physiological responses to AII and may contribute to the pathogenesis of vascular dysfunction in diabetes.

CONCLUSION

As discussed in the preceding sections, several key signaling components are activated in response to hyperglycemia in VSMC which include PKCs, MAPK, JAK, STAT as well as several transcription factors (Fig. 1). Stimulation of these signaling components is believed to mediate growth, migration, hypertrophy and proliferation of VSMC. The precise mechanism by which hyperglycemia activates the pathway shown in Fig. 1 is not clear. However, based on accumulated evidence, generation of reactive oxygen species (ROS), such as superoxide anion and H_2O_2, in response to hyperglycemia appears to be among the first events in this process. It has been suggested that ROS modulate cell signaling by inhibiting protein tyrosine phosphatase (PTPase) activity.[50] This is accomplished by oxidation of a catalytically-essential cysteine residue in the active site of PTPases.[51] Inhibition of cellular PTPase by ROS shifts the equilibrium of the phosphorylation-dephosphorylation cycle in favor of phosphorylation, enabling the basal activity of non-receptor and receptor protein tyrosine kinase (PTK) to enhance the tyrosyl phosphorylation of substrate proteins, triggering relevant signaling events and leading to activation of the MAPK pathway and transcription factors. H_2O_2 has also been shown to phosphorylate some PKC isoforms in tyrosine residues, eliciting their activation.[52] However, a role of PTKs in mediating hyperglycemic responses in VSMC has not yet been established. Moreover, there are also no studies to indicate that the PI3-K pathway is stimulated in response to hyperglycemia, whereas ROS have been reported to activate this pathway in VSMC.[53] PI3-K, through the generation of 3-phosphoinositides, such as phosphatidylinositol 3,4,5 triphosphate, can activate 3-phosphoinositide-dependent kinases (PDK-1/2).[54] PDKs are known to activate several downstream protein kinases, including PKC-zeta, PKB, mTOR and p70[s6k], which are involved in the regulation of cell growth, proliferation and survival[55] and, thus, can also contribute to abnormalities in VSMC associated with diabetes and hyperglycemia.

In summary, the signaling components activated in response to hyperglycemia (Fig. 1) are capable of triggering cellular processes which, if not appropriately regulated, can lead to abnormal growth, migration and proliferation of VSMC and thereby vascular dysfunction in diabetes (Fig. 2).

Acknowledgments

Studies in the author's laboratory are funded by grants from Heart and Stroke Foundation of Quebec and the Medical Research Council of Canada. Thanks are due to Susanne Bordeleau-Chénier for her excellent secretarial work and Ovid Da Silva of the Bureau d'aide à la recherche, Centre de recherche, CHUM, for his expert editorial assistance.

REFERENCES

1. J.A. Colwell, Vascular thrombosis in type II diabetes mellitus, *Diabetes* 42:8 (1993).
2. D. Givgliano and A. Ceriello, Oxidative stress and diabetic vascular complications, *Diabetes Care* 19:257 (1996)
3. J.W. Baynes, and S.R. Thorpe, Role of oxidative stress in diabetic complications, A new perspective on an old paradigm, *Diabetes* 48:1 (1999).
4. D. Koya, and G.L. King, Protein kinase C activation and the development of diabetic complications, *Diabetes* 47:859 (1998).
5. N. Natarajan, N. Gonzales, L. Xu, and J.C. Nadler, Vascular smooth muscle cells exhibit increased growth in response to elevated glucose, *Biochem. Biophys. Res. Commun.* 187:552 (1992).
6. K. Yasunari, K. Kohno, H. Kano, K. Yokokawa, M. Minami, and J. Yoshikawa, Antioxidants improve impaired insulin-mediated glucose uptake and prevent migration and proliferation of cultured rabbit coronary artery smooth muscle cells induced by high glucose, *Circulation* 99:1370 (1999).
7. S.E. Bursell, and G.L. King, Can protein kinase C inhibition and vitamin E prevent the development of diabetic vascular complications? *Diabetes Res. Clin. Pract.* 45:169 (1999).
8. B. Frei, On the role of vitamin C and other antioxidants in atherogenesis and vascular dysfunction, *Proc. Soc. Exp. Biol. Med.* 222:196 (1999).
9. R.A. Kowluru, R.L. Engerman, and T.S. Kern, Diabetes-induced metabolic abnormalities in myocardium: effect of antioxidant therapy, *Free Radic. Res.* 32:67 (2000).
10. T. Finkel, Oxygen radicals and signaling, *Curr. Opin. Cell Biol.* 10:248 (1998).
11. S. Chakraborti, and T. Chakraborti, Oxidant-mediated activation of mitogen-activated protein kinases and nuclear transcription factors in cardiovascular system: A brief overview, *Cell. Signal.* 10:675 (1998).
12. H. Kamata, and H. Hirata, Redox regulation of cellular signaling, *Cell. Signal.* 11:1 (1999).
13. Y. Nishizuka, Protein kinase C and lipid signaling for sustained cellular responses, *FASEB J.* 9:484 (1995).
14. W.S. Liu, and C.A. Heckman, The seven-fold way of PKC regulation, *Cell. Signal.* 10:529 (1998).
15. A.C. Newton, and J.E. Johnson, Protein kinase C: a paradigm for regulation of protein function by two membrane targeting modules, *Biochim. Biophys. Acta* 1376:155 (1998).
16. N. Nakanishi, K.A. Brewer, and J.H. Exton, Activation of zeta isozyme of protein kinase C by phosphatidylinositol 3,4,5-trisphosphate, *J. Biol. Chem.* 268:13(1993).
17. P.A. Ccraven, F.R., and DeRubertis, Protein kinase C is activated in glomeruli from streptozotocin diabetic rats, *J. Clin. Invest.* 83:1667 (1989).
18. T. Inoguchi, R. Battan, E. Handler, J.R. Sportsman, W. Heath, and G.L. King, Preferential activation of protein kinase C isoform bII and diacylglycerol levels in the aorta and heart of diabetic rats: differential reversibility to glycemic control by islet cell transplantation, *Proc. Natl. Acad. Sci. USA* 89:11059 (1992).
19. M. Kunisaki, S.-E. Bursell, F. Umeda, H. Nawata, and G.L. King, Normalization of diacylglycerol-protein kinase C activation by vitamin E in aorta of diabetic rats and cultured rat smooth muscle cells exposed to elevated glucose levels, *Diabetes* 43:1372 (1994).
20. I.K. Lee, D. Koya, H. Ishi, H. Kanoh, and G.L. King, d-Alpha-tocopherol prevents the hyperglycemia-induced activation of diacylglycerol (DAG)-protein kinase C (PKC) pathway in vascular smooth muscle cell by an increase of DAG kinase activity, *Diabetes Res. Clin. Pract.* 45:183 (1999).
21. T. Inaba, S. Ishibashi, T. Gotoda, M. Kawamura, N. Morina, Y. Nojima, M. Kawakami, Y. Yazaki, and N. Yamada, Enhanced expression of platelet-derived growth factor-β receptor by high glucose, *Diabetes* 45:507 (1996).
22. B. Williams, B. Gallacher, H. Patel, and C. Orme, Glucose-induced protein kinase C activation regulates vascular permeability factor mRNA expression and peptide production by human vascular smooth muscle cells in vitro, *Diabetes* 46:1492 (1997).

23. H. Ishii, M.R. Jirousek, D. Koya, C. Takagi, P. Xia, A. Clermont, S.E. Bursell, T.S. Kern, L.M. Ballas, W.F. Heath, L.E. Stramm, E.P. Feener, and G.L. King, Amelioration of vascular dysfunction in diabetic rats by an oral PKC beta inhibitor, *Science* 272:728 (1996).

24. N.A. Patel, C.E. Chalfant, M. Yamamoto, J.E. Watson, D.C. Eichler, and D.R. Cooper, Acute hyperglycemia regulates transcription and post-transcriptional stability of PKC βII mRNA in vascular smooth muscle cells, *FASEB J.* 13:103 (1999).

25. R. Seger, and E.G. Krebs, The MAPK signaling cascade, FASEB J. 9:726 (1995).

26. C. Widman, S. Gibson, M.B. Jarpe, and G.L. Johnson, Mitogen-activated protein kinase: conservation of a 3-kinase module from yeast to human, Physiol. Rev. 79:143 (1999).

27. Y.T. Ip, and R.J. Davis, Signal transduction by c-Jun N-terminal kinase (JNK) from inflammation to development, *Curr. Opin. Cell Biol.* 10:205 (1998).

28. T. Force, and J.V. Bonventre, Growth factors and mitogen-activated protein kinases, *Hypertension* 31(Part II):152 (1998).

29. C. Widmann, S. Gibson, M.B. Jarpe, and G.L. Johnson, Mitogen-activated protein kinase: conservation of a three-kinase module from yeast to human, *Physiol. Rev.* 79:143 (1999).

30. R.J. Davis, The mitogen-activated protein kinase signal transduction pathway, J. Biol. Chem. 268:14553 (1993).

31. R.M. Denton, and J.M. Tavare, Does mitogen-activated protein kinase have a role in insulin action? The cases for and against, *Eur. J. Biochem.* 227:597 (1995).

32. Y. Tan, J. Rouse, A. Zhang, S. Cariati, P. Cohen, and M.J. Comb, FGF and stress regulate CREB and ATF-1 via a pathway involving p38 MAP kinase and MAPKAP kinase-2, *EMBO J.* 15:4629 (1996).

33. X. Wang, and D. Ron, Stress-induced phosphorylation and activation of the transcription factor CHOP (GADD 153) by p38 MAP kinase, *Science* 272:1347 (1996).

34. S. Gupta, D. Campbell, B. Derijand, and R.J. Davis, Transcription factor ATF-2 regulation by the JNK signal transduction pathway, *Science* 267:389 (1995).

35. R. Zinck, M.A. Cahill, M. Kracht, C. Sachsenmaier, R.A. Hipskind, and A. Nordheim, Protein synthesis inhibitors reveal differential regulation of mitogen-activated protein kinase and stress-activated protein kinase pathways that converge on Elk-1, *Mol. Cell Biol.* 15:4930 (1995).

36. M. Frodin, and S. Gammeltoft, Role and regulation of 90 kDa ribosomal S6 kinase (RSK) in signal transduction, *Mol. Cell. Endocrinol.* 151:65 (1999).

37. R. Natarajan, S. Scott, W. Bai, K. Kumar, V. Yeneni, and J. Nadler, Angiotensin II signaling in vascular smooth muscle cells under high glucose conditions, *Hypertension* 33 (Part II):378 (1999).

38. M. Igarashi, H. Wakasaki, N. Takahara, H. Ishii, Z.-Y. Jiang, T. Yamauchi, K. Kuboki, M. Meier, C.J. Rhodes, and G.L. King, Glucose or diabetes activates p38 mitogen-activated protein kinase via different pathways, *J. Clin. Invest.* 103:185 (1999).

39. M.J. Lenardo, and D. Baltimore, NF-kβ: a pleiotropic mediator of inducible and tissue-specific gene control, *Cell* 58:227 (1989).

40. D. Thanos, and T. Maniatis, NF-kβ: a lesson in family values, *Cell* 80:529 (1995).

41. M.J. May and S. Ghosh, Signal transduction through NF-Kappa β, *Immunol. Today* 19:80 (1998).

42. K. Kumar, V. Yerneni, W. Bai, B.V. Khan, R.M. Medford, and R. Natarajan, Hyperglycemia-induced activation of nuclear transcription factor kβ in vascular smooth muscle cells, *Diabetes* 48:855 (1999).

43. T. Colline, Endothelial nuclear factor-Kβ and the initiation of atherosclerotic lesions, *Lab. Invest.* 68:499 (1993).

44. K. Brand, S. Page, G. Rogler, A. Bartsh, R. Brandi, R. Knuechel, M. Page, C. Kaltschmidt, P.A. Baeuerle, and D. Neumeier, Activated transcription factor-Kβ is present in the atherosclerotic lesions, *J. Clin. Invest.* 97:1715 (1996).

45. M.V. Autieri, T.L. Yue, and G.Z. Ferstein, E. Ohlstein, Antisense oligonucleotides to the p[65] subunit of NF-kβ inhibit human vascular smooth muscle cell adherence and proliferation and prevent neointima formation in rat carotid arteries, Biochem. Biophys. Res. Commun. 213:827 (1995).

46. H. Matsubara, Pathophysiological role of angiotensin II type 2 receptor in cardiovascular and renal disease, *Circ. Res.* 81:1182 (1998).

47. F. Amiri, V.J. Chema, X. Wang, R.C. Venema, and M.B. Marrero, Hyperglycemia enhances angiotensin II-induced Janus-activated kinase/STAT signaling in vascular smooth muscle cells, *J. Biol. Chem.* 274:32382 (1999).

48. B. Williams, and P. Tsai, R.W. Schrier, Glucose-induced down regulation of angiotensin II and arginine vasopressin receptor in cultured rat aortic vascular smooth muscle cells, *J. Clin. Invest.* 90:1992 (1992).

49. M.L. Vignasis, H.B. Sadowski, D. Watling, N.C. Rogers, and M. Gilman, Platelet-derived growth factor induces phosphorylation of multiple JAK family kinase and STAT proteins, *Mol. Cell. Biol.* 16:1759 (1996).

50. J.-I. Abe, and B.C. Berk, Reactive oxygen species as mediator of signal transduction in cardiovascular disease, *Trends Cardiovasc. Med.* 8:59 (1998).

51. K.L. Guan, and J.E. Dixon, Evidence for protein tyrosine phosphatase catalysis proceeding via a cysteine-phosphate intermediate, *J. Biol. Chem.* 266:17026 (1991).

52. H. Konishi, M. Tanaka, Y. Takemura, H. Matsuzaki, Y. Ono, V. Kikkawa, and Y. Nishizuka, Activation of protein kinase C by tyrosine phosphorylation in response to H_2O_2, *Proc. Natl. Acad. Sci. USA* 94:11233 (1997).

53. A.K. Srivastava, and S.K. Pandey, Stimulation of mitogen-activated protein kinases ERK 1 and ERK 2 by H_2O_2 in vascular smooth muscle cells, in: *Hypertrophied Heart*, N. Takeda, M. Nagano, and N.S. Dhalla, eds., Kluwer Academic Publishers, Boston (2000).

54. B. Vanhaesebroeck, and M.D. Watefield, Signaling by distinct classes of phosphoinosites 3-kinases, *Exp. Cell Res.* 253:239 (1999).

55. E.S. Kandel, and N. Hay, The regulation and activities of multifunctional serine/threonine kinase AKT/PKB, *Exp. Cell Res.* 253:210 (1999).

REGULATION OF MYOCARDIAL AND SKELETAL MUSCLE NA,K-ATPase IN DIABETES MELLITUS IN HUMANS AND ANIMALS

Henning Bundgaard, and Keld Kjeldsen

Medical department B 2142
The Heart Centre, Rigshospitalet
National University of Copenhagen
2100 Copenhagen, Denmark.

INTRODUCTION

Na,K-ATPase actively translocates potassium (K) into and sodium (Na) out of the cell in a 2:3 relationship, which contributes to the electrical properties of the cells. The influence of the Na,K-ATPase on the membrane potential is essential for excitability and contractility in skeletal muscles and myocardium. The transmembraneous gradients of Na and K also serves as a source of energy storage for secondary active transport of nutrients and other ions including glucose, amino acids, vitamins, Ca and H. The Na and K gradients are also of major importance for maintenance of osmotic balance and cell volume, since cations are of major importance for maintaining osmolarity of mammalian cells. In animals as well as in humans diabetes is associated with reduced skeletal muscle Na,K-ATPase function. On this basis a variety of muscular disturbances seen in diabetes may be related to regulation of muscular Na,K-ATPase.

The quantitative studies of muscular Na,K-ATPase regulations have become possible by means of assays for measurements of ^{3}H-ouabain binding to intact samples and K-dependent 3-O-methylfluorescein phosphatase (3-O-MFPase) or K-dependent para-nitrophenyl phosphatase (pNPPase) activity measurements in crude homogenates. These methods ensures high recovery of enzyme, accuracy and precision and can be performed on animal as well as human muscular tissue samples and biopsies.

In general, vanadate-facilitated ^{3}H-ouabain binding is used for complete quantifications in tissues with Na,K-ATPase with high ouabain affinities, and K-dependent pNPPase or K-dependent 3-O-MFPase activity measurements are useful in tissues with low or mixed ouabain affinities.

RESULTS AND DISCUSSION

Animal studies

In general, induction of experimental diabetes in animals leads to reduced body

Diabetes and Cardiovascular Disease: Etiology, Treatment and Outcomes
Edited by Aubie Angel et al., Kluwer Academic/Plenum Publishers, 2001

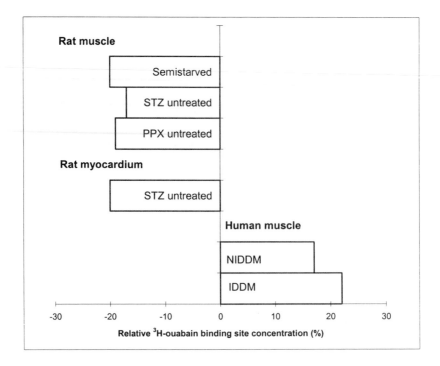

Figure 1. Overview of relative changes in skeletal muscle and myocardial Na,K-ATPase concentrations in relation to diabetes mellitus. STZ; Streptozotocin treated, PPX; Partial pancreatectomy, NIDDM; Non-insulin dependent diabetes mellitus, IDDM; Insulin dependent diabetes mellitus.

weight gain. It is well known that reduced body weight gain caused by semistarvation is associated with reduced skeletal muscle Na,K-ATPase concentration.[1] Thus, the evaluation of the effect of diabetes on skeletal muscle Na,K-ATPase need in addition to be compared to standard fed controls also to be compared to measurements obtained in weight matched control animals. Furthermore, age dependent changes in muscular Na,K-ATPase[2] necessitates comparisons with carefully age matched controls.

Figure 1 gives an overview of changes in muscular Na,K-ATPase in animals and humans in various conditions associated with changes in insulin levels or insulin sensitivity. In the animal models diabetes was induced by streptozotocin (STZ) treatment or partial pancreatectomy (PPX).[3] As previously observed semistarvation caused a 20% (p<0.05, n=9) reduction in ³H-ouabain binding site concentration in the rat soleus muscle. Compared to fed controls STZ (8 weeks) or PPX (10 weeks) induced diabetes was associated with reductions in soleus muscle ³H-ouabain binding site concentrations of 23% (p<0.05, n=9) and 19% (p<0.05, n=15), respectively. However, compared to weight matched control rats changes of similar order of magnitude were seen. In STX treated animals daily administration of insulin was associated with a 23% (p<0.05, n=9) increase above the level in age matched controls.

Few days after STZ treatment, rat myocardial K-dependent pNPPase activity was reduced by 11% (p<0.05, n=11-12) as compared to weight matched controls. Furthermore, the duration of diabetes was of importance for the myocardial Na,K-ATPase regulation, as a 22% (p<0.05, n=5-6) decrease was observed few weeks after induction of diabetes.

Human studies

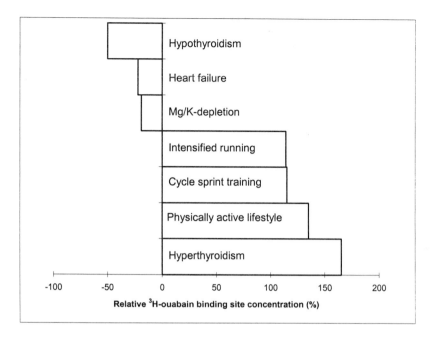

Figure 2. Overview of relative changes in human skeletal muscle Na,K-ATPase concentrations in relation to a number of diseases and conditions.

Human skeletal muscle Na,K-ATPase concentration changes in relation to a number of diseases and conditions (Fig. 2).[4]

In patients with diabetes changes in muscular Na,K-ATPase concentration measured by ^{3}H-ouabain binding to biopsies obtained from the vastus lateralis muscle are seen in Figure 1. Patients with NIDDM were treated with diet and / or oral antidiabetics and patient with IDDM were treated with insulin.[3] Compared to healthy control subjects, NIDDM was associated with a 17% (p<0.05, n=24) higher skeletal muscle Na,K-ATPase concentration and IDDM with a 22% (p<0.05, n=7) higher level. Furthermore, a highly significant positive correlation between plasma-insulin level and skeletal muscle Na,K-ATPase concentration was observed.

The present data indicates that insulin is a regulator of skeletal muscle as well as myocardial Na,K-ATPase concentrations. The reductions seen in skeletal muscle Na,K-ATPase concentration in untreated IDDM bears similarities with undernourishment. This downregulation may not only be corrected by insulin treatment, but physical conditioning that has previously been shown to induce an upregulation of skeletal muscle Na,K-ATPase concentration in healthy subjects[5] may also be of importance in the management of the disease.

It is well know that the skeletal muscle Na,K-ATPase plays a crusial role in the extrarenal K homeostasis.[6,7,8] Thus, dysregulation of skeletal muscle Na,K-ATPase mediated K uptake capacity have been shown to affect plasma K regulations during physical exercise.[9] This may be of importance for development of muscle fatigue and may influence physical performance capacity, important aspects of diabetes.

Diabetes is well known to be associated with ischaemic as well as cardiomyopathic heart disease. Human studies have documented a highly significant positive linear correlation between left ventricular systolic function (ejection fraction) and myocardial Na,K-ATPase concentration.[10] It has not been established whether a primary downregulation of myocardial Na,K-ATPase leads to compromised left ventricular systolic function or vice versa. On this basis it may be speculated that alterations in myocardial

Na,K-ATPase induced by diabetes may independently affect cardiac contractile function. Furthermore, compromised intramyocardial K homeostasis by reduced Na,K-ATPase mediated K uptake capacity may predispose diabetic patients to development of arrhythmia.

Acknowledgement

Løvens Kemiske Fabriks Fond is thanked for financial support.

REFERENCES

1. KJELDSEN, K., EVERTS, M.E. & CLAUSEN, T. (1986). Effects of semi-starvation and potassium deficiency on the concentration of [^{3}H]ouabain-binding sites and sodium and potassium contents in rat skeletal muscle. *Br.J.Nutr.* **56**, 519-532.
2. KJELDSEN, K., NØRGAARD, A. & CLAUSEN, T. (1984). The age-dependent changes in the number of ^{3}H-ouabain binding sites in mammalian skeletal muscle. *Pflugers Arch.* **402**, 100-108.
3. SCHMIDT, T.A., HASSELBALCH, S., FARRELL, P.A., VESTERGAARD, H. & KJELDSEN, K. (1994). Human and rodent muscle Na$^+$-K$^+$-ATPase in diabetes related to insulin, starvation, and training. *J.Appl.Physiol.* **76**, 2140-2146.
4. SCHMIDT, T.A. (1997). Human myocardial and skeletal muscular Na,K-ATPase in relation to digoxin therapy of heart failure. *Dan.Med.Bull.* **44**, 499-521.
5. MCKENNA, M.J., SCHMIDT, T.A., HARGREAVES, M., CAMERON, L., SKINNER, S.L. & KJELDSEN, K. (1993). Sprint training increases human skeletal muscle Na$^+$-K$^+$- ATPase concentration and improves K$^+$ regulation. *J.Appl.Physiol.* **75**, 173-180.
6. CLAUSEN, T. (1986). Regulation of active Na$^+$-K$^+$ transport in skeletal muscle. *Physiol.Rev.* **66**, 542-580.
7. BUNDGAARD, H., SCHMIDT, T.A., LARSEN, J.S. & KJELDSEN, K. (1997). K$^+$ supplementation increases muscle [Na$^+$,K$^+$-ATPase] and improves extrarenal K$^+$ homeostasis in rats. *J.Appl.Physiol.* **82(4)**, 1136-1144.
8. NØRGAARD, A. & KJELDSEN, K. (1991). Interrelation of hypokalaemia and potassium depletion and its implications: a re-evaluation based on studies of the skeletal muscle sodium, potassium-pump [editorial]. *Clin.Sci.* **81**, 449-455.
9. SCHMIDT, T.A., BUNDGAARD, H., OLESEN, H.L., SECHER, N.H. & KJELDSEN, K. (1995). Digoxin affects potassium homeostasis during exercise in patients with heart failure. *Cardiovasc.Res.* **29**, 506-511.
10. NØRGAARD, A., BAGGER, J.P., BJERREGAARD, P., BAANDRUP, U., KJELDSEN, K. & THOMSEN, P.E. (1988). Relation of left ventricular function and Na,K-pump concentration in suspected idiopathic dilated cardiomyopathy. *Am.J.Cardiol.* **61**, 1312-1315.

FOOD STRATEGIES FOR DIABETES AND HEART HEALTH

Kathryn Camelon

Toronto General Hospital
Toronto, Ontario

APPROACH TO NUTRITION CARE

Historically diet prescriptions for the management of diabetes and heart disease had many nutrient targets describing the appropriate daily amounts and types of fat and carbohydrate, as well as specific carbohydrate distributions through the day in defined numbers of meals and snacks. Predetermined nutrient prescriptions required the dietitian to perform detailed nutrient calculations to meet all the specified requirements. In contrast, the latest Canadian Diabetes Association (CDA) Guidelines for the Nutritional Management of Diabetes (1) are based on the principle that for most people with diabetes, the dietary recommendations are the same as those for the general population as outlined in Canada's Food Guide to Healthy Eating (2). The CDA guidelines are based on the premise that the dosage and timing of medications to help control diabetes should be worked around a healthy lifestyle and not vice-versa.

Implicit in the guidelines is the understanding that the composition of the diet should be individualized to the needs of each person considering several factors including other medical conditions. Thus for the person with diabetes and dyslipidemia, dietary adjustments are made to these healthy eating recommendations taking into account the nature of the lipid abnormality without losing sight of the need for optimal glycemic control.

Counseling clients to adopt the dietary guidelines usually means that behavioral changes are required. The goal with any dietary change is to get the best outcome for the client's effort expended in making the change. Every person's needs are individual. Negotiation of practical and realistic food plans becomes the core activity of the dietitian's interaction with the client. There is the need to have assurances that nutrition advice given reflects nutrient intakes in desirable ranges and the use of computer spreadsheet calculations has allowed dietitians to do this work in a fraction of the time from hand calculated meal patterns of the past. The dietitian assesses usual eating styles and determines with the client the key dietary changes which will improve metabolic control without unnecessarily disrupting a favored lifestyle.

Diabetes and Cardiovascular Disease: Etiology, Treatment and Outcomes
Edited by Aubie Angel et al., Kluwer Academic/Plenum Publishers, 2001

DIETARY ASSESSMENT

Some of the common factors taken into consideration in nutrition counseling are the client's age, gender, occupation, retired or active status, financial situation, food accessibility, sensory perception, food handling skills and knowledge and interest in food preparation. These factors shape the individual messages given about food and eating as well as how those messages are delivered.

Another part of assessment is to find out which faucets of today's food environment most influence our clients. The following are questions which can be used to evaluate food selection behaviors:
1. How often do they choose low fat or sugar free foods?
2. Do they use alternative therapies?
3. How often do they visit health food stores?
4. Do they read the detailed label information on foods?
5. How often do they use prepared foods?

Food Portion Sizes

In addition to understanding the influences on eating, it is important to find out what, when and how much food the client eats. This is vital information both for glycemic control and control of total energy intake. Determining food portion sizes is a crucial yet increasingly difficult aspect of assessing dietary intake (3).

Research has shown that most people, including health professionals, cannot accurately estimate portion sizes of commonly consumed foods. Compounded to this problem is the finding in United States that standard portions as defined by the Food Guide Pyramid (4) are considerably smaller than portions typically consumed by the public. Several of the dietary teaching materials including the portions in Canada's Good Health Eating Guide (5) make reference to small, or medium portions. Young and Nestle examined how people view qualitative terms such as small, medium, and large and found that people generally ignore the amounts associated with the term "medium" on food frequency questionnaires and consider the portion they eat as medium, regardless of its actual size (3).

To examine perceptions of "medium-sized" portions, Young and Nestle conducted a study in which university students were asked to bring to class at least one sample of a bagel, muffin, baked potato, apple or cookie that they considered to be medium sized. The foods were weighed and compared to the portion sizes recommended by United States Department of Agriculture. The mean weights of several of the medium samples brought in by the students were twice the size of a medium portion defined by the national food guide, and in all cases there was a wide variation perceptions of medium portion sizes. The conclusion from this study is that reliance on a description using terms small, medium or large for assessing dietary intake likely to result in a large underestimation of intake (3).

In view of such variability in perceptions of usual portion sizes, some studies have investigated whether the use of food models and visual aids assists with estimation of intake. A study conducted in Sweden evaluated the use of three types of models and compared results to using no models for accuracy of portion size determination (6). The types of models tested were photocopies of food items, plastic models, and geometric abstract models. The conclusions were: each model must come in different sizes to allow the respondent to discriminate among sizes shown; it must be easy to transport the models and handle them in interviews and there must be a key to the models but it must be concealed from clients (6).

One tool which meets these criteria is the publication Portion Photos of Popular Foods (7). This book contains life size photos of commonly eaten food items. Each food in the book is displayed in three portion sizes, the smallest size usually being equivalent to the portions defined in the diabetes exchange lists, and the other portions equal to the Food Guide Pyramid, or the portion defined on the food label - a common point of reference for many clients or it many be none of these. On each photo there is a coding system for identifying standard portions which assists the nutrition counselor but is not obvious to the client. Food portion sizes are presented randomly and not always shown in order from small to large. A reference table is provided which states gram weights and standard measures of portions and indicates equivalency of the photos to reference portions used in other food guides (7).

Food portions that are twice as large as those on a calculated meal plan represent a significant amount of extra energy, and affect glycemic control. Some clients may be convinced to measure food more carefully if they are aware of the wide range of portion sizes in the market.

Qualitative Description of Food Eaten

An integral part of any dietary assessment for the person with diabetes and dylipidemia is to find out what food and when the client eats. The food diary has been used extensively for assessing food intake. However the extent of under reporting of intake that has been well documented (8,9) has made us look at other methods. While any method of evaluating dietary intake has limitations, one method which is receiving increasing attention is the food frequency questionnaire. Because of its low cost, fairly modest demands on the client and the speed with which results can be obtained from the scanner readable format, this method is being used with increasing acceptance (10). Another practical advantage is that the food frequency questionnaire can be done at one time compared to the food diary which is recorded over a period of time, typically a minimum of three days. Food frequencies questionnaires are useful for identifying proportional trends in macronutrient intake.

Food diaries are excellent for showing the patterns of eating. Even in the presence of under reporting and imprecise documentation, one can obtain useful counseling information about the type, frequency and relative size of eating episodes and lifestyle in general. Food diaries are useful for problem solving in conjunction with the results of self-monitoring of blood glucose levels. No one assessment method answers all questions, but each method has advantages for answering different questions or describing different elements of the usual eating pattern.

Considerable time is spent in assessment, yet if this work is done carefully, priorities for individualized counseling become easy to identify and this allows the dietitian to focus on promoting two to three key dietary changes rather than presenting an entire new eating scheme.

DIETARY GOALS FOR DIABETES AND HEART DISEASE

The factors to consider in setting dietary goals for persons with diabetes and dyslipidemia are glycemic control, management of blood lipids, and healthy weight management. There are several interrelationships among these factors with the most encompassing being that of weight management.

A priority for any dietary guidelines is to strive for nutritional adequacy. While this may be assumed to be a dietary goal, over attention to some of the other goals, especially relating to fat intake, can preclude attention to nutrient adequacy. For many persons an increase in fruit and vegetables and fibre rich starchy foods are the dietary changes that are needed to achieve nutritional adequacy. If these dietary changes are made, other aspects of the diet frequently fall into place, such as reduced saturated fat intake and reduced energy intake.

There is some variation in targets for total fat intake in the Canadian and American guidelines for diabetes care (1,11). However there is agreement on the restriction in saturated fat intake to less than 10 % of energy and to a greater extent (less than 7%) if LDL cholesterol levels are high. In practicality many clients can readily achieve a restriction of 10 % of energy from saturated fat yet may not be consistently able to lower fat intake to less than 7 % of energy. Target levels can be individually determined based on extent o. change from usual intake. Trans fatty acids should be included in the restriction on saturated fat because of their similar deleterious effect on LDL cholesterol and in addition on HDL cholesterol. Another reason for restricting trans fat acids is that this type of fat often resides in foods that are calorically dense and nutrient poor and are not part of a healthy diet in any large amount. Dietary cholesterol levels usually decline with a reduction in saturated fat intake and a target intake of less than 300 mg per day is a reasonable goal.

Carbohydrate proportions in the diet can be determined by individual food preferences and glycemic response to different types and amounts of this nutrient. The 1998 position of American Diabetes Association is to have carbohydrate and fat provide 80% of energy thus giving wide leeway on an individual basis to the energy distribution between these nutrients (11). The Canadian guidelines recommend that approximately 55% of the individual's daily energy intake be derived from carbohydrates (1). Many clients have demonstrated success in being able to incorporate added sugars in small amount in their meals and this is consistent with recommendations in existing Canadian and American guidelines (1,11). However in cases of elevated triglyceride levels, caution with large fructose and sucrose intakes is advised (12).

Alcohol recommendations are comparable to those for the general population. There are individuals who have triglyceride levels that are extremely sensitive to alcohol and these people are identified by trial and error. Alcohol is a source of energy which is a consideration for those persons who are overweight.

MEAL PLANNING

One could pose the question, " If we are promoting healthy eating comparable to that for all Canadians, is a meal plan necessary?" Evidence for the value of a meal plan comes from the Diabetes Control and Complications Trial (DCCT) (13). In this study, the diet behaviors associated with improved glycemic control in persons with Type 1 diabetes were: adherence to a prescribed meal plan and prompt treatment of hyperglycemia. On the other hand overtreating hypoglycemia and consuming extra snacks beyond the meal plan were associated with higher glycosylated hemoglobin levels (13).

A meal plan is helpful as a master plan for diet therapy. The meal plan may be as useful for establishing consistent meal and snack spacing as it is for describing meal composition. The medication regimen should be worked around the meal plan and not vice versa. Thus establishing a healthy meal plan is an important first step in therapy. Any meal plan that is established is up for review depending on the results of self monitoring of blood glucose.

Another lesson learned from DCCT with relevance to weight management is the importance of avoidance of frequent hypoglycemia. Frequent hypoglycemia needs to be addressed either by adjustment of medications, or meal and snack spacing. Weight loss may be impeded by hypoglycemia if medications are not adjusted or snacks are eaten a little too late to prevent the hypoglycemia.

In designing the meal plan one may consider increasing the frequency of eating and reducing the size of feedings. This has metabolic advantages. In a study conducted by the Jenkins group in Toronto, less insulin was required to produce lower glucose concentrations when the same food is taken hourly as opposed to three meals over 10 hours. Additionally, in the long term, there was a reduction in serum triglycerides (14). The distribution of food intake through the day and avoidance of excessive carbohydrate at one eating episode requires negotiation with the client in establishing a model meal plan.

TEACHING METHODS

Once dietary goals and a master meal plan are established, the next step in nutrition care is determining the method of translating those goals into healthy eating messages. Some commonly used methods are described below.

Food Exchanges or Groups

A classic method for teaching healthy eating to persons with diabetes is by the use of the exchange system (12). This system is based on food groups , each of which has a list of foods and portion sizes that constitute a serving. Using this system, sources of carbohydrate are readily identified and one can promote nutritional adequacy, variety and balance in daily meals through the use of all food groups. Many food labels and recipes are coded according to the exchange system, thus making it possible for these prepared products to be satisfactorily incorporated into the meal plan. Disadvantages of the exchange system are that some stated portion sizes are unrealistically small and that combination foods may be difficult to classify into food groups. The complexity of the exchange system may limit its use with certain clients.

Plate Model

Another approach is the plate model method for teaching meal planning (15). This method is used extensively in the Nordic Countries for counseling persons with diabetes and dyslipidemia. The Plate Model is a visual method of promoting healthy eating through the use of charts or pictures. This key piece of the model is the dinner plate which serves as a pie chart to show the proportions of the plate that should be covered by foods from different food groups. The plate is divided into three sections, with 1/3 to 1/4 of the plate covered by meat, fish , poultry, or other protein source and the remainder split between grain products including bread, rice, pasta and potatoes and vegetables and fruit. It is a simple approach - in fact simplicity is seen as its distinguishing characteristic.

An advantage of using the Plate Model is that showing whole meals consisting of familiar foods translates general dietary advice into specific suggestions for eating. Meal components can be selected to match client preferences. The Plate Model helps the client make the connection between nutrition theory and food practice. Pictures of meals that are appealing provide a positive approach to meal planning. This helps to keep the interest in food which is an important feature for our aging population as senses of smell and taste decline.

While exact control of portion sizes may be beyond the scope of the model, improvements in proportions of foods relative to each other on the plate can correct major nutrient imbalances without the need to use scales and measures. Once initial dietary goals are met, the counselor can move on to using more complex methods if necessary to improve glycemic and serum lipid control. If a language barrier exists between the counselor and client, the pictorial Plate Model method assists in bridging the communication gap.

Sample Menu

The sample menu remains a useful guide for persons who desire an easy to follow approach to meal planning and can be quickly prepared and altered using computer templates. A sample menu represents the combined results of decision making about choice of foods appropriate for management of dyslipidemia, timing of eating for blood glucose control, portion sizes for carbohydrate distribution and energy control all in the context of familiar favorite foods of the client. It may seem like a simple approach from the health professional's perspective but it exemplifies a large amount of expertise and eliminates the need for many decisions by the client. One disadvantage cited by clients after initial use is that it is too confining unless variations are added to the basic menu.

Carbohydrate Counting

Carbohydrate counting is a teaching method where emphasis is solely on controlling the carbohydrate content of meal and snacks (16). While it is a useful technique to enhance glycemic control by focusing attention on the one nutrient that has the greatest effect on blood glucose, it does not promote eating healthy balanced meals, the achievement of nutrient adequacy or weight management. Carbohydrate counting is useful to introduce variety to meal and snack choices once healthy eating patterns have been established.

Each method of teaching meal planning has its advantages and disadvantages and some are more suited to targeting different types of food behavior change than others. The choice is dictated by client needs. Often one method may suit at one point in counseling, and another later on when priorities change or throughout the follow up period. Varying teaching approaches over time provides novelty in reinforcing dietary habits which is necessary for maintaining new health behaviors.

MAINTENANCE OF HEALTHY HABITS

Maintaining healthy eating habits is as difficult a task as making the changes in the first place. The weight management literature gives us evidence for more success if follow up is provided and that amount and duration of weight loss is proportional to amount of follow up (17). The practice guidelines for medical nutrition therapy for persons with type 2 diabetes published by the American Dietetic Association recommend that after initial counseling and follow up, patients receive ongoing dietary follow up every 6 to 12 months (18). In an environment where the nutritional characteristics of foods are strongly promoted and healthy eating is a common public health message our challenge becomes to work within this favorable environment to promote maintenance of nutritional health in people with diabetes.

REFERENCES

1. Wolever T, Barbeau M-C, Charron S, Harrigan K, Leung S, Madrick B, Taillefer T, Seto C. Guidelines for the nutritional management of diabetes mellitus in the new millenium; a position statement by the Canadian Diabetes Association. *Canadian Journal of Diabetes Care* 23(3):56-69 (1999).

2. Health Canada. *Canada's Food Guide to Healthy Eating*. Minister of Supply and Social Services. Ottawa, Canada (1992).

3. Young L., Nestle M. Variation in perceptions of a 'medium' food portion: Implications for dietary guidance. *J Am Diet Assoc* 98: 458-9 (1998).

4. *The Food Guide Pyramid*.: US Dept of Agriculture, Human Nutrition Information Service;. Home and Garden Bulletin No. 252 Hyattsville, Md (1992).

5. The Canadian Diabetes Association, *Good Health Eating Guide Resource*. Toronto (1994).

6. Karlström B, Abrahamsson L, Hädell K, Skoog E, Barkeling B, Wirfält E. Användning av livsmedelsmodeller i kostintervjuer. Naringsforskning 29:52-59 (1985).

7. Hess MA, editor. *Portions Photos of Popular Foods*. The American Dietetic Association and Center for Nutrition Education University of Wisconsin - Stout, Chicago. (1997).

8. Schoeller DA. How accurate is self-reported dietary energy intake? *Nutrition Reviews* 48: 373-378 (1990).

9. Hirvonen T, Männistö S, Roos E, Pietinen P. Increasing prevalence of under reporting does not necessarily distort dietary surveys. *European Journal of Clinical Nutrition* 51: 297-301 (1997).

10. Jain M. Culture-specific food frequency questionnaires: development for use in a cardiovascular study. *Can J Diet Prac Res.* 60:27-36 (1999).

11. American Diabetes Association. Nutrition recommendations and principles for people with diabetes mellitus. *Diabetes Care* 21(Supplement 1):S32-S35 (1998).

12. Kalergis, M., Pacaud, D., Yale, J-F. Attempts to control the glycaemic response to carbohydrate in diabetes mellitus: Overview and practical implications. *Canadian Journal of Diabetes Care* 22:20-29 (1998).

13. Jenkins DJA, Ocana A, Jenkins AL, Wolever TMS, Vuksan V, Katzman L, Hollands M, Greenburg G, Corey P, Patten R, Wong G, Josse RG. Metabolic advantages or spreading the nutrient load: effects of increased meal frequency in non-insulin dependent diabetes. *Amer J Clin Nutr* 55: 461-467 (1992).

14. Delahanty, L.M., Halford, B.N. The role of diet behaviors in achieving improved glycemic control in intensively treated patients in the Diabetes Control and Complications Trial. *Diabetes Care* 16:1453-7 (1993).

15. Camelon KM, Hådell K, Jämsén PT, Ketonen KJ, Kohtamäki HM, Mäkimatilla S, Törmälä MJ, Valve RH. The plate model: A visual method of teaching meal planning. *J Am Diet Assoc.* 98:1155-1158 (1998).

16. The DCCT Research Group. Nutrition interventions for intensive therapy in the Diabetes Control and Complications Trial. *J Am Diet Assoc* 93:768-72 (1993).

17. Perri MG, Sears SF, Clark JE. Strategies for improving maintenance of weight loss. Toward a continuous care model of obesity management. *Diabetes Care* 16 (200-209 (1993).

18. Monk A, Barry B, McClain K, Weaver T, Cooper N, Franz M. Practice guidelines for medical nutrition therapy provided by dietitians for persons with non-insulin-dependent diabetes mellitus. *J Am Diet Assoc* 95:999-1006 (1995).

THE ATHEROSCLEROSIS REVERSAL CLINIC:
THE WAY OF THE FUTURE

K. J. Kingsbury, J. Frohlich*

Healthy Heart Program
St. Paul's Hospital
Vancouver, British Columbia

*On behalf of the ARC team: S. Barr, A. Brozic, S. Chan, J. Frohlich, A. Ignaszewski, F. Johnson, K. J. Kingsbury, W. Linden.

INTRODUCTION

Clinical trials have demonstrated the effectiveness of rigorous exercise[1], diet[2] or aggressive drug therapy[3] to facilitate the regression of atherosclerosis. We hypothesized that an intensive, integrated approach to cardiovascular risk reduction utilizing strict dietary and exercise requirements, and, when necessary, adjunctive pharmacotherapy to aggressively reduce all modifiable risk factors is a more effective way to induce regression of atherosclerosis and achieve normalization of endothelial function than diet, exercise, or drug therapy alone. To test this hypothesis, we implemented the Atherosclerosis Reversal Clinic (ARC) program in January, 1998.

ARC – OVERVIEW

ARC is designed for individuals with coronary artery disease who want to go beyond conventional treatment standards to aggressively modify their cardiovascular risk. In order to test our hypothesis, we estimate 150 ARC participants will be needed to detect a significant change in carotid intima-media thickness (IMT) and brachial artery reactivity, our measures for evaluating regression of atherosclerosis and normalization of endothelial function, respectively. To accommodate a 10% non-completer/drop-out rate, we are seeking to enroll 165 participants into ARC. The length of participation for each individual enrolled in ARC is two years. Each week we enroll two new participants into ARC; the goal for 165 participants should be achieved by November 1999.

Because of the rigorous lifestyle intervention involved, we screen potential participants for self-efficacy and compliance intentions prior to enrollment and only enroll individuals who are willing and able to undergo extensive lifestyle modification and also willing and able to accept pharmacological intervention, if required. Individuals who are over the age of 65 years, diabetics requiring insulin, high-risk individuals with low-

Diabetes and Cardiovascular Disease: Etiology, Treatment and Outcomes
Edited by Aubie Angel et al., Kluwer Academic/Plenum Publishers, 2001

Table 1. ARC Goals for Risk Factor Management

Lipids:		
LDL-cholesterol ≤ 2.1 mmol/L	HDL-cholesterol ≥ 1.3 mmol/L	Triglycerides ≤ 1.1 mmol/L
Homocysteine		
Male ≤ 9.2 mmol/L	Female ≤ 7.8 mmol/L	
Glucose		
Maintain glycosylated hemoglobin < 0.065		
Body Weight		
Achieve and maintain BMI ≤ 25kg/m^2		
Blood Pressure		
Systolic blood pressure ≤ 120 mmHg	Diastolic blood pressure ≤ 80 mmHg	
Maintain "ARC" diet		
Total fat 15 – 20 % / Saturated fat ≤ 6%	Cholesterol ≤150mg/d	High fibre
Exercise		
Caloric Expenditure ≥ 2000 kcals/week		
Smoking		
Complete smoking cessation		

threshold exercise induced ischemia or arrhythmia, current smokers not contemplating complete smoking cessation, and individuals with limited ability to exercise are not enrolled in ARC.

ARC PROTOCOL

Participants are seen at regular intervals: monthly for the first four visits, bi-monthly for the next four visits, then once every three months for a total participation duration of two years. At each visit the participant is seen by a nurse, dietitian and exercise specialist for goal setting and evaluation. A cardiologist is available for consultation as required. An individualized approach to risk factor modification includes specific dietary and exercise recommendations as well as stress management and social support sessions. Goals for cardiovascular risk factors are shown in Table 1.

MEASURES

Standard lipid testing is done at baseline and at 6 month intervals (TC, LDL-C, HDL-C, triglycerides); other laboratory tests done at baseline and repeated as required include total homocysteine; apo B, lipoprotein (a), fasting glucose, glycosylated hemoglobin (if diabetic), TSH, AST, Creatinine, and Uric Acid. Anthropometic measures (weight, BMI, waist circumference, waist to hip ratio, sum of skin folds) are done at baseline and at 3-month intervals. Reports of smoking cessation are confirmed by exhaled carbon monoxide analysis. Maximal exercise stress testing is conducted at baseline, 1 and 2 years to determine functional capacity. To elicit specific self-reported information, we

Table 2. Participant Profile

Sex	Diagnosis	
	MI	**Angina**
Male (n=91)	50	41
Female (n=15)	7	8
Sex	**Intervention**	
	PTCA	**CABG**
Male (n=91)	30	26
Female (n=15)	6	1

administer the following assessment tools at baseline and at various evaluation points during participation:

- Nutrition related Quality of Life Questionnaire
- Diet history
- Three-day food records
- Minnesota Leisure Time Physical Activity Questionnaire
- Self-efficacy screening tool (developed for ARC)

VASCULAR OUTCOME ANALYSIS

At baseline and at 1 and 2 years, vascular studies are done, including brachial artery flow mediated dilation (FMD) with high resolution ultrasound to determine endothelial and smooth muscle response to shear stress, and B-mode ultrasound of carotid IMT to determine atherosclerotic burden. ARC vascular outcome analysis between baseline and year 1 and 2 will include the following:

- Change in carotid IMT
- Change in brachial artery FMD
- Relation and sequence of change in carotid artery IMT and brachial FMD
- Correlation between change in carotid artery IMT and brachial artery FMD with change in cardiovascular risk factors

ARC PARTICIPANTS

The goal for enrollment is 165 participants and to date 106 individuals are enrolled in the ARC clinic. Each participant has a cardiac history (see Table 2); cardiovascular risk factor history and baseline measures (lipids, carotid IMT and brachial FMD) are shown in Tables 3 - 5.

As of January 1998, only 7 individuals have discontinued participation in ARC. The decision to discontinue was based on the following:

- Absence of coronary artery disease (3)
- Newly diagnosed diabetic requiring insulin (1)
- Unable to accommodate ARC visits and prescribed regimen into personal schedule (3)

Prior to enrollment, interested individuals are invited to attend an information session explaining the ARC protocol (diet, exercise, medications, visit schedule; the fact that participants are responsible for the costs of medications, etc.) so that individuals are

Table 3. Baseline Risk Factor Profile

Sex	Age (yrs)	BMI (kg/m²)	HTN	Diabetes	FamHx
M (n=91)	57 +/- 6	27.9	34 (37%)	7 (8%)	56 (62%)
F (n=15)	58 +/- 4	29.6	11 (73%)	1 (7%)	10 (67%)

Table 4. Average Lipid Profile (SD) - Baseline

Sex	TC*	LDL-C*	HDL-C*	TG*	Lp(a)**
M (n=91)	4.6 (0.8)	2.8 (0.7)	1.1 (0.2)	1.7 (0.9)	437 (445)
F (n=15)	5.2 (0.9)	2.9 (0.9)	1.5 (0.3)	1.8 (0.7)	585 (494)

*mmol/L **U/L

Table 5. Baseline Measures

	Mean	Minimum	Maximum
Carotid IMT (mm)	0.87	0.63	1.27
Brachial FMD (%)	5.0	-0.40	12.30

Table 6. Baseline – 6 months (Male, n=91)

Lipid Profile (mmol/L)				Blood Pressure (mmHg)	
TC**	LDL-C*	HDL-C**	TG**	Systolic**	Diastolic***
-.35 (6%)	-.30 (8%)	+.05 (6%)	-.22 (4%)	-8.8 (5%)	-3.9 (5%)

*p=.001; **p<.05; ***p<.001

informed about ARC expectations prior to agreeing to participate in the clinic. Not only is the ARC population self-selected in that they volunteer for participation, we also screen the pool of volunteers for self-efficacy and compliance intentions. Only individuals reporting higher levels of self-efficacy and confidence about implementing behavior changes to their lifestyle are invited to participate in ARC. Once enrolled, time is spent with each participant to describe the process of atherosclerosis (both atherosclerotic disease progression and reversal) relative to their own medical history. The basis for each ARC intervention is thoroughly explained and prompt feedback on all test results is provided. When the use of medications is indicated, an explanation of the rationale for use, dosage, and potential side effects is given in conjunction with close monitoring for untoward effects and follow-up to ensure compliance with prescribed regimen.

PRELIMINARY FINDINGS

Overall, the response to ARC and adherence to the ARC regimen have been very good. In part, we attribute this to the pre-screening that is done to ensure the participants have higher levels of self-efficacy and motivation to undertake the intervention protocol. Adherence to the prescribed regimen is also enhanced by regular follow-up, telephone reminders to re-book missed appointments, availability of staff for support and assistance and close monitoring for adverse effects relating to exercise or use of medications.

Preliminary data showing results between baseline and 6 months (Table 6) suggest objective benefit in lipids and blood pressure.

FUNDING

ARC is funded by an unrestricted grant from Merck Frosst Canada. Annual staffing costs approximate $80,000 and includes staff equivalent of 1.0 FTE (nurse, exercise specialist, dietitian) and sessional physician and psychologist fees. Test and ultrasound evaluation costs are approximately $30,000 per year.

CONCLUSION

Designed as an experimental clinic, ARC is feasible and relatively easy to implement within an existing cardiac rehabilitation program/lipid clinic setting. For this group of volunteer participants, pre-selected for higher levels of self-efficacy and motivation, the ARC intervention protocol is carried out independently with follow-up visits scheduled at regular intervals. Preliminary data suggest objective benefit in lipids and blood pressure, however we await the results of carotid IMT and brachial FMD studies to evaluate our hypothesis that aggressive risk factor modification will result in the regression of atherosclerosis and normalization of endothelial function.

REFERENCES

1. Schuler, G., Hambrecht, R., Schlierf, G., Niebauer, J., Hauer, K., Neumann, J., Hoberg, E., Drinkmann, A., Bacher, F., Grunze, M., & Kubler, W. (1992). Circulation, 1992; 86: 1-11.
2. Ornish, D., Brown, S., Scherwitz, L.W., Billings, J.H., Armstrong, W.T., Ports, T.A., McLanahan, S.M., Kirkeeide, R.L., Brand, R.J., & Gould, K.L. (1990). Lancet, 1990; 336: 129-33.
3. Quinn, T.G., Alderman, E.L., McMillan, A., & Haskell, W. (1994). J Am Coll Cardiol 1994; 24:900-8.

LIPID CLINICS / CARDIOVASCULAR RISK REDUCTION CLINICS CURRENT STATE AND FUTURE CONSIDERATION

J. Frohlich, Kori Kingsbury

Healthy Heart Program
Lipid Clinic
St. Paul's Hospital
Vancouver, B.C.

THE OBJECTIVES OF A LIPID CLINIC

There are three primary objectives:
1. Specialty care for both primary and secondary prevention of coronary artery disease (CAD)
2. Education for public and health professionals
3. Research centered on the understanding of the role of lipids in cardiovascular disease.

Specialty Care

Specialty care includes diagnosis and recommendations for treatment of patients (and, where appropriate, their family members) with metabolic risk factors for atherosclerosis; in particular about their absolute and relative risks of CAD and how their risk is influenced by lifestyle changes and/or drug treatment. Education of patients and their families about their disorders is also an important component of this specialty care.

Furthermore, the clinics should be able to demonstrate patient outcomes with data on mortality and morbidity or at least record changes in patients' risk factors through follow up.

In our Healthy Heart Program Lipid Clinic we use a referral form (Table 1) which is reviewed by a clinic nurse and the referred patients are either accepted to the program or a letter is written to the referring physician with reasons why the referral appears inappropriate.

The criteria for lipid clinic referral include:
- difficulty with diagnosis or treatment of the lipid/metabolic disorder
- severe, premature or unusual clinical presentation of vascular disease
- a need for second opinion regarding initiation of (a potentially lifelong) drug treatment for lipid abnormalities.

All new patients have a series of laboratory tests (unless done by the referring physician within the previous 3 months) aimed at excluding secondary causes of lipid

Diabetes and Cardiovascular Disease: Etiology, Treatment and Outcomes
Edited by Aubie Angel et al., Kluwer Academic/Plenum Publishers, 2001

Table 1. Healthy Heart Program, St. Paul's Hospital

● Phone 604-806-8591
● Fax 604-806-8590

LIPID CLINIC REFERRAL

PATIENT INFORMATION

Patient's Name _____ _____
First Name   Last Name

PHN# _____

Patient's _____
Street

Date of _____

_____ _____
City   Postal Code

Phone (home) (____) _____

☐ Male ☐ Female

Phone (work) (____) _____

MEDICAL HISTORY

Risk Factors. Check if positive:

Known artery disease: ☐ Coronary ☐ Cerebrovascular ☐ Peripheral vascular

☐ Strong family history (in 1st degree relative <60yrs of age) ☐ Hypertension
☐ Smoker

☐ Diabetes ☐ Post-menopausal ☐ Other _____

Comments

_____

CURRENT MEDICATIONS & DOSE

For lipid disorders _____

Others _____

LABORATORY RESULTS (attach results)

Date (d/m/y) _____

HDL-cholesterol _____

Cholesterol _____

LDL-cholesterol _____

Triglyceride _____

Other _____

PHYSICIAN INFORMATION

Date Referred _____

Referring _____
          print

Physician's _____

Physician's _____

For Administrative Use only

☐ Complete Lipid   ☐ GLU/BUN/CREAT
☐ Apo E   ☐ AST/GGT/CPK
☐ Chol/Trig   ☐ TSH/UA
☐ HDL/LDL   ☐ ALK/TP/ALB
☐ Lp(a)   ☐ TBIL
☐ Homocysteine   ☐ Other
☐ WBC/HGB   _____

338

Table 2. Lipid Clinic Bloodwork - NEW PATIENTS

Criteria	Test to order:
Most recent lipid profile > 3months prior to time of LC appointment	• TC • LDL-C • HDL-C • TG
Fasting Glucose > 3months prior to time of LC appointment	• FBS • Hgb A1C if FBS abnormal
+ family history (1 relative <55♂ ; < 65♀)	• Lp(a) • tHcy
Suspect FCH or Type III disease (↑LDL-C + ↑TG; ↑TC + ↑TG)	• apo B
For women	• TSH if not on referral • repeat if TSH on referral abnormal • Alk Phos • AST if Rx with medication likely
For men	• AST if Rx with medication likely
Children	• Order "usual" (as above) • Order tHcy & Lp(a) if + Fam H$_x$
Low HDL	• If TG normal, order Apo A1
Other	• Uric Acid if ↑ in past or H$_x$ of gout

disorders and aiding in the diagnosis (Table 2). Tests are ordered selectively; test results accompanying the patient's referral are not repeated if done within the last 3 months.

In the clinic the patient is first seen by a Lipid Clinic nurse/patient educator who fills in the relevant history, assesses cardiovascular risk factor profile (Table 3) and records family history (with emphasis on vascular disease and risk factors). The patient is then seen by the dietitian and a lipid specialist (endocrinologist, clinical pathologist, cardiologist or clinical geneticist in our clinic). In the consultation letter the emphasis is on assessment of overall risk for vascular disease, diagnosis, targets for lipids and recommendations how to reduce cardiovascular risk (Table 4a). A shorter consult letter with several of the above parameters is mailed to the referring physician (Table 4b) for patients coming for follow up visit.

In many of the lipid disorders the knowledge of serum lipid values in first degree relatives is necessary for a more accurate diagnosis but such data are rarely available. Thus we use three degrees of certainty for diagnosis of lipid disorder: possible, probable and definite. Table 5 shows the criteria for possible, probable and definite diagnosis of familial

Table 3. Lipid clinic history / CV risk review

2.0 (a) History of Abnormal Lipids: ❏ ↑TC ❏ ↑LDL ❏ ↑TG ❏ ↓HDL ❏ Other:

Treatment prior to LC visit: ❏ none ❏ diet ❏ *past visit O/P dietitian* ❏ exercise ❏ medication (specify):

3.0 PAST MEDICAL HISTORY   ❏ *No prior illness* ❏ *No prior hospitalization*

❏ **CAD** (angina, MI, CABG, PTCA)
❏ **PVD** (stroke, claudication, TIA)
❏ **OTHER**

CNS   ❏ *no problems* ❏ *dizziness* ❏ *headache* ❏ *syncope* ❏ *visual disturbance* ❏ *speech/swallowing disorder*

CVS   ❏ *no problems* ❏ palpitations ❏ arrhythmia ❏ chest pain:

RESP ❏ *no problems*

GI   ❏ *no problems*

GU   ❏ *no problems*

MENOPAUSE age @ onset _____ yrs. ❏ **premature**: ❏ *hysterectomy* ❏ *oophorectomy*
❏ HRT:

4.0 ALLERGY ❏ NKDA ❏ Allergy to:	**5.0 MEDICATIONS** (Lipid) ❏ **HMG CoA Reductase Inhibitor**: ❏ **Fibrate**: ❏ **Resin**: ❏ **Niacin**:	Other Medications/Supplements:

8.0 CV RISK REVIEW

7.0 FAMILY HISTORY ❏ 1 : ❏ mother ❏ father ❏ sister ❏ brother
❏ 2 : ❏ *MAT* ❏ grandmother ❏ grandfather ❏ aunt ❏ uncle
   ❏ *PAT* ❏ grandmother ❏ grandfather ❏ aunt ❏ uncle

(a) SMOKING HX: ❏ lifelong nonsmoker ❏ ex-smoker ❏ current smoker ❏ wants to quit ❏ not interested in quitting
Smoking Cessation Plan:

(b) DIABETES: ❏ no ❏ yes age @ onset:_____ yrs ❏ NIDDM ❏ IDDM   Glucose Control: ❏ stable ❏ labile
❏ unknown

(c) ABDOMINAL CIRCUMFERENCE _____ **cm**

(d) HYPERTENSION ❏ yes ❏ no ❏ unknown age @ onset:_____ yrs BP Control: ❏ stable ❏ labile ❏
unknown

(e) PATTERN OF EXERCISE:
Frequency (times per week): ❏ none ❏ <1-2x/wk ❏ 3-5x/wk ❏ >5x/wk ❏ seasonal
Intensity ❏ Low ❏ Mod ❏ High   Time:
Type of Exercise:
Recommendations made:

(f) ALCOHOL ❏ no ❏ yes: average # drinks per week: ❏ ↓ recommended as
Rx

(g) STRESS ❏ low ❏ medium ❏ high *related to*: History of: ❏ sleep disturbance ❏ anxiety ❏ depression	Marital Status: ❏ S ❏ M ❏ D ❏ W Occupation:

Table 4a. Consultation letter.

Date:
Referred by:
Consultant:

Thank you for referring your patient to the Healthy Heart Program – Lipid Clinic for initial assessment and recommendations. Your patient was evaluated by Lipid Clinic R.N., a dietitian and myself, and the findings and recommendations are outlined below:

CURRENT COMPLAINT:
HISTORY OF ABNORMAL LIPIDS:

OTHER:

PAST HISTORY:

ALLERGIES:

MEDICATIONS:

DIETARY ASSESSMENT:

FAMILY HISTORY:

OTHER CV RISK REVIEW:
SMOKING:

DIABETES:

ABDOMINAL OBESITY:

HYPERTENSION:

EXERCISE:

ALCOHOL:

STRESS (SOCIAL):

PHYSICAL EXAMINATION

LABORATORY RESULTS:

DIAGNOSIS:

TREATMENT GOALS/RECOMMENDATIONS:

NEXT SCHEDULED VISIT:

Once again, thank you for asking us to assess your patient.

Table 4b. Consult letter mailed to the referring physician for patients coming for a follow up visit.

Date:

Your patient <> was seen in a follow-up visit in the Healthy Heart Program – Lipid Clinic.

PROGRESS:
GENERAL HEALTH:

TREATMENT GOALS/COMPLIANCE WITH PREVIOUS RECOMMENDATIONS:

WEIGHT, BLOOD PRESSURE, ABDOMINAL CIRCUMFERENCE (WHEN APPROPRIATE):

DIET AND LIFESTYLE:

DRUGS:

RECOMMENDATIONS:

NEXT VISIT:
This patient is well controlled on the current regiment. Unless you think it necessary, no follow-up visits are needed.

Once again, thank you for the opportunity to participate in the care of your patient.

---

hypercholesterolemia and familial combined dyslipidemia. Similar criteria have been established for the diagnosis of other lipoprotein disorders, such Type III disease, hypoalphalipoproteinemia, etc.

Our recommendations for treatment are based on the current Working Group on Dyslipidemia criteria which are summarized in Table 6. Discharge criteria have also been formulated and are summarized in Table 7.

Clinic Role in Education

Education is aimed at:
- patients and public at large
- students
- healthcare professionals

A weekly series of lectures for patients of lipid and cardiac rehabilitation and prevention program cover a variety of topics from diet and exercise to dyslipidemias and other risk factors as well as talks dealing with different classes of medications

Graduate students working towards their M.Sc. or Ph.D. degrees in experimental pathology are supervised by faculty members while medical and nursing students, clinical clerks and residents from various subspecialties of internal medicine participate in the daily operation of the clinic.

Over the past few years we have established a program for healthcare professionals called Healthy Heart Experience whereby a group of family physicians or other healthcare professionals play the role of a patient: undergo an exercise stress test, have an interview

Table 5. Guidelines for the Diagnosis of Dyslipidemias in the St. Paul's Hospital Healthy Heart Program Lipid Clinic

Three "Degrees of certainty" are used to classify diagnosis of dyslipidemia in the Lipid Clinic:

1. Possible
2. Probable
3. Definite

The following 2 examples illustrate how these terms should be applied.

HETEROZYGOTE FAMILIAL HYPERCHOLESTEROLEMIA:

1. Possible	LDL Cholesterol > 5 - 6 for Age/Sex (LRC criteria) No physical findings and no data on relatives *Example: A patient presents with total cholesterol of 11, LDL of 8, more or less normal triglycerides and HDL, no knowledge of lipid values (or history of cardiovascular disease) in family, and no physical signs of FH. In this case secondary causes would have to be excluded first.*
2. Probable.	As 1, but also 1st degree relative (parent/sibling/child) with TC or LDL > 95th Percentile
3. Definite.	As 2, but • Either the patient has or a 1st Degree relative has definite tendon xanthomas • Pediatric relative with ↑ TC and LDL-C

FAMILIAL COMBINED DYSLIPIDEMIA:

1. Possible	• ↑Trigs and/or LDL-C > 95th Percentile • Anyone who does not have distinctive physical findings but has mixed dyslipidemia and high apoB.
2. Probable.	• As 1, but also 1st degree relative has either mixed dyslipidemia or hypercholesterolemia or hypertriglyceridemia (↑Trigs and/or LDL-C > 95th percentile; proband with ↑Trigs must have a relative with ↑ LDL-C)
3. Definite.	Where lipid profile is known on numerous members of the family where definite pattern for FCH emerges: 1/3 of the affected relatives have mixed hyperlipidemia, 1/3 have hypercholesterolemia alone and, 1/3 have hypertriglyceridemia alone.

The above examples illustrate a degree of certainty of the diagnosis. In most cases of FCH, we will probably end up with a "possible" or "probable" diagnosis because we rarely study very large families. In other cases such as Type 3 disease, the definite diagnosis is clinched when we have, in addition to dyslipidemia and/or typical clinical findings, results of apoE genotype (or phenotype). In other cases such as lipoprotein lipase deficiency and a whole host of other rare monogenic disorders only genotyping and finding the specific genetic defect (this also applies for FH and FCH to a degree) yield the "definite" diagnosis.

with a dietitian, exercise specialist and physician. Participants' risk factors are assessed and a lecture on current issues in cardiology/lipidology ends the program. Over 140 physicians have participated so far and the response has been very positive. A number of visiting physicians, dietitians, nurses and students from other parts of Canada and the world also participate in our educational activities.

Table 6.

LEVEL OF RISK	TARGET VALUES		
	LDL-C level, mmol/L	Total cholesterol: HDL:C ratio	Triglyceride level mmol
1- VERY HIGH * (10-yr risk > 30% or history of CVD or diabetes mellitus)	<2.5	<4	<2.0
2- HIGH * (10-yr risk 20-30%)	<3.0	<5	<2.0
3- MODERATE ** (10-yr risk 10-20%)	<4.0	<6	<2.0
4- LOW ** (10-yr risk < 10%)	<5.0	<7	<3.0

* start medication and lifestyle changes concomitantly if above targets
** start medication if targets not achieved after 3 months of lifestyle modification
***start medication if target values are not achieved after 6 months of lifestyle modification.

Research

Basic and clinical research and clinical trials form an important part of the clinic function. The rationale for having a clinical research laboratory attached to the clinic has been well described by Dr. Jean Davignon[1]; the benefits of a research laboratory within the clinic are clear: investigation of interesting/unusual patients leads frequently to new discoveries.

Many lipid clinics participate in national and international clinical trials assessing new lipid lowering medications and also, increasingly, new nutraceuticals such as phytosterols. This allows the clinic to stay on the forefront of advances in the treatment of lipid disorders.

LIPID CLINIC TEAM

Program coordinator, clinical clerks, nurses, dietitians, physicians and a data manager are usually needed to run an active academic program. We have also established Lipid Clinic Outreach branches in B.C. over the last 10 years and have formed an integrated computerized network. Data have been collected on close to 2,000 patients by the outreach physicians thus adding significantly to the central clinic's database of approximately 10,000 individuals.

LIPID CLINIC MANUAL OF OPERATIONS

This should include functional aspects of the lipid clinic "start-up checklist"[2].

Table 7.

Healthy Heart Program
Proposed Patient Discharge Guidelines

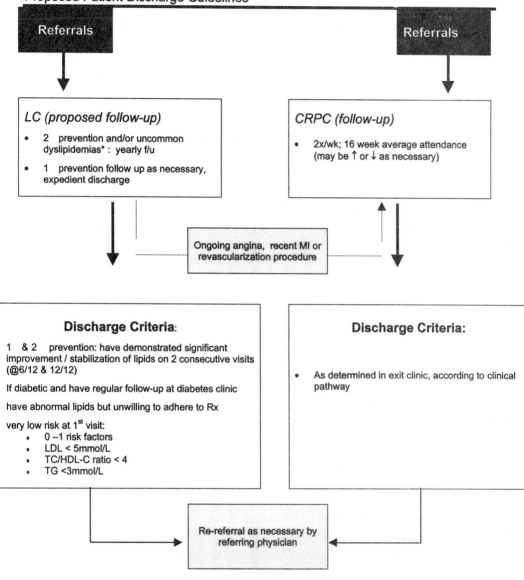

*FH, sitosterolemia, hyperchylomicronemia, etc.

FUTURE: COMPREHENSIVE CARDIOVASCULAR DISEASE RISK MANAGEMENT IN CLINICAL AND COMMUNITY-BASED SETTING

This topic has been well summarized by Dr. N.F. Gordon[4]. Currently two types of such programs exist: one aimed at patients with established disease as established by the SCRIP investigators[5] which includes a comprehensive lifestyle intervention, appropriate pharmacotherapy and takes place in a physician-supervised nurse-managed clinic. In the original SCRIP program there was a very impressive 40% reduction in hospitalizations for cardiac events over the study period of 5 years.

Table 8 summarizes the sequence of events in a secondary prevention program[3].

In patients without symptomatic disease guidelines formulated by professional bodies such as Canadian Cardiovascular Society should be followed[6].

In both types of programs (1° and 2° prevention) the key components are:

Lifestyle intervention which usually consists of regular exercise prescription (the most common of which is walking daily 2 miles in 30 minutes - (or 2 x 1 mile in 15 minutes) and a diet low in saturated fat (7% of total calories) and limited in total fat usually to below 30% of total calories with higher monounsaturated fat content. Use of complex carbohydrates and additional fibre is also emphasized as is sufficient quantity of omega 3 fatty acids. Medications are used where necessary to treat hypertension, dyslipidemia and in some cases as an aid to smoking cessation. Referrals to a specialist (such as exercise specialist, dietitian or smoking cessation expert) are part of the program.

In addition to the above, dealing with psychosocial factors such as stress reduction, social integration for those who are lonely, treatment of depression and anger management are of major importance.

Table 8.
Sequence of Events

Figure 1	Figure 2
Step 1 Patient with cardiovascular disease referred to preventive cardiology program after hospitalization for acute cardiac event, office visit to cardiologist or other physician, or following identification by other means (e.g. via completion of health risk appraisal by patients enrolled in a managed care plan).	**Step 1** Individual with cardiovascular disease risk factors enrolls in program. Participant is either: a) self-referred or b) referred after hospitalization, physician office visit, or identification by other means (e.g. completion of health risk appraisal by individuals enrolled in managed care plan or worksite health promotion program).
Step 2 Initial consultation with MD, RN and other program staff (e.g. dietitian, exercise physiologist). Risk stratification status is determined, cardiovascular disease risk management goals are set and action plan for achieving these goals is formulated and initiated. Focus on lifestyle modification and appropriate use of medications to optimize risk factors.	**Step 2** Participant completes baseline medical history and health habits questionnaire. Initial evaluation performed by appropriately qualified non-physician health care professional. Computerized data used to generate: a) cardiovascular disease risk management goals; b) action plan for achieving goals; and c) referrals to participant's physician for medication changes to either health care professionals/programs (e.g. psychologist, physician) or for additional laboratory testing if clinically indicated.
Step 3 Lifestyle modifications are initiated in: a) Phase II cardiac rehabilitation program at cardiovascular disease risk management facility; b) Phase II cardiac rehabilitation program at a satellite facility; or c) home or community based program (depending on variables including risk stratification status, place of residence, available resources, insurance coverage, personal preferences).	**Step 3** Comprehensive lifestyle modification program is initiated. Focus on correct nutrition, physical activity and exercise training, smoking cessation, stress management and weight management. Use of state-of-the-art behaviour modification techniques, including assessment of stage of readiness for change and single concept learning theory. Individualized counselling/guidance by health care professional.
Step 4 Long-term follow up (lifelong) via mail, telephone contact, and office visits to evaluate progress in achieving and/or maintaining cardiovascular disease risk management goals and to revise action plan as indicated.	**Step 4** Long term follow up (lifelong) including: a) ongoing individualized counseling/guidance; b) support group meetings; c) evaluation of progress in achieving and/or maintaining cardiovascular disease risk management goals; d) revision of action plan; e) additional physician or other referrals as indicated; f) monitoring of compliance with lifestyle interventions and medications; and g) outcomes assessment. Follow up conducted via visits to program, telephone, computer and mail using computerized tracking system.

Am. Coll. Sports Med Vol 8, No. 3, December 1998

It has been shown that compliance can be improved by office visit recalls, telephone and mail contact, support group meetings and by organizing special events.

There is little doubt that cost effectiveness of nurse-managed and physician-supervised risk reduction clinics exceeds that of a specialized lipid clinic. Furthermore, compliance may be better in such settings as shown by precedents in the management of diabetes.

What is needed (and currently gathered in a number of these programs) are outcome data that will provide proof of the programs' overall effectiveness and particularly their cost effectiveness. Apart from the SCRIP secondary prevention study few data are available to demonstrate the effectiveness of global risk reduction clinics in managing patients with symptomatic vascular disease and none for the primary prevention population. This is an important area of future research.

REFERENCES

1. Davignon J. A Lipid Clinic associated with a Research Laboratory working on dyslipoproteinemias and atherosclerosis. Can J. Cardiol 1996:12:885-890
2. Mason C. How to organize and manage a lipid clinic. J. Cardiovasc. Management Sept/Oct 1996
3. Am. Coll. Sports Med Vol 8, No. 3, December 1998
4. Cordon NF. Comprehensive cardiovascular disease risk management in clinical and community-based settings. Certified News 1998;8:1-4.
5. Haskell WL, Alderman EI, Fair JM et al. Effects of intensive multiple risk reduction on coronary atherosclerosis and clinical events in men and women with coronary artery disease. The Sanford Coronary Risk Intervention Project (SCRIP).
6. Canadian Cardiovascular Society 1998 Consensus Conference on the Prevention of Cardiovascular Diseases: The Role of the Cardiovascular Specialist. Can J Cardio 1999;15 Suppl G

AMPUTATION PREVENTION AND REHABILITATION IN DIABETES

John M. Embil
Consultant, Infectious Diseases
Director, Infection Control Unit
Coordinator, Diabetic Foot and Complicated Wound Clinic
Assistant Professor, Internal Medicine, Infectious Dieseases
And Medical Microbiology

Departments of Internal Medicine,
Infectious Diseases and Medical Microbiology
Health Sciences Centre
Winnipeg, Manitoba

INTRODUCTION

Diabetes is a multi-system disease which can lead to complications such as peripheral neuropathy and peripheral vascular disease. These two complications can synergistically lead to the formation of ulcerations in the feet and lower extremities of persons with diabetes (PWD). Should an ulceration develop, it may be a self limited process healing spontaneously or it may lead to more serious complications such as infection of the skin, soft tissue, bone, sepsis, and possibly amputation of toes, foot, or lower extremity. For the year 1991, 57% of all amputations involving lower extremities in Manitoba were in PWD. Lower extremity amputations were 10 times higher amongst PWD than those without diabetes. In 1991, the prevalence of diabetes in adult Manitobans was as follows: First Nations individuals - 12% males, 20% females, non-First Nations individuals - 7% male, 6.4% females. The Manitoba Health Services Commission records for 1993 - 1994 show 16% of lower extremity amputations in Manitoba were amongst First Nations individuals, and 84% in non-First Nations individuals.[1]

Despite great advances made in the treatment of diabetes, significant morbidity and mortality still occurs with this disease. Factors which influence the predisposition for amputation include neuropathy which may lead to ulcerations, autonomic insufficiency leading to dry, cracked skin serving as a portal for infection, vasculopathy leading to ischaemia and decreased wound healing capacity, and immunopathy as a consequence of altered neutrophil function. These factors combined with a lack of or inadequate knowledge of diabetes can lead to serious complications. It is thus critical to identify PWD at risk of foot complications and prevent the complications. Unfortunately, some individuals present with a foot complication as their first presentation of diabetes. In all individuals, it is important to quickly and effectively treat the underlying infection, be it skin, soft tissue, and/or bone. The goal is to minimize the risk of amputation. The

Diabetes and Cardiovascular Disease: Etiology, Treatment and Outcomes
Edited by Aubie Angel et al., Kluwer Academic/Plenum Publishers, 2001

349

summary and recommendations that follow address the major risk factors for lower extremity ulcerations in the feet of PWD. The major risk factors include neuropathy, ischemia, and infection.

INFECTIONS IN THE LOWER EXTREMITIES OF PWD

Infections in the lower extremities of PWD can be divided into those which are mild, moderate and severe and may involve skin, soft tissue, and/or bone. Numerous reports outline the management of infections in the lower extremities of PWD.[2,3,4,5,6,7,8,9,10,11] Uncomplicated lower-extremity infections in PWD are usually caused by aerobic gram-positive cocci, and responded well to oral outpatient therapy.[5] A variety of antibiotics exist that are well tolerated orally and can achieve suitable serum and bone levels for the treatment of deep seated infections.[12] The management of osteomyelitis in the foot of PWD is more complicated, and numerous approaches have been recommended ranging from prolonged parenteral therapy to initial parenteral therapy followed by oral antimicrobial therapy (OAT) or exclusively OAT.[6,7,8,9,10,11]

It is important to differentiate between wound infection and colonization. Infections are usually associated with purulent discharge, edema, erythema, and occasionally pain, and bacteria may be recovered from the wound base. With colonization bacteria will be recovered from swabs of the wound base but the other signs of infection are absent. Superficial skin and soft tissue infections may arise as a consequence of direct trauma and contiguous spread of organisms. If the infection is not controlled and the ulceration progresses, the underlying bone may become involved.

Initially, aerobic gram positive bacteria such as *Staphylococcus aureus* and Streptococcus species are the most frequently isolated organisms. As the ulceration persists, more necrotic tissue is present and gram negative and anaerobic bacteria soon predominate in the wound.

Specimens for culture are best obtained from infected tissue that does not communicate with the skin surface. The ideal specimen for culture assessment of infection is a curettage specimen from the base of the ulcer or bone biopsy specimens if osteomyelitis is suspected. If such specimens are not available, cultures of purulent exudate from within the ulcer base or sinuses may be an alternative.

Before appropriate therapy can be provided, it is important to establish the status of the lower extremity of the PWD as it relates to infection. Issues that must be considered are:

1. Extent of infection - mild, moderate, severe
2. Presence of underlying ulcerations
3. Presence of neuropathy
4. Adequacy of circulation
5. Presence of underlying osteomyelitis
6. Adjunctive measures

The suggestions that follow for investigations, dressings and therapeutic interventions have been kept as simple as possible. The suggestions are to be used in conjunction with appropriate management of the underlying diabetes and other metabolic abnormalities:

EXTENT OF INFECTION

Table 1 summarizes the classification of infections in the lower extremities of PWD and provides treatment suggestions. It is important to recall that it is advisable to use wound or bone cultures to help guide antimicrobial choices. Figure 1 provides a simplified algorithm to help determine the most appropriate treatment regimens for patients presenting with diabetic foot infections.

Table 1. Antibiotic Therapy for Infected Ulcerations in the Lower Extremity of PWD

Type of Infection	Medication	Dosage [2]	Daily Cost [3]	Total Daily Cost [4]
Mild Infections: These are deemed to be neither limb nor life threatening processes. They are usually associated with cellulitis surrounding an ulceration. A small amount of purulent material may be present at the base of the ulcer. The most likely organisms are aerobic gram positive cocci. Patients with these infections can frequently be treated as outpatients with oral therapy.	Cloxacillin	500 mg po qid	$1.03	As per daily cost.
	Cephalexin	500 mg po qid	$1.50	
	Tmp/Smx*	1 ds po bid	$0.27	
	Clindamycin	300 mg po qid	$7.51	
	Amoxicillin-clavulinic Acid	500 /125 mg po tid	$4.57	
Moderate Infections: These can range from plantar abscesses to more significant cellulitis with tissue necrosis and deep seated infection. Antimicrobial regimens should be effective against staphylococci, streptococci, anaerobes, and common Enterobacteriaceae species.				
• **Patients who are not toxic**: can be treated with local incision and drainage and oral antimicrobial therapy.	Tmp/Smx* and Metronidazole	1 ds po bid 500 mg po tid	$0.27 $0.24	$0.51
	Tmp/Smx* and Clindamycin	1 ds po bid 300 mg po qid	$0.27 $7.51	$7.78
	Ciprofloxacin and Clindamycin	500 mg po bid 300 mg po qid	$5.01 $7.51	$12.52
	Ciprofloxacin [4] and Clindamycin	750 mg po bid 300 mg po qid	$13.33 $7.51	$20.84
	Amoxicillin-clavulinic acid	500 /125 mg po tid	$4.57	$4.57
• **Patients who are critically ill or toxic:** best treated with parenteral therapy until stable, then switch to oral therapy.	Managed as per severe infections, see below.			
Severe Infections: Patients with severe diabetic foot infections have limb or life threatening infections requiring immediate hospitalization and parenteral antimicrobial therapy. Early surgical debridement and drainage of abscesses is critical	Clindamycin and Gentamicin	IV 600 mg Q8H IV 80 mg Q8H	$40.00 $12.00	$52.00
	Cefotetan	IV 2gm Q12H	$60.00	As per daily cost
	Cefazolin and Metronidazole	IV 2gm Q8H IV 500mg Q8H	$18.00 $4.59	$22.59
	Piperacillin and Tazobactam	IV 3.375g Q6H	$63.60	$63.60
	Clindamycin and Ceftriaxone	IV 600mg Q8H IV 1gm Q24H	$40.00 $34.00	$74.00
	Imipenem/Cilistatin	IV 500/500 mg Q6H	$97.52	$97.52
	Meropenem	IV 1 gm Q8H	$141.84	$141.84

Table 1: Antibiotic Therapy for Infected Ulcerations in the Lower Extremity of PWD (continued)

Type of Infection	Medication	Dosage[2]	Daily Cost[3]	Total Daily Cost[4]
Osteomyelitis: is a frequent complication of diabetic foot ulcerations. Antimicrobial choices must be guided by culture data. Monotherapy may be used based upon clinical assessment and culture results.	Tmp/Smx* and Metronidazole	1 ds po bid 500 mg po tid	$0.25 $0.40	$0.65
	Tmp/Smx* and Clindamycin	1 ds po bid 300 mg po qid	$0.25 $6.05	$6.30
• **Oral Therapy**: Osteomyelitis may be managed with long term oral antimicrobial therapy with agents that are well absorbed from the gastrointestinal tract and have good distribution to bone and tissue.	Amoxicillin-clavulinic acid	500/125 mg p tid	$4.20	$4.20
	Ciprofloxacin and Metronidazole	500 mg po bid 500 mg po tid	$5.02 $0.40	$5.42
	Ciprofloxacin and Clindamycin	500 mg po bid 300 mg po qid	$5.02 $6.05	$11.07
	Ciprofloxacin[4] and Clindamycin	750 mg po bid 300 mg po qid	$9.48 $6.05	$15.53
	Cefazolin and Metronidazole	IV 2 gm Q8H IV 500 mg Q8H or 500 mg po tid	$18.00 $4.59 $0.40	$22.59 $18.40
• **Parenteral Therapy**: In some cases, parenteral therapy may be necessary. Although multiple parenteral regimens exist, only those which may be easily administered through a community intravenous therapy program are noted here. Aminoglycoside based regimens are avoided for prolonged treatment courses because of potential complications. The duration of parenteral therapy is guided by clinical response and every attempt should be made to use oral regimens when possible.	Cefotetan	IV 2 gm Q12H	$60.00	$60.00
	Piperacillin and Tazobactam	IV 3.375 gm Q6H	$63.60	$63.60
	Clindamycin and Ceftriaxone	IV 600 mg Q8H IV 1 gm Q24H	$40.00 $34.00	$74.00
	Ceftriaxone and Metronidazole	IV 1 gm Q24H IV 500mg Q8H or 500 mg po tid	$34.00 $4.59 $0.40	$38.59 $34.40

* Tmp/Smx = Trimethoprim/sulfamethoxazole

[1]If in doubt about the most appropriate antibiotic for the management of the diabetic foot infection, discussion with an Infectious Disease consultant may be prudent.

[2] Before antimicrobials are used in the PWD, an evaluation of renal function must be undertaken to best guide appropriate dosing. This is particularly important with the aminoglycosides. Dosages shown are for normal renal function. If using aminoglycosides it is imperative that the renal function and drug levels be monitored closely.

[3] Approximate daily cost for oral therapy excludes the dispensing fee. These are 1998 costs based upon the Manitoba Drug Benefits and Interchangeability Formulary and the Manufacturer's recommended dosing regimen and listed price.

[4] In some instances, a higher dose of ciprofloxacin may be necessary. Other quinolone antimicrobial agents may be considered as alternatives, but a review of product monographs is necessary to establish optimal doses.

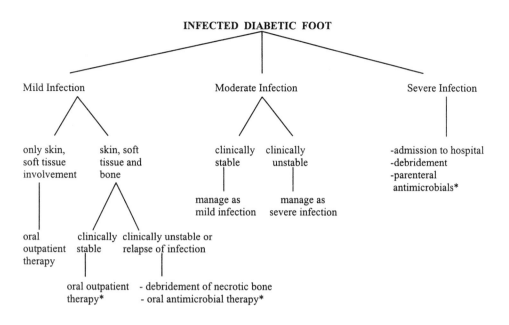

INFECTED DIABETIC FOOT

Mild Infection   Moderate Infection   Severe Infection

only skin,   skin, soft   clinically   clinically   -admission to hospital
soft tissue   tissue and   stable   unstable   -debridement
involvement   bone   -parenteral
                                    manage as   manage as   antimicrobials*
                                    mild infection severe infection

oral   clinically clinically unstable or
outpatient stable   relapse of infection
therapy

            oral outpatient   - debridement of necrotic bone
            therapy*   - oral antimicrobial therapy*

*See Table 1 for antimicrobial choices.

Figure 1: Algorithm for the Selection of Antimicrobial Therapy

NEUROPATHY

A history of foot numbness, lack of sensation, prior amputation of the contralateral lower extremity or toes on either extremity, and prior foot ulcerations should raise the suspicion that an individual lacks protective sensation. Callouses may result from unrelieved pressure and may also lead to ulcerations due to undermining of the underlying skin. The loss of pain perception due to neuropathy leads to increased susceptibility to mechanical and thermal trauma. Injury, ulcerations and subsequent infection may go unnoticed in the insensate foot. At every office visit, the PWD should be asked whether they are inspecting their feet regularly, and whether they have a current ulceration of their feet.

ADEQUACY OF CIRCULATION

For resolution of infection and promotion of wound healing, adequate circulation is necessary. If pulses are not palpable in the lower extremity, it is important to obtain an estimate of the adequacy of circulation. The "ankle brachial index" (ABI) is a non-invasive method where comparison of either the dorsalis pedis or posterior tibial blood pressure is made to the brachial artery blood pressure. Ankle brachial indices below 0.5 indicate significant reduction in large blood vessel flow, corresponding with severe peripheral vascular disease.[13] Ratios of < 0.3 are associated with rest pain and limb threatening ischaemia.[14] In some clinical presentations, ischaemia is suspected even where an adequate ABI has been documented. This may be due to non-compressible vessels as a consequence of calcification.[15] It may be prudent to proceed to angiography in these situations.

STATUS OF BONE

The diagnosis of osteomyelitis in the PWD with a foot infection is difficult as it may be difficult to use standard clinical criteria. Individuals with soft tissue infections or skin ulcerations that have been present for several weeks are at high risk of contiguous bone involvement particularly if these lesions are located over a bony prominence[6]. Clinical findings which can be used to determine the presence of osteomyelitis are that the larger and deeper an ulceration is, the more likely an underlying osteomyelitis will be present.[16] In another study, all ulcers in which bone was exposed either visibly or by probing had underlying osteomyelitis.[17] Imaging techniques for the diagnosis of osteomyelitis are varied with a wide range of sensitivity, specificity, and positive predictive value. The plain radiograph, for instance, will only demonstrate bony abnormalities related to osteomyelitis 10 - 20 days after the bone infection has occurred and 40 - 70% of the bone has been resorbed.[6] Although the plain radiograph findings are not pathognomonic for infection, a diagnosis of probable osteomyelitis can be made when classic radiologic findings are noted[6]. If plain radiographs are being used for the diagnosis of osteomyelitis, it is important to obtain a baseline radiograph and then follow it in 10 - 21 days with another plain radiograph to determine whether the typical bony abnormalities are present. Table 2 demonstrates the available imaging techniques for identifying osteomyelitis in the foot of PWD. Initial screening investigations for osteomyelitis include the erythrocyte sedimentation rate, and a plain radiograph of the affected area. A three phase technetium bone scan (Tc-99m MDP) is sensitive for diagnosing osteomyelitis, but suffers from poor specificity in diabetic foot infections due to frequent false positives from overlying soft tissue hyperaemia.[18] The simplest approach is to obtain a baseline x-ray and then repeat it in two to three weeks. In that intervening period, osteomyelitis should be visible radiographically. If clinical suspicion persists, a bone scan combined with a gallium scan, or white blood cell study, if equivocal, may be warranted.[18] The addition of gallium or white blood cell scanning to the three phase bone scan yields improved specificity while maintaining sensitivity.

Adjunctive Therapy

In addition to the antimicrobial therapy outlined in Table 1, ongoing care of the wound or foot ulcer is necessary. Table 3 demonstrates some suggestions for the management of these wounds. It is not clear what role, if any, topical antimicrobials play in the management of foot lesions of PWD. There is insufficient, well controlled data to support the routine use of topical enzymatic debriding agents such as collagenase at this time.

Table 2. Imaging Techniques for identifying osteomyelitis in the foot of PWD

Test Modality	Mean (Range) Sensitivity (%)	Mean (Range) Specificity (%)	Positive Predictive Value (%)
Plain Radiography	60 (28-93)	60 (50-92)	74-87
Technicium Bone Scan	86 (68-100)	45 (0-79)	43-87
Indium WBC* Scan	89 (45-100)	78 (29-100)	75-85
MRI	99 (29-100)	83 (71-100)	50-100

Modified from references 6, 16, 18, 19, 20

*WBC = White Blood Cell

TABLE 3. Management Suggestions for Ulcerations in the Foot of the PWD

GRADE	WAGNER CLASSIFICATION	MANAGEMENT SUGGESTION
Grade 0	Skin intact, no open lesions. Callus may be present under weight bearing areas. Calluses may act as abnormal pressure point leading to ulceration of underlying skin. Non-blanching erythema may be present as a consequence of unrelieved pressure.	• Pare calluses • Footwear properly fitted for weight displacement
Grade 1	Superficial skin ulceration, often seen under high pressure areas (metatarsal heads, toes).	• Pare calluses to expose ulcer base • Deep swabs or curettage specimen from ulcer base for bacterial culture to determine of underlying infection if one is present • Saline cleansing for 5 to 10 minutes with dressing changes daily • A hydroactive gel covered by a clean gauze is the simplest approach, saline wet to dry dressings are an alternative. • Should necrotic tissue be present or the wound be dirty, sharp debridement to remove this material should be undertaken. Alternatively, a gauze moistened with ¼ strength Eusol can be packed into the wound with dressing changes bid. If Eusol is used, petroleum jelly should be applied to wound edges to protect healthy skin. • Once the wound is clean and provided that granulation tissue is present, hydroactive gel should be substituted for the Eusol. • Infected ulcers (cellulitis) will require systemic antibiotics. Antibiotic choice can be guided by appropriately collected swabs for culture. • Radiographs should be obtained to exclude unsuspected bone infection (if this is detected, the ulcer should be considered a Grade 3 lesion). • Pressure relief is critical for the healing of these lesions. Pressure relief can be accomplished by appropriate footwear, crutches, wheelchairs and casting. If casting is considered, it must be applied by an experienced individual and monitored on a regular basis.
Grade 2	Deeper ulceration, usually associated with infection/cellulitis. The ulceration is deeper and may reach bone or joint capsule.	• These ulcers are deeper and often penetrate to subcutaneous tissue with local infection but no bony involvement. These ulcerations are managed in a fashion similar to Grade 1 lesions.

TABLE 3. Management Suggestions for Ulcerations in the Foot of the PWD (continued)

GRADE	WAGNER CLASSIFICATION	MANAGEMENT SUGGESTION
Grade 3	The ulceration has extended to deeper tissue layers such as bone. If bone can be probed at the base of an ulceration, osteomyelitis is very likely to be present. Osteomyelitis, tendinitis, tenosynovitis and deep space abscesses may be present.	• Some advocate aggressive surgical debridement of all infected bone. • Appropriate systemic antimicrobials must be administered for a prolonged period. Antimicrobials may be administered orally in most patients. Only in very rare instances is a home intravenous therapy program necessary for the management of osteomyelitis in individuals with diabetes. • Non-invasive assessment of the adequacy of peripheral circulation (ankle brachial index). • Radiographs should be obtained of the affected foot to rule out foreign bodies, gas, and to establish the magnitude of bony involvement. • Surgical opinion may be necessary if vascular insufficiency is present, or resection of infected bone and gangrenous material is necessary.
Grade 4	Localized gangrene (toes, forefoot, heel). The gangrene may be dry or wet, and infection may or may not be present	• Management should be as for a Grade 3 ulceration. • An urgent non-invasive assessment of a peripheral circulation and vascular surgical opinion is indicated, an angiogram may be needed. Angioplasty or by-pass surgery may be required if a suitable stenotic lesion is demonstrated on angiography. • Some individuals may have vascular disease which is not amenable to any revascularization procedure. Local surgery to remove gangrenous tissue may be attempted, however, single ischaemic toes should be kept dry and may be left to mummify and auto-amputate.
Grade 5	Gangrene of entire foot	• Patients with more extensive gangrene require urgent assessment as outlined for Grade 4 lesions. • These individuals will require control of diabetes and infection and will require foot-preserving surgery or amputation, guided by the level and adequacy of circulation.

Duration of Therapy

Based upon the preceding considerations, antimicrobial therapy can be initiated as outlined in Table 1. The vast majority of mild infections can be treated with a 2 week course of appropriately culture guided oral antimicrobial therapy.[5] If a culture is not available, empiric therapy will be needed. If an infection is acute and the ulcer has been present for less that two to three weeks, the most likely pathogens are *S aureus* and Streptococcus species (Group A and B). Therapy with a β-lactam such as cloxacillin or cephalexin would be appropriate (Table 1). If the lesion has been present for a more prolonged period, the presence of a mixed flora of microorganisms is likely and empiric therapy with trimethoprim/sulfamethoxazole or cephalexin would be appropriate (Table 1). Treatment choices are shown in Table 1. Moderate infections range from those in which the patients are not toxic which can be treated with local incision and drainage and oral antimicrobial therapy to those who are critically ill or toxic who will require incision, drainage, debridement and parenteral therapy.

In those individuals with severe infections, parenteral therapy is necessary. Once the acute infection has been stabilized and an assessment of whether an underlying bone infection is present, it is prudent to step down the patient's care to oral therapy if possible. If an underlying osteomyelitis is present, in the vast majority of cases, the infection can be treated with a prolonged course of antimicrobial therapy appropriately guided by culture data as outlined in Table 1.

The ideal duration of therapy for the treatment of osteomyelitis in the lower extremities of PWD has not been precisely established. Surgical debridement, where necessary, must be adequate to remove devitalized tissue. It has been traditionally recommended that 4 - 6 weeks of parenteral therapy is sufficient. These recommendations have been based upon experimental animal models.[21] However, combined regimens of parenteral therapy followed by prolonged oral therapy have had good results as have prolonged courses of OAT.[22] Prolonged appropriate OAT may be an alternative to parenteral therapy for osteomyelitis.[7,8,9,10,11,12] We have recently performed a retrospective cohort study with a prospective follow up examining the records of 327 PWD who were assessed and managed for lower extremity ulcerations at our multi-disciplinary foot clinic. There were 128 foci of osteomyelitis involving 141 bones, and data was available for the exclusive use of OAT in 101, with healing of 80.2% of the foci. The mean duration of OAT was 37 ± 28 weeks with 3 foci later relapsing.[8] The decision that remains is whether to use parenteral antimicrobial therapy administered at home or whether the patient should receive an oral antimicrobial which is well absorbed from the gastrointestinal tract and which achieves high serum levels.[12,23] Selecting the most appropriate antimicrobial is important because prolonged duration of therapy will be required.[24] It is believed that for most antimicrobials, the concentrations achieved in bone are similar to those achieved in serum.[21,23,24] The decision to use oral antimicrobial therapy for the treatment of osteomyelitis must take into account that regular follow up of the patient with regards to their lower extremity is critical. It is important to follow the erythrocyte sedimentation rate as a marker of decreasing inflammation and serial plain radiographs to ensure that bone healing and remodeling is occurring. These measures can help guide the total duration of therapy and detect relapses.

If the patient does not improve or deteriorates after the initiation of oral antimicrobial therapy, re-evaluation of the treatment is critical to ensure that the appropriate therapy has been selected according to the culture data or perhaps aggressive debridement of the bone is necessary as is ensuring adequacy of circulation.

CONCLUSIONS

Diabetes is a multi-system disease and the lower extremity ulceration in the foot of the PWD arises as a consequence of multiple factors. The ulceration may be the first lesion in the continuum to amputation. Aggressive interventions to heal the ulceration and treat infection are essential to arresting the process which may ultimately lead to amputation. Table 1 summarizes frequently used antibiotic choices according to the magnitude of infection. Figure 1 provides a simple algorithm for the selection of antimicrobial therapy.

In table 2, adjunctive measures are summarized for the management of foot ulcerations in the PWD.

REFERENCES

1. Blanchard J. Manitoba Epidemiology of Lower Extremity Complications in diabetes (personal communication). September 1997.
2. Grayson ML, Silvers J, Turnidge J. Home intravenous antibiotic therapy: A safe and effective alternative to inpatient therapy. Med J Aust 1995; 162: 249-253.
3. Milkovich G. Cost and benefits. Hosp Pract 1993 (supplement) 39 - 43.
4. Eisenberg JN, Kitz DS. Savings from outpatient antibiotic therapy for osteomyelitis: Economic analysis of a therapeutic strategy. JAMA 1986; 225: 1584-1588.
5. Lipsky BA, Pecoraro RE, Larson SA, et al. Outpatient management of uncomplicated lower-extremity infections in diabetic patients. Arch Intern Med 1990; 150: 790-797.
6. Lipsky BA. Osteomyelitis of the foot in diabetic patients. Clin Infect Dis 1997; 25: 1318-1326.
7. Pittet D, Wyssa B, Herter-Clavel C, et al. Outcome of diabetic foot infection treated conservatively. A retrospective cohort study with long-term follow-up. Arch Intern Med 1999; 159: 851-856.
8. Embil JM, Rose G, Duerksen F, et al. Oral antimicrobial therapy (OAT) for osteomyelitis of the foot in diabetic patients. Submitted Clin Infect Dis 1999.
9. Wilson KH, Kauffman CA. Oral antibiotic therapy for osteomyelitis of the foot in diabetic patients. South Med J 1985; 78: 223-224.
10. Venkatesan P, Lawn S, MacFarlane RM, et al. Conservative management of osteomyelitis in the feet of diabetic patients. Diabetic Med 1997; 14: 487-490.
11. Peterson LR, Lissack LM, Canter K, et al. Therapy of lower extremity infections with ciprofloxacin in patients with diabetes mellitus, peripheral vascular disease or both. Am J Med 1989; 86: 801-808.
12. MacGregor RR, Graziani AL. Oral administration of antibiotics: A rational alternative to the parenteral route. Clin Infect Dis 1997; 24: 457-467.
13. Orchard TJ, Strandness DE Jr on behalf of the participants. Assessment of peripheral vascular disease in diabetes. Report and recommendation of an International Work Shop sponsored by the American Heart Association and the American Diabetes Association 18 – 20 September 1992. NewOrleans, Louisiana. Circulation 1993; 88: 819 – 828.
14. Barner MG, Kaiser GC, William VL. Blood flow in the diabetic leg. Circulation 1971; 43: 391-394.
15. Takolander R, Rauwerda JA. The use of non-invasive vascular assessment in diabetic patients with foot lesions. Diabetic Med 1996; 13: 539-542.
16. Newman LG, Waller J, Palestro CJ et al. Unsuspected osteomyelitis in diabetic foot ulcers: Diagnosing and monitoring by leukocyte scanning with indium In[111] oxyquinonlone. JAMA 1991; 226: 1246-1251.
17. Grayson ML, Gibbons GW, Balogh K, et al. Probing to bone in infected pedal ulcers. JAMA 1995; 273: 721-723.
18. Keenan AM, Tindel NL, Alavi A. Diagnosing pedal osteomyelitis in diabetic patients using current scintigraphic techniques. Arch Intern Med 1989; 149: 2262 – 2266.
19. Schauwecker DS. Osteomyelitis: diagnosis with In-111-labled leukocytes. Radiology 1989; 171: 141 – 146.
20. Shults DW, Hunter GC, McIntyre KE, et al. Value of radiographs and bone scans in determining the need for therapy in diabetic patients with foot ulcers. Am J Surg 1989; 158: 525 – 530.
21. Norden CW. Lessons learned from animal models of osteomyelitis. Rev Infect Dis 1988; 10: 103-109.
22. Bamberger DM, Duas GP, Gerding DM. Osteomyelitis in the feet of diabetic patients. Am J Med 1987; 83: 653-659.
23. Fitzgerald RH. Antibiotic distribution in normal and osteomyelitic bone. Orthop Clin North Am 1984; 15: 537-446.
24. Gentry LO, Rodrigues GG. Oral ciprofloxacin compared with parenteral antibiotics in the treatment of osteomyelitis. Antimicrob Agents Chemother 1990; 34: 40-43.

LABORATORY TESTING IN DIABETES MELLITUS

Michael Leroux

Department of Clinical Chemistry
Health Sciences Centre
820 Sherbrook Street
Winnipeg, Manitoba   R3A 1R9

INTRODUCTION

Diabetes is a common chronic and serious disease with the estimate that as many as 10% of Canadian adults have diabetes (1).   All definitions of diabetes include some measure of hyperglycemia.   Laboratory tests are used to screen for, diagnose and monitor diabetes.   The test menu includes blood (plasma) measurement of glucose, ketone bodies and glycated proteins and urine glucose ketone bodies and microalbumin.   This paper will discuss the use of these tests in screening for, diagnosis and monitoring of diabetes.   Test characteristics such as cost, ease of use etc, to be considered in test selection will also be discussed.   The patient populations to be considered are Type 1 and Type 2 diabetics.

SCREENING FOR DIABETES

The purpose of screening is to detect people with diabetes who are unaware of having it, with the intention of intervention.   Earlier detection and treatment may reduce the occurrence or slow the progression of diabetic complications.

Test characteristics to be considered in test selection are listed in Table 1.   A screening test intended for widespread use should be easy to use, inexpensive, convenient and acceptable to both the subjects and the health care providers and provide acceptable detection sensitivity and specificity.

Screening healthy children for Type 1 diabetes is not considered feasible due to; low incidence (<0.5% of children considered "prediabetic" would be detected), acute onset of symptoms and lack of consensus as to what action should be taken when a positive auto antibody test is obtained (2).

It is estimated that as many as 50% of Type 2 diabetics go unrecognized (3).   To be cost-effective it is recommended that screening for Type 2 diabetes be limited to high risk subjects (2).   Testing may be performed in a central laboratory or, for some tests, as point-of-care testing.

Diabetes and Cardiovascular Disease: Etiology, Treatment and Outcomes
Edited by Aubie Angel et al., Kluwer Academic/Plenum Publishers, 2001

Table 1.   TEST CHARACTERISTICS

- Diagnostic Sensitivity/Specificity
- Precision/Accuracy
- Simple/Rapid/Available
- Practical/Sample Type
- Convenient/Acceptable
- Assay Standardization
- Clinical Data Base for Interpretation
- Inexpensive

URINE TESTING

Ketone Bodies

The so-called ketone bodies include acetoacetate, beta-hydroxybutyrate and acetone. The main ketone body, quantitatively is beta-hydroxybutyrate which is not detected by the routine testing procedures (4). As well, since Type 2 diabetics are not ketosis prone, urine ketone body detection is not considered a useful test for screening for Type 2 diabetes.

Glucose

Glucose appears in the urine when the renal threshold for glucose is exceeded which for most people is approximately 10 mmol/L. The test is relatively inexpensive and easy to perform. However, although the test gives a rough estimate of the prevailing blood glucose, it gives no information about blood glucose levels below 10 mmol/L. Knowler et al (5) report the test is highly sensitive in detecting severe hyperglycemia but is less useful in screening fasting subjects.

Microalbumin

This test is not used as a screening test for diabetes. The test is used to monitor patients diagnosed as diabetic to detect early progressive nephropathy. The goal is to detect diabetes before nephropathy develops.

BLOOD (PLASMA) TESTING

Blood Glycated Proteins
Fructosamine (glycated serum proteins)

This test is not used as a screening test due to the lack of assay standardization, lack of agreed to reference range and limited clinical data base.

HbA1c

HbA1c is not used as a screening test due to lack of standardization, cost and limited availability compared to testing such as plasma glucose.

Blood (plasma) Glucose

Plasma glucose may be measured as fasting (fpg) casual (non-fasting) or as an oral glucose tolerance test (OGTT).

A casual plasma glucose is not standardized as to the time and composition of the last meal. The selection of a decision level used for screening purposes will therefore be somewhat arbitrary. However in some circumstances, for example, screening in a remote community or patients presenting for other medical reasons, a casual plasma glucose may be the only sample readily available.

The OGTT is standardized both as to patient preparation and sampling times and has a large clinical data base for interpretation. The disadvantage is the inconvenience of having the patient remain, resting in the test area for 2 hours.

The fasting plasma glucose is standardized for patient preparation and also has a large clinical data base for interpretation. The fpg is more convenient and practical compared to the OGTT. Table 2 shows the recommended cut off values for screening (6). Some states in the U.S. allow use of Food and Drug Administration approved glucose meters for diabetes screening. Thus the table includes whole blood results which are 10-15% lower than plasma values. However in Canada, Table 3 the current glucose meters report plasma equivalent values.

The recommended screening test is the fpg (1,2).

Table 2. Cut-off values for screening tests that warrant additional testing and evaluation by a physician.

FPG ≥ 7.0 mmol/L

or

Fasting capillary whole blood glucose

≥ 6.1 mmol/L

or

Casual plasma glucose ≥ 8.9 mmol/L

or

Casual capillary whole blood glucose

Result ≥ 7.8 mmol/L

Table 3   GLUCOSE METERS

METER	COMPANY	CALIBRATED TO:
Advantage	Roche	Capillary plasma
Elite	Bayer	Venous plasma
Surestep	Lifescan	Capillary plasma
Medisence	Abbott	Venous plasma

Laboratory Testing in the Diagnosis of Diabetes

Laboratory tests used in the diagnosis of diabetes describe plasma glucose only (1,2). Urine glucose, ketone bodies, microalbumin, plasma fructosamine and HbA1c are not included.

In 1979, classification and diagnostic criteria for diabetes were introduced by the United States National Data Group (7). Most populations show a frequency distribution curve for plasma glucose, fasting and 2 h post-load glucose, that is skewed to the high end but becomes a bell-shaped curve on a logarithmic axis (8). Populations with a high prevalence of diabetes such as the Pima Indians, show a bimodal frequency distribution curve of plasma glucose both in the fasting and 2 h post-load glucose (9). Based on the approximate antimode of the frequency distribution curves of plasma glucose and the prevalence of complications, the plasma glucose concentrations of 7.8 mmol/L (fasting) and 11.1 mmol/L (2 h post-load glucose) were chosen as the diagnostic cut-off points for diabetes (7). However the 2 decision levels are not equivalent in detecting diabetes (10). The decision level for fpg has been lowered to 7.0 mmol/L to make it approximately equivalent in diagnostic sensitivity/specificity to the 2 h post-load glucose for detecting diabetes (2).

Fasting plasma glucose shows better reproducibility (11), is considered more convenient and practical compared to the OGTT and is the recommended test for diagnosing diabetes (2).

The analytical precision and accuracy required for diagnosis are more stringent than that required for screening or monitoring of diabetes. Glucose meter measurements are not as accurate or precise as plasma glucose measured in a central laboratory and are not accepted for use in diagnosis of diabetes.

Laboratory Testing in Monitoring of Diabetes

The Diabetes Control and Complication Trial (DCCT) established the relationship between mean blood glucose and the development and progression of complications in diabetic patients (12). Laboratory tests used in monitoring diabetes include, urine glucose, ketone bodies and microalbumin and blood glucose and glycated proteins.

URINE TESTING

Urine Glucose

Urine glucose testing (dipstick) is relatively inexpensive and easy to perform, but has limitations (13) and has now been largely replaced by patient self-monitoring of capillary blood glucose (SMBG). The ADA recommends use of urine glucose testing only for patients who are unable or unwilling to perform SMBG (14).

Urine Ketone Testing

Testing for urine ketones is considered important, particularly for Type 1 diabetics to monitor for impending or established keto acidosis, especially under certain conditions outlined by the ADA (15).

Urine Microalbumin

An increase of albumin excretion in the urine, not detectable by usual urine screening techniques such as dipsticks, is defined as microalbuminuria. The decision level defining microalbuminuria is different in Canada (1) and the U.S. (16). Elevated microalbuminuria is considered the earliest reliable and clinically detectable sign of progressive diabetic nephropathy. The Canadian Diabetes Association has published recommended guidelines for monitoring diabetic patients for microalbuminuria (1). Measurement of microalbuminuria may be performed using a random, spot urine (measured as albumin/creatinine ratio) or as a timed collection, 24 h or 4 h (measured as ug albumin/min.). The random urine is the most widely used specimen since it is the most convenient and generally provides accurate information (16)

BLOOD (PLASMA) TESTING

Blood (Plasma) Glucose

Measurement of blood (plasma) glucose, performed either in a central laboratory or by self-monitoring is now a well-established tool for short term monitoring of glucose control. The CDA has published recommended guidelines for diabetes management (1).

Blood Glycated Proteins

Glycated proteins are the products of a nonenzymatic reaction between the free aldehyde group of glucose or other sugars and the free, unprotonated form of amino group of proteins. The percentage of glycated protein in blood depends on the concentration of glucose, duration of glucose exposure to the proteins and the half-life of the proteins.

Fructosamine (Glycated serum proteins)

Since albumin, with a half-life of 15-20 days is quantitatively the main serum protein, measurement of fructosamine gives, primarily a measure of glycemia over the previous 2 to 3 weeks. However fructosamine assays are not standardized, lack a common reference range, do not have a large clinical data base for interpretation, and may require correction for changes in serum albumin/protein concentration which can occur in a variety of conditions such as liver disease.

HbA1c (HbA glycated at one or both N-terminal valines of the β chains)

Quantitatively the main adult Hb is HbA, making up approximately 97% of the blood Hb.

In 1958, Allen et al (17) noted, using ion exchange chromatography that HbA had three minor components which were named HbA1a, HbA1b and HbA1c according to their sequence of elution. In 1968, Rahbar et al (18,19) noted that these minor fractions of HbA were elevated in diabetic patients. Measurement of glycated Hb, using a variety of assays became widespread.

In 1993 the DCCT results (12) established the clinical importance of HbA1c measurement. Erythrocyte half-life is approximately 60 days so measurement of HbA1c reflects the mean plasma glucose over the previous 6-8 wks. However the lack of assay standardization became apparent. In 1993 the American Association for Clinical Chemistry Standards Committee established a Glycated Hemoglobin Standardization Subcommittee. The recommendation of this committee was that, since there is no purified glycated hemoglobin standard and no definitive method, that the cation exchange resin, high performance chromatography method used for HbA1c measurement in the DCCT be used as the interim reference method. In 1996 the National Glycated Standardization Program (NGSP) was established to implement standardization of HbA1c measurements with the goal of having all results traceable to the DCCT method, where the relationship to mean blood glucose and risk for complication had been established. Methods are certified as traceable to the DCCT based on measures of precision and bias of fresh sample results compared with the DCCT reference using a network of reference laboratories established by the NGSP.

In the author's own laboratory, HbAlc was measured using the Abbott IMX, affinity chromatography method, factored to report HbAlc equivalent values. Comparison of HbAlc measurements with two certified methods (Fig. 1 & 2) showed that the IMX shows a low bias for HbAlc values greater than 7.0%.

Our laboratory now measures HbAlc at an adolescent diabetes clinic using a Bayer DCA 2000 Analyzer and in the central laboratory, the Hitachi 917 with Roche reagents. Both methods are NGSP certified and are based on the turbidimetric inhibition immunoassay for hemolyzed whole blood. It is important for laboratories to use a method where results are traceable to the DCCT and to notify health care providers, using the results, when a method change is made, especially when patient results will show a shift from their previous pattern. It should be noted that the Abbott IMX method has now been NGSP certified. However, the new reagents will not be available to Canadian sites until the fall of 1999.

The DCCT established the importance of long term monitoring of diabetic blood glucose control using HbAlc. It is recommended that laboratories use only GHb assay methods that are certified by the NGSP (20).

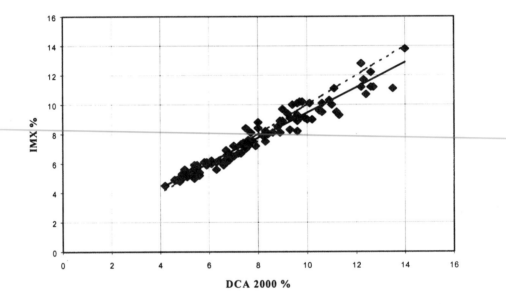

Figure 1: Correlation between whole blood HbAlc levels measured by the Abbott IMx affinity chromatography method and the Bayer DCA 2000 turbidimetric inhibition immunoassay method. Regression equation y = 0.8553x + 0.9122 R^2 = 0.9404 n=98 Regression analysis was carried out using Microsoft Excel for Windows '95, version 7.0.
Dashed line (-----) = Identity Line; Solid line (——) = Trend Line

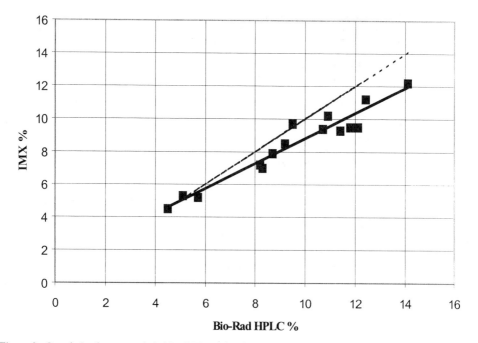

Figure 2: Correlation between whole blood HbA1c levels measured by the Abbott IMX affinity chromatography and the Bio-Rad Variant HPLC system. Regression equation y = 0.7667x + 1.1512 R^2 = 0.9328 n=15 Regression analysis was carried out using Microsoft Excel for Windows '95, Version 7.0. Dashed line (-----) = Identity Line; Solid line (——) = Trend Line

REFERENCES

1. Canadian Diabetes Association: *Clinical Practice Guidelines for the Management of   Diabetes in Canada, CMAJ:* 159 (8 suppl.) (1998).
2 American Diabetes Association: *Report of the Expert Committee on the Diagnosis and Classification of Diabetes Mellitus, Diabetes Care:* 20:1183-1197 (1997).
3 M.I. Harris, W.C. Hadden, W.C. Knowler, P.H. Bennett, *Prevalence of Diabetes and Impaired Glucose Tolerance and Plasma Glucose Levels in the U.S. Population Aged 20-74 yrs, Diabetes:* 36: 523-534 (1987).
4. B.S. Sacks, *Carbohydrate In,* C.A. Burtis, E.R. Ashwood, eds., Tietz Textbook of Clinical Chemistry, W.B. Saunders Company, Philadelphia, Pennsylvania: p. 972 (1994).
5. R.L. Hanson, R.G. Nelson, D.R. McCance, J.A. Beart, M.A. Charles, D.J. Pettitt, W.C. Knowler, *Comparison of Screening Tests for Non-Insulin Dependent Diabetes Mellitus, Arch. Intern Med:* 153: 2133-2140 (1993).
6. American Diabetes Association: *Screening for Type 2 Diabetes (Position Statement), Diabetes Care:* 22 (1 suppl) (1999).
7. National Diabetes Data Group: *Classification and Diagnosis of Diabetes Mellitus and Other Categories of Glucose Intolerance,* Diabetes: 28: 1039-1057 (1979).
8. B.S. Sacks, *Carbohydrate In,* C.A. Burtis, E.R. Ashwood, eds., Tietz Texbook of Clinical Chemistry, WB Saunders Company, Philadelphia, Pennsylvania: p 947 (1994).
9. D.R. McCance, R.L. Hanson, D.J. Pettitt, P.H. Bennett, D.R. Hadden, W.C. Knowler, *Diagnosing Diabetes Mellitus: Do We Need New Criteria?*; Diabetologia: 40: 247-255 (1997).
10. M.I. Harris, W.C. Hadden, W.C. Knowler, P.H. Bennett, *Prevalence of Diabetes and Impaired Glucose Tolerance and Plasma Glucose Tolerance and Plasma Glucose Levels in the U.S. Population Aged 20-74 yrs., Diabetes:* 36: 523-534 (1987).

11. J.M. Mooy, P.A. Gootenhuis, H. De Uries, P.J. Kostense, C. Popp-Snijders, L.M. Bouter, R.J. Heine, *Intra-Individual Variation of Glucose, Specific Insulin and Proinsulin Concentrations Measured by Two Oral Glucose Tolerance Tests in General Caucasian Populations: the Hoorn Study, Diabetologia*: 39: 298-305 (1996).

12. Diabetes Control and Complications Trial Research Group: *The Effect of Intensive Treatment of Diabetes on the Development and Progression of Long-Term Complications in Insulin-Dependent Diabetes Mellitus, N Engl J Med:* 329: 977-986 (1993).

13. D.E. Goldstein, R.R. Little, *Monitoring Glycemia in Diabetes: Short-Term Assessment, Endocr. and Metab. Clinics of N.A.*: 26:475-486 (1997).

14. American Diabetes Association: *Tests of Glycemia in Diabetes (position statement) Diabetes Care:* 20 (1 suppl): 518 (1997).

15. American Diabetes Association: *Standards of Medical Care for Patients with Diabetes Mellitus (position statement), Diabetes Care:* 20 (1 suppl): 55 (1997).

16. American Diabetes Association: *Diabetic Nephropathy (position statement), Diabetes Care:* 22 (1 Suppl): 66-69 (1999).

17. D.W. Allen, W.A. Schroeder, J. Balog, *Observations on the Chromatographic Heterogeneity of Normal Adult and Fetal Human Hemoglobin, J Am Chem Soc:* 80: 1628-1634 (1958).

18. S. Rahbar, *An Abnornal Hemoglobin in Red Cells of Diabetics, Clin Chem Acta:* 22:296-298 (1968).

19. S. Rahbar, O. Blumenfeld, H.M. Ranney, *Studies of An Unusual Hemoglobin in Patients with Diabetes Mellitus, Biochem Biophys Res Commun:* 36: 838-843 (1969).

20. American Diabetes Association: *Test of Glycemia in Diabetes. (position statement) Diabetis Care:* 22 (1 Suppl): 77-79 (1999).

DIABETES AND CARDIOVASCULAR DISEASE

Brian O'Connor
North Shore Health Region
Vancouver, British Columbia

THE CANADIAN HEART HEALTH INITIATIVE

The Canadian Heart Health Initiative (CHHI) is a countrywide cardiovascular disease (CVD) prevention program that emphasizes a public health approach. All 10 provinces are in partnership with the Federal Government (through the respective Health Ministries). The Heart & Stroke Foundation, both nationally and at the provincial level, is a key partner. As well, several hundred organizations, agencies and professional associations have been involved in delivering this interdisciplinary set of strategies, primarily at the community level.

The Initiative was the consequence of an appreciation that cardiovascular disease is the leading cause of death in Canada, accounting for 37% or about 80,000 of the annual deaths. It is also a major cause of illness and disability. It is a disease which is costly to the system. It accounts for 5,600,000 hospital days annually, 13% of all prescriptions, 17% of health expenditures and has significant indirect costs as well.

There has been marked progress in achieving a decline in CVD mortality and morbidity over the last 40-50 years. This success is attributable to both the lifestyle improvement of Canadians in reducing their use of tobacco, improving their nutritional choices and undertaking physical activity, as well as to better interventions in those with demonstrable disease in terms of medical and surgical treatments and pharmaceuticals.

It is interesting to consider what we would be experiencing if this downward trend had not occurred. It is projected that 40,000 more Canadians would have died from coronary heart disease in 1997 and that 14,000 more Canadians would have died from stroke in 1997, if we maintained the CVD death rates of 1970. Thus, 54,000 fewer Canadians died of CVD in 1997 as a result of the downward trend from the 1970s.

There is still considerable room for improvement. For instance, France has one of the lowest rates for CVD in the world. If Canada was able to achieve the French rate, then about 25,000 fewer Canadians would die annually from coronary heart disease. Within Canada, if the remainder of the country could achieve British Columbia's rates for coronary heart disease, then there would be about 7,000 fewer Canadians who would die annually of this disease. Canada fares much better with respect to stroke, having one of the best rates in the

Diabetes and Cardiovascular Disease: Etiology, Treatment and Outcomes
Edited by Aubie Angel et al., Kluwer Academic/Plenum Publishers, 2001

world; yet if the rest of Canada could achieve Quebec's rates, then 2,000 fewer Canadians would die each year.

Policy Development

In light of this evidence, the Federal and Provincial Governments in 1986 placed a priority on the development of a comprehensive strategy for Cardiovascular Disease. A Working Group was struck; a broad countrywide consultation was held; a policy document entitled "Promoting Heart Health in Canada" was developed and, ultimately, the Canadian Heart Health Initiative was launched.

The main elements of the policy paper were as follows:
- CVD is a preventable disease in that the major risk factors can be modified but, to that point (1986), it had been dealt with solely as a clinical issue.
- A population public health strategy was necessary and because so many were at risk, it is impossible to deal with it individually through a health care provider.
- It is multifactorial in its etiology and so requires integrated approaches.
- Partnerships are important because of the vast array of stakeholders, the broad scope of the CVD issue and its multifactorial nature.
- There has been a significant appreciation that population approaches demand the involvement of the community and its leadership as partners.

Additionally, the Initiative was built upon the strong epidemiological and interventional base of programs such as North Karelia, Stanford, Minnesota and Pawtucket.

From this policy base, the CHHI was launched. The Initiative consists of the following phases, with a 15-20 year timeframe:
- The Heart Health Surveys
- The Demonstration Programs
- The Evaluation
- The Dissemination Phase
- The Deployment Phase

In 1988, the Federal and Provincial Departments of Health agreed to co-fund the Initiative. On the part of Health Canada, the National Health Research Development Program (NHRDP) provides research contributions which are matched by the provinces.

Surveys The Heart Health Surveys were conducted in each of the 10 provinces between 1986-1991. There were some 24,000 participants who were surveyed as to their awareness and knowledge of the risk factors to CVD; their behaviours and risks; and had their individual risk parameters assessed, including blood lipids, blood pressure and height and weight.

All of the protocols and methodologies were standardized and common to the provinces, including the use of a common laboratory for analysis of the lipids. This ensured the comparability of the data.

Some highlights from the survey data include:
- 2/3 of Canadians have one or more of the major risk factors (smoking, elevated BP, elevated serum cholesterol).
- One in six Canadian adults has high BP (above 140/90)
- 43% of Canadians have high blood cholesterol levels (above 5.2 mmol/L).
- 1/3 of Canadians are sedentary.
- One quarter of Canadians are regular smokers.
- 48% of Canadians have a BMI >25.

across the country to the Atlantic provinces which generally demonstrate the highest rates.

This data base has proven to be an excellent tool for planning and evaluation; has helped the CHHI build epidemiological research capacity; has aided in the development of coalitions and has enabled the public health practitioners to link with researchers and scientists in other disciplines.

Demonstration Phase   The Demonstration Phase was characterized by projects which each province tailored to its specific needs. The projects consisted of programs designed to influence individuals to modify risk; to initiate community action and to influence public policy.   The research at the community level was particularly interesting and challenging. The CHHI researchers became familiar with a variety of theoretical frameworks (social learning theory, social marketing, community organization, community development) in learning how to mobilize community, develop coalitions and partnerships and deliver effective programs.

The Demonstration Phase was intended to be characterized by interventions:
*   that were directed at the population at large as well as at high risk groups
*   were multifactorial in nature - addressing tobacco, nutrition, physical activity, etc.
*   were community based
*   demonstrated intersectoral partnerships, e.g., health, recreation, education, not-for-profits.

The Demonstration Phase positioned the leadership for heart health in the public health system in an attempt to expand the interest of public health beyond its traditional focus on communicable diseases to the whole range of potentially preventable chronic diseases. Some of the key strategies were:
*   Health promotion and public education.
*   Advocacy for healthy public policy (e.g., tobacco, recreation, nutrition)
*   Community development and community mobilization through the selection of community leaders and champions and the development of partnerships with community agencies and organizations. This type of work is very difficult and takes much time and patience. A strategy that is very important, yet one which the Initiative has not developed well, is the enhanced partnership with professionals in strengthening preventive practices.

The Demonstration Programs were conducted in many communities right across Canada. The key linkages were the relationship of the Provincial Heart Health Programs to Health Canada (via financial and mutual support agreements) and between the Provincial level and communities. This was a very unique way to deliver a national health policy.

The Demonstration Programs varied from location to location - targeting tobacco, nutrition, physical activity, etc., in sites that ranged from schools, hospitals, small businesses and the community at large.

Some of the limitations of the Demonstration Phase included:
*   The very limited reach - there were insufficient resources to deliver a "preventive dose."
*   Few programs were targeted specifically to those at high risk.
*   There were only limited partnerships with the clinical sector.
*   And little action was taken on the biomedical risk factors.

Dissemination Phase   The Dissemination Phase will be discussed in greater detail by subsequent speakers in this session. This phase focuses on taking the learnings and successes of the Demonstration Phase and research how to have these successes actively taken up by other communities. The aim of the research component is to identify variables and factors that mediate the uptake of interventions by health jurisdictions, organizations and communities. Much of the research in this phase will focus on organizational capacity, organizational development and capacity building. Most of the provinces are currently in the Dissemination Phase.

Deployment Phase The next phase is the Deployment Phase. Ontario may be the first province to enter this phase. The challenge for the Deployment Phase is to develop the systems infrastructure and create the political will so that every Canadian has access to health promotion and disease prevention just as every Canadian has access to health care and hospital care. This universal "access to health" would ensure that the preventive dose is administered population-wide. It is interesting that access to health is not seen as an entitlement by policy makers - or for that matter, by the public at large.

The research will focus on:

- The methods, tools, systems, that will enable and cause the timely application of scientific knowledge on a scale large enough to make a difference.
- What is the "preventive dose" and what is its cost?
- What system can be developed for the management and accountability of promotion and prevention interventions?
- Are there creative financing options - other partnerships?
- What are the optimal organizational configurations to deliver scaled-up heart health programs?

The Canadian Heart Health Initiative is the pre-eminent example of a successful Federal/Provincial partnership which has expanded into broad coalitions at community, provincial, national and international levels.

The CHHI has been a key partner and influence in International Heart Health endeavours, notably, the International Heart Health Conferences (Victoria, 1992; Barcelona, 1995; Singapore, 1998) and the resulting declarations (Victoria, Catelonia, Singapore) which have outlined the strategic framework for CVD; catalogued the wisdom of investing in heart health through highlighting successful strategies from around the world; declared that our knowledge base was sound and abundant, and now we needed to forge the will, build the infrastructure and take personal responsibility for advancing the CVD prevention agenda.

CONCLUSION

The Canadian Heart Health Initiative has proven to be a successful platform on which Canadian Health policy can build a universal expectation that heart disease and stroke are preventable, and not inevitable.

REFERENCES

Advisory Board, International Heart Health Conference (1992). The Victoria Declaration on Heart Health. Ottawa: Health and Welfare Canada.

Advisory Board of the Second International Heart Health Conference (1995). The Catalonia Declaration: Investing in Heart Health. Barcelona: Government of Catalonia, Spain, 1996.

Advisory Board of the Third International Heart Health Conference (1998). The Singapore Declaration: Forging the Will for Heart Health in the Next Millennium. (in print).

Federal-Provincial Working Group on Cardiovascular Disease Prevention and Control. <u>Canadians and Heart Health</u>. Ottawa:Health and Welfare Canada, 1995.

Working Group on the Prevention and Control of Cardiovascular Disease. Report to the Federal Provincial Advisory Committee on Community Health. <u>Promoting Heart Health in Canada</u>. Ottawa, 1987.

PREVALENCE OF CARDIOVASCULAR RISK FACTORS IN CANADIANS WITH DIABETES MELLITUS

David R. MacLean[a], Michel R. Joffres[a], Meng H.Tan[b], Andres Petrasovits[c]

[a]Department of Community Health & Epidemiology, Dalhousie University
[b]9741 Winter Way, Zionsville, Indiana
[c]CVD Prevention Unit, Programs Division, Health Canada, Ottawa, Ontario

INTRODUCTION

Cardiovascular disease is the leading cause of mortality and morbidity among people with diabetes mellitus. Epidemiological studies have shown that individuals with diabetes are at increased risk of premature coronary heart disease and stroke.[1,2,3,4] People with non-insulin dependent diabetes mellitus (NIDDM) have age-specific mortality rates which are about double those of the non-diabetic population[5]. Most of the excess mortality is attributable to coronary heart disease.[6] Poor glycemic control in people with diabetes has been demonstrated to lead to higher rates of cardiovascular events[7,8,9].

The major modifiable risk factors for CVD in general are, apart from diabetes, high blood pressure, smoking, dyslipidemias, obesity, and sedentary living. People with diabetes share many of these established risk factors with the non-diabetic population.[10] Although the importance of these risk factors for the development of atherosclerosis in the general population has been widely documented, the same is not the case in individuals with diabetes. However, there are some studies[11,12] which conclude that the established CVD risk factors are also important for people with diabetes with respect to the onset of atherosclerosis and that people with diabetes benefit from the treatment of these risk factors[13,14,15].

The purpose of this paper is to report the prevalence of the established modifiable CVD risk factors in a sample representative of Canadians with self reported diabetes mellitus.

METHODS

The data presented in this paper are from the Canadian Heart Health Surveys database that has been assembled as part of the Federal-Provincial Canadian Heart Heath Initiative[16]. The risk factor data were collected in the ten provinces from 1986 to 1992 using a common survey protocol that was originally developed in Nova Scotia. A probability sample of approximately 2200 individuals was selected in each Province. Trained public health nurses collected data during a home interview and a clinic visit. The specifics concerning the design of the database, methods of data collection, data analysis and response rates have been

Diabetes and Cardiovascular Disease: Etiology, Treatment and Outcomes
Edited by Aubie Angel et al., Kluwer Academic/Plenum Publishers, 2001

373

Table 1: Prevalence of a positive response to the question 'Have you ever been told by a doctor that you have diabetes?', by age and sex.

Sex\Age	N	%
Men		
18-24	14	0.8
25-34	32	1.8
35-44	36	2.2
45-54	58	5.9
55-64	98	10.6
65-74	249	12.9
All Men*	487	4.5
Women		
18-24	31	1.4
25-34	119	2.8
35-44	62	3.1
45-54	52	5.8
55-64	79	7.7
65-74	236	9.8
All Women*	579	5.6
Total	1066	4.5

*Age standardized to the 1986 Canadian population

published previously.[17] Estimates of prevalence have been calculated using probability weights. Total prevalence estimates for each sex have been age-standardized using the direct method and the 1986 Canadian population as a standard. The standard errors of the estimates have been obtained using the Jackknife method.

The information given in this paper concerning the prevalence of diabetes, age of diagnosis, treatment status and type of treatment, smoking status and levels of education and income is self-reported. Blood pressure, blood lipid, height and weight measurements were carried out following standardized protocols. In nine of the ten provinces individuals were asked if they had "been ever told by a doctor or nurse that you had diabetes"; if yes, they were further asked the age at diagnosis and the treatment being followed. The methodology for these procedures and for the analysis of the blood for plasma lipids have been described elsewhere.[18]

RESULTS

The Canadian Heart Health Data Base includes 1066 individuals between 18 to 74 years of age who report they had been told by a doctor or a nurse they had diabetes mellitus.

Prevalence of self reported diabetes by age and sex is given in Table 1. The overall prevalence is 4.5%. There were no significant regional differences across the country (data not shown). Overall the prevalence is similar in both men and women and generally increases with age. However men over the age of 55 years have a higher diabetes prevalence than women in the same age group.

Prevalence of diabetes by self reported age at diagnosis and sex is presented in Table 2. The pattern for men and women differs. Among women there is suggestion of a bimodal distribution for prevalence by age of diagnosis. The first peak occurs in the second and third decades of life and the second in the fifth and sixth decades. Among men the distribution appears more unimodal with the peak prevalence occurring between the fourth and fifth decades of life.

The age-standardized prevalence of individuals in each of three levels of education is presented in Table 3 by sex and diabetes status. In both men and women there was a lower

Table 2: Distribution of self-reported diabetes by reported age of diagnosis and sex.

Age of diagnosis years	N	Men	N	Women
<=5	7	0.7	6	0.7
6-10	6	1.9	5	0.4
11-15	6	2.4	12	2.6
16-20	16	3.7	38	4.9
21-25	16	1.8	60	14.2
26-30	24	6.6	55	7.4
31-35	23	6.3	42	13.3
36-40	34	17.9	34	9.9
41-45	49	13.5	33	5.9
46-50	42	9.9	33	7.3
51-55	47	13.9	40	5.9
56-60	63	7.1	61	10.2
61-65	69	7.9	80	13.8
66-70	63	5.5	45	2.9
71-74	11	0.7	12	0.7

Table 3: Age standardized[1] percentage of individuals with different levels of education by sex and diabetes status

Sex/Educational Status[2]	Diabetes		No diabetes	
	%	se[3]	%	se
Men;				
Elementary or less	8.9	2.71	5.1	0.43
Some Secondary	30.7	4.72	24.6	1.66
Secondary Completed	44.9	5.69	47.1	0.65
University Degree	15.4	4.23	23.2	1.43
Women;				
Elementary or less	11.7	2.45	5.8	0.71 *[4]
Some Secondary	26.8	2.74	22.2	2.48
Secondary Completed	52.4	4.84	53.9	1.12
University Degree	9.1	2.41	18.1	2.85 *

[1] Age standardized to the 1986 Canadian population

[2] Elementary or less - 0-6 years of education

 Some Secondary - 7-11 years of education

 Secondary Completed - 12-15 years of education

 University Degree - 16+ years of education

[3] se=standard error obtained by the Jackknife method

[4] * Prevalence significantly different between diabetes and no diabetes at the 0.05 level

proportion of individuals who attained university education among individuals with diabetes than those without diabetes (9% vs. 18%). Conversely there was a higher proportion of individuals with elementary or less education among people with diabetes than those without (12% vs.6%).

Table 4 shows treatment status and type of treatment by age. Overall 28% of adults report not being on any treatment for their diabetes. This percentage varies with age declining from 41% in those 18 to 34 years to 19% in those 65 to 74 years. Diet is the most common form of reported treatment, followed by oral hypoglycaemic agents and insulin. The use of insulin declines with age from a high of 26% in individuals 18 to 34 years to 16% in those 65 to 74 years. The use of oral hypoglycaemic agents varies markedly with age ranging from less than 1% in those 18 to34 years to 44% in individuals 65 to 74 years.

Table 4: Distribution of self-reported treatment status among individuals reporting diabetes by age group.

Treatment Status	Age Group			
	18-34 n=196	35-64 n=385	65-74 n=485	All n=1066
Some treatment[1]	59.0	72.3	80.6	72.2
Insulin	25.5	21.4	15.5	20.6
Pills	0.7	27.4	43.7	27.1
Diet	33.8	42.7	43.0	41.3
Weight Loss	1.5	8.5	4.0	6.3
Other	9.0	5.8	3.1	5.6
No treatment	41.0	27.7	19.4	27.8

[1] Individuals may be one or more treatments at the same time

Individuals under age 35 used dietary measures less frequently. Thirty-four percent of individuals in this category reported being on a diet to control their diabetes. This percentage increased to 43% in the older age groups. Overall 6% of individuals reported trying to lose weight as part of the treatment for their diabetes. The highest prevalence of use of weight loss was in the 35 to 64 year age group at 9%, with the lowest prevalence at less than 2% in the group under 35 years of age.

The age-standardized prevalence of the established modifiable risk factors for cardiovascular disease[a] in both men and women with diabetes as compared to non-diabetics is presented in Table 5. Prevalence of all risk factors is higher in people with diabetes - one third of people with diabetes smoke; approximately one-half have elevated blood cholesterol; one-half are over weight; almost one-half lead a sedentary life style; and more than one third have high blood pressure.

Prevalence of multiple risk factors for CVD in people with diabetes as compared to the non-diabetic population is given in Table 6. Eighty-nine percent of people with diabetes have one or more of the modifiable risk factors for cardiovascular disease. This compares to 78% for the general population. Forty-three percent of individuals with diabetes have three or more risk factors for cardiovascular disease, which is more than double the prevalence found in the non-diabetic population at 20%.

DISCUSSION

The data presented here come from only nine provinces, but it is reasonable to assume that results may apply to ten provinces since we have seen no variation in diabetes prevalence by province in separate analysis. The population prevalence of diabetes reported in this paper is approximately 5% and is higher than previous estimates for the disease.[19] As these data are

---

[a] Risk factors are defined as: high blood pressure: BP ≥ 140/90 mm Hg and/or on treatment; elevated blood cholesterol ≥ 5.2 mmol\L; smoking one or more cigarette\day; obesity BMI ≥ 27; and sedentary living - leisure time activity less that once per week.

Table 5: Age-standardized[1] prevalence of modifiable risk factors for cardiovascular disease by self-reported diabetic status.

Risk Factor[2]	Diabetes		No Diabetes	
	%	se	%	se
Smoking	32.1	2.65	26.7	1.35
Hypercholesterolemia	49.8	3.48	42.6	1.29 *[3]
Sedentary	47.1	2.23	36.8	1.90 *
Obesity	49.9	4.02	29.7	2.00 *
Hypertension	37.8	3.06	19.5	0.75 *

[1] Age standardized to the 1986 Canadian population
[2] Smoking - currently smoke 1 or more cigarettes/day
Hypercholesterolemia - Total Cholesterol ≥ 5.2mmol/l
Sedentary - do not exercise at least once/week
Obesity – BMI ≥ 27
Hypertension BP ≥ 140/90mm Hg and/or on treatment
[3] * Prevalence significantly different between diabetes and no diabetes at the 0.05 level

Table 6: Age standardized[1] prevalence of selected[2] risk factors by number of risk factors and self-reported diabetes status

Number of Risk Factors	Diabetes[3]		No diabetes	
	%	se	%	se
0	11.0	2.64	21.3	0.66
1	16.9	2.26	32.4	0.70
2	29.3	2.93	26.2	0.93
>= 3	42.9	3.98	20.1	1.28

[1] Age-standardized to the 1986 population
[2] Smoking - currently smoke 1 or more cigarettes/day
Hypercholesterolemia - Total Cholesterol ≥ 5.2mmol/l
Sedentary - do not exercise at least once/week
Obesity – BMI ≥ 27
Hypertension- BP ≥ 140/90mm Hg and/or on treatment
[3] All prevalence estimates significantly different at the 0.05 level between diabetes and no diabetes.

self reported it is not possible to determine the type of diabetes i.e. IDDM or NIDDM being reported. In addition, self reported diabetes also includes those who previously had gestational diabetes and who were not diabetic at the time of the survey.

It has been estimated that at any given time, for white Americans at least, only about half of the people with diabetes are aware they have the disease[20]. Consequently, the true prevalence of diabetes in Canada could be as high as 10% of the population. This suggests that approximately 1,800,000 Canadians 18 to 74 years old may have diabetes, making this condition a major public health problem. The prevalence appears to be quite uniform across the country making diabetes a significant issue in all regions of Canada.

As one of the major independent risk factors for the development of cardiovascular disease, diabetes contributes significantly to the burden of this condition on the Canadian population. Design of the database does not allow calculation of diabetes prevalence in specific sub-populations that are known to be at increased risk to develop diabetes e.g. First Nation Canadians. In terms of education, a higher prevalence of diabetes mellitus in Hispanic Americans and white Americans with less education has been reported[21].

Prevalence of diabetes reported here is similar in men and women. However when the age of diagnosis is considered it appears there is an appreciable increase in prevalence among women of childbearing age (the first peak). This is a trend not observed in men of comparable age. The data suggest that childbirth (gestational diabetes) may have a significant influence on the prevalence of diabetes in women and that the childbearing years may present important opportunities for the prevention of diabetes in women.

Lower levels of education are associated with higher levels of mortality, disability and increased prevalence of risk factors, particularly risk factors for the development of chronic diseases[22]. Other risk factors associated with lower educational attainment may explain some of the differences in the levels of risk factors between people with diabetes and the non-diabetic population reported above. In particular the higher prevalence of reported diabetes among those with lower levels of education parallels the higher prevalence rates of obesity that are also found in this group.

The finding that over one quarter of people with diabetes do not appear to be on any treatment is surprising. There are several possible reasons, not mutually exclusive, including:

(a) The question was not understood. It is possible for example that some individuals who are not on insulin or oral hypoglycaemic medications feel that they are not on any treatment for their diabetes when in fact they regularly consult their physician and perhaps follow a diet.

(b) It has been estimated that only about one third of people with diabetes are followed regularly by diabetes education centres[23]. The sample reported upon here is a representative sample of people with self-reported diabetes and suggests that a significant proportion of people with diabetes in Canada may not have received the appropriate education concerning their diabetes. This lack of diabetes education may lead to misconceptions about the treatment of diabetes.

(c) The question that was asked during the survey was "Have you ever been told by a physician that you have diabetes?" It is possible that a certain percentage of the participants were told they had diabetes in the past and no longer had the disease at the time of the survey. This would include those women with gestational diabetes who did not have diabetes at the time of the survey and the people who had diabetes previously, especially those who were previously obese and diabetic, and no longer had diabetes as a result of treatment (e.g. weight reduction).

(d) It is possible that the data reflect the fact that a significant number of people with diabetes in Canada are not on any treatment.

From the perspective of diabetic complications, macrovascular disease produces significant problems for people with diabetes. It is the major cause of morbidity and mortality, particularly for those with NIDDM. It has now been widely accepted that glycemic control of diabetes reduces the risk of developing microvascular complications[24]. Major progress has been made in this regard over the last number of years. However glycemic control of diabetes has not been shown to have such an impact on the development of macrovascular complications of diabetes[24]. This fact has lead to increased attention to the risk factors for large vessel disease in people with diabetes, particularly those for the major modifiable risk factors to coronary heart disease and stroke.

CONCLUSIONS

The fact Canadians with diabetes smoke as much as the general population is particularly disheartening. The percentage of people with diabetes in an unhealthy weight range and with a sedentary lifestyle is much higher than that in non-diabetics. This is of special importance because obesity and sedentary living are now major public health problems in the general population[25]. The risk of CVD among people with diabetes is also increased because these individuals have higher levels of hypercholesterolemia and high blood pressure.

Cardiovascular disease is a multiple factor disease. The presence of multiple risk factors acts synergistically to increase the risk of acquiring the disease to a much greater level than is the case with the sum of the individual risk factors acting alone[26]. As reported here people with diabetes in Canada are much more likely to suffer from multiple risk for CVD than the non-diabetic population. This is a particular matter for concern because in Canada multiple risk for CVD among the general population is already high[27].

The presence of significant multiple risk to the development of CVD in people with diabetes in Canada is likely to account for some of the excess mortality observed in this population. This speaks not only to the need but also to the potential for prevention of macrovascular complications in people with diabetes. If this potential is to be realised greater attention is required by policy makers, health professionals and most importantly by people with diabetes themselves, to preventing the onset of or reducing the level of the known modifiable risk factors to cardiovascular disease.

REFERENCES

1.. W.B. Kannel, D.L. McGee, Diabetes and cardiovascular disease: the framingham study. JAMA; **241**:2035-38 (1979).
2. R.J. Jarrett, M.J. Shiply, Type 2 (non-insulin dependent) diabetes mellitus and cardiovascular disease. Diabetologia; **31**:737-40 (1988).
3. A. Rosengren, L. Welin, A. Tsipoganni, L. Wilhelmsen, Impact of cardiovascular risk factors on coronary artery disease and mortality among middle-aged diabetic men; a general population study. Br Med J; **299**:1127-31 (1989).
4. M.I.J, Uusitupa, L.K. Niskanen, O. Siitonen, E. Voutilainen,K. Pyorala, 5-year incidence of atherosclerotic vascular disease in relation to general risk factors, insulin level, and abnormalities in lipoprotein composition in non-insulin dependent diabetics and non-diabetic subjects. Circulation; **82**:27-36 (1990).
5. G. Panzram, Mortality and survival in type 2 (non-insulin dependent) diabetes mellitus. Diabetologia; **30**:123-31 (1987).
6. R.J. Jarrett, Epidemiological and public health aspects of non-insulin dependent diabetes mellitus. Epidemiol Rev; **11**:151-71 (1989).
7. M. Coutinho, H.C. Gerstein, Y. Wang, S. Yusuf, The relationship between glucose and incident cardiovascular events. A metaregression analysis of published data from 20 studies of 95,783 individuals followed for 12.4 years. Diabetes Care; **22**:233-240 (1999).
8. H.C. Gerstein, S. Yusuf, Dysglycaemia and risk of cardiovascular disease. Lancet; **347**:949-950 (1996).
9. H.C. Gerstein, Glucose: a continuous risk factor for cardiovascular disease. Diabetic Med; **14** (Suppl 3):S25-S31 (1997).
10. N.J. Morrish, K.L. Stevens, H.J. Fuller, Risk factors for macrovascular disease in diabetes mellitus: the London follow-up to the WHO Multinational Study of Vascular disease in Diabetes. Diadetologia; **34**:590-594 (1991).
11 N.J. Morash, L.K. Stevens, J. Head, A prospective study of mortality among middle-aged diabetic patients (the London cohort of the WHO multinational study of vascular disease in diabetics). 1. Causes and death rates. Diabetologia; **33**:538-41 (1990).
12. J.S. Yudkin, C. Blauth, P. Drury, Prevention and Management of Cardiovascular Disease in Patients with Diabetes Mellitus: An Evidence Base. Diabetic Medicine; **13**:S101-121 (1996).
13. J.D. Curb, S.L. Pressel, J.A Cutler, P.J. Savage, W.B. Applegate, H. Black, Effect of diuretic-based antihypertensive treatment on cardiovascular disease risk inolder diabetic patients with isolated systolic hypertension. Systolic Hypertension in the Elderly Program Cooperative Research Group. JAMA; **276**:1886-1892 (1996).
14. UK Prospective Diabetes Study (UKPDS) Group. Tight blood pressure control and risk of macrovascular and microvascular complications in type 2 diabetes: UKPDS 38. Br Med J; **317**:703-713 (1998).
15. K. Pyorala, T.R. Pedersen, J. Kjekshus, O. Faergeman, A.G. Olsson, G. Thorgeirsson, Cholesterol lowering with simvastatin improves prognosis of diabetic patients with coronary heart disease. Diabetes Care; **20**:614-620 (1997).
16. The Federal-Provincial Heart Health Initiative: Canadian Heart Health Surveys: A profile of Cardiovascular Risk. Editorial. Can Med Assoc J; **146** (11 suppli.): 1967-1968 (1992).
17. D.R. Maclean, A. Petrasovits, M. Nargundkar, Canadian Heart Health Surveys: a Profile of Cardiovascular Risk: Survey methods and data analysis. Can Med Assoc J; **146** (11 suppli.): 1969-

1974 (1992).

18. P.W. Connelly, D.R. MacLean, L. Horlick, B. O'Connor, A. Petrasovits, J.A. Little, Plasma lipids and lipoproteins and the prevalence of risk of coronary heart disease in Canadian adults. Can Med Assoc J; **146** (11 suppli.): 1977-1987 (1992).

19. J. Warram, S. Rich, A. Krolewski, Epidemiology and genetics of diabetes mellitus: In Joslin's diabetes mellitus, 13th Edition, Kahn and Weir Eds., Lea & Febiger, **1994**, 201-215.

20. M.I. Harris, Undiagnosed NIDDM: Clinical and Public Health Issues. Diabetes Care; **16**:642-52 (1993).

21. S.M. Haffner, H.P. Hazuda, B.D. Mitchell, J.K. Patterson, M.P. Stein, Increased incidence of type 11 Diabetes mellitus in Mexican Americans. Diabetes Care; **14**:102-08 (1991).

22. W.J. Millar, D.T. Wigle, Socio-economic Disparities in Risk Factors for Cardiovascular Disease. Can Med Ass J; **134**:127-32 (1986).

23. M.H. Tan, Unpublished data. Nova Scotia Diabetes Care Program. Nova Scotia Department of Health, Halifax, N.S. Canada. **1995**.

24. The Diabetes Control and Complications Trial Research Group. The effect of intensive treatment of diabetes on the development and progression of long term complications in insulin-dependent diabetes mellitus. N Engl J Med; **329**:977-86

G7 PROJECT PROMOTING HEART HEALTH

Jennifer L. O'Loughlin[1,2], Alison C. Edwards[3], Susan Elliott[4], and Andres Petrasovits[5*]

[1]Direction de santé publique
Régie régionale de la santé et des services sociaux de Montréal-Centre
1301 Sherbrooke E.
Montreal, Quebec H2L 1M3

[2]Epidemiology and Biostatistics
McGill University, Montreal, Quebec

[3]Memorial University
St-John's, Newfoundland

[4]McMaster University
Hamilton, Ontario

[5]WHO Collaborating Centre for Policy Development in the Prevention of Noncommunicable Diseases
Health Canada, Ottawa, Ontario
* On behalf of the G7/G8 Group on Promoting Heart Health Telematics Project which includes D. Cianflone, D. Vanuzzo, L. Pilotto, W. Scheuermann, E. Nuessel, V. Moltchanov, H. Korhonnen, P. Puska, I. Glasunov, A.T. Kamardina, M. Wilkinson, R. Cameron, D. MacLean, J. Lariviere, M. Lalonde

In cardiovascular disease (CVD), as in other chronic and acute diseases, one important challenge is to integrate lessons learned from previous intervention experiences, to improve future primary, secondary and tertiary prevention interventions. The purpose of the *G7 Project Promoting Heart Health* is to establish, maintain, and evaluate a telematics database for the timely dissemination through the INTERNET, of knowledge and experience gained from the implementation of heart health interventions in a wide variety of contexts and settings across G7 countries. Others who wish to implement similar interventions in different contexts and settings can therefore build upon successes and failures from previous implementation experiences.

The *G7 Project Promoting Heart Health* is one component project of the G7 Sub-project #3 that aims to improve the prevention, early detection, diagnosis, and treatment of CVD in G7 countries. It contributes a public health and health promotion perspective to

Diabetes and Cardiovascular Disease: Etiology, Treatment and Outcomes
Edited by Aubie Angel *et al.*, Kluwer Academic/Plenum Publishers, 2001

Sub-project #3, and as well, it reflects the G7 commitment to further the utilization of information technology in projects related to CVD. The project is coordinated by Health Canada with collaborating centers in Italy, Germany, the Russian Federation, the United Kingdom, and Finland. The Pan American Health Organization (PAHO), and the Countrywide Integrated Noncommunicable Disease Intervention Program (CINDI) are also active participants.

The purpose of this article is to describe the pilot work undertaken in Canada to develop the INTERNET database which houses descriptions of a wide variety of CVD-related interventions which have been implemented in participating countries. The specific objectives were to develop and pre-test a standardized methodology to collect data systematically on experiences implementing CVD interventions, to incorporate these project descriptions into a mixed qualitative and quantitative database, and to make the database accessible to potential users through the INTERNET. The following paragraphs describe each of these steps in detail.

DEVELOPMENT OF DATA COLLECTION METHOD

The data collection method was developed in three steps. The first task was to enumerate descriptors that adequately tapped important dimensions of project implementation experiences, that would be useful to persons wanting to implement CVD interventions, and for which reliable and valid data collection was feasible. Because data collection was likely to be retrospective, potential problems with recall and with obtaining detailed information on each descriptor had to be considered. A first list of 30 descriptors was eventually expanded to include approximately 60 descriptors which incorporated items describing the project anatomy (objectives, project structure, target group(s), risk factor(s), channels of delivery, resource needs, etc.), "how to" descriptors (initiate, plan and develop, champion, acquire resources, recruit and train volunteers, recruit target group, etc.), evaluation descriptors (goal attainment, barriers and facilitators to implementation, utility of evaluation, etc.), outcome and impact descriptors (reach, capacity-building, change in behavior, risk factors or health achieved, policy development, coalition/network building, etc.), sustainability achieved, and finally whether and how the project was disseminated to other settings. Publications and reports pertaining to the projects, as well as any intervention print materials developed for the project are also listed in the questionnaire, as well as contact information for persons directly involved in project implementation. Questions to collect data on each descriptor were formulated and incorporated into a first version of a mixed closed and open-ended questionnaire intended for telephone administration. A key respondent who had either managed the project or who had been directly involved in its implementation was to be identified, contacted and invited to provide data.

In the second step, this first version of the G7 questionnaire and its method of administration over the telephone were pre-tested in a convenience sample of six respondents across Canada. These interviews showed that telephone administration was not feasible - the questionnaire took far too long (two hours on average) and was difficult to administer because the respondent had to refer to documentation that was not necessarily immediately accessible. Based on this experience, the questionnaire was shortened considerably and revised into a self-administered version that included a mix of "check the box" and "short-answer narrative" questions.

Next, the new streamlined version of the questionnaire was tested across Canada in all ten provinces. The "source organizations" approached in Canada to provide data included the 10 demonstration projects, one per province, which had participated in the demonstration phase of the Canadian Heart Health Initiative. To solicit participation, each provincial principal investigator was contacted to explain the project, request their province's participation, identify projects for inclusion in the database, and identify key respondents who were familiar enough with the projects selected to provide complete and accurate data. This was usually a project manager or a field practitioner with hands-on experience implementing the project. Key respondents were then sent copies of the questionnaire with a cover letter explaining the project, as well as instructions on how to complete the self-administered form. Questionnaires took approximately two hours to complete. To supplement recall, respondents were encouraged to consult colleagues as well as any written documentation on the project, such as in-house reports, annual reports to the funding agencies, and journal publications. A glossary of terms was included with the questionnaire to standardize understanding of terminology. To facilitate completion of the questionnaire as well as data entry, a diskette version of the questionnaire has recently been developed and is now available from the author for those wishing to add data on their own projects to the database.

G7 HEART HEALTH PROJECTS DATABASE

Data for the next phase of the pilot work were collected from January to March 1998, on a total of 45 Canadian projects from 15 key respondents. Projects addressed a wide range of risk factors and target groups and used many diverse intervention strategies and channels of delivery. Projects included, among others, risk factor screening programs, national and provincial education campaigns, health professional education programs, preventive clinical guidelines, and cardiac rehabilitation programs. Data for these projects were entered into an MS Access database that accommodates both quantitative and narrative data, in preparation for entry onto the Canadian Heart Health Database Center Website. This website, which was created and is maintained at Memorial University in Newfoundland, also houses data from the Canadian Heart Health Surveys which were conducted in each province from 1986-92, as well as data from the national process evaluation of the Canadian Heart Health Initiative Demonstration Projects. After entry of the data for each project, data files were returned to the key respondent for verification and correction. Respondents signed a release form to permit inclusion of the project in the website database.

WEBSITE ACCESS TO THE DATABASE

The website which houses the G7 Heart Health Database is available at http://www.med.mun.ca/chhdbc/. Both static and dynamic options are available to users. For example, users can view a listing of all projects housed in the database and link to a narrative text that describes the project. They can view all or select only specific variables collected in the questionnaire, pertaining to a single project. They can identify and then view data from all projects according to a specific descriptor(s) (i.e., all projects related to tobacco; all school-based projects; all projects targeting low-income women, etc.). Alternatively they can run queries of the database. Examples of queries now available to users include: (i) select projects where smoking is a risk and list project information; (ii) select projects where delivery channel = school and list projects; (iii) search by country, risk factor, target group and delivery channel and list project information (iv) select project by prevention type and list primary risk factors; (v) select project by main activity type and list project information; (vi) select project by target group focus and list project information; (vii) select projects where health professionals are the target and list project information; and (vii) select projects by country and list project information. Eventually it is planned that users will be able to run their own queries of the database to solicit information specific to their own needs, and then leave these queries on the website for others to use. Another option available to users is to enter data on new projects or to update data on a previously entered project . Finally users can view a list of variables in the database, view a glossary of terminology, or view table definitions.

CONCLUSION

Dissemination of knowledge to those who need it to build new and better heart health interventions is a formidable challenge for the new millennium. An international project involving G7 countries is currently underway to develop and test a method for disseminating data on practical experiences and lessons learned from the implementation of heart health promotion and CVD prevention interventions. The intent of the *G7 Project Promoting Heart Health* is to explore the utility of the INTERNET for diffusing this kind of information to program planners, field practitioners, and policy makers so that knowledge acquired from these implementation experiences can be built upon and used to design better interventions. In 1998 Health Canada, as coordinator of this project, undertook pilot work in Canada to develop and test a method for collecting data on implementation, to create a database with the data collected, and to make the database available through the INTERNET. This pilot work will be built upon so that dissemination of knowledge on hearth health implementation experiences is facilitated. Also, from a broader perspective, this project contributes to our knowledge base on the methodologies of effective dissemination.

FUTURE DIRECTION

Based on the results of the pilot work, the following developmental steps are planned or underway: (i) more Canadian and international projects are being added to the database; (ii) a study funded by the Population Health Fund is being undertaken to evaluate the perceived utility of the database to potential users; (iii) a method to tag "best practices" in heart health intervention implementation is being developed; (iv) a marketing strategy to increase awareness and use of the database is planned; and (v) an on-line tutorial on how to use the database will be developed.

Acknowledgements

This project is supported by the Heart Health/WHO Collaborating Centre, Adult Health Division, Health Canada.

CANADIAN HEART HEALTH INITIATIVE: RESEARCH REVIEW

Dexter Harvey
Faculty of Education
University of Manitoba
Winnipeg, Manitoba Canada

The Canadian Heart health Initiative (CHHI) was designed to address the cardiovascular disease epidemic in Canada. The Initiative, a Federal-Provincial partnership, encompasses policy, research, and collaboration within and across sectors at the national, provincial, and local levels in the delivery of community-based heart health promotion activities [1,2].

The CHHI is jointly funded by the Federal and Provincial Health departments. Health Canada, through the National Health Research and Development Program, provides the research funding while the Provincial health departments provide the program support funding.

Since its inception in 1986, the CHHI has moved through five phases. Policy Development was the first phase. This involved policy development work at the Federal and Provincial levels between 1986 and 1988 laying the foundation for subsequent phases. The second phase involved the conduct of the Provincial Heart Health and Nutrition surveys in each of the ten provinces (1986-99) by their respective Provincial Health departments. The surveys have made possible the creation of an epidemiological cardiovascular risk factor data base containing risk profiles of 23,120 individuals. A similar data base for nutrition will follow.

Following the heart health surveys, phase three Research Demonstration was initiated in all ten provinces. This phase saw each province complete a 5 year research demonstration project to examine the implementation of integrated level approaches to reducing cardiovascular disease risk factors. The primary goal of this phase was to develop best practices at a community level for dissemination to the wider heart health community. The research demonstration phase resulted in more than 311 provincial and community projects in 35 demonstration areas across Canada. The fourth phase is a process evaluation of the research demonstration phase [3] resulting in qualitative and quantitative information on indicators of inputs, process, impacts and outcomes of the work emanating from this phase. The design, collection and analysis of the Evaluation Phase was a joint effort of national, provincial and community stakeholders.

In 1996, the fifth phase Dissemination Research was initiated. This phase is a series of research initiatives aimed at understanding the factors affecting capacity to undertake community based heart health promotion activities. The following is the process used during the dissemination research phase to build research team capacity and to ensure quality research protocols.

There is a dearth of research literature on dissemination, or the transfer and uptake of

Diabetes and Cardiovascular Disease: Etiology, Treatment and Outcomes
Edited by Aubie Angel *et al.*, Kluwer Academic/Plenum Publishers, 2001

385

knowledge and practice in both individuals and organizations. Most of the available literature on dissemination is anecdotal or descriptive at best. The CHHI focuses on research that will provide comparative, analytic and explanatory data about dissemination, which will be a foundation for advancing the dissemination of heart health promotion initiatives. In Canada, there is limited funding available so it precludes large research endeavors related to transfer and uptake. This has posed a major challenge in the design of dissemination research that will lead to changes in practice. While funding is limited, the National Health Research Development Program (NHRDP) and Provincial departments of health should be commended for their long-term support of research in the area of transfer and uptake. Also, CHHI member projects should be commended for their endeavor to maximize the use of available funding to produce quality research.

NHRDP appointed Site-Visit Panels to provide a peer review of each of the CHHI dissemination research protocols submitted to NHRDP. Each Panel consists of 4 or 5 members including the chair. In total, there are 8 persons who have served on one or more panels. A total of 10 research protocols, one for each province in Canada, have been reviewed by a Site-Visit Panel. Each research protocol requested funding for a five year time frame.

Site-Visit Panel membership is drawn from the international community. Members are researchers who have the expertise and record to judge the quality of the research proposals. The Site-Visit Panel is unique in the review of NHRDP research requests for funding. It serves a dual function: On the one hand it aids in the building of capacity to engage in dissemination research in the respective provincial heart health research team; and on the other hand, it provides a peer review.

Each dissemination research proposal goes through two stages with a Site-Visit Panel. The first stage is a consultation site-visit with the respective research team, to discuss a "consultation proposal" submitted to NHRDP. The major purpose of the consultation site-visit is the enhancement of the capacity of the research team to prepare a quality research proposal. The consultation proposal is a comprehensive presentation detailing research plans. The consultation proposal is really a "first attempt" at the final proposal. The consultation proposal is critically reviewed by the Site-Visit Panel, and they provide the research team with both an oral and written formative review including recommendations for strengthening the research. The consultation stage has proven effective, as none of the consultative proposals were sufficient to recommend tentative approval without revisions. Recommendations emanating from the consultation stage have ranged from outright rejection, suggestions on how to strengthen the research team with additional members with specific research skills, to major changes in the focus of the research and the research design.

The second stage is the Peer Review of the final proposal and application submitted to NHRDP. The Site-Visit Panel reviews this final proposal, and at a second site-visit discusses the proposal with the research team. At the conclusion of this Peer Review site-visit, the Panel presents a report with recommendations about the research, including funding to NHRDP. Even with the two-stage process, all peer reviews have resulted in further recommendations for modifications to the research protocol before receiving the final approval by the Site-Visit Panel.

This means that each research team gets two opportunities: One at the consultation stage and the other at the peer review stage. The two-stage process has resulted in an enhancement of the capacity of all research teams, as evidenced by the quality of the final proposals. It is worth noting that not all research protocols have been recommended for funding.

Another unique action of the CHHI is its plans to evaluate the research being conducted by the 10 provincial research teams. A major objective of the CHHI is to make a contribution to the knowledge and practice on the transfer and uptake of heart health promotion across Canada. A coordinating committee, independent of the CHHI, has been formed to plan and guide the evaluative research process. The committee consists of persons with the knowledge and experience to understand the quality of the applied research, and its connection to public and agency goals. The evaluation will be an Expert (peer review) Review, with a focus on two kinds of review; Relevance and Quality [4].

A Relevance Review addresses the question "What contribution does the research make to local and national governments and agencies, as well as to the state of knowledge about dissemination?" A Relevance Review will bring together potential users, who will be joined by experts to assess the appropriateness of the research to make a contribution to its intended users. A Quality Review focuses on the question "How good is the current research, compared with other work being conducted in the respective field?"

A third review, called Benchmarking will be considered. A benchmark review addresses the question: "Is the research being performed at the forefront of scientific knowledge?" In the first instance, benchmarking will be done by a panel of experts who have sufficient recognition and perspective to assess the Canadian standing of research. It is in the plans to benchmark CHHI research to an international standing.

A final focus of the research review will be on the opportunities the research has offered to the training and education of young scientists.

The procedures for the evaluation of the dissemination research projects will commence in June 1999 with all the principal investigators or their designates meeting in Winnipeg, Manitoba, Canada as a first step in a process to identify evaluation indicators and the mechanisms to initiate the assessment process. The research evaluation will focus on the contribution that the research being conducted by CHHI members is making to local and national settings, as well as to the transfer and uptake literature at large.

The dissemination research protocols developed by the CHHI members are quite different yet have some commonalities. All the proposals have some form of capacity building as an intervention. Capacity as defined in most of the protocols reflects the Singapore Declaration, 1998. Capacity consists of two key elements - Infrastructure and Will to Act. Leadership which is included in the Will to Act is essential to drive change whether in a community, organization, coalition or health region or district. The development of capacity is seen as a crucial element in the enabling of any group or organization to implement heart health initiatives. The focus of the research is varied. Two of the protocols are applying interventions to communities to study capacity building and its impact on the transfer and uptake of heart health promotion. Two protocols are applying interventions to organizations and/or coalitions to examine capacity building on the transfer and uptake of heart health promotion initiatives and five protocols are examining the impact of capacity building on health regions/districts to examine organizational change leading to the implementation of heart health promotion initiatives. At the time of this presentation, one provincial program has completed its dissemination research and their findings have important implications for increasing the transfer and uptake of heart health promotion initiatives in health districts.

If research is to be a drive engine in the promotion of heart health, it is important that the research findings are disseminated. The CHHI has been most active in dissemination: Collectively since 1987, the 10 Provincial Heart Health Programs have produced 105 peer reviewed publications; 34 non-peer reviewed publications; 56 reports; 19 theses and dissertations; 89 international conference presentations; 141 national conference presentations; 82 poster presentations; and 85 local area presentations.

REFERENCES

1. Stachenko, S. The canadian heart health initiative :Dissemination perspectives. Canadian Journal of Public Health 1996; 87: Supp 2: S57 - S59
2. Health and Welfare Canada. The canadian heart health initiative. Health Promotion 1992; 30:Supp. 1-20.
3. Stachenko, Sylvie. *Evaluation Guideline for Heart Health Programs.* Ottawa, Ontario: Health Canada 1991.
4. National Academy Press. *Evaluation Federal Results: Research and the Government Performance and Results Act,* Washington: Academy Press 1999.

PUTTING POLICY INTO ACTION

Sharon M. Macdonald

The International Conference on Diabetes & Cardiovascular Disease is an interesting mix of basic sciences, clinical management, prevention activities and a successful public forum. During the conference the posters and papers reported the costs of medical care for chronic disease; addressed the cost effectiveness of hypertension monitoring and control; identified the cost of diabetes on coronary artery bypass surgery; and examined the cost of diabetes on a population basis. The social impact of diabetes has been measured in Hawaiian populations and it is documented that depression in groups with type II diabetes is more prevalent amongst the poorest. Other researchers revealed lower employment rates and income levels amongst those with complicated diabetes. Forecasting is being done through the establishment of a National Diabetes Surveillance System. The predictions are that one in four persons will have diabetes by the year 2016 if we continue on this same pathway.

How do we address the challenges posed by such research? The interrelationship of diabetes with other disease processes highlights the complexity of the issue. It is fitting that the discussion of policy concludes the program. Problem solving in today?s world is not an easy task. Policy development can be a strategic approach. But moving from policy to action through clinical and public health interventions can take months and years to unfold. Pathways to action are not straightforward. In theory, the scientific information presented here is the foundation for healthy public policy. Such policy should extend well beyond the traditional boundaries of health. The forces which drive or impede the introduction of new programs and new strategies vary from one issue to another.

What is public policy? Thomas Dye defines public policy as ?whatever governments choose to do or not to do?. Public policy has a broad framework. The ideas, values and ethics of our society are the underpinning of decisions made by governments. Policy is the guiding principle that forms the basis for action or inaction by government. Programs are the most concrete aspects of public policy. Programs bring to life the activities needed to target the expenditure of public revenue. If an issue is not on the public agenda, government is unable to pursue public policy pertaining to it.

There are identifiable stages in developing public policy. There is a science to it. An issue can be identified and defined. There is a search for alternative strategies. A choice is made about which resources to commit. Finally there is a process of evaluation with feedback to modify the programs and activities that developed from policy directions. The techniques of policy analysis can be identified. Cost-benefit analysis measures the relative merits of alternative actions. A social and environmental impact assessment should take into account the demographic, socioeconomic and psychological affects of specific actions. The potential

Diabetes and Cardiovascular Disease: Etiology, Treatment and Outcomes
Edited by Aubie Angel *et al.*, Kluwer Academic/Plenum Publishers, 2001

services and structures must be appropriate to the population served. Forecasting predicts the future as social and economic indicators are detailed in an effort to measure the potential impact of services. The ethical issues regarding resource allocation need to be considered. Will resources be allocated to those in greatest need? If higher costs pertain to rural and remote areas of Canada, will they be given equal weight in the formulas developed? Are we as a society (or government as our representative) prepared to pay the costs of culturally appropriate services?

Those close to the development of public policy realize that planning and logical coherence are not prerequisites. It may be difficult to connect actions of the state with innovative policy ideas developed in academic settings. Evidence-based recommendations can be generated by civil servants, but implementation faces many challenges. There is an old adage that you do not want to see how sausages or legislation is made. This applies equally to policy in health-care. It is not a clean process.

The environment of public policy-making is complex in and of itself. There are a vast number of special interest groups organized specifically to influence the behavior of government. Pressure groups compete for resources. In Canada they are well organized, have designated spokespersons and may be capable of financing their own activities. The media plays an important role and has a direct and indirect effect on public policy. Effective communication campaigns about diabetes were launched recently by voluntary organizations. In the public health sector, projects related to prevention of cardiovascular disease have garnered high profile spokespersons and media attention.

Diabetes has become a concern for provincial and federal governments, primarily because of the costs generated by the outcomes of complications ? dialysis, loss of vision, and cardiovascular disease. We are in a quandary about how to allocate resources to deal with these consequences of disease. Hence, prevention seems a safe harbour for Health Canada in its 1999 ?Strategy of Diabetes Prevention and Control?. It may be achievable but not without the development of strong and healthy public policy.

What are the provinces doing? Health-care issues have been on the election agendas most recently in Quebec and Ontario. The focus has been on hospital closures and layoffs. In a recent Maclean?s magazine article about provincial health care ?First-Ranking: the Health Report? (June 7, 1999), the focus was on health-care services. Curative care - hip replacements and heart transplants - dominates the pages. The closest any of the review comes to a population or prevention or public health focus is on two pages referring to the two-tiered nature of the health services in Canada. The opinion expressed is that rural Canada is the second tier. Are the federal and provincial governments in tune? There have been diabetes reports released in several provinces. The focus appears to be on a broad range of issues.

Lessons about effective public policy for diabetes and cardiovascular disease can be learnt from the fight against tobacco use. The science was in place about 40 years before effective public health interventions appeared. Education, coalitions, advocacy, and legislation were used to change behavior at the corporate and individual level. Though the fight goes on, we now have smoke-free workplaces, schools, airplanes and public places. Science, human interest and policy have changed our perception and use of tobacco.

Policy and evidence-based guidelines have been less effective when we examine cervical cancer programs. We see excessive rates and mortality in disenfranchised and disadvantaged populations. This exists despite the fact that cervical screening and early intervention can clearly prevent death and disease. Where are the obstacles to developing new caregivers and to target programs? Are there vested interests that impede progress?

Public policy has not successfully addressed other issues such as medical manpower for rural Canada a problem for at least 50 years. Recently politicians moved to decrease the numbers of doctors in Canada based on evidence in part from academics. So doctors left and the rural ones seem to have left first! Depletion of rural physicians, estimated to be 15% over the last four years, has led to crisis management. Physician recruitment plans are prepared.

Recommendations are made to increase the size of medical school classes, initiated by policy makers who reduced those class sizes just a few years ago. The Canadian Medical Association and the Royal College of Physicians of Canada released action statements. What has been the result? Less doctors to serve rural and remote areas. For the thirtieth consecutive year northern health programs are recruiting doctors from overseas. Basic health services for some of the highest risk groups are threatened. How will residents of rural areas seek health care?

Can the primary health-care system be sustained in rural Canada? How will the new Diabetes Clinical Guidelines be implemented by doctors who have not trained in Canada? Where there are no doctors who will provide primary care? The medical profession has not agreed to share primary health-care with other providers such as nurse practitioners. Experience shows that nurse practitioners and dietitians can help persons with cardiovascular disease and diabetes manage their disease. What about physical education trainees who can develop relevant exercise programs and psychologists to address motivation? Will the primary health-care system be re-oriented to include these providers?

These examples highlight the difficulties and successes of public policy. Effective public policy and interventions take a long time to emerge ? despite the importance of the issue. Policy proponents need to find implementers and allies to advance the agenda. What and who will drive healthy public policy in relationship to diabetes and cardiovascular disease?

Diabetes was declared to be a world-wide epidemic by the National Institutes of Health in the USA and by the World Health Organization in 1997 with the publication of their document Obesity: Prevention and Management of the Global Epidemic. However, in 1990, aboriginal people were already worried and convened a conference on Diabetes and Aboriginal Peoples in Minneapolis, Minnesota. There an Assistant Deputy Minister for Health and Welfare Canada indicated in his speech that a diabetes program for aboriginal people in Canada would be implemented within a few short months. Those of us who worked in aboriginal health were delighted! There was some money allocated to research. But it was not until 1999 that the Government of Canada dedicated funds through the Canadian Diabetes Prevention and Control Strategy. Fifty-five million dollars in new funding over three years was announced. Some of this money will be directed towards diabetes in aboriginal people. But before aboriginal programs unfold there will be environmental assessment, forecasting, culturally appropriate programs developed and establishment of social and economic indicators to support an evaluation. One wonders what has been happening in the nine years between the first announcement of the initiative and the dedication of funds!

Now the challenge is before us. How will we recommend that the Canadian government move forward its new strategy for the prevention and control of diabetes? Are the advocates for diabetes prepared to be partners with those working on cardiovascular disease? Will effective coalitions be formed? What will the message be? The tobacco reduction initiative had an impact. But, the message was simple. It was ?do not use tobacco?. When we look at the issues surrounding cardiovascular disease and diabetes there are not many yes-no answers. What are the priority areas for public policy? Is it to increase physical activity, to improve the quality of diet, or to address the hard-to-reach high-risk groups most affected by chronic disease? What are the priority policies and programs for the prevention, detection and control of diabetes?

Interventions directed to chronic disease are difficult to define as discreet programs or activities addressing each risk factor. Physical activity and diet are inextricably linked with many other factors in the causal web. For years industrial nations have been caught up in a process of urbanization and displacement from the traditional knowledge base and activities.

Consider this example as it relates to aboriginal people. During the development of the James Bay Hydroelectric Projects, a number of community consultations were undertaken. The Cree and Inuit residents of Hudson and James Bay region identified a food web. It contained 138 animal and 36 plant types linked together in a food web. How do we replace that knowledge with a map of a Safeway or Loblaws store? How do we construct a food policy as intricate as this food web? How do we replicate the tastes of and traditions in gathering country food?

Are we prepared to challenge and work with the manufacturers of food, many of whom are multinational companies? Whoever thought governments would sue tobacco companies? Who are the allies for setting the healthy public policy for improved food and nutrition? Can we alter the distribution and marketing of food products? Can we define the role of regulation by government in food content?

Urbanization has affected not only the food sources but also levels of physical activity. What impact do urban transport policies have on an active lifestyle and indirectly on the management of diabetes? Will urban municipalities ensure urban green areas, safe cycling and walking routes, and transport policies which support active lifestyles beginning during childhood? What about schools boards? How are physical education and good nutrition valued within the context of education policies in the provinces?

What about improving detection? How can we identify those at risk of diabetes and obesity-related morbidity? The height-weight charts have been useful to some degree but a body mass index is a more complicated to do in an office setting. How about measuring waist circumference? We know that for men 102 cm. and for women 88 cm. is the criterion for ideal waist circumference. Distribution of body fat and waist circumference predicts cardiovascular disease and diabetes. Why not simplify primary care approaches by introducing waist circumference as a predictor of disease? Should measuring-tapes measures replace weigh scales in doctors? offices? Could we agree on a simple message such as ?100 cm of waist is enough??

Turning to control of chronic disease, a number of myths exist in the practice of clinical medicine and public health. Look at the myth of individuals returning to an ?ideal body weight?. This has been considered by health-care providers to be a reasonable and even mandatory target for obese people and those with cardiovascular disease and diabetes. This misperception is promoted to the public and reinforced by mass media. But what does the science show? Some studies show that relatively small weight loss can decrease mortality while others demonstrate that weight loss can also lead to increased mortality. Do we clearly understand the link between eating disorders, such as bulimia and anorexia and obesity? It is difficult to explain the science to the public and the policy makers.

What we do know is that the physiological response of our bodies limits our ability to lose weight. The literature is burgeoning with evidence showing repeated failures of weight loss programs, both in the commercial venue and in the medical therapeutic milieu. Organizations such as Weight Watchers understand very well that it is hard to sustain weight loss. Nonetheless, advertising about weight loss programs is deceptive and there are few objective assessments of outcomes. The next myth is that drugs work; that drugs can help in weight loss. The recent Fenphenamine debacle illuminates the problem of this approach. Are the drug therapy costs justified by the therapeutic outcomes?

We have undertaken the easy parts of chronic disease prevention and control. The message is clear for tobacco-? no?. It is more complicated for serum cholesterol and hypertension ?? lower is better?. But, for food intake and physical activity, what is the simple message? What is achievable in our environments? What should healthy public policy tackle? How will we ever be able to replicate in the urban setting the understanding the people of Hudson Bay have of their food web and what it take to fill their food basket?

The policy agenda must move forward. There needs to be debunking of the myths. To implement public health interventions we must address policy-making across government sectors such as transportation, education, and health. New partners must be found to address the issues. The corporate sector must be engaged in the discussion and participate in the solutions. The federal government has put money on the table in their latest health initiative-$55 million for diabetes. How will we respond to the challenge? Let us begin to discuss the options and clarify healthy public policy for chronic disease.

NATIONAL AND INTERNATIONAL STRATEGIES TO PREVENT OBESITY AND DIABETES

Bruce A. Reeder

University of Saskatchewan
Saskatoon, Saskatchewan

INTRODUCTION

In recent years, obesity and diabetes mellitus have rapidly become major health issues throughout the world. They lead often to premature death, diminished quality of life, and increased health care expenditures in those affected and compromise the present and future well-being of national populations.

Obesity and Type 2 diabetes mellitus share common risk factors and health consequences. Genetic and nutritional factors as well as physical inactivity predispose individuals to the development of both conditions, whereas coronary heart disease, stroke, peripheral vascular disease, hypertension, dyslipidemia, and gallbladder disease result from them. It is estimated, for example, that 50-70% of Type 2 diabetes mellitus is attributable to overweight and obesity (Body Mass Index ≥ 25) and hence could theoretically be prevented by weight normalization (WHO 1998). In view of this overlap of risk factors for, and health consequences of, the two conditions, a joint preventive approach is appropriate (Tuomilehto et al 1992).

To present a broad view of the prevention of obesity and diabetes, this paper will first describe current and projected international trends in the occurrence of these two conditions. A conceptual framework for the design of preventive programs will be outlined and selected examples given. Finally, the paper will conclude by examining the lessons that have been learned which help point to future directions and priorities.

INTERNATIONAL TRENDS IN OBESITY AND DIABETES

Until recently, global comparisons of trends in obesity have been hampered by the lack of a standard method of measurement. The growing international adoption of the WHO classification system (WHO 1998) is helping to rectify this situation. Body Mass Index (BMI), calculated as weight in kilograms divided by height in metres squared, is used to define weight categories (Table 1).

Type 2 diabetes comprises about 90% of all cases of diabetes mellitus and will be exclusively dealt with in this paper. As with obesity, there is growing international acceptance of standard classification and diagnostic criteria, those of the American Diabetes Association

Diabetes and Cardiovascular Disease: Etiology, Treatment and Outcomes
Edited by Aubie Angel et al., Kluwer Academic/Plenum Publishers, 2001

(Expert Committee 1997)(Table 2).

The prevalence of overweight and obesity is increasing in both developed and developing countries (WHO 1998). Striking increases have been reported in the United Kingdom and central Europe, with more modest changes in Sweden and the Netherlands. In the Americas during the past 20 years the prevalence of obesity has risen in the USA (from 12% to 20% in men, and from 16% to 25% in women), in Canada (from 7% to 13% in men, and from 10% to 14% in women) and in Brazil (from 3% to 6% in men, and from 8% to 13% in women). The trend appears to be similar elsewhere in the Americas, especially in those countries undergoing a more rapid rate of development and urbanization. In many countries, obesity is more prevalent among certain ethnic groups. In the USA, for example, Afro- and Hispanic-Americans are more likely to be obese than white Americans. In early stages of development, obesity tends to be more common in the higher socio-economic strata, while in later stages of the 'nutrition transition' that accompanies development, the reverse is true (Monteiro 1995).

It is estimated that 4% of the adult population, or over 135 million people worldwide, have diabetes (King 1998). The prevalence ranges from as high as 40% in several populations of North American Indians and Pacific Islanders to less than 1% among rural Melanesians and Bantu-Africans (Hales 1997). In the Americas, Canada, Argentina, Brazil and Chile have prevalence rates of 5 - 7%, while Jamaica, Trinidad and Tobago and Mexico City have rates

Table 1. Classification of weight in adults according to Body Mass Index (BMI)

Classification	BMI (kg/m^2)
Underweight	< 18.5
Normal range	18.5 - 24.9
Overweight	≥ 25
Pre-obese	25 - 29.9
Obese Class I	30 - 34.9
Obese Class II	35 - 39.9
Obese Class III	≥ 40

Source: WHO. *Obesity: Preventing and managing the global epidemic.* Geneva: WHO. 1998

Table 2. Glucose levels for the diagnosis of diabetes mellitus and related disorders

Category	FPG (mmol/L)	PG 1 h after 75 g glucose load (mmol/L)	PG 2 h after 75 g glucose load (mmol/L)
Impaired fasting glucose (IFG)	6.1 - 6.9	NA	NA
Impaired glucose tolerance (IGT)	< 7.0	NA	7.8 - 11.0
Diabetes mellitus (DM)	≥ 7.0	NA	≥ 11.1
Gestational Diabetes mellitus (GDM)	≥ 5.3	≥ 10.6	≥ 8.9

FPG=fasting plasma glucose; PG=plasma glucose; NA=not applicable
Source: Report of the expert committee on the diagnosis and classification of diabetes mellitus. *Diabetes Care* 1997;20:1-15.

up to 14% (Llanos 1994). Within the USA, the prevalence of diabetes is lowest among whites (6%), higher among Afro-Americans (10%) and Hispanic-Americans ((13%), and highest among the Pima Indians (50%). Projections conducted by WHO indicate that diabetes is expected to affect 300 million people, or 5.4% of the world's population, by the year 2025 (King 1998). The rate of increase in diabetes will be greatest in developing countries where the disease will be more prevalent in the age group 45-64 years than, as in the developed countries, in the group 65 years and older. In developing countries, diabetes will be increasingly concentrated in urban areas.

A CONCEPTUAL FRAMEWORK FOR THE PREVENTION OF OBESITY AND DIABETES

A conceptual framework can aid the design of interventions to prevent obesity and diabetes. Let us consider one such framework having the following dimensions: level of prevention, intervention objective, and target population.

Prevention has traditionally been considered to have three levels: primary prevention - the reduction of disease incidence through action on risk factors; secondary prevention - the reduction of disease prevalence and recurrence through early identification and management; tertiary prevention - the reduction of disability resulting from disease by means of therapy and rehabilitation. A fourth level, primordial prevention, has also been described to refer to the prevention of the social conditions and lifestyle habits that lead to the development of the risk factors and disease. Gill (1997) has argued that this scheme applies poorly to conditions such as obesity and diabetes that are multifactorial in origin and that lead to a diversity of non-communicable disease outcomes. Instead he recommends that we adapt the 'population'/ 'high risk' approach first proposed by Geoffrey Rose (1992). Doing so, we might instead envision three levels of prevention:

> *Universal prevention* - the use of population, or public health, strategies in the entire population.
> *Selective prevention* - the use of population, or public health, strategies in high risk population subgroups.
> *Indicated or Individual prevention* - the use of clinical strategies with high risk individuals.

To reduce the health burden of obesity in a population, we should consider that a spectrum of objectives may be acceptable for certain groups in particular circumstances. For some, an appropriate objective may be obesity prevention, for others weight loss, while for others weight maintenance and the management of co-morbidities. The appropriateness of the objective will depend upon the population's age, weight and weight loss history, current co-morbidities, and level of motivation for change (WHO 1998).

Target populations should be selected according to risk for the development of obesity and diabetes, as well as the feasibility, effectiveness, and ideally, cost-effectiveness of proposed interventions in that group. Life stages during which the risk for the development of obesity is high include (Gill 1997):

> Prenatal period. Hales (1997), Barker and colleagues have argued that undernutrition in the prenatal and early postnatal period leads to relative insulin resistance and underdevelopment of the pancreas, which, if the individual is exposed to a positive energy imbalance in later life, may lead to the development of obesity, diabetes and cardiovascular disease.
> The period of 'adiposity rebound' (5 - 7 years).
> Adolescence
> Early adulthood (18 - 30 years)
> Pregnancy/post-partum
> Menopause

Similarly, certain population subgroups are at high risk for the development of obesity:

Genetically susceptible individuals with a strong family history of obesity.
Ethnic groups which include North American Indians, South Asians, Afro-
and Hispanic-Americans.
Lower socioeconomic groups
Individuals who have recently quit smoking, lost weight, or are taking
certain medications such as corticosteroids and beta-blockers.

As a result of their risk for the development of obesity, these groups are also at risk for
the development of diabetes. Yet, in addition, other population groups are at high risk for
diabetes: children with diabetes in a first degree relative, children of mothers with gestational
diabetes, women with gestational diabetes, individuals with impaired glucose tolerance, older
individuals (> 45 years), and those with clinical conditions associated with diabetes such as
dyslipidemia, hypertension and coronary artery disease (Meltzer 1998).

Using these three dimensions: level of prevention, intervention objective, and target
population, one can construct a graphic framework for the design of interventions to prevent
and control obesity and diabetes in populations (Table 3). One might propose , for example,
a program to prevent obesity by targeting the prenatal stage in the genesis of the disease. This
might include a public education campaign through the mass media to promote the
consumption of a healthy diet during pregnancy (a universal level of prevention), as well as
a community garden and kitchen program for mothers in the urban slums (a selective level of
prevention). Such a program may have several merits, but these would include the potential
for the prevention of obesity and diabetes. The use of such a framework can help to ensure that
an appropriate and comprehensive approach is taken in the design of interventions.

SELECTED INTERVENTIONS TO PREVENT OBESITY AND DIABETES

The international scientific literature points to several promising interventions. As
shown in Table 4, these include obesity prevention programs for youth, obesity and diabetes
prevention programs in North American aboriginal communities, screening programs for
impaired glucose tolerance, and community-wide programs promoting weight loss and
maintenance.

As it is believed that approximately 30% of obese children go on to become obese
adults, the prevention of obesity in children has considerable potential value. In view of the
long term follow-up and compliance required to evaluate the merits of youth programs,
however, relatively few studies have been conducted. The experience of Epstein (1990)
indicates that comprehensive behavioral treatments of obese children and their families can
reduce the risk of obesity in adulthood. The goal in managing obesity in children is not weight
loss, but rather weight maintenance. Since children experience an increase in lean body mass
as they grow, maintenance of body weight will reduce fat mass. The practical objectives in
promoting weight maintenance in obese children, and prevention of obesity in normal weight
children, are: 1.) a reduction in energy by limiting portion sizes, modest reductions in dietary
fat, and compensatory *ad lib* intact of fruit and vegetables, 2.) an increase in physical activity
through an increase in general living and play activity rather than by means of competitive
sports and standardized exercise, 3.) a reduction in sedentary behaviors including the watching
of television, use of computers, and the playing of video games. Yet programs for the
prevention of obesity in childhood need to attend to the special nutritional requirements of
children for growth and development, avoid the induction of eating disorders by their focus on
eating habits, and avoid stigmatization of the obese by other children. Successful programs
in Australia (Dwyer 1983), USA (Epstein 1995) and Singapore (Ministry of Health 1996) have
included one or more of the following components: 1.) Identification, behavioral counseling
regarding diet and physical activity, and follow-up provided in a primary care setting by a
nurse or doctor, 2.) Family-based support through the involvement of at least one parent,
3.) School-based programs for primary school children that involve not only educational
curriculum but also compulsory physical activity of up to 50 minutes daily.

Table 3. Framework for interventions to prevent obesity and diabetes

Objective	Level of Prevention		
	Universal	Selective	Individual
Prevention of Obesity			
Prenatal			
Childhood			
Adolescence			
Adult Life Stages			
Ethnic groups			
Low socio-economic groups			
Prevention of Diabetes			
Impaired glucose tolerance (IGT) screening and intervention			
Weight maintenance			
Weight loss			

Table 4. Selected interventions for the prevention of obesity and diabetes

Objective	Level of Prevention		
	Universal	Selective	Individual
Prevention of Obesity			
Prenatal			
Childhood		PREVENTION IN YOUTH	
Adolescence			
Adult Life Stages			
Ethnic groups		ABORIGINAL PROGRAMS	
Low socio-economic groups			
Prevention of Diabetes			
Impaired glucose tolerance (IGT) screening and intervention		SCREENING AND INTERVENTION FOR IGT	
Weight maintenance	COMMUNITY-WIDE PROGRAMS		
Weight loss			

As an example of programs for specific ethnic populations, I will refer to several of those currently underway in aboriginal communities in North America. The Kahnawake

Schools Diabetes Prevention Project is a three year community-based project in a Mohawk community of 6700 near Montreal, Canada (Macaulay 1997). A community advisory board provides direction to the project and the day-to-day decisions regarding interventions and evaluation are made by aboriginal staff. During the three years it has been operative, 63 distinct interventions has been carried out that range from 1.) a grade 1-6 educational curriculum (10 sessions of 45 minutes each per year) which incorporates traditional foods and activities, to 2.) the development and implementation of a school nutrition policy which requires the students to bring healthy lunches and snacks and the school canteen to offer only low-fat, low-sugar, high-fibre foods, through to 3.) community awareness and activities including the construction of a public walking and cycling path. Qualitative results suggest improved levels of physical activity and healthy dietary change, but the outcome evaluation is not yet reported. The Sandy Lake Health and Diabetes Program in northern Ontario, Canada has similar features to the Kahnawake Project, and is also yet to report its findings (Harris 1998). The 'Pathways' project is a multi-center obesity prevention program for American aboriginal schoolchildren funded by the National Institutes of Health. The rationale and design of this project have been recently described in a special issue of the American Journal of Clinical Nutrition (April 1999). Forty-one schools in seven communities have been randomized to one of several arms of the study. The interventions focus upon schoolchildren in grades 3 - 5 (ages 8 - 10 years) and comprise educational curriculum, increased physical activity, a school meal program and a family intervention component. Evaluation will be conducted by a two-year follow-up of the school cohorts, with one of the outcome measures being percent body fat. This promises to be an instructive study on the merits of specific components of a youth obesity prevention program in an ethnic population.

Screening for impaired glucose tolerance (IGT) coupled with intervention appears promising as a strategy for the prevention of diabetes. Screening is recommended for the high risk population groups (listed above) with a fasting plasma glucose measurement. In those whose level is between 6.1 -6.9 mmol/L, this is followed by a plasma glucose measurement 2 hours after a 75 g glucose load. IGT is diagnosed as outlined in Table 2. Studies from Sweden and China suggest that the rate of progression from IGT to diabetes can be reduced in these individuals through dietary regimens and enhanced physical activity. The Malmo Preventive Trial (Eriksson 1991, 1998) was a non-randomized cohort study which followed 6956 middle-aged Swedish men over 12 years to assess the effect of a modest program of annual diet and exercise counseling. 288 of those with IGT participated in the intervention program, while 135 with IGT did not. After six years 10% of those in the intervention program had progressed to diabetes, compared to 28% in the control group. In the Da Qing IGT and Diabetes Study (Pan et al 1997) 577 men and women with IGT were randomized by local health clinic (33) to one of four arms of treatment: 1.) Diet only. Initial counseling was provided by a physician with ongoing group counseling and support. A healthy diet (consistent with the USA/Canada Food Guide) was recommended, and, for those with a BMI $\geq$ 25, a weight loss of 0.5-1.0 kg/month by means of caloric restriction, 2.) Exercise only. Initial physician counseling followed by group support to increase physical activity by one 'unit' per day, 3.) Both diet and exercise, 4.) A control group received general instruction regarding diet and leisure-time physical activity. At the end of six years of follow-up each of the intervention groups had experienced an incidence of diabetes of approximately 45% compared to 66% in the control group. To confirm this promising study, the NIH funded Diabetes Prevention Trial is currently underway in the USA.

As a final example of opportunities for the prevention of obesity and diabetes, one might examine community-wide programs. Some, such as those in Singapore and Minnesota, have targeted the prevention of obesity, while others, such as those in Canada, California and North Karelia have targeted the prevention of cardiovascular disease. The Trim and Fit Program in Singapore (Ministry of Education 1996) which has a school, community education and an environmental component, has demonstrated a reduction in the prevalence of obesity in primary and secondary schools from 14% to 10% between 1992 and 1996. Obesity interventions carried out as part of the Minnesota Heart Health Project included adult education classes, a worksite weight control program, a weight loss program by home correspondence, and a financial incentive weight gain prevention program (Jeffery 1995). These programs produced a modest weight loss (1-3 kg) which was maintained for up to one year among participants, however strong temporal trends of weight gain precluded any significant difference in the prevalence of obesity between intervention and control communities. Cardiovascular disease prevention projects such as the Stanford Five City Project, as well, encountered a strong temporal trend of increase in obesity during the 1970's and 1980's, although the rate of weight gain was less in the intervention than the control communities (Farquhar 1990).

CONCLUSIONS

Effective prevention of obesity and diabetes will require the use of multiple strategies in any population. The selection of approaches should be based on evidence derived from clinical and community trials, but such evidence is present in only a minority of the potential areas of intervention. Research effort and funding need to be directed to address these gaps.

The social and environmental influences promoting over-consumption of an energy-rich diet and physical inactivity are pervasive and strong in developed countries, and becoming so in many developing countries as well. Community-wide prevention programs have demonstrated that risk factor change is slow, and that the stages of behavior change related to diet and physical activity are complex. Public education and skill development are insufficient by themselves to prevent the development of obesity and diabetes; changes in our social and physical environments are vital. Economic and other incentives should be developed to promote the production and consumption of healthy food and the engagement in physical activity. Regulation and legislation may be required in areas such as food labeling and advertising. Advocacy by professionals and community groups will be essential in order to change such public policy.

The epidemic wave of obesity and diabetes is upon us. Coherent, comprehensive national strategies as proposed by the WHO (1998) and PAHO in the Declaration of the Americas on Diabetes (1996) are urgently needed worldwide.

REFERENCES

Dwyer T et al. An investigation of the effects of daily physical activity on the health of primary school students in South Australia. *International Journal of Epidemiology* 1983;12:308-313.

Epstein LH et al. Ten-year follow-up of behavioral, family-based treatment for obese children. *Journal of the American Medical Association* 1990;264:2519-2523.

Epstein LH. Exercise in the treatment of childhood obesity. *International Journal of Obesity* 1995;19(suppl 4):S117-S121.

Eriksson KF, Lindgarde F. Prevention of Type 2 (non-insulin-dependent) diabetes mellitus by diet and physical exercise: the 6-year Malmo feasibility study. *Diabetologia* 1991;34:891-898.

Eriksson KF, Lindgarde F. No excess 12-year mortality in men with impaired glucose tolerance who participated in the Malmo Preventive Trial with diet and exercise. *Diabetologia* 1998;41:1010-1016.

Expert committee on the diagnosis and classification of diabetes mellitus. Report of the expert committee on the diagnosis and classification of diabetes mellitus. *Diabetes Care* 1997;20:1-15.

Expert panel on the identification, evaluation and treatment of overweight in adults. Clinical guidelines on the identification, evaluation and treatment of overweight and obesity in adults: executive summary. *American Journal of Clinical Nutrition* 1998;68:899-917.

Farquhar JW et al. Effects of community-wide education on cardiovascular disease risk factors: the Stanford Five-City Project. *Journal of the American Medical Association* 1990;264:359-365.

Gill TP. Key issues in the prevention of obesity. *British Medical Bulletin* 1997;53:359-388.

Hales CN. Non-insulin-dependent diabetes mellitus. *British Medical Bulletin* 1997;53:109-122.

Harris SB. What works? Success stories in Type 2 diabetes mellitus. *Diabetic Medicine* 1998;15 (Suppl 4):S20-S23.

Jeffery RW. Community programs for obesity prevention: the Minnesota Heart Health Program. *Obesity*

Research 1995;3 (suppl 2):283s-288s.

King H, Aubert RE, Herman WH. Global burden of diabetes, 1995-2025. *Diabetes Care* 1998;21:1414-1431.

Knowler WC, Narayan KMV, Hanson RL et al. Preventing non-insulin-dependent diabetes. *Diabetes* 1995;44:483-488.

Llanos G, Libman I. Diabetes in the Americas. *Bulletin of PAHO* 1994;28:285-301.

Macaulay AC, Paradis G, Potvin et al. The Kahnawake Schools Prevention Pproject: intervention, evaluation, and baseline results of a diabetes primary prevention program with a native communtiy in Canada. *Preventive Medicine* 1997;26:779-790.

Manson JE, Spelsberg A. Primary prevention of non-insulin-dependent diabetes mellitus. *American Journal of Preventive Medicine* 1994;10:172-184.

Meltzer S, Leiter L, Daneman E et al. 1998 clinical practice guidelines for the management of diabetes in Canada. *Canadian Medical Association Journal* 1998;159 (8 Suppl)S1-S29.

Ministry of Education. *Update on trim and fit programme.* Singapore: Ministry of Education 1996.

Monteiro CA et al. The nutrition transition in Brazil. *European Journal of Clinical Nutrition* 1995;49:105-113.

Pan X, Li G, Hu Y et al. Effects of diet and exercise in preventing NIDDM in people with impaired glucose tolerance. *Diabetes Care* 1997;20:537-544.

Pan American Health Organization. *Declaration of the Americas on Diabetes.* Washington: PAHO 1996.

Rose GA. *The strategy of preventive medicine.* Oxford: Oxford University Press 1992.

Tuomilehto J, Knowles WC, Zimmet P. Primary prevention of non-insulin-dependent diabetes mellitus. *Diabetes/Metabolism Reviews* 1992;8:339-353.

World Health Organization. *Obesity - preventing and managing the global epidemic: report of a WHO consultation on obesity, Geneva, 3-5 June 1997.* Geneva: WHO 1998.

THE DIABETES COUNCIL OF CANADA (DCC): COORDINATING NATIONAL DIABETES STRATEGIES

N.W. Rodger

Chair, Diabetes Council of Canada
University of Western Ontario
London, Ontario   N6A 4V2

This report describes the membership, background, activities and future plans of the Diabetes Council of Canada. The roles, goals and successes will be reviewed.

There are 13 members of the DCC including 6 from the volunteer health charity sector: Association Diabète Québec (ADQ), Canadian Diabetes Association (CDA), Juvenile Diabetes Foundation of Canada (JDFC), Canadian National Institute for the Blind (CNIB) and The Kidney Foundation of Canada (KFC). The Assembly of First Nations (AFN) and National Aboriginal Diabetes Association (NADA) are well represented. The Canadian Pharmacists Association has recently been joined by a representative from Canada's Research-Based Pharmaceutical Companies. We have recently appointed a member from the diabetes Lay Community. From government, Health Canada and the Medical Research Council of Canada (MRC) are represented. The Council has been gratifyingly stable, is cohesive, and works productively.

The mandate of the DCC is to promote the health of Canadians by influencing and coordinating strategies that address diabetes mellitus as a serious, costly and growing public health issue and concern.

The origin of the DCC goes back to 1985 with report of the National Diabetes Task Force chaired by Dr. J. L. Chaisson which made a number of recommendations published as a book "Status of Diabetes in Canada" (1986). As a result of these deliberations the Canadian Diabetes Advisory Board (CDAB) was established, chaired by Dr. M.H. Tan. Notable activities of the CDAB included sponsorship of a workshop resulting in the publication of " Diabetes in Canada : Strategies Towards 2000" which has been an invaluable source of guidance. In 1995 the CDAB was transformed under Dr. Tan's direction to form the Diabetes Council of Canada which he initially chaired.

As constituted the DCC fulfils the first "minimum essential short-term national target" of the Declaration of the Americas (1996) which has been acknowledged by Canada. Target number 1 recommends a national focal point for diabetes program development with the identification of organizational partners, and the formation of a national planning and consultative group, to be recognized by the Ministry of Health. The three further sequential targets include an assessment of the national burden of diabetes, the development of a strategic plan for the control and prevention of diabetes and the implementation of local and regional activities consistent with the strategic plan. The Declaration of the Americas was sponsored

Diabetes and Cardiovascular Disease: Etiology, Treatment and Outcomes
Edited by Aubie Angel et al., Kluwer Academic/Plenum Publishers, 2001

by the Pan American Health Organization and the International Diabetes Federation in the face of an estimated 28 million people with diabetes in the hemisphere (1994).

The DCC operates with the assistance of support staff and funding from the Adult Health Division of Health Canada. At inception it was clear that the impetus for the formation and continuation of the operation of the DCC should be derived from a "buy-in" of the member organizations. Health Canada recommended that Aboriginal and Lay members be included. CDA volunteered to provide some infrastructure including the management of funds initially contributed by member organizations for the use mainly of secretarial services and travel by the Chair. It was apparent that the DCC should facilitate communications with the Federal Government on matters important to diabetes permitting the organizations around the table to speak with "one voice". Nevertheless organizations are free to deliver messages to government individually, recognizing that support of the DCC would add strength to such an approach.

Activities of the DCC have included a visit in early 1998 to the Ministry of Health permitting the CDA to draw attention to the forthcoming Clinical Practice Guidelines for the Management of Diabetes in Canada and to the National Forum on Diabetes being organized for May 1998. JDFC emphasized the importance of matching research funds with the MRC. KFC and NADA/AFN pointed to the burgeoning incidence of renal failure in aboriginal communities. ADQ discussed its program of community diabetes care.

Dr. Cindy Bell of the MRC has been and is continuing to develop a research database using MRC programs. It was recognized that in the U.S. Dr. Kahn of the Joslin Clinic has chaired a Congressionally Established Diabetes Research Working Group: A Strategic Plan for the 21st Century. A similar approach is indicated in Canada. The DCC has provided input and advice to the Laboratory Centre for Disease Control (LCDC) which has produced a report "Diabetes in Canada" (1999) summarizing presently available statistical data. DCC was represented (NWR) at formative meetings of the National Health Surveillance Infostructure, which proposes to provide technical resources to groups and regions interested in developing health-related databases. DCC urged that non-governmental organizations eg. from the voluntary health sector be represented.

To date the major project of the DCC has been in facilitating the development of the National Diabetes Surveillance System (NDSS). The National Diabetes Surveillance System is envisioned as a multi-sectoral initiative of non-governmental agencies, government and industry committed to reducing the incidence of complications of diabetes through leadership in the development, implementation and national coordination of provincial and territorial diabetes surveillance systems. We have learned that the federal government is now committed to providing major funding for this initiative. In addition the CDA is in the final stages of obtaining financial commitments from the private sector. The presently conceived 5 year budget is approximately 8 million dollars. Sheila Chapman acting on behalf of the Diabetes Division, LCDC, presented a paper describing the NDSS in detail earlier in this meeting. The initial operations of the NDSS have been funded by a competitively obtained grant from the Health Infostructure Support Plan (HISP) to epidemiologists representing Alberta, Saskatchewan and Manitoba who are now developing the necessary tools to combine administrative databases and supply information to the LCDC. Partners in the grant application included LCDC and the three Provincial Ministries concerned.

Other partnering activities have included support of the long standing relationship between MRC and JDFC which have matched research funds. The Chair described the activities of the DCC at a recent meeting of the Cardio/Cerebrovascular Research Advisory Council at which it became apparent that members of cardiology community, eg. The Canadian Cardiovascular Society, would be interested in corresponding with the CDA in relation to the CDA Clinical and Scientific Section Annual Meeting with respect to shared grants and communications. Partnership is occurring between CDA and Health Canada for NDSS funding, and between DCC and Health Canada for NDSS operations (the DCC Chair chairs the NDSS Steering Committee). Health Canada has used the DCC model to develop with the CNIB a Council "Prevent Blindness Canada", now in its formative stages.

In the future there are challenges for all. The 1998 Clinical Practice Guidelines for the Management of Diabetes in Canada require implementation and should stimulate the development of new patient care resources, and models of care, the education of health care professionals and the facilitation of screening programs for diabetes and complications. The implications of the United Kingdom Prospective Diabetes Study with respect to the current management of hypertension and type 2 diabetes have yet to be completely thought through. Again, new models of clinical care are required. The identification of gaps in research must be a continuing task. For example at this meeting it has come apparent that we must examine the role of near-normoglycemia in patients with diabetes undergoing such interventions for coronary artery disease as stenting, and angioplasty. Fruitful interactions for example among cardiologists and endocrinologists must continue to be developed.

The health care system must be reconfigured to include elements of population health, preventative medicine with appropriate screening, and long-term risk management. Decisions based on information available from such sources as the NDSS must be rational, and thought out by health care economists. Cost effectiveness considerations must apply in terms of access to limited resources and funds.

Finally there must be implementation of the recently announced federal Canadian Diabetes Prevention and Control Strategy, which has over a 3 year period assigned 55 million dollars to the Canadian Diabetes Prevention and Control Initiative, and the Aboriginal Diabetes Initiative. The DCC has formed a task group chaired by Mr. Jim O'Brien, CEO of the CDA to develop a rational process for the development of a strategy to ensure that these funds are spent as productively as possible. Components of the 1.4 billion dollars described by Hon. Mr. Duhamel (Minister of State for Science and Technology) at the outset of this Health Policy Forum, include the funding of the Canadian Institutes for Health Research which we envision as being the main sponsor of Diabetes Research in widest interpretation, in the foreseeable future.

Extrapolating from 1997 U.S. data (in the absence of our own), the annual cost both indirect and direct of diabetes in Canada is estimated to be as high as 10 billion dollars. Clearly the task before us is monumental, but we are enthusiastic that now we are preparing to develop the tools and processes to achieve the long-term goal for which we all strive.

Acknowledgments

This paper was presented at the Health Policy Forum. Tara Griffin expertly prepared the report. Dr. W.P. Mickelson, Manager, Disease Prevention Section, Adult Health Division, Health Canada, provided valuable assistance.

Dr. Rodger's term as Chair, D.C.C. ended on June 25, 1999.

THE FEDERAL GOVERNMENT AND DIABETES
AN INCREMENTAL PROCESS

W. Phillip Mickelson

Health Canada
Ottawa, Ontario

IMPACT OF DIABETES

Diabetes mellitus is a serious and growing public health problem in the developed world, including Canada. It is the seventh ranking cause of premature death at about 5,500 per year, and is estimated to contribute to 25,000 deaths per year through its complications.

This disease costs the Canadian economy an estimated $9 billion annually.

This presentation will review the way in which federal health programs relate to the problem of diabetes by subdividing the government activities into three categories:
*   general programs -- not diabetes specific
*   projects related to diabetes
*   diabetes specific activities

GENERAL PROGRAMS

There are a number of general federal programs which benefit the diabetes community. Foremost among these is medicare. The national health insurance program ensures that all medically required medical practitioners' and hospital care are covered without direct charge. While there is much that still needs to be done in the diabetes field, just imagine how much worse things would be without medicare in place.

Other points of intersection involve the federal government's *regulatory functions* under the Food and Drug Act and Regulations, and other related statutes. This includes the review of pharmaceuticals and biologicals for safety and efficacy. Affected are such critical products as: newer insulin formulations, oral hypoglycemics; lipid lowering agents; and antihypertensives.

The regulatory process also includes medical devices. All medical devices, including insulin pumps, glucometers and other *in vitro* diagnostic test kits are regulated by the Food and Drugs Act and the Medical Devices Regulations. The regulations are intended to ensure that Canadians are able to access safe, effective and quality medical devices. Effective July 1, 1998 all devices, except for those of very lowest risk, such as tongue depressors and bandaids, are subject to a degree of premarket evaluation by Health Canada. The degree of scrutiny is dependent on the class of a device which, in turn is linked to the risk of a device as established

Diabetes and Cardiovascular Disease: Etiology, Treatment and Outcomes
Edited by Aubie Angel *et al.*, Kluwer Academic/Plenum Publishers, 2001

by a series of rules. These new rules mean a greater degree of premarket review is being given to glucometers and external infusion pumps than was seen prior to July 1, 1998. Also within the regulations are provisions for mandatory problem reporting, manufacturing quality system audits and record keeping requirements.

Federal regulation of food and nutrition labelling is currently under review, with public consultation underway. I understand consultation kits were provided at the Health Canada booth, they are also available on the Health Canada website: http://www.hc-sc.gc.ca/

Nutrition labelling is intended to assist us in making informed food choices that support healthy eating. However, the selections made by many Canadians result in inadequate amounts of some essential nutrients, and excess amounts of energy, fat and saturated fat, thereby contributing to the high incidence of nutrition-related chronic diseases, including diabetes and heart disease.

The consumer research conducted as a component of the policy review on nutrition labelling included a subsample of those with diabetes, or heart disease. The study reported that Canadians with diabetes attribute significantly greater levels of importance to the role of nutrition, and nutrition related information on food packages, than do Canadians in general. They are more frequent users of the information on the nutrition information panel on packaged foods; but report lower levels of understanding.

Canadians with heart disease report more often (17% vs 8%) that they dislike the insufficient nutrition information currently provided on foods.

Federal support for *research* is important in addressing the problem of diabetes. The Medical Research Council is consistently the largest single contributor to diabetes research, providing some $4-6 million annually. MRC is also working with partners such as the Juvenile Diabetes Foundation in jointly supported activities. Future federal involvement will largely revolve around the actions of the soon to be created *Canadian Institutes of Health Research*.

Many of the investigator driven research applications under the National Health Research and Development Program (NHRDP) had pertained to diabetes. In a five year initiative, launched in 1992, there was a specific call for proposals under NHRDP in respect of aboriginal diabetes. There were 11 projects which were funded for $2.1 million, and these were designed to promote education programs within selected aboriginal communities. These communities were involved in the evolution of the projects, and were not simply subjects.

There have also been incidental projects under various children's and seniors programs. For example, in March 1998, the National Indian and Inuit Community Health Representatives Organization (NIICHRO)published a *Resource Kit on Diabetes and Aging in Aboriginal Communities*. The kit is a collaborative project of NIICHRO, the Lifescan Education Institute and Health Canada. It was funded by the population health fund through Health Canada's division of aging and seniors.

The project was designed as a train-the-trainer package to raise awareness and develop education programs for elders and community members in diabetes prevention, treatment and care. It was delivered to community health workers in First Nation and Inuit communities across Canada.

The kit is available through NIICHRO at their offices in Kahnawake, Quebec. You can e-mail niichro@total.net .

With respect to children, the Aboriginal Head Start Program has projects which involve feeding children nutritious food, and nutrition education for parents and children, both activities are highly relevant to diabetes prevention.

Finally, in this review of general federal programs, we should mention the Canada Pension Plan in relation to persons with diabetes who are totally and permanently disabled.

RELATED PROGRAMS

Health Canada, in conjunction with a variety of partners, has, and has had, a number of activities which are *closely related* to diabetes. These include: the Canadian Heart Health Initiative (HHI) which was launched in 1986 and is still ongoing. HHI has gathered and analysed data on diabetes, and other risk factors for cardiovascular disease. Its findings, and demonstration projects on community-based interventions to reduce cardiovascular risk are highly regarded nationally and internationally.

In 1988, a departmentally sponsored expert committee published the *Canadian Guidelines For Healthy Weights*, which have provided a solid reference standard for over a decade. This was followed in 1991 by the *Report of the Task Force on the Treatment of Obesity* which outlined the safe management of excess weight in both medical and non-medical situations.

With regard to the non-nutritional causes of obesity, in 1997, federal and provincial territorial Ministers responsible for fitness, recreation and sport set a policy goal of reducing the number of inactive Canadians by 10% by the year 2003.

DIABETES SPECIFIC ACTIVITIES

With respect to programs specifically directed to diabetes, these began during the mid 1980's. A representative from the Medical Services Branch will be reporting on diabetes among aboriginal people.

From 1984-87 a National Diabetes Task Force was in place which, in 1985, held a major conference in Montebello, Quebec, organized along the themes of: epidemiology, complications, treatment, education and research. Some 111 recommendations emerged from this event. Subsequently, in 1987, the task force tabled a report to the Minister of Health and Welfare which distilled the 1985 recommendations down to ten, which can be abbreviated as follow:

1. National surveys with biological measures must be organized to determine the prevalence of diabetes and its impact on the Canadian health care system.

2. Studies on the prevalence of diabetes and associated specific characteristics among special populations are required; these include ethnic groups, rural versus urban population, age and sex.

3. Registries should be created to collect reliable health care statistics on hospital admissions, mortality and survival rates of diabetics, physician usage, and medical costs.

4. Case control and cohort studies are needed to identify risk factors for diabetes and its complications.

5. Governments, health authorities, universities and health professionals must recognize patient education as an integral part of the treatment of diabetes, and make a corresponding commitment to providing resources and access to services.

6. A system of evaluation for diabetes education and treatment centres should be developed and funded by the governments.

7. Steps should be taken to rectify the shortage of health professionals trained to treat diabetes mellitus in Canada.

8. More funds for personnel awards in the form of scholarships and fellowships should be made available for young investigators and trainees pursuing diabetes related research.

9. Additional funds should be made available to support research projects in diabetes related fields.

10. It is recommended that a "Canadian Diabetes Advisory Board" be established to oversee the progress made in implementing the various recommendations of the national diabetes task force.

Subsequently, the Canadian Diabetes Advisory Board (CDAB) was established in 1988, and remained in existence until 1995. CDAB was made up of representatives from the Canadian Diabetes Association, the Juvenile Diabetes Foundation, L'association du Diabète du Québec, Health Canada, and ten other members agreed to by the parent organizations.

The federal conditions for support were not stringent. They specified that there was to be public representation on the CDAB, that it not be solely a body of experts, and that there be appropriate representation for the problem of diabetes among aboriginal people. That role was filled by two aboriginal physicians who were consecutive members of the CDAB.

CDAB activities were organized along three areas of interest: epidemiology; education and treatment; and research. In its seven years the Canadian Diabetes Advisory Board was active and had its accomplishments:

*it regularly monitored and reported on the status of diabetes in Canada;

*it met regularly with Ministers of Health and Welfare;

*it identified the extent of support for diabetes research in Canada, and along with MRC developed an agenda for diabetes research, which was subsequently subsumed by other events;

*it produced the first clinical practice guidelines for the management of diabetes in Canada, and fostered a national implementation program;

*it provided interim support for the diabetes educator accreditation process. Subsequently a national accreditation body was established;

*it reviewed Income Tax Act provisions with Revenue Canada with a view to encouraging industry support for the training of diabetes clinical scientists.

In 1994, CDAB convened a multi-sectoral national workshop which ultimately led to the publication of *Diabetes in Canada: Strategies Towards 2000* in 1997, and the establishment of the *Diabetes Council of Canada* on the premise that CDAB had outlived its mandate, and it was time for a more comprehensive consortium to address the problem of diabetes on a national basis.

Diabetes in Canada: Strategies Towards 2000, contains six main conclusions:

1. Diabetes is a common, growing, serious, costly public health problem

2. Diabetes has many serious, disabling, and debilitating consequences

3. Acute and long-term complications can be prevented and minimized through integrated diabetes care

4. Research can help to prevent and cure diabetes

5. An up-dated focus on diabetes-related societal issues is needed to address quality of life problems experienced by people with diabetes

6. There is a need for a national diabetes advocacy group to lobby for improvements in diabetes research, diagnosis, prevention, treatment and education.

The spirit behind the last recommendation led to the formation of the *Diabetes Council of Canada* which is a consortium of diabetes agencies, organizations concerned with the target organ complications of diabetes, and others, including the private sector. Its mandate is to promote the health of Canadians by influencing and coordinating strategies that address diabetes mellitus as a serious, costly, and growing public health issue and concern. The chair of the DCC, Dr. Wilson Rodger, is scheduled to talk about the council.

The February 1999 federal budget announced the Government of Canada's commitment to a Canadian Diabetes Strategy (CDS), amounting to $115 over five years for this purpose. The strategy is not a solution, but a means for enabling stakeholders, and building capacity in the country. Its development and operation is premised on the principle of citizen engagement.

The CDS has as its long term objectives:

*a reduction in the incidence of diabetes and its complications;

*a decrease in the deaths attributable to diabetes;

*improvement in the quality of life of those living with diabetes by working with provinces and territories, aboriginal and NGO partners in respect of four elements:

National Coordination, Surveilllance, the Aboriginal Diabetes Initaitve, and Prevention & Promotion.

The overall strategy has three interlinked components:

1. directly addressing the problem of diabetes in the aboriginal population, emphasising cultural relevance and on reserve services;

2. enhancing existing efforts for the rest of the population; and,

3. supporting both of these efforts by the development the *National Diabetes Surveillance System* (NDSS) as the source of strategic data upon which to plan and evaluate activities. The NDSS was the topic of a session earlier in this international conference.

Research is expected to be addressed by the launching of the Canadian Institutes of Health Research and other research initiatives announced in the budget, which amount to $550 million. This development, and the other recent federal investments in scientific research were already referred to in the speech by the Honourable Mr. Duhamel.

Next steps for the strategy involve widespread consultations. Consultations with aboriginal stakeholders are well advanced, having been set in motion by the announcement of an aboriginal diabetes focus in the 1997 speech from the throne.

In addition, consultations with the Diabetes Council of Canada, provinces and other stakeholders with respect to the NDSS have been ongoing for two years, and well preceded the budget announcement. Consultations with the not for profit sector, and the provinces about the remaining aspects of the budget strategy have already begun and will intensify in the near future.

CONCLUSION

Diabetes, and awareness about diabetes, as a growing national public health problem has coincided with incremental federal government involvement in efforts to reduce the toll of this disease.

This trend has recently culminated in the $155 million Canadian Diabetes Strategy, originally announced in the February 1999 Federal Budget.

INDEX